2nd edition

INTRODUCTION TO

COMMUNICATION DISORDERS

A Life Span Perspective

Robert E. Owens, Jr. 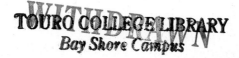 **Dale E. Metz** **Adelaide Haas**

State University
of New York
at Geneseo

State University
of New York
at Geneseo

State University
of New York
at New Paltz

Boston   New York   San Francisco
Mexico City   Montreal   Toronto   London   Madrid   Munich   Paris
Hong Kong   Singapore   Tokyo   Cape Town   Sydney

Executive Editor and Publisher: Stephen D. Dragin
Editorial Assistant: Barbara Strickland
Editorial-Production Administrator: Joe Sweeney
Editorial-Production Service: Walsh & Associates, Inc.
Composition Buyer: Linda Cox
Manufacturing Buyer: Megan Cochran
Cover Administrator: Linda Knowles
Photo Research: PoYee Oster

Library of Congress Cataloging-in-Publication Data
Owens, Robert E.
    Introduction to communication disorders : a life span approach / Robert E. Owens, Jr.,
Dale E. Metz, Adelaide Haas.—2nd ed.
      p. ; cm.
    Includes bibliographical references and index.
    ISBN 0-205-36012-2
    1. Communicative disorders.   I. Title: Communication disorders.   II. Metz, Dale Evan.
III. Haas, Adelaide.   IV. Title.
    [DNLM: 1. Communication Disorders.   WL 340.2 097i 2002]
RC423.095 2002
616.85'5—dc21

                                    2002066661

Printed in the United States of America

10 9 8 7 6 5 4   06   05   04

Photo Credits: p. xviii, Patrick Ward/Corbis; p. 11, Laura Dwight/Photo Edit; p. 26, Rachel Epstein/The Image Works; pp. 46, 138, 261, 433, Michael Newman/Photo Edit; p. 54, Mary Kate/Photo Edit; p. 61, Terry Wild Studio; pp. 84, 420, Robert Brenner/Photo Edit; p. 108, Peter M. Fisher/Corbis Stock Market; p. 118, Rhoda Sidney/Photo Edit; p. 160, Elizabeth Crews/The Image Works; p. 167, Richard Lord/Photo Edit; p. 206, Jeff Greenberg/The Image Works; p. 229, Spencer Grant/Stock Boston; p. 250, Roger Ressmeyer/Corbis; p. 278, Larry Mulvehill/The Image Works; pp. 306, 384, 506, Bob Daemmrich/The Image Works; p. 337, Ray Stott/The Image Works; p. 348, Phil Schermeister/Corbis; p. 381, Carl Glassman/The Image Works; p. 410, Kevin Redford/ Superstock; p. 452, Jack Kurtz/The Image Works; p. 480, Richard T. Nowitz/Corbis; p. 498, Harry Sieplinqa/HMS Images/Getty Images

Contents

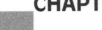

CHAPTER 2

TYPICAL AND DISORDERED COMMUNICATION 27

CHAPTER 3

ANATOMY AND PHYSIOLOGY RELATED TO SPEECH, HEARING, AND LANGUAGE 55

CHAPTER 4

COMMUNICATION DEVELOPMENT   85

CHAPTER 5

ASSESSMENT AND INTERVENTION   119

CHAPTER 6

CHILDHOOD LANGUAGE IMPAIRMENTS   161

CHAPTER 7

ADULT LANGUAGE IMPAIRMENTS   207

CHAPTER 8

FLUENCY DISORDERS 251

CHAPTER 9

THE VOICE AND VOICE DISORDERS 279

CHAPTER 10

DISORDERS OF ARTICULATION AND PHONOLOGY 307

CHAPTER 11

CLEFT LIP AND CLEFT PALATE 349

CHAPTER 12

NEUROGENIC SPEECH DISORDERS   385

CHAPTER 13

DISORDERS OF SWALLOWING

CHAPTER 14

AUDIOLOGY AND DISORDERS OF HEARING 453

CHAPTER 15

AUGMENTATIVE AND ALTERNATIVE COMMUNICATION   499

AN AFTERWORD: FUTURE OF THE PROFESSIONS   524

Preface

We hope this book will serve as a good introduction to the fields of speech-language pathology and audiology. Our goals have been to be informative and interesting, to provide enough information without overwhelming the reader, and to be scholarly in our production of a challenging text. Unlike edited texts, we have attempted to speak with one voice and to provide an overview, not to force-feed the reader with our pet approaches to assessment and intervention. This does not mean that our text is without perspective. It has been our objective to follow models of good practice and approaches that represent the best of our own clinical experience.

Within each chapter, we have attempted to describe a specific disorder and related assessment and intervention methods. In addition, we have included life span issues to provide the reader with added insights. Each disorder is also illustrated by the personal story of an individual with that disorder. Reader interest and reflection are stimulated by thought questions placed throughout each chapter and by margin notes. Further knowledge can be gained by the suggested readings and the Internet locations provided at the conclusion of each chapter.

Students will find the accompanying CD-ROM helpful as a learning device and study tool. Many disorders are also presented in sound and video format on this disk. In addition, self-study questions follow the outline of each chapter and highlight important information.

No book of this magnitude is prepared without the cooperation and aid of a great number of individuals. We are especially indebted to Jim Feuerstein, Ph.D., audiologist and chair of the Department of Communication Disorders and Sciences, Nazareth College, for his expertise in the preparation of the audiology chapter.

ACKNOWLEDGMENTS

ROBERT OWENS

I would like to thank the faculty of the Department of Communicative Disorders and Sciences at State University of New York at Geneseo for their forbearance and assistance with this book. Dr. Nicholas Schiavetti and Dr. Kathlyn Jones, who both have taught introductory courses, were especially helpful in their review of the manuscript and their insistence that the text adhere to high standards of inclusiveness and content coverage. A clinical perspective, especially with young children, was provided by Ms. Linda Deats. Finally, my and Dr. Metz's chair, Dr. Linda House, has been extremely helpful both with her expertise and her understanding of the magnitude of our writing task. She has provided a genial atmosphere in which to create.

My most personal thanks goes to my partner at O and M Education, Byung, who supported me throughout this project. He made the job much easier and I'm looking forward to our future collaborations.

DALE EVAN METZ

I gratefully acknowledge Dr. Donald Warren, University of North Carolina, Chapel Hill, for the photographs of children with cleft lip and palate, and Dr. Robert Orlikoff, Memorial Sloan-Kettering Cancer Center, New York City, for the photographs of laryngeal pathology and for the audio samples of voice disorders. I also greatly appreciate Dr. Bridget Russell for contributing the CD-ROM video segments of vocal fold behavior.

Ms. Janice Masterson kindly contributed video fluoroscopic samples of swallowing which can be seen on the book's CD-ROM. Kelly Julian and Julie Klejdys were invaluable to the development of the book's CD-ROM and they also, along with Shanna Wiech, were significant contributors to selected tracks of the CD-ROM. We are especially appreciative of the videotape segments supplied for the CD-ROM by the Prentke-Romich Company of Wooster, Ohio, a developer of augmentative and alternative communication equipment.

Kay Elemetrics, Inc., Pine Brook, New Jersey, kindly provided pictures of some of their clinical instruments, and we thank them for their cooperation. I deeply appreciate the efforts of my wife, Wendy, for her tireless reading of this book at all stages of development and for her love and boundless forbearance with me.

ADELAIDE HAAS

I wish to thank former and current members of the Department of Communication Disorders State University of New York at New Paltz; Anne Balant, Wendy Bower, Gretchen Brassard, Wendell Brooks, James Dembowski, Helen Hook, Patricia Mullins, Stella Turk, Sandy Vayo, Robert Volin, and Donald Wildy. They each offered assistance within their own areas of expertise. Professor Phillip Schneider of Queens College, City University of New York, remains a steady source of inspiration. Hong Lee dos Reis was helpful in defining sociolinguistic and multicultural issues. Professor Loek Helminck of North Carolina State

University, Tony dos Reis and Linda Smith of SUNY New Paltz, and Joseph M. Haas and Carma Haas were consistently available to solve computer problems. Librarians and staff of the Sojourner Truth Library at SUNY New Paltz extended every courtesy to help me obtain needed source material. I am indebted to speech-language pathologist Nadine Rod who permitted me to follow her in her work with clients with dysphagia and to Cathy Augello who shared information regarding her work with prescholers. Professor Emerita Susan L. Puretz and Michael Lecesse offered encouragement and insights at various stages of the project. Suggestions and recommendation from students in my classes who used the first edition as a text are incorporated in this second edition. Thanks go to SLPs Louisa Finn, Andrea Thompson, and John Trembley for arranging for tapes of their clients for the CD-ROM.

My husband Kurt, who enticed me to collaborate with him on a textbook many years ago and honed my writing skills, receives my special thanks. Our adult children Ruth and Joseph, both teachers themselves, listened, encouraged, and advised as I strove to make complex material accessible to introductory-level students.

The following reviewers of this edition diligently questioned chapter organization and content in conscientious detail and offered many fine suggestions for improving the original manuscript. Their efforts are sincerely acknowledged: John W. Oller, Jr., Univeristy of Louisiana–Fayette; Kathryn N. Polmanteer, Eastern Kentucky University; Mary H. Purdy, Southern Connecticut State University; and Kathryn Chezik, Marshall University.

We especially appreciate Professor John W. Oller's thoughtful review of the 1st edition and his many helpful suggestions. He called to our attention that an omission of authorship was made in Table 4.2 of the first edition. We note in Table 5.3 of the present edition that the pragmatic criteria listed were adapted from Damico JS, Oller JW, & Storey ME (1983), The diagnosis of language disorders in bilingual children: surface-oriented and pragmatic criteria. Journal of Speech and Hearing Disorders, 48, 388; as well as from Nelson (1993) and others, as originally stated. We regret this earlier oversight.

Finally, we appreciate Steve Dragin's positive appraisal of our abilities and the energetic work of the entire Allyn and Bacon team that helped to make this book a reality.

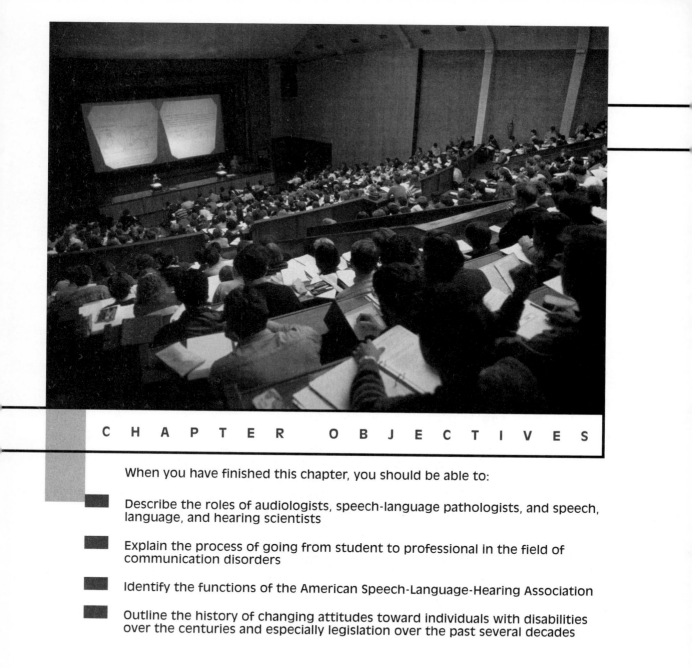

C H A P T E R   O B J E C T I V E S

When you have finished this chapter, you should be able to:

- Describe the roles of audiologists, speech-language pathologists, and speech, language, and hearing scientists

- Explain the process of going from student to professional in the field of communication disorders

- Identify the functions of the American Speech-Language-Hearing Association

- Outline the history of changing attitudes toward individuals with disabilities over the centuries and especially legislation over the past several decades

A Journey:
From Student
to Professional

Can you imagine life without communication? No talking, no listening, no interacting with others? Communication is part of what makes us human. Even minor or temporary problems with communication are often frustrating.

Many individuals who choose to study communication disorders have experienced a problem in speaking or listening at some time in their lives, or someone close to them is in this situation. Perhaps your impetus in reading this book is largely personal: to better understand yourself, a friend, or a relative. On the other hand, whatever your own experience, you may be embarking on a first step toward a possible career objective of becoming a speech-language pathologist or audiologist.

For all readers, we hope to provide a book that offers some insights into the nature of **communication disorders** and that is interesting and easy to read. We have attempted to establish a solid basis for further learning and provide in these pages sufficient detail that you will feel knowledgeable about major principles and issues.

In this first chapter, we take you on a journey from student to professional. We outline the steps for becoming an audiologist, speech-language pathologist, or speech scientist. These and other professional team members who work with people who have speech and language problems, where they work, and what they do are explained.

You will learn about the various types of credentials that are needed in different employment settings and about the organizations through which professionals can address issues, learn, and advocate for the people they serve. This first chapter also provides a historical perspective and outlines the laws that mandate appropriate care for those in need. Along the way, we'll find out why people choose these careers.

HELPING OTHERS TO HELP THEMSELVES

Why do people decide to become speech-language pathologists or audiologists? It is mostly because of the satisfaction that they receive from helping others to live a fuller life. Box 1.1 contains excerpts from student applications to communication disorders programs. Many students cite a personal or family encounter with a communication disorder. Almost all write about a desire to be useful to society.

THE PROFESSIONALS

Opportunities for speech-language pathologists and audiologists include serving individuals of all ages from infancy through the aged with varied disorders, from mild to profound, in a wide assortment of settings.

Today, professionals who serve individuals with communication disorders come from several disciplines. They often refer clients to one another or work together to provide optimal care. Specialists in communication disorders are employed by preschools, schools, colleges, universities, hospitals, independent clinics, nursing care facilities, research laboratories, and home-based programs. Many are in private practice. Speech-language pathologists and audiologists receive similar basic training but in their advanced study concentrate on one profession or the other.

AUDIOLOGISTS

Audiologists are specialists who measure hearing ability and identify, assess, manage, and prevent disorders of hearing and balance. They use a variety of instruments to measure and appraise hearing in people from infancy through old age. Audiologists evaluate and assist individuals with central auditory processing disorders. Audiologists select, fit, and dispense hearing aids and other amplification devices, and they provide guidance in their care and use. They work within educational settings to improve communication and programming for people with hearing disabilities. Audiologists contribute to the prevention of hearing loss by recommending and fitting protective devices and by consulting to government and industry on the effects and management of environmental noise. Licensed audiologists are independent professionals who practice without a prescription from any other health care provider (ASHA, 2001b). Box 1.2 contains an audiologist's comments on some of the challenges and rewards of the profession. As you will note, being a good detective, or problem solver, is one of the skills that is needed.

CREDENTIALS FOR AUDIOLOGISTS

At the present time, the entry-level requirement for audiologists is a master's degree. Prospective audiologists have studied hearing science, the assessment and remediation of hearing loss, anatomy and physiology, and related subjects, and they have obtained supervised clinical experience (see Table 1.1: Steps to becoming a speech-language pathologist or audiologist).

Beginning in the year 2012, individuals wishing to work as audiologists will need three to five years of education beyond the bachelor's degree. Their studies will culminate in a doctoral degree that may be an audiology doctorate (Au.D.), doctor of philosophy degree (Ph.D.), or doctor of education degree (Ed.D.). Preparation will include additional emphasis on hearing science and disorders, as well as assessment, treatment, and professional issues. The number of hours and types of settings used for preprofessional clinical experience will also increase. Some universities have already implemented an Au.D. program, a relatively new concept; others are in various stages of planning.

After a person has earned either a master's degree (prior to 2012) or a doctorate (after 2012), obtained the required preprofessional as well as paid clinical experience, and passed a national examination, she or he is eligible for the Certificate of Clinical Competence in Audiology (CCC-A) awarded by the American Speech-Language-Hearing Association (ASHA). ASHA CCC-A (sometimes referred to as ASHA "Cs") is the generally accepted standard for most employment opportunities for audiologists. In addition, most states require audiologists to obtain a state license. The requirements tend to be the same or very similar to the ASHA standards (ASHA, 2001a, b).

Beginning in the year 2012, a doctorate degree will be required for professional employment as an audiologist.

SPEECH-LANGUAGE PATHOLOGISTS

Speech-language pathologists (SLPs) are professionals who provide an assortment of services that relate to communicative disorders. The distinguishing role of the SLP is to identify, assess, treat, and prevent speech and language disorders both receptively and expressively in all modalities (including spoken, written, pictorial, and manual). This includes attention to physiological, cognitive, and social aspects of communication. Speech-language pathologists also provide services for disorders of swallowing and may work with individuals who choose

BOX 1.1

Reasons for Selecting a Major in Communication Disorders

Students who applied to major in communication disorders were asked to write a brief essay explaining their motivation. Some excerpts from these essays follow:

Erika B.: When I was a little girl I can painfully remember being picked on by the other children about the way I spoke. My once cute lisp was no longer cute at 8. I was told that "I talked like a baby" or sometimes the kids would mimic what I said in an exaggerated way. At age 10, my family moved to a new school district. A speech-language pathologist there worked with me on my lisp and other articulation problems. People who meet me today can hardly believe that I ever had a problem! I want to help people who are in similar situations. I know the hurt that accompanies the humiliation of being teased because you can't communicate properly.

Dana C.: One of my best friends was born with a complete bilateral cleft lip and palate. After thirteen operations and over nine years of speech therapy, a stranger would never know that my friend ever had a communication problem. I want to have the opportunity to help to make a similar difference in someone's life.

Victoria F.: All of her life, my cousin Jackie's family had been told that she had a common disfluency problem and that she would outgrow it. How-

ever, Jackie was a teenager and continued to be dysfluent. Finally Jackie's parents took her to a speech-language pathologist in private practice. The speech therapy resulted in transforming Jackie from a shy child with a reluctance to speak to a gregarious adolescent. At her Sweet 16 party, Jackie took the microphone and read her own speech of thanks and recognition and everyone cried. That's when I realized that I wanted to be a speech pathologist.

Tara F.: My interest in speech science began soon after I graduated from our local community college with a business degree. I knew this would result in a monotonous desk job, and I wanted my career path to take a different direction but I did not yet know what. That August my grandmother had quadruple heart bypass surgery and a stroke followed. I entered the world of speech science three days after she slipped into a semi-coma. When she awoke, she couldn't speak at all. I went to my library and checked out a book about strokes and read it cover to cover that night. I learned that even though she couldn't express herself through spoken word, she might be able to do so in writing, and she did. Each day was frustrating, but my grandmother improved and was soon able to grunt. From grunting, she moved to words

to modify a regional or foreign dialect. Like audiologists, licensed speech-language pathologists are independent professionals who practice without a prescription from any other health care provider (ASHA, 2000a, b, c). Box 1.3 contains reflections by two speech-language

like "No!" and she laughed aloud. Often words would come out, but they did not make sense. It was as though she was speaking a foreign language. She eventually recovered, but not fully. Although she regained her ability to speak, she speaks more slowly and more thought is required than before the stroke. My grandmother is the motivation behind my anticipated speech pathology career choice.

Denise F.: I had always considered attending college after completing my high school education, but due to unfortunate financial circumstances at that time, I was unable to do so. I took a job with an insurance agency and through eighteen years of employment developed a satisfying career. About twelve years ago, at the age of 2, my oldest son was classified as Speech Impaired and Learning Disabled. He is now in the ninth grade and has made tremendous progress. He is mainstreamed for all subjects with only minimal Resource Room time. He is no longer classified as Speech Impaired. Although I tried to help him at home, I know my son would never have made the progress that he has without the professional services of special educators. I want the opportunity to provide these services and benefits to other families and their children.

Devon T.: My mother is hard-of-hearing. She has less than 50 percent hearing in each ear. Growing up was a little bit different because of this. I had to repeat myself most of the time while talking to her. I had to speak clearly, and most of all, I could not cover my mouth. My mother reads lips. Whenever the phone rings in my house, a lamp in my mother's room lights up. My mother bought her first hearing aid several years ago and cried all night. The only thing I could think of was how amazing that this little machine could help her hear better. I loved looking at it, and I admired my mother for overcoming her hardships and handicap.

John T.: I am a 40-year-old successful pastry chef. Since I have a family, a career change took lots of planning and the beginning of a dream being fulfilled. When my son was 3 years old, he still was only babbling. His doctor was wonderful, but from Korea and did not see any problems with Jimmy's speech. Since my wife and I were worried, we had Jimmy evaluated by a speech-language pathologist. He was diagnosed with language and articulation difficulties. We took him to the clinic at St. John's University. The therapy made a difference in my son's life. It also crystallized my desire to work with children in a helpful and meaningful way.

pathologists; the first one has been in private practice as a clinician for about twenty-five years. Although sometimes frustrated by the lack of support within his work setting, he believes in setting his imagination free and not giving up in the challenge to help others. The other

BOX 1.2

An Audiologist Reflects

Stella T.: I love the detective work of diagnostic procedures and the closure of rehab. I am given the clues from case history and my test findings. My job is to quickly and efficiently come up with an accurate diagnosis, recommendations, and rehabilitative plan. I have to be able to explain these in terms my patients can understand. I have to have completed all of this in less than one hour before moving on to save the rest of the world. I get closure by being able to measure the success of my rehabilitative plan within a relatively short span of time (a few weeks) and make adjustments in my plan as needed. I love making another person's life a little easier.

SLP, similar to the audiologist quoted earlier, notes the detective-like work and satisfaction of helping others.

CREDENTIALS FOR SPEECH-LANGUAGE PATHOLOGISTS

Speech-language pathologists have a master's or doctoral degree and have studied typical communication and its development in children, anatomy and physiology of the speech and hearing mechanisms, phonetics, and speech and hearing science.

Three types of credentials are available for speech-language pathologists:

1. Public school certification normally stipulates basic and advanced coursework, clinical practice within a school setting, and a satisfactory score on a state or national examination. At the least, prospective school SLPs need a bachelor's degree, although in an increasing number of states, a master's degree either is the entry-level requirement or is mandated after a certain number of years of employment. The exact requirements to become a school SLP vary from state to state. If you plan to move to another state after completing your education as a speech-language pathologist, you should investigate the specifics through that state's education department. The American Speech-Language-Hearing Association does not endorse the lower degree and encourages the same standards for SLPs in all employment settings, as described in the following paragraph.

2. The American Speech-Language-Hearing Association issues a Certificate of Clinical Competence in Speech-Language Pathology

TABLE 1.1

Steps to becoming a speech-language pathologist or audiologist

1. Obtain a B.S. or a B.A., preferably with a major in communication disorders.
   a. Complete the general studies or general education requirements of your college or university.
   b. Complete 27 semester hours or more in basic science (some may overlap with 1a above):
      - 3 semester hours or more in biological or physical science
      - 3 semester hours or more in college level mathematics (e.g., calculus, statistics, computer science with a large mathematical component)
      - 6 semester hours or more in behavioral and/or social sciences (e.g., psychology, sociology, gerontology)
      - 3 semester hours or more in anatomy and physiology of the speech and hearing mechanism
      - 3 semester hours or more in physical bases and processes of the production and perception of speech, language, and hearing (e.g., acoustics, physics of sound, phonetics, speech/hearing science)
      - 3 semester hours or more in normal development of speech, language, and hearing (e.g., linguistics, psycholinguistics, language and speech acquisition)
2. Obtain an M.A. or M.S. with a major in communication disorders from an ASHA-accredited college or university.
   a. Complete 36 semester hours or more in professional coursework:
      - 30 semester hours or more in major area of speech-language pathology or audiology
      - 6 semester hours or more in minor area of speech-language pathology or audiology
      - Courses must cover:
        Specific types of disorders
        Evaluation skills
        Management procedures
        Prevention
        Information on culturally diverse populations
        Communication disorders across the life span.
   b. If you plan to work within a public school system, take courses that lead to certification by your state to teach students with speech and language disabilities.
   c. Complete 25 hours of clinical observation and 350 (375 beginning in 2005) hours of clinical practicum.
3. Pass the National Examination in Speech-Language Pathology or Audiology.
4. Complete a clinical fellowship equivalent to 36 weeks (9 months) of full-time professional employment for speech-language pathology or 12 months for audiology, within seven years of completion of academic and practicum education.
5. For audiology, earn a doctoral degree, if applying for certification in 2012 or later.
6. Apply for certification and licensure.
7. Demonstrate continuing education.

Source: Adapted from ASHA (2001a, b).

BOX 1.3

Two Speech-Language Pathologists Reflect

Phillip S.: Gladys was 12 when I met her. She had NO voice, no laugh, no cry, no moan, no words and no song. The administrators of the school for multiply handicapped children said not to work with her because she could not be helped—after all, she had no voice. Why? Why no voice? Why no way to help? Why such pessimism? Against the will of the institution, we began to explore and she sang in the school show five months later. It was not until the following fall that she began to speak normally, as though she had been doing it all her life. It was experiencing the birth of Gladys's voice that sent me back to school for my doctoral studies. Was this a miracle? I guess a miracle is when something is possible, and does happen, but it was beyond your imagination. In our work we must first see something that is not yet there and believe in it long enough to become a partner in making it come about.

Robert O.: For me, the exciting part of my job is the problem solving and the satisfaction of helping others. Similar to a fictional detective who collects all the clues, synthesizes the information, and deduces the guilty party, I evaluate each client and determine the best course of intervention. The more severe the impairment, the greater the challenge, and I love a challenge. How can I help a young man who attempted suicide and is now brain injured to access the language within him? How can a young child with autism begin the road through communication to language? How can I help parents communicate with their infant who has deafness, blindness, and cerebral palsy? When is the best time to introduce signing with a nonspeaking client? These are all challenges for me and the children and adults I serve. We work together as I try to solve each communication puzzle and propose and implement possible intervention strategies. Sometimes I'm very successful and sometimes I have to reevaluate my methods, but as I said, I love a challenge.

(CCC-SLP) to individuals who have obtained a master's degree or doctorate in the field with at least 25 hours of clinical observation and 350 clock hours of supervised clinical practicum. In addition, certificate holders must have a year of paid professional experience and have passed a national examination.

Beginning January 1, 2005, 375 clock hours of direct patient contact during supervised practicum will be required, and ongoing professional development will have to be demonstrated through any of a variety of continuing education options (ASHA, 2000a).

3. Many states have licensure laws for speech-language pathologists, audiologists, and other professionals that are independent of the state's department of education certification requirements. A license might be needed if you plan to engage in private practice or work in a hospital, clinic, or other setting apart from a public school. Most states accept a person with ASHA CCC-SLP as having met licensure requirements, although you will need to check with your state licensing board and be prepared to submit documentation and pay a fee.

Table 1.2 shows the credentials that are needed in the professions of audiology and speech-language pathology.

SPEECH, LANGUAGE, AND HEARING SCIENTISTS

Individuals who are employed as speech, language, or hearing scientists typically have earned a doctorate degree, either a Ph.D. or an Ed.D. They are employed by universities, government agencies, industry, and research centers to extend our knowledge of human communication processes and disorders. Some may also serve as clinical speech-language pathologists or audiologists.

The professions of speech-language pathology and audiology require life-long learning. Clinicians need to be able to intelligently use relevant research findings in their practice. Conventions, short courses, journals, the World Wide Web, as well as lively personal and on-line exchanges among colleagues foster growth and dedication to the fields. By 2005, continuing education must be demonstrated by those who intend to maintain their credentials.

TABLE 1.2

Credentials for speech-language pathologists and audiologists

Credentialing Organization	Speech-Language Pathologist	Audiologist
American Speech-Language-Hearing Association	Certificate of Clinical Competence in Speech-Language Pathology (CCC-SLP)	Certificate of Clinical Competence in Audiology (CCC-A)
State department of education	Certification as Teacher of Students with Speech and Language Disabilities*	—
State professional licensing board	License as Speech-Language Pathologist	License as Audiologist

*The title for the school-based speech-language pathologist varies from state to state.

WHAT SPEECH, LANGUAGE, AND HEARING SCIENTISTS DO

Speech scientists may be involved in basic research exploring the anatomy, physiology, and physics of speech-sound production. Using spectrographs, speech synthesizers, computers and the like, these researchers strive to learn more about typical and pathological voice and articulation. Their findings help clinicians to improve service to clients with speech disorders. Recent advances in knowledge of human genetics provide fertile soil for continuing investigation into the causes, prevention, and treatment of various pathologies. Some speech scientists are involved in the development of computer-generated speech that may be used in telephone answering systems, substitute voices for individuals who are unable to speak, and many new purposes. Box 1.4 contains some observations by a speech-language scientist who enjoys the interdisciplinary nature of his work. His current research involves the study of tongue placement in the production of speech sounds.

BOX 1.4

A Speech-Language Scientist Reflects

James D.: What I like best about speech-language science is the way it combines disciplines. When I was in high school, my favorite subjects were English and biology. Studying speech-language science is like studying English and biology at the same time. To be a good speech-language scientist, or a good speech-language pathologist, or a good neuro-linguist, you have to know about BOTH language and physiology. It is not enough to be just a linguist or just a physiologist. And you have to know how these two things, one primarily a product of the "mind" (however one chooses to define that) and the other a function of the body, interact. Furthermore, the physiology of speech and language encompasses a broad range of bodily systems, including the neurologic, respiratory, laryngologic (or phonatory), and upper vocal tract articulatory. As if that wasn't enough in itself, you must know something about the physics of sound to really understand speech and its production. If you choose to explore speech modeling or have a clinical interest in augmentative communication systems, you could even touch on areas that we normally think of as associated with engineering. Thus, the study of speech-language science is a truly interdisciplinary study, in any number of ways. In that respect, it is a continual challenge, intellectually, and provides an opportunity to interact with a tremendously broad range of other professionals.

Language scientists, also called **linguists,** may investigate the ways in which children learn their native tongue. They may study the differences and similarities of different languages. Over the past half a century or so, the United States has become increasingly linguistically and culturally diverse; this provides an excellent opportunity for cross-cultural study of language and communication. Some language scientists explore the variations of modern-day English (dialects) and how the language is changing. Others are concerned with language disabilities and study the nature of language disorders in children and adults. An in-depth knowledge of typical language is critical to understanding language problems.

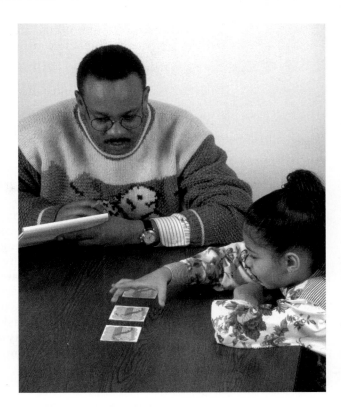

Simple props are often used to elicit language in a nonthreatening way.

T H O U G H T   Q U E S T I O N

What language and cultural groups were represented in your elementary and high school? Were issues regarding bilingualism or cultural diversity raised? What important research might a language scientist conduct in this environment?

Hearing scientists investigate the nature of sound, noise, and hearing. They may work with other scientists in the development of equipment to be used in the assessment of hearing. They are also involved in the development of techniques for testing the hard-to-test, such as infants or those with severe physical or psychological impairments. Hearing scientists develop new and improved ways to help people who have limited hearing, including assistive listening devices such as hearing aids and telephone amplifiers. They are concerned with conservation of hearing and are engaged in research to measure and limit the impact of environmental noise.

PROFESSIONAL AIDES

Professional aides, sometimes referred to as paraprofessionals or speech-language pathology or audiology assistants, are individuals who work closely with an SLP or audiologist. The title, requirements, and responsibilities of these individuals vary from state to state. Some two- and four-year colleges have special programs that lead to credentialing of support personnel.

Speech-language pathology assistants (SLPAs) typically participate in screenings. They often engage in routine therapy tasks that have been structured by an SLP. They may engage in clerical tasks and assist the SLP in the preparation of assessment and treatment materials. SLPAs may work in any of the settings in which a fully credentialed SLP is found. Audiology assistants are supervised by an audiologist and may conduct screenings, participate in calibration of audiological instrumentation, and engage in a variety of clerical tasks.

Support personnel may work only with supervision and are not permitted to perform such tasks as interpretation of test results, service plan development, family/client counseling, or determination of when to discharge a client from treatment (ASHA, 1995b; Paul-Brown & Goldberg, 2001).

Paraprofessionals usually have an associate's or bachelor's degree; they work closely with and are supervised by professionals with more training and experience.

RELATED PROFESSIONS: A TEAM APPROACH

Specialists in communication disorders do not operate in a vacuum. They work closely with family members, regular and special educators, psychologists, social workers, doctors and other medical personnel, occupational, physical, and music therapists. They may collaborate with physicists and engineers. Box 1.5 contains a speech-language pathologist's schedule, showing a tremendous amount of teamwork.

SERVICE THROUGH THE LIFE CYCLE

Individuals with communication disorders may be of any age, and professionals address their needs from birth through old age. Infants may be screened for hearing loss and a host of other disabilities soon after birth. About 2 percent of all children born in the United States have some disabling condition, and hearing loss occurs more often than any other physical problem (U.S. Census Bureau, 1997). Babies and toddlers may exhibit developmental delay and mental retardation. They may have physical problems including those involving movement, hearing,

BOX 1.5

A Team Approach

Alicia is the senior speech-language pathologist in a community-based rehabilitation center in New York state. During the mornings, Alicia works with infants, preschoolers, and school-age children at the center. In the afternoons, she directs the Augmentative/Alternative Communication Program and assists severely impaired individuals of all ages to improve their communication abilities. The schedule outlined below has a bit more collaboration than is normally found in any one day, but it suggests the kinds of activities that are typical within a workweek.

8:30 A.M. Education staff meeting for preschool children: classroom teacher, psychologist, social worker, occupational therapist, physical therapist.

9:00 Preschool class activity: eight children ages 3–4, one classroom teacher, two aides.

10:00 Individual half-hour therapy sessions with children in the preschool and school programs.

11:30 Combined physical and speech therapy for Jeramy, age 4, diagnosed with spastic cerebral palsy; work with physical therapist.

noon Lunch

12:30 P.M. Prepare for the afternoon.

1:00 Consult with engineer on wheelchair switch for Lucretia, age 7, who is multiply handicapped.

1:30 Outpatient, David, aged 24, had been in a motorcycle accident and experiences some speech and language difficulties.

3:00 Conference with Sally Brown, Bettina's foster mother, and Barbara Sloane, the social worker for the family.

3:30 Communication Disorders Department Meeting. Malcolm, an audiologist, reports on three-hour course he took on Saturday on cochlear implants.

4:30 The workday is officially over, but Alicia stays until 5:00 to read the professional journal *Language, Speech, and Hearing Services in the Schools,* which arrived today. Alicia is especially interested in the article about using children's books in working with preschoolers and photocopies it to share with other staff members.

and vision. These disabilities may be due to a wide range of causes, discussed later in this text, and may impact the youngster's communication and feeding abilities. An interdisciplinary approach is necessary in the assessment and treatment of children, and an Individualized Family Service Plan (IFSP), developed for each child treated, must be directed at the entire family with sensitivity to its language and culture. Early intervention has been demonstrated to be highly valuable in facilitating optimum results and potentially preventing later difficulties.

Preschoolers with communication difficulties must also be identified and helped. For some, services begun earlier may now be handled by different agencies. The youngster may be placed in a special preschool; professionals may continue to assist the family in addressing the child's needs. Parents may voice concerns about preparing their child for the challenges of first grade.

Almost half of all speech-language pathologists are employed by school systems. They work with youngsters in all grades, addressing a full range of communication problems. These are described in the chapters that follow. School-age children with communication difficulties often also suffer academically and socially, thereby adding additional urgency to the work of communication experts.

Some young adults such as those who were identified earlier as being developmentally delayed or with physical disabilities may continue to receive certain services until they are 21 years old. At this point some of these women and men may enter day-treatment programs, and/or find employment in sheltered workshops where speech-language pathologists and audiologists may be available to serve their needs.

Other individuals may find themselves in need of communication services for the first time later in life. More than 5 million Americans are reported to have suffered traumatic brain injury (see Chapter 12) stemming from bicycle, motorcycle, or car accidents or from falls. As a result, they may have cognitive and/or motor problems that interfere with their ability to communicate and/or eat normally. The speech-language pathologist may play an important role in rehabilitative efforts.

Among those over age 65, stroke, neurological disorders, and dementia may interfere with effective communication and swallowing. Hearing loss may affect at least one in four, creating a need for assessment and treatment. Speech-language pathologists and audiologists work directly with older people. They often also work with spouses and children, as well as staff members of nursing homes and other adult facilities in providing counseling and guidance directed at improving quality of life in these later years (Lubinski & Masters, 2001).

PROFESSIONAL ORGANIZATIONS

AMERICAN SPEECH-LANGUAGE-HEARING ASSOCIATION

The American Speech-Language-Hearing Association (ASHA) is a nonprofit organization of speech-language pathologists, audiologists, and speech and hearing scientists that was founded in 1925. In 2001, it had a membership of more than 100,000 professionals from throughout the

United States and the world. It is the largest association for those concerned with communication disorders. ASHA's mission is to "promote the interests of and provide the highest quality services for professionals in audiology, speech-language pathology, and speech hearing science, and to advocate for people with communication disorders" (ASHA, 2002). Toward these ends, ASHA promotes scientific study, encourages quality clinical services, supports high ethical principles, and advocates for those with communicative disorders.

SCIENTIFIC STUDY OF THE PROCESSES AND DISORDERS OF HUMAN COMMUNICATION

ASHA encourages study of typical and disordered communication by mandating a curriculum of study for prospective speech-language pathologists and audiologists that specifies appropriate coursework. This is outlined in Table 1.1. In addition, ASHA provides financial grants to individuals who are engaged in research that furthers our knowledge of communication and assessment, treatment, and prevention of pathologies. ASHA works closely with governmental agencies that may sponsor relevant scientific investigation.

To dispense knowledge among professionals, ASHA publishes several scholarly periodicals: *Journal of Speech, Language, and Hearing Research*; *Language, Speech, and Hearing Services in Schools*; *American Journal of Speech-Language Pathology: A Journal of Clinical Practice*; and *American Journal of Audiology: A Journal of Clinical Practice*. ASHA also holds an annual convention at which members and others share information and learn through scientific sessions, exhibits, seminars, and short courses. Additional institutes, workshops, conferences, and teleseminars are held throughout the year. Continuing education for professionals is fostered through these activities, and an Award for Continuing Education (ACE) is granted to individual speech-language pathologists and audiologists as recognition of accomplishment.

Students who join the National Student Speech-Language-Hearing Association (NSSLH) receive professional journals and may attend conferences at reduced rates.

CLINICAL SERVICE IN SPEECH-LANGUAGE PATHOLOGY AND AUDIOLOGY

Programs that provide clinical services to people with communicative disorders may be accredited by ASHA. This means that representatives of ASHA will review the procedures that are used in diagnosis and treatment. A site visit will ensure that equipment, materials, and record keeping adhere to the highest professional standards. Clinical service will be the responsibility of individuals who meet ASHA standards for the CCC-SLP or CCC-A (see Table 1.1).

MAINTENANCE OF ETHICAL STANDARDS

To ensure that the highest moral and ethical principles are followed within the professions of speech-language pathology and audiology,

Ethical questions pervade our lives as individuals and professionals. New technology requires that speech-language pathologists and audiologists continually update their skills so as to safely and accurately address patient needs. Managed care or other administrative leadership may tempt a clinician to spread her- or himself too thin. A student clinician may observe what she or he believes to be unethical behavior. At all times, it is up to each individual to know the code of ethics and to seek consultation in assuring adherence to the highest possible standards.

ASHA provides a code of ethics, which is in the appendix to this chapter. The basic principles are as follows:

1. The welfare of the persons served by communication disorders specialists is paramount. If you observe in a clinical center as part of your coursework, what you see is to be treated with confidentiality. Client records are privileged documents. Your observations must not interfere with the clinical service being provided. If student clinicians are engaging in therapy, supervisors must consider the clients' needs as primary.

2. Each professional must achieve and maintain the highest level of professional competence. The ASHA Certificates of Clinical Competence (CCC) are considered the minimal achievement for independent professional practice. Clinicians should provide service only within their own areas of competence. Professional development and continuing education should be ongoing.

3. Professionals must promote understanding and provide accurate information in statements to the public. In a college or university center, you'll note that the qualifications of student clinicians as well as the nature of their supervision are explained to clients.

4. Professionals are responsible for assuring that ethical standards are maintained by themselves, colleagues, students, and members of allied professions. All members of ASHA are responsible for the monitoring and maintaining of ethical standards throughout the profession (American Speech-Language-Hearing Association, 2001).

T H O U G H T   Q U E S T I O N

Why must clinical supervisors consider the welfare of their clients of primary importance? Does this impinge on student learning?

ADVOCACY FOR INDIVIDUALS WITH COMMUNICATIVE DISABILITIES

The American Speech-Language-Hearing Association is active in encouraging members of Congress and state legislatures to pass legislation that provides for appropriate services for communication-impaired individuals. Bills such as the Individuals with Disabilities Education Act and the Americans with Disabilities Act became law in part because of the extensive promotional activities of organizations such as ASHA.

The needs and characteristics of people with speech, language and hearing disabilities are clarified and publicized by ASHA on radio, on television, and through print media. In May, which is "Better Speech and Hearing Month," you are especially likely to hear public service announcements that advocate for understanding, prevention, and treatment of communication disorders.

RELATED PROFESSIONAL ASSOCIATIONS

Although ASHA is the largest organization for communication disorder professionals, other groups are also active and worthwhile. Some speech-language pathologists and audiologists belong to several associations. Table 1.3 lists some of those most closely affiliated.

COMMUNICATION DISORDERS IN HISTORICAL PERSPECTIVE

Disorders are nothing new. However, the terminology, identification, and treatment of people with disabilities have changed dramatically through the years. Handicaps of any type were viewed harshly in days of old. Society was built on a survival-of-the-fittest mentality, and less able individuals were shunned. Primitive peoples are reported to have abandoned those who could not keep up with the rest of the group. Children who were malformed were often abandoned, and the aged who could no longer contribute were sometimes deprived of food or even killed.

Over the centuries attitudes changed somewhat and by the 1700s in many parts of the world, societal efforts were being made to help those who were unable to care for themselves. Individuals began to be classified and grouped according to their disorder. Special residences for

Prospective speech-language pathologists and audiologists are advised to take courses in related areas such as psychology and sociology in order to better understand their clients and work more effectively with professionals from other disciplines.

TABLE 1.3

Selected professional associations relevant to communication disorders

Academy of Dispensing Audiologists	American Auditory Society	National Hearing Conservation Association
Academy of Rehabilitative Audiology	American Speech-Language-Hearing Association	National Student Speech-Language-Hearing Association
American Academy of Audiology	Audiology Foundation of America	Orton Dyslexia Society
American Academy of Otolaryngology–Head and Neck Surgery	Canadian Association of Speech-Language Pathologists	Stuttering Foundation of America
	Council on Education of the Deaf	

---

individuals with deafness, blindness, mental illness, and intellectual limitations were established. However, some were little more than warehouses providing no services other than what was necessary to keep the residents alive (Karagiannis, Stainback, & Stainback, 1996).

Eventually, improvement was made, and during the 1960s in the United States and elsewhere, intense energy was directed toward the advancement of civil rights for all people. Just as the rights of women, ethnic minorities, gays, and lesbians were recast, the status of individuals with disabilities was reevaluated, and bold reforms were initiated. The American Coalition of Citizens with Disabilities was created in 1974; legislative action on behalf of all Americans with handicapping conditions began in earnest around the same time. In many cases, people who were disabled occupied leadership roles in the push for change. As

---

TABLE 1.4

It's the law: Major provisions of important federal legislation affecting people with communicative disabilities

1965: *Elementary and Secondary Education Act (Public Law 89-10)*
- States were provided federal funds so that students with special needs, including the gifted, would be evaluated and educated.

1966: *Handicapped Children's Early Education Act (Public Law 90-247)*
- Model programs for educating children with disabilities were federally funded.

1973: *Section 504 of the Vocational Rehabilitation Act (Public Law 93-112)*
- Forbids discrimination of services or employment to people with disabling conditions.

1975: *Education of All Handicapped Children Act (EAHCA) (Public Law 94-142)*
- All school-age children with disabilities must be provided a free, appropriate public education in the least restrictive environment.
- All related services (including speech-language therapy, physical therapy, and occupational therapy) that are needed for the child to benefit from the education must be provided.

- To benefit from this law, children must be evaluated and found to have a disabling condition as defined in the law.
- An Individual Education Plan (IEP) must be written for each child and must stipulate:
  Present level of performance;
  Annual long-term goals and short-term objectives;
  Designated instruction, services, and placement;
  Date services are to be initiated and anticipated duration of services.
- A Committee on Special Education (CSE) composed of the child's parents (or person designated by them), school administrator, and relevant educators and teachers must meet to review and endorse the IEP.
- Parents must agree to the initial evaluation in writing and approve and sign the IEP.
- The IEP must be reviewed each year.

1986: *Education of the Handicapped Amendments (Public Law 99-457)*
- Federal funds were provided to states that want to develop programs for disabled infants and toddlers from birth through age 2.

---

a result of this work, providing opportunities for individuals with disabilities to develop to their full potential was no longer simply an ethical position. It became federally mandated through a series of laws.

Congress enacted the Education for All Handicapped Children Act (EAHCA) as Public Law Number 94-142 in 1975. It mandated that a free and appropriate public education must be provided for all handicapped children between the ages of 5 and 21. Several years later, Public Law 99-457 extended the age of those served to cover youngsters between the ages of birth and 5. In 1990, Congress reauthorized the original law and renamed it the Individuals with Disabilities Education Act (IDEA). IDEA addressed the multicultural nature of U.S. society. The needs of individuals with limited English proficiency and those from racial and ethnic minorities were targeted for special consideration. Table 1.4

A series of laws passed by the United States Congress over the past fifty years mandate appropriate treatment for individuals with disabilities.

1986: *Education of the Handicapped Amendments (continued)*

- The provisions of P.L. 94-142 were extended to disabled children between the ages of 3 and 5 years.

- Services must be provided by qualified personnel who meet the criteria for licensure stipulated by the state. (The intent was to end the double standard with one set of requirements needed to provide services in a school setting and another set needed to work in hospitals or private agencies.)

- An Individualized Family Service Plan (IFSP) must be written for each child with special needs that may include home-based instruction and therapy and parent education.

1988: *Technology-Related Assistance for Individuals with Disabilities (Public Law 100-407)*

- Included funding for centers to serve children and adults who may benefit from augmentative and alternative communication (AAC).

- Additional technological support became available.

1990: *Individuals with Disabilities Education Act (IDEA)*

- Reauthorized and renamed the 1975 EAHCA.

- Recognized and made provisions for increasing diversity of U.S. population.

1990: *Americans with Disabilities Act (ADA) (Public Law 101-336)*

- Mandated improved access to buildings and facilities that provide goods or services to the public through provision of ramps, parking facilities.

- Mandated accessible rest rooms.

- Provided for effective communication with people with disabilities, including use of interpreters, appropriate signage; and telecommunication devices for the deaf (TDDs).

- Included reasonable modifications of policies and practices that may be discriminatory.

Sources: Rosenfeld (1999), U.S. Department of Justice (2000), Zantal-Wiener, K. (1988).

summarizes major federal legislation that has implications for individuals with communication disorders.

SUMMARY

Speech-language pathologists, audiologists, and other specialists work together to assist those with communicative impairments. They work in a variety of settings and with people of all ages. They are rewarded by contributing to the well-being of others. Professionals who are engaged in clinical service for those with communication disorders have a minimum of a master's degree and supervised clinical experience. They generally have earned the American Speech-Language-Hearing Association Certificate of Clinical Competence (ASHA-CCC) in their area of specialization. Speech, language, and hearing scientists usually have doctorate degrees and are dedicated to advancing knowledge regarding typical and disordered communication processes. Professional aides may work with a two- or four-year college degree, but are limited in the tasks that they may perform and work only with supervision. Services are provided to individuals from birth through old age. The American Speech-Language-Hearing Association (ASHA) is the largest organization of professionals in communication disorders. ASHA's missions include the scientific study of human communication, provision of clinical service in speech-language pathology and audiology, maintenance of ethical standards, and advocacy for individuals with communication disabilities. Federal legislation currently mandates services for people with disabilities.

REFLECTIONS

- What do speech-language pathologists and audiologists do?
- What do speech, language, and hearing scientists do?
- What are the requirements for becoming a professional in the fields of communicative disorders?
- What services might be needed for individuals at different ages?

- What are the missions of the American Speech-Language-Hearing Association?
- How have attitudes toward people with disabilities changed through the centuries?

SUGGESTED READINGS

Nicolosi, L., Harryman, E., & Kresheck, J. (1996). *Terminology of communication disorders: Speech, language, hearing* (4th ed.). Baltimore: Williams & Wilkins.

Nolan, C. (1987). *Under the eye of the clock: The life story of Christopher Nolan.* New York: St. Martin's Press.

Peterson's Guides. (Ed.). (2000). *Peterson's graduate & professional programs 2001: An overview.* Princeton, NJ: Peterson's (published annually).

Singh, S. (Ed.). (2000). *Singular's illustrated dictionary of speech-language pathology.* San Diego: Singular.

ON-LINE RESOURCES

http://www.acoustics.org/   Acoustical Society of America.

Of special interest to hearing scientists and audiologists.

http://www.audiology.org/   American Academy of Audiology.

Consumer and professional information regarding hearing and balance disorders as well as audiological services.

http://professional.asha.org/   American Speech-Language-Hearing Association.

Information for professionals, students, and others who are interested in careers in speech-language pathology, audiology, or speech, language, or hearing science.

http://nidcd.nih.gov/   National Institute on Deafness and Other Communication Disorders (NIDCD).

The U.S. governmental agency site containing relevant health and research information.

http://iiswinprd01.petersons.com/   Peterson's Guide to Graduate and Professional Education.

Links to a list and descriptions of institutions offering programs in communication disorders.

APPENDIX 1.1: AMERICAN SPEECH-LANGUAGE-HEARING ASSOCIATION CODE OF ETHICS

Last Revised November 16, 2001

PREAMBLE

The preservation of the highest standards of integrity and ethical principles is vital to the responsible discharge of obligations in the professions of speech-language pathology and audiology. This Code of Ethics sets forth the fundamental principles and rules considered essential to this purpose.

Every individual who is (a) a member of the American Speech-Language-Hearing Association, whether certified or not, (b) a nonmember holding the Certificate of Clinical Competence from the Association, (c) an applicant for membership or certification, or (d) a Clinical Fellow seeking to fulfill standards for certification shall abide by this Code of Ethics.

Any action that violates the spirit and purpose of this Code shall be considered unethical. Failure to specify any particular responsibility or practice in this Code of Ethics shall not be construed as denial of the existence of such responsibilities or practices.

The fundamentals of ethical conduct are described by Principles of Ethics and by Rules of Ethics as they relate to responsibility to persons served, to the public, and to the professions of speech-language pathology and audiology.

Principles of Ethics, aspirational and inspirational in nature, form the underlying moral basis for the Code of Ethics. Individuals shall observe these principles as affirmative obligations under all conditions of professional activity.

Rules of Ethics are specific statements of minimally acceptable professional conduct or of prohibitions and are applicable to all individuals.

PRINCIPLE OF ETHICS I

Individuals shall honor their responsibility to hold paramount the welfare of persons they serve professionally.

RULES OF ETHICS

A. shall provide all services competently.

B. Individuals shall use every resource, including referral when appropriate, to ensure that high-quality service is provided.

C. Individuals shall not discriminate in the delivery of professional services on the basis of race or ethnicity, gender, age, religion, national origin, sexual orientation, or disability.

D. Individuals shall not misrepresent the credentials of assistants, technicians, or support personnel and ahll inform those they serve professionally of the name and professional credentials of persons providing services.

E. Individuals who hold the Certificates of Clinical Competence shall not delegate tasks that require the unique skills,

Source: American Speech-Language-Hearing Association. (2001, December 26). Code of ethics. (revised). *Asha Leader*, 6 (23), 2.

knowledge, and judgment that are within the scope of their profession to assistants, technicians, support personnel, or any nonprofessionals over whom they have supervisory responsibility. An individual may delegate support services to assistants, technicians, support personnel, or any other persons only if those services are adequately supervised by an individual who holds the appropriate Certificate of Clinical Competence.

F. Individuals shall fully inform the persons they serve of the nature and possible effects of services rendered and products dispensed.

G. Individuals shall evaluate the effectiveness of services rendered and of products dispensed and shall provide services or dispense products only when benefit can reasonably be expected.

H. Individuals shall not guarantee the results of any treatment or procedure, directly or by implication; however, they may make a reasonable statement of prognosis.

I. Individuals shall not provide clinical services solely by correspondence.

J. Individuals may practice by telecommunication (for example, telehealth/e-health), where not prohibited by law.

K. Individuals shall maintain adequate records of professional services rendered and products dispensed and shall allow access to these records when appropriately authorized.

L. Individuals shall not reveal, without authorization, any professional or personal information about the person served professionally, unless required by law to do so, or unless doing so is necessary to protect the welfare of the person or of the community.

M. Individuals shall not charge for services not rendered, nor shall they misrepresent,[1] in any fashion, services rendered or products dispensed.

N. Individuals shall use persons in research or as subjects of teaching demonstrations only with their informed consent.

O. Individuals whose professional services are adversely affected by substance abuse or other health-related conditions shall seek professional assistance and, where appropriate, withdraw from the affected areas of practice.

PRINCIPLE OF ETHICS II

Individuals shall honor their responsibility to achieve and maintain the highest level of professional competence.

RULES OF ETHICS

A. Individuals shall engage in the provision of clinical services only when they hold the appropriate Certificate of Clinical Competence or when they are in the certification process and are supervised by an individual who holds the appropriate Certificate of Clinical Competence.

B. Individuals shall engage in only those aspects of the professions that are within the scope of their competence, considering their level of education, training, and experience.

---

[1]For purposes of this Code of Ethics, misrepresentation includes any untrue statements or statements that are likely to mislead. Misrepresentation also includes the failure to state any information that is material and that ought, in fairness, to be considered.

C. Individuals shall continue their professional development throughout their careers.

D. Individuals shall delegate the provision of clinical services only to: (1) persons who hold the appropriate Certificate of Clinical Competence; (2) persons in the education or certification process who are appropriately supervised by an individual who holds the appropriate Certificate of Clinical Competence; or (3) assistants, technicians, or support personnel who are adequately supervised by an individual who holds the appropriate Certificate of Clinical Competence.

E. Individuals shall prohibit any of their professional staff from providing services that exceed the staff member's competence, considering the staff member's level of education, training, and experience.

F. Individuals shall ensure that all equipment used in the provision of services is in proper working order and is properly calibrated.

PRINCIPLE OF ETHICS III

Individuals shall honor their responsibility to the public by promoting public understanding of the professions, by supporting the development of services designed to fulfill the unmet needs of the public, and by providing accurate information in all communications involving any aspect of the professions.

RULES OF ETHICS

A. Individuals shall not misrepresent their credentials, competence, education, training, or experience.

B. Individuals shall not participate in professional activities that constitute a conflict of interest.

C. Individuals shall refer those served professionally solely on the basis of interest in those being referred and not on any personal financial interest.

D. Individuals shall not misrepresent diagnostic information, services rendered, or products dispensed or engage in any scheme or artifice to defraud in connection with obtaining payment or reimbursement for such services or products.

E. Individuals' statements to the public shall provide accurate information about the nature and management of communication disorders, about the professions, and about professional services.

F. Individuals' statements to the public—advertising, announcing, and marketing their professional services, reporting research results, and promoting product—shall adhere to prevailing professional standards and shall not contain misrepresentations.

PRINCIPLE OF ETHICS IV

Individuals shall honor their responsibilities to the professions and their relationships with colleagues, students, and members of allied professions. Individuals shall uphold the dignity and autonomy of the professions, maintain harmonious interprofessional and intraprofessional relationships, and accept the professions' self-imposed standards.

RULES OF ETHICS

A. Individuals shall prohibit anyone under their supervision from engaging in any practice that violates the Code of Ethics.

B. Individuals shall not engage in dishonesty, fraud, deceit, misrepresentation, or any form of conduct that adversely reflects on the professions or on the individual's fitness to serve persons professionally.

C. Individuals shall not engage in sexual activities with clients or students over whom they exercise professional authority.

D. Individuals shall assign credit only to those who have contributed to a publication, presentation, or product. Credit shall be assigned in proportion to the contribution and only with the contributor's consent.

E. Individuals shall reference the source when using other persons' ideas, research, presentations, or products in written, oral, or any other media presentation or summary.

F. Individuals' statements to colleagues about professional services, research results, and products shall adhere to prevailing professional standards and shall contain no misrepresentations.

G. Individuals shall not provide professional services without exercising independent professional judgment, regardless of referral source or prescription.

H. Individuals shall not discriminate in their relationships with colleagues, students, and members of allied professions on the basis of race or ethnicity, gender, age, religion, national origin, sexual orientation, or disability.

I. Individuals who have reason to believe that the Code of Ethics has been violated shall inform the Ethical Practice Board.

J. Individuals shall cooperate fully with the Ethical Practice Board in its investigation and adjudication of matters related to this Code of Ethics.

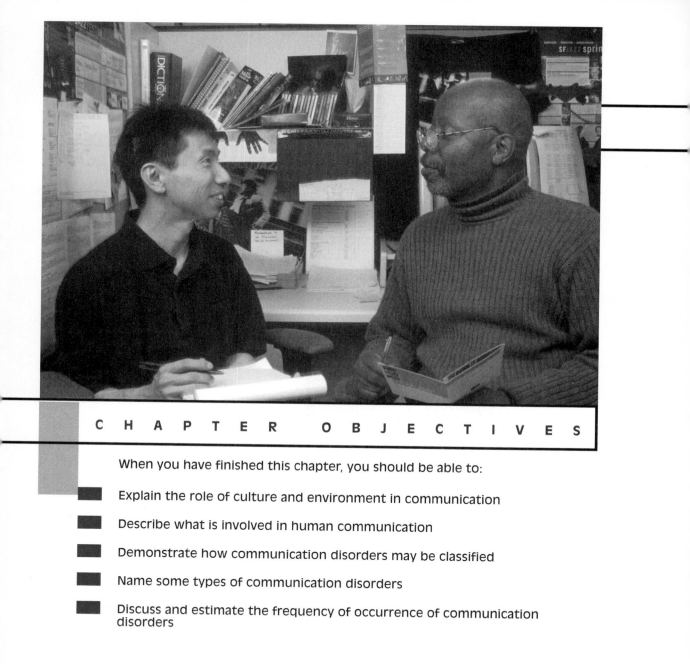

When you have finished this chapter, you should be able to:

Explain the role of culture and environment in communication

Describe what is involved in human communication

Demonstrate how communication disorders may be classified

Name some types of communication disorders

Discuss and estimate the frequency of occurrence of communication disorders

2

Typical and Disordered Communicaton

HUMAN COMMUNICATION

THE SOCIAL ANIMAL

Possibly the worst punishment that can be given to a prisoner is to be sentenced to isolation. Discipline for a teenager might include limitations on telephone or email use. These restrictions are punitive because we humans are social beings. We have powerful drives to be with and to communicate with others.

What is **communication?** In general, we can say that communication is an exchange of ideas between sender(s) and receiver(s). It involves message transmission and response or feedback. "Someone does or says something, and others think or do something in response to the action or the words as they understand them" (Beebe, Beebe, & Redmond, 1996, p. 6). We communicate to make contact, to reach out and touch others. We communicate to satisfy our wants, to reveal feelings, to share information, and to accomplish a host of purposes. If your mother ever said, "Talking to you is like talking to the wall," you recognized that she was unhappy because you did not respond. Communication is interactive; it is a give-and-take. The importance of effective communication is highlighted in Box 2.1.

It is axiomatic to say, "We cannot *not* communicate" (Watzlawick, Beavin, & Jackson, 1967, p. 48). Lack of response to someone who is speaking to you sends a message to the speaker, which might simply mean "leave me alone."

Several variables affect communication and its success or failure. These include cultural identity, setting, and participants. The study of these influences on communication is called **sociolinguistics.**

CULTURAL IDENTITY

Each of us is a member of a language community. The more you understand about your own culture and that of the people with whom you communicate, the more effective your interaction will be. If this text were written in perfectly good Mandarin Chinese and you could not read that language, it would communicate nothing meaningful to you. Speakers and listeners must share competence in a common language if they are to communicate fully.

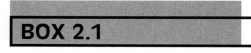

BOX 2.1

Mundo Pax

Mundo pax means "world peace " in Latin. A school superintendent we know uses this as his email address. As an educator, he deeply believes that peace on earth comes through education. As communication specialists, we suggest that the key element of education that may lead to peace is effective communication. Visualize a 2-year-old child, whom we'll call Donna. Unable to use language well enough to express her needs, she will push, hit, cry, grab, and engage in temper tantrums. If Donna were older and had words to ask for what she craved, all that fussing might have been avoided. This might be especially true if she had the words "please" and "thank you" to open opportunities for her. If what Donna wants was possessed by another child who was not easily swayed by polite requests, Donna, if able to use sophisticated language, could trade, negotiate, or bargain. She could offer a toy that she had in exchange for the one she wanted, or she might suggest taking turns or playing together. Now picture nations that are greedy for wealth, building up military might to enable them to attack to obtain what they desire. Could improved communication skills spare us warfare? Can effective communication lead to mundo pax?

Perhaps you have traveled to a country in which a language that you did not know was spoken. You might have been able to communicate by gesture and pantomime; however, you would have to agree that while you could exchange some meaning, it fell far short of optimal communication. Even when two people come from the same language background, "perfect" communication is rare. This is because successful communication depends on related factors such as age, socioeconomic status, geographical background, ethnicity, and gender.

Babette and John were college sweethearts with thoughts of eventual marriage. However, they recognized significant differences in ways of relating that stemmed from childhood. When Babette was growing up, her family openly discussed issues and disagreements, often to the point of forceful argumentation and yelling. These heated discussions sometimes led to tears, but eventually they typically terminated in hugs. John's family was more reserved. When two people did not agree, it was considered polite to keep your thoughts to yourself. Males neither cried nor hugged. In her relationship with John, Babette soon learned that she could not criticize him without his becoming sullen and hurt. On the other hand, she often wished that he would comment more frankly on decisions she was making. They both recognized that each would have to make major adjustments if their future marriage was to succeed.

T H O U G H T   Q U E S T I O N S

How do the sociolinguistic factors that describe you influence your communication? What variations in communication may be due to age, gender, and ethnicity? Are these differences perfectly predictable?

SETTING AND PARTICIPANTS

The location of communication influences its nature and is also usually considered a sociolinguistic factor. Where you interact affects how and what you'll say. You communicate differently at home, in school, in a noisy restaurant, and at a ball game. Similarly, you might speak quite differently to your best friend, your mother, your father, your boss, your grandmother, and large audiences.

T H O U G H T   Q U E S T I O N S

How might your speech change as you communicate with different people, in different settings, and with large or small groups? How might you communicate with someone who stutters or has another type of communication disorder?

MEANS OF COMMUNICATION

Communication takes many forms. It can involve any or a combination of our senses including sight, hearing, smell, and touch. We often think of good communication skills as a sign of intelligence: Humans have used this premise to search for life beyond the earth. Long the province of science fiction, this question has been investigated by physicists and astronomers since 1960. The Search for Extraterrestrial Intelligence (SETI) League has major search sites around the United States and in Australia, Canada, Argentina, Puerto Rico, and Russia, where optical and radio telescopes hooked to supercomputers scan the skies for intelligent signals. In addition, SETI@home is a screen saver program, available since 1999, that taps into home computers and has the potential to provide additional search techniques.

What are they looking for? Researchers admit that they are not really sure, but the basic task is to find patterns or signals that go beyond random noise. Whether the signals are deliberate messages from aliens trying to contact us or signs of an environment that has been altered by intelligent beings, the search goes on (Owen, 2001).

T H O U G H T   Q U E S T I O N S

If you were to send messages into the cosmos for intelligent beings to receive, what form would they take? What do you think a signal from space might be like? How would you judge the effectiveness of the communication?

LANGUAGE

The primary vehicle of human communication is **language.** Language may be defined as "a socially shared code or conventional system for representing concepts through the use of arbitrary symbols and rule-governed combinations of those symbols" (Owens, 2001, p. 472). Language is a tool for relating to others and for accomplishing a variety of objectives.

Taking this definition apart, we see, as we pointed out earlier, that others must share the code if communication is to occur. When an infant utters, "ga da da ka," we cannot call this language, since this "code" is not shared.

Many people are so accustomed to their own language that they fail to recognize its arbitrary nature. Is there anything in the sound combination or the written letters of the word "water" that resembles the wet stuff? Is the French word "l'eau" or the Italian "l'acqua" any more or less moist? A comparison of different languages rapidly confirms this very arbitrary nature. The equivalent of the English word "butterfly"

Parents often assume that their infant's earliest "ma ma" or "da da" are uttered in reference to themselves. These sound combinations are not considered true words unless there is evidence that they are used meaningfully.

is "farfalla" in Italian, "mariposa" in Spanish, and "Schmetterling" in German—four very different renditions of that graceful creature.

Each language, in addition to being composed of arbitrary but agreed upon words, consists of rules that dictate how these words are arranged in sentences. In English, an adjective precedes a noun; for example, we say, "brown cow." In French, as in many other languages, this sequence is reversed, and they say, "le vache brun" ("the cow brown"). The rules of a language make up its **grammar.** Interestingly, you do not have to be able to explain the rules to recognize when they have been broken. Take, for example the sentence, "The leaves of the maple green tree in the breeze swayed." Most American students will simply know that the sentence is wrong and say, "It doesn't sound right." This recognition of "wrong" and "right" grammar is called **linguistic intuition** and is possessed by native speakers of a language.

Language is **generative;** this means that each utterance is freshly created. We do not just quote or repeat what has been heard. We paraphrase and modify and present our own ideas in an individual way. Imagine a conversation if all we could do was imitate one another.

Languages are also **dynamic;** they change over time. The famous Academie Française has tried to keep French "pure" and true to its origins. The Academie still attempts to keep "foreign" words from infiltrating French. For example, it has tried to ban the English words "jet" and "drugstore." But "le jet" is apparently easier to use than the French "l'avion de reaction," and so it stays. No academy, no school, no law, and no army can keep languages from being modified. In American English, we add five or six new words each day. Pronunciation, grammar, and ways of communicating also change. Some characteristics of language follow:

- Socially shared tool
- Rule-governed system
- Arbitrary code
- Generative process
- Dynamic scheme

T H O U G H T   Q U E S T I O N S

In what ways has English changed since your grandmother was a child? Do you use words that she doesn't understand?

While all are important, it is the use or purpose of communication that dictates form and content.

All human languages consist of similar basic ingredients, although the specifics mark their differences. The primary components have been labeled in various ways. The most generally accepted method highlights form, content, and use (American Speech-Language-Hearing Association [ASHA], 1993; Bloom, 1970).

FORM Form is the perceivable aspect of language, and consists of phonology, morphology, and syntax. The sound system, or **phonology,** of English consists of about forty-three phonemes (unique speech sounds). Although different languages use many of the same phonemes, variations exist. Spanish and German, to name only two, do not use the English "th." As a consequence, since this sound is not learned as a child, it is difficult for some nonnative English speakers to produce.

Phonotactic rules specify how sounds may be arranged in words. Like rules of grammar, phonotactic rules are not universal. For example "k" and "n" cannot be blended in spoken English, though this combination is acceptable in German. For this reason the "k" in "knife" and "Knoxville" is silent for native English speakers but might be pronounced by Germans speaking English as a second language.

T H O U G H T   Q U E S T I O N S

Which of the following nonsense words violates a phonotactic rule of English: sprell, framble, ngopi? Do you know what rule was broken? Can you make up some "acceptable" nonsense words?

Morphology involves the structure of words. A **morpheme** is the smallest grammatical unit within a language. Words contain both **free morphemes** and **bound morphemes.** A free morpheme may stand alone as a word. For example, "cat," "go," "spite," "like," and "magnificent" are all free morphemes. If you attempt to break them into smaller units, you lose the meaning of the word. On the other hand, "cats," "going," "spiteful," "dislike," and "magnificently" each contain one free and one bound morpheme. The bound morphemes (-s), (-ing), (-ful), (dis-), and (-ly) change the meanings of the original words by adding their own meanings but can be used only as attachments to free morphemes.

Syntax pertains to how words are arranged in a sentence. In an English declarative sentence, the subject comes before the verb: "John is going to the opera." When we reverse the order of the subject and the auxiliary or helping verb, we change the meaning of the sentence and end up with a question: "Is John going to the opera?" In the sentence "Mary was kissed by John," who is doing the kissing? Even though "John" comes after the verb, he is the actor because this sentence is in the passive voice. Although you probably don't consciously know and can't recite the rules for active and passive sentences, your linguistic intuition makes it easy for you to comprehend their meaning (Chomsky, 1965, p. 19).

In addition to phonemes, morphemes, and syntactic units, language form also contains **suprasegmental** features such as loudness, rate, and intonation. "Supra-" means above or beyond, so suprasegmental features go beyond individual speech sound segments and are applied to whole phrases or sentences. Suprasegmentals, gestures, facial expression, and other **nonverbal** (meaning nonword) aspects of communication will be discussed later in this chapter.

CONTENT   Since language is used to communicate, it must be about something, and that is its content, meaning, or **semantics. Semantic features** are the pieces of meaning that come together to define a particular word. For example, "girl" and "woman" share the semantic features of *feminine* and *human*, but *young* is generally considered a feature in "girl" and not in "woman." You'll notice that we said "generally" because, while most of us think of a "girl" as being young, it is quite common among some groups of people to refer to any woman as a "girl." Each word has multiple meanings, as you can quickly verify by looking in the dictionary. It is the other aspects of language, such as use and form, that determine the appropriate definition in context.

If you are beginning to think that this is complicated and nothing is definite, you are right. As we said earlier, social and cultural factors influence the way language is used. The more two people know about one another, the more effectively they will be able to communicate.

USE   Use, or **pragmatics,** is the driving force behind all aspects of language. We speak for a reason. It is the purpose of our utterance that primarily determines its form and content. For example, if you are with a friend and are hungry, you might say, "Let's get something to eat." If function was a simple biological drive, then "eat" grunted out might suffice. But who and where you are, whom you are with, and the time of day also influence what you say. If you are at your home and you have invited the friend to dinner, you might say, "Dinner is ready." If you are working with someone as noon approaches, you might suggest, "Let's break for lunch."

Pragmatic rules of communication have been identified (Grice, 1975), some of which vary with culture (Gumperz & Hymes, 1972). For example, in the United States, business meetings tend to be very task oriented. Very little time is spent on social exchanges; the work to be done has center stage. On the other hand, in Saudi Arabia when two people meet for the first time for business purposes, they might spend the entire session talking about family and friends and not get to the meat of the business until the second meeting. The rules for business conversations in each of these societies are different. A few general rules for speakers of American English are presented in Table 2.1.

TABLE 2.1

A sampling of pragmatic rules for speakers of American English

1. Only one person speaks at a time. Each person should contribute to the conversation.
2. Speakers should not be interrupted.
3. Each utterance should be relevant.
4. Each speech act should provide new information.
5. Politeness forms reflect the relationship of the speakers.
6. Topics of conversation must be established, maintained, and terminated.
7. The speaker should be sensitive to successfully communicating the message, avoiding vagueness and ambiguity.
8. The listener should provide feedback that reflects comprehension of the message.

SPEECH

Speech may be defined as spoken language, and it is the primary modality or pathway for language. The words and grammar of a language also may be expressed in writing or in sign. When speech is used, interconnected features such as articulation, fluency, and voice influence the final product.

ARTICULATION   Articulation refers to the way in which speech sounds are formed. How do we move our tongue, teeth, and lips in order to produce the specific phonemes of a language? How do we combine these individual sounds to form words? After all we don't speak in a series of isolated sounds such as "h-e-ll-o" or we'd sound like robots. Chapter 10 explains the nature of speech sound production and describes the problems that may occur.

FLUENCY   Fluency is influenced by the rhythm and rate of speech. Every language has its own rhythmic pattern; we often think of rhythm as timing. Do we pause after each word that we speak? Do we pause after each sentence? If we do, how long do the pauses last? What is our phrasing? You'll note that timing is not an isolated feature of speech. A word or syllable that is held tends to be emphasized and said more loudly. A skilled storyteller uses pauses and rhythmic variations for dramatic effect.

The speed at which we talk is our **rate.** Overall rate can reveal things about us. It may provide clue as to where we come from. For example, people from New York usually speak more rapidly than those from Georgia. On the other hand, if you habitually speak very quickly, it may suggest that you are in a hurry, are impatient, or have a great deal to say. By contrast, slow speech may connote a relaxed or casual personality.

The rate and rhythm of speech are sometimes referred to as vocal **prosody.** When it is smooth and relatively free of disruptions, we say that the speech is **fluent.**

Although most of the time we attempt to use a clear, sufficiently loud voice, sometimes our meaning may be more effectively communicated by a whisper, a whine, or a throaty rasp. When you are upset, your voice might sound angry to the point where someone says, "Don't use that tone of voice with me." Clearly, tone communicates information.

T H O U G H T Q U E S T I O N

What different meanings can you convey by saying the sentence "I love you," with varying suprasegmental features?

Voice can reveal things about the speaker as well as about the message. A woman with a hoarse voice might (correctly or not) communicate to others that she smokes. A person with a soft, high-pitched voice might be communicating youth or immaturity. A deep, throaty voice might connote masculinity or authority.

Both the overall level of loudness and the loudness pattern within sentences and words are important. A generally loud voice may communicate strength, while a soft one may suggest timidity. By stressing different words within a sentence, you are also conveying different meanings. Say the following sentence in each of the ways listed below, with the emphasis or increased loudness on the underlined word. Notice how the meaning changes.

I got an "A" on my Physics final.
I got an "A" on my Physics final.
I got an "A" on my Physics final.
I got an "A" on my Physics final.

Placing the stress on different syllables within certain words also changes the meaning. Contrast the following:

record/record
recess/recess
present/present

The symbols /ɛ/, /ə/, and /I/ represent phonemes or speech sounds to be described in more detail in Chapter 10, "Disorders of Articulation and Phonology."

You might have noticed that as you vary the stress, the pitch, rhythm, and pronunciation of different speech sounds may also change. The pitch tends to go up as the loudness is increased. Similarly, you are likely to prolong the syllable that receives stress. The first vowel in the noun "<u>record</u>," meaning a log or old-fashioned musical platter, is usually pronounced /ɛ/, as in "bed," while in the verb "re<u>cord</u>," as in the act of jotting something down or making a tape or CD, that "e" is more likely a schwa, /ə/, the sound in "above," or an /I/, as in "bid."

T H O U G H T   Q U E S T I O N S

What are the different meanings of the words "recess" and "present" with the stress patterns suggested above? Can you think of other words that have a single spelling but change in meaning with variations in stress?

Some adolescent boys are eager for their voices to lower so that they will sound more grown up.

Pitch is a listener's perception of how high or low a sound is; it can be physically measured as frequency or cycles per second, called hertz. **Habitual pitch** is the basic tone that an individual uses most of the time. Women usually have higher-pitched voices than men, and children have higher voices than adults of both sexes. So our habitual pitch tells something about who we are.

Pitch movement within an utterance is called **intonation.** A rising intonation turns a statement into a question. First say the following sentence by bringing your pitch down for the last word, then say it by raising your pitch at the end:

I want to do the dishes.

You'll notice that intonation influences meaning. You should also observe that as you alter intonation, your rhythm and loudness patterns also change.

NONVERBAL COMMUNICATION

Punctuation and type and size of print or handwriting may contribute to the meaning perceived by a reader. A century ago, perfumed letter paper was intended to add to the written word.

Although most humans rely heavily on spoken communication, some researchers report that about two-thirds of human exchanges of meaning take place nonverbally (Zeuschner, 1997). The term "nonverbal" encompasses both the suprasegmental aspects of speech that we described in the previous section and the **nonvocal** (without voice) message exchange that we present in the following paragraphs.

ARTIFACTS   The way you look and the way you have decorated your personal environment communicate something about you. Even the car that you drive can deliver a message. One young man we know impressed a woman he was dating for the first time by correctly selecting her car out of thirty in a municipal parking lot. He did this by evaluating the make and year as well as the items on the seat and dashboard. An easier experiment to carry out is to walk into the best hotel in your area dressed in a business suit and ask for the restroom. Repeat this wearing shabby jeans and looking unkempt. Chances are you'll be asked to leave in the second situation. Assumptions are made about our personalities and trustworthiness on the basis of our possessions, clothing, and general appearance.

Music, art, architecture, and furniture are also artifacts that communicate. They communicate messages from the artists who designed and produced them and also from the people who purchase, patronize, or in some way support them.

T H O U G H T   Q U E S T I O N

What might the music you listen to communicate about you?

KINESICS **Kinesics** refers to the way we move our bodies, or *body language.* This includes overall body movement and position as well as arm, hand, and foot gestures, and facial expression. While there is some overlap with signing and gesturing, kinesics typically lack **explicit** (clearly defined) lexical and syntactical movements. In signing, the meanings of particular movements are well specified; for example, in American Sign Language (ASL), a thumb stroke down the cheek means "girl." Kinesics tend to be more general, subtle, or **implicit;** as a gesture, that same thumb stroke might mean "I'm thinking" or simply "I have an itch." While gestures such as the hitchhiker's thumb or a cutting movement across the neck have explicit meanings, they simply support and contribute to the larger speech system. By contrast, signing is a primary means of communication that is used by many people who are deaf. ASL is described in greater detail in Chapter 14, "Audiology and Hearing Loss," and Chapter 15, "Augmentative and Alternative Communication."

T H O U G H T   Q U E S T I O N S

Are there some conversations that you would rather have in person than over the telephone? Why? What can a person's facial expression or body movement tell us?

SPACE AND TIME The study of the physical distance between people as it affects communication is called **proxemics.** Four zones—intimate, social, formal, and public—describe the progressively increasing distance of communicators from one another (Hall, 1966). Proxemics not only reflects the relationship between people, but is also influenced by age and culture. Infants, children, people from Middle Eastern and Latin cultures, and those with strong emotional attachments, such as lovers, tend to interact in intimate or close proximity, very near one another. One young U.S. student we know reported feeling "backed into a corner" by an exchange student from Spain whom she had just met at a social gathering. It is likely that the Spanish woman felt that the American was "too distant."

Tactiles are touching behaviors. Who touches whom and how and where on the body the touch occurs can reveal a great deal. For example, some friends hug and kiss, others shake hands, and still others simply greet with a smile and a nod. Children in our society learn that touching others is usually not appropriate and are told early on to "keep your hands to yourselves." In contrast, infants' earliest interactions normally include considerable parental and caretaker touch.

Chronemics is the effect of time on communication. Again cultural and age factors influence this nonvocal aspect of communication. People from German and Scandinavian backgrounds tend to be exactingly prompt, while those from Latin and African cultures may permit greater time flexibility. When two individuals come from cultures with different time rules, conflicts can easily arise. Status and context also affect chronemics (Poyatos, 1983). You might not be surprised to be kept waiting at the doctor's office, but your doctor does not expect to have to wait for you. Promptness is part of the U.S. work ethic. If you are routinely late to class or to a job, you've violated a chronemic norm and might have to pay a price in terms of a lowered grade or lost employment.

Young children operate in the here and now. When infants cry to be fed, they do not accept "Dinner will be ready in half an hour." Most toddlers do not normally patiently wait to have their needs and desires fulfilled. During these years, their communication is also only about the present. With increasing maturity, youngsters learn to tell time, to wait, and to talk about past, future, and nonpresent events, people, and things.

Age, sex, education, and cultural background influence every aspect of communication. It is essential to highlight that these variations in communication are not impairments. Communication dialects are differences that reflect a particular regional, social, cultural, or ethnic identity and are not a disorder of speech or language (ASHA, 1993). Table 2.2 on pages 40 and 41 offers a sampling of typical communication features at different life stages. We describe communication impairments in the next section.

T H O U G H T   Q U E S T I O N

Do you think a person can have a disorder of chronemics? If so, what might be some symptoms and implications?

COMMUNICATION IMPAIRMENTS

Now that we have an idea of the complexity and varied nature of communication, it should be easy to see that much can go wrong. The American Speech-Language-Hearing Association (ASHA) defines "communication and related disorders: Disorders of speech (articulation, voice, resonance, fluency), orofacial, myofunctional patterns, language, swallowing, cognitive communication, hearing, and balance" (ASHA, 1997, p. I-64iii). You will notice that this definition does not confine itself to speech and hearing; also included are reading and writing, as well as manual and other communication systems, in addition to processes such as swallowing and balance that share anatomy and physiology with parts of the communication mechanism. Communication disorders may be categorized on the basis of whether reception, processing, and/or expression is affected. Is the problem primarily one of hearing, comprehending and manipulating language, or speaking? In fact, the three dimensions may be intertwined, reflecting the "interaction and interdependence among the processes of speech, language, and hearing" (ASHA, 2001a, Standard 3.4). Table 2.3 on page 42 presents systems for categorizing communication disorders.

Etiology, the cause or origin of the problem, may also be used to classify a communication problem. Disorders may be due to faulty learning, neurological impairments, anatomical or physiological abnormalities, cognitive deficits, hearing impairment, or damage to any part of the speech system.

Sometimes a dichotomy is made between **congenital** and **acquired** problems. Congenital disorders are present at birth; acquired ones are the result of illness, accident, or environmental circumstances anytime later in life. Finally, disorders may range from borderline or mild to profoundly severe. A possible system of classification is presented in Table 2.2.

It is essential to highlight that variations in communication output are not impairments. Communication **dialects** are differences that reflect a particular regional, social, cultural, or ethnic identity and are not disorders of speech or language (ASHA, 1993).

In this text, we provide a **holistic** approach to diagnosis and treatment of people with communicative impairments. While we have separate chapters that discuss speech characteristics such as voice, fluency, and phonology, we also provide chapters that are organized on the basis of etiology such as neurogenic and craniofacial disorders. Within each chapter, we examine the interconnectedness of age, time of onset, social and cultural factors, and cause on the presenting disorder. We observe that it is common for an individual who demonstrates difficulties with one aspect of communication to be affected in other areas as well. We demonstrate that differences and dialects do not constitute disorders,

TABLE 2.2

A lifespan view of typical communication

Age Range	Receptive Communication	Expressive Communication							Nonverbal Communication	
		Language			Speech					
		Form	Content	Use	Articulation	Fluency	Voice	Artifacts	Kinesics	Space/Time
Infancy	Quiets/turns to human voice; Distinguishes speech sounds	Prelinguistic sound-making	No "true" speech; vocalizations, body movement focus on here and now	Obtain assistance; imitate, respond to others	Gurgles, coos, babbles	Rhythm and rate begin to resemble that of surrounding language toward end of year	Varies volume, rate, pitch	Toys, materials given to child, may "give" objects to others	Gestures precede meaningful spoken language	Close proximity/ immediacy
Toddler	Responds to some verbal commands	Vocabulary growth from 4 to 300 words; moves from single word to short utterances	Familiar names, actions	Imitate, greet, protest, question	Simplified phonology		High (childish) pitch, more variability than adults	Toys, begins to construct things, start of imaginary play	Gestures slowly take second place to spoken language	Proximity decreases, begins to comprehend "now" "later"
Pre-school	Comprehension far exceeds expression; enjoys stories, books; follows increasingly complex commands; comprehends simple humor	Vocabulary grows from 1000 to more than 2000 words; uses complete sentences	Immediate to imaginary, includes past, present, and future	Greet, request, protest, inform, pretend, entertain	Almost all speech sounds correctly produced by the end of this period	Part-word, whole word, and phrase repetition not uncommon	Adjusts to listener; often used effectively to enhance verbal communication	Tremendous variability, reflects social/ cultural background	Gestures used to enhance verbal communication	Begins to understand personal space

Age									
School-Age	Reading skills improve; receptive language grows to 50,000 words by 6th grade, 80,000 words end of high school; comprehension becomes adult-like	Vocabulary grows to 25,000-30,000 words; slang important; written language more complex than spoken language	Very broad, includes distant as well as near and abstract concepts	Many enjoy talking, sharing thoughts, raising and answering personal as well as abstract questions; narrative skills expand	Speech sounds correctly produced	Rate may be rapid, fluency is good	Pitch drops to adult levels with puberty, voice used to supplement verbal message	Clear indication of what is wanted, reflect peer group, gender	Gestures used in wide array of means to supplement speech	Becomes territorial, mature understanding of space and time
Early and Middle Adulthood	Comprehension increases	Education and occupation may be reflected in vocabulary	Full range of topics; written language continues in importance and sophistication	Instructing, directing others may be added if not there earlier	Mature articulation	Use of rhythm and rate to enhance message	Mature pitch, full-bodied vocal quality	Tremendous variety dependent on sociocultural and individual variables	Body movement and gesture continue to supplement verbal communication	Space may reflect relative "importance" in environment as well as cultural factors
Old Age	Comprehension may decrease	Vocabulary may reflect "older" generation	May focus more on past than future	May have limited communication partners, speech may be major way to achieve companionship	Normally not impaired	Rate may slow	Pitch may increase, vocal quality become "thinner"	Old/familiar items may become increasingly treasured	Body movement may be less forceful	May crave touch, as significant others become less available

Sources: Owens, 2001; Shadden & Toner, 1997.
Note: This is a sampling of communication behaviors. Variability within each age group is the norm.

TABLE 2.3

Classification of speech communication disorders

Reception	Expression	Etiology	Time of Onset
Hearing Acuity:	*Speech:*	Neuromotor abnormalities	Congenital
Conductive	Articulation		Acquired
Sensorineural	Fluency	Hearing impairment	
Mixed	Voice	Environmental/ learning factors	*Severity*
			Borderline
Central Auditory Processing:	*Language:*	Cognitive deficits	Mild
Decoding	Form	Anatomical or physiological impairments	Moderate
Integration	Phonology		Severe
Organization	Morphology		Profound
Understanding speech under adverse conditions	Syntax		
	Content		
Short-term memory	Lexicon		
Multiple categories	Use		
	Pragmatics		

and we examine the sometimes perplexing contrast between "typical" and "impaired."

LANGUAGE DISORDERS

DISORDERS OF FORM

As we explained earlier, the form of language includes phonology, morphology, and syntax. We speak in sounds (phonemes) that are combined into words (morphemes), which in turn are combined into phrases and sentences (based on syntactical rules). Errors in sound use, such as not producing the ends of words ("hi shir i too sma" for "his shirt is too small), constitutes a disorder of phonology. Incorrect use of past tense or plural markers ("the girl wented home" for "the girls went home"), is an example of a disorder of morphology. It should be noted that these patterns are sometimes a reflection of a particular speech dialect. The SLP must distinguish between dialectal variations, which do not signify impairment, and disorders. (See Chapter 5, "Assessment and Intervention.") Syntactical errors include incorrect word order and run-on sentences (for example, "I want to go mall and go skate and buy peanuts and you come with me 'cause I want you to but not Jimmy 'cause he's not big enough to go skate"). These errors in school-age children may affect academic achievement and social well-being.

Disorders of form may be due to many factors, including sensory limitations such as hearing problems or perceptual difficulties such as learning disabilities. Limited exposure to correct models may also handicap a child's language development. For many children who are delayed in their production of mature language forms, the cause is not apparent.

T H O U G H T   Q U E S T I O N

What type of error has occurred when a 6-year-old child says, "John and Mary is my best friends"? What might be the cause?

DISORDERS OF CONTENT

Children and adults with limited vocabularies, those who misuse words, and those with word-finding difficulties may have disorders of content or semantics. Similarly limited ability to understand and use abstract language as in metaphors, proverbs, sarcasm, and some humor suggests semantic difficulties. A persistent pattern of avoiding naming objects and referring instead to "the thing" is another indication of a disorder of content. Limited experience or a concrete learning style may contribute to this problem in youngsters. Among older people, cerebrovascular accidents (strokes), head trauma due to accidents, and certain illnesses may result in word-retrieval problems and other content-related difficulties.

DISORDERS OF USE

Disorders of use, or pragmatics, involve inappropriate or inadequate communication. From the birth cry through the first few months of cries, coos, smiles, and awkward movements, the responsibility for communication rests primarily with people other than the infant. As children mature, the responsibility for communicating their intention through speech and nonverbal means becomes increasingly theirs.

Pragmatic language problems may stem from poor or in some way unacceptable conversational, social, and narrative skills; limited spoken vocabulary; and/or immature or disordered phonology, morphology, and syntax. The group affiliations, setting, and participants that we described earlier in this chapter play a major role in judgments of pragmatic competence.

Speech-language pathologists are concerned with both verbal and nonverbal disorders of communication.

SPEECH DISORDERS

Disorders of speech may involve articulation (the production of speech sounds), **fluency** (rhythm and rate), or **voice** (vocal tone and resonance). They may affect people of all ages, be congenital or acquired, be due to numerous causes, and reflect any degree of severity.

It is not uncommon for an individual to have an impairment in more than one aspect of communication.

DISORDERS OF PHONOLOGY AND ARTICULATION

Production of speech requires perception and conceptualization of the speech sounds in a language as well as motor movements to form these sounds in isolation and in context. You must have both a mental/auditory image of the sound you are going to say and the neuromuscular skills to produce the sound. The cognitive and theoretical concepts of the nature, production, and rules for producing and combining speech sounds in language is known as *phonology*. The actual production of these sounds is called **articulation.**

It is not always possible to determine whether an individual's speech-sound errors indicate an impairment of phonology or articulation. To sort this out, speech-language pathologists (SLPs) identify the phonemes that are incorrectly produced and look for error patterns that may point to phonological disturbances. The sound system of a language is usually fully in place by age 7 or 8. Children with multiple speech-sound errors past age 4 may have *phonological* difficulties. The causes are often not known but may be the result of faulty learning due to illness, such as ear infections, hearing impairments, or other problems in the early years.

The SLP also assesses the client's ability to move the structures needed in speech, such as the tongue and lips; poor coordination may suggest articulatory difficulties. The causes for articulation disorders include neuromotor problems such as cerebral palsy, physical anomalies such as cleft palate, and faulty learning. When paralysis, weakness, or poor coordination of the muscles for speech result in poor speech articulation, the disorder is called **dysarthria.** Speech **apraxia** is similarly poor articulation due to neuromotor difficulties; however, the difficulty appears to be in programming the speech mechanism while muscle strength is normal. Dysarthria and apraxia can affect children as well as adults. Assessment and treatment of phonological and articulatory disorders are described in Chapter 10, "Disorders of Articulation and Phonology."

DISORDERS OF FLUENCY

As we described earlier, fluency refers to the rate and rhythm of language. Certain types of fluency disruptions are fairly common at different ages. For example, many 2-year-olds repeat words: "I want-want-want a cookie." Around age 3, youngsters often make false starts and revise their utterances: "Ben took . . . he broked my crayon." Because these speech patterns are so common, they are sometimes referred to as **developmental disfluency.** Typically fluent adults occasionally use **fillers** ("er," "um," "ya know," and so on), **hesitations** (unexpected pauses), **repetitions** ("g-g-go"), and **prolongations** ("w-w-well"). However, when these arhythmic patterns exceed or are qualitatively different from the norm or are accompanied by excessive tension or struggle behavior, they may be identified as **stuttering.** Appropriate diagnosis and intervention when warranted are the task of the SLP (Yairi, Watkins, Ambrose, et al., 2001).

Fluency disorders are generally first noticed before 6 years of age. If remediation efforts are not made or are unsuccessful, this condition might continue and even worsen by adulthood. In contrast, some individuals find the problem gradually disappearing even without treatment. Adult onset of disfluency also occurs. Advancing age, accidents, and disease can all disrupt the normal ease, speed, and rhythm of speech. The causes of nonfluent speech are typically unclear; this is explored further in Chapter 8, "Fluency Disorders."

Speech-language pathologists use several indices to differentiate developmental disfluency from early stuttering.

VOICE DISORDERS

As in other areas of speech, voice matures as the child gets older. From uncontrolled cries to carefully modulated whispers, shouts, and variations in pitch, the development of voice follows a predictable pattern. Although occasionally children are born with physiological problems that interfere with normal voice (such as a congenital laryngeal web; to be described in Chapter 9, "The Voice and Voice Disorders"), more common is the pattern of **vocal abuse.** It is characterized by excessive yelling, screaming or even occasional loud singing that resuls in **hoarseness** or another voice disorder.

Habits such as speaking with physical tension, yelling, coughing, throat clearing, smoking, and alcohol consumption can disrupt normal voice production. These behaviors may result in pathology to the vocal folds such as polyps, nodules, or ulcers. Disease, trauma, allergies, and neuromuscular and endocrine disorders may also affect voice quality. For example, individuals with Parkinson's disease, a progressive neurological disorder, often have a soft voice with limited vocal variety.

HEARING DISORDERS

According to ASHA, a hearing disorder "is the result of impaired auditory sensitivity of the physiological auditory system" (ASHA, 1993, p. 40). It may affect the ability to detect sound, to recognize voices or other auditory stimuli, to discriminate between different sounds, such as mistaking the phoneme /s/ for /f/, and to understand speech.

DEAFNESS

When a person's ability to perceive sound is limited to such an extent that "the primary sensory input for communication [is] other than the auditory channel," the individual would be considered deaf (ASHA, 1993, p. 41). Deafness may be congenital or acquired.

Many hospitals have instituted universal neonatal hearing screening. In this way, congenital deafness can be identified and addressed very early.

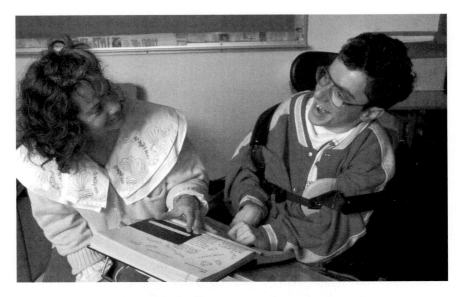

Good humor adds sparkle to the
therapeutic relationship.

Total communication, including sign, speech, and speechreading,
is often considered most effective intervention. **Assistive listening devices, cochlear implants,** and **auditory training** may be helpful. These
are explained in Chapter 14.

T H O U G H T   Q U E S T I O N

What differences might you expect in someone who was born
deaf compared to someone who lost hearing at an older age?
Why?

HARD OF HEARING

A person who is hard of hearing, in contrast to one who is deaf, depends primarily on audition for communication. Hearing loss may be
temporary due to an illness, such as an ear infection, or permanent,
caused by disease, injury, or advancing age. Hearing loss is usually categorized in terms of severity, laterality, and type. The severity of a hearing loss may range from mild to severe. It may be **bilateral,** involving
both ears, or **unilateral,** affecting primarily one ear. Finally, the loss may
be **conductive, sensorineural,** or **mixed.** A conductive loss is caused by
damage to the outer or middle ear; people with this type of loss usually report that sounds are generally too soft. A sensorineural loss in-

volves problems with the inner ear and/or auditory nerve; this type of damage is likely to affect a person's ability to discriminate and consequently understand speech sounds, although they may "hear" them. A typical pattern is that of older people who report that they hear just fine but wish others would not mumble. Mixed hearing loss, as the name implies, is a combination of both conductive and sensorineural loss. (See Chapter 14 for further discussion.)

T H O U G H T   Q U E S T I O N S

Do you know anyone with a hearing loss? How does he or she cope with this situation? Is that person's speech affected? How do you modify your communication when speaking with him or her?

CENTRAL AUDITORY PROCESSING DISORDERS

An individual with a **central auditory processing disorder (CAPD)** may have normal conductive and sensorineural hearing but still have difficulty understanding speech. People with CAPD may have difficulty "keeping up with the flow of conversation," "understanding speech under adverse conditions," and integrating what they hear with non-verbal aspects of communication (Stecker, 1998). These problems are sometimes traced to tumors, disease, or injury to the brain, but more often the cause is unknown. CAPD ranges in severity from mild to severe; it can be present in both children and adults. Special tests are required in the diagnosis of CAPD; routine hearing tests are capable of indicating only sensitivity to sound and middle ear function. CAPD is often implicated in speech, language, and learning disabilities; it may co-occur with attention deficit hyperactivity disorder (ADHD).

HOW COMMON ARE COMMUNICATION DISORDERS?

Before we attempt to estimate the numbers of people who have disorders of communication, we examine the concepts of normalcy and patterns of disability.

WHAT IS "NORMAL"?

A recent cartoon showed an empty room and a sign reading "Meeting of Members of Functional Families." The implication was that there are no functional or "normal" families. Is anybody normal? If anything, variability is the norm. We humans are remarkable in our diversity. Just as no two snowflakes are identical, no two individuals, even twins, are exactly alike. Our faces, fingerprints, and manner of communication are unique.

The bell-shaped normal curve graphs measurements that are used to distinguish those who are average from those who perform above and below others of the same population (see Figure 2.1). Many language tests use a scoring system comparable to IQ scores. Most people (a little over 68%) of those tested will score between 85 and 115. Higher or lower scores are above or below average. An individual who performed in the lowest 5–10 percent achieved a score that is significantly below average (Haynes & Pindzola, 1998).

T H O U G H T   Q U E S T I O N S

Does being like your peers make you "normal"? If everyone on a boat, including you, is seasick, is this normal or does everyone have a problem? If fifty students in your Intro to Communication Disorders class take an exam and only one person gets more than 65% of the questions correct, should all but that one person fail? Do you believe that exams should be graded on a curve? Why or why not?

Since the word "normal" suggests "without problems," we prefer to use the term "typical" when we mean "like most others of the same

FIGURE 2.1   The normal curve, percentile equivalents, and IQ scores.
Source: Adapted from Nuttall, E. V., Romero, I., & Kalesnik, J. (1992). *Assessing and screening preschoolers.* Boston: Allyn and Bacon and Wiig, E. H., & Secord, W. A. (1991). *Measurement and assessment.* Chicago: Riverside Publishing Co.

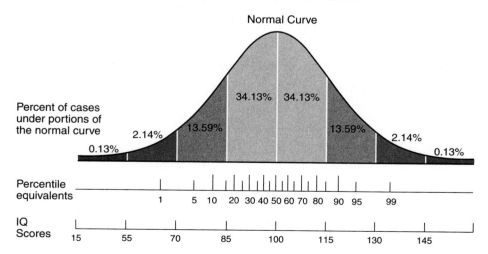

age and group." Classifying people on the basis of a bell curve, using a statistical percentage cutoff, may be little more than disability "by decree" (Lubker, 1997, p. 4). A more valid approach requires clear definitions of speech and language disorders. We discuss this further in Chapter 5, "Assessment and Intervention."

COMMUNICATION DISORDERS AS SECONDARY TO OTHER DISABILITIES

The term **specific language impairment (SLI)** is used when communication alone is impaired; however, if people with SLI are the only ones counted, we have a significant underestimate of the commonality of communication disorders (Lubker, 1997). Most communication disorders are secondary to other disabilities. For example, children with a cleft palate will have physical health problems as well as voice and articulation disorders. Children with learning disabilities are especially likely to have language difficulties. They may also have articulation, voice, fluency, and/or hearing deficits (Gibbs & Cooper, 1989).

ESTIMATES OF PREVALENCE

Prevalence refers to the number or percentage of people within a specified population who have a particular disorder or condition at a given point in time. It is computed by taking the number of people with the condition, dividing by the total number of individuals in the specified population, and multiplying by 100 to get a percent. If you determined the prevalence of stuttering in the entire U.S. population, among first grade children, among college seniors, among U.S. males, or among U.S. females, you would get different prevalence figures in each case. For this reason, prevalence statistics must specify the population on which they are based.

The terms "incidence" and "prevalence" are often confused. Incidence refers to the number of *new* cases of a disease or disorder in a particular time period. Prevalence is the number of *new and old* cases in a particular time period.

Current estimates suggest that about 17 percent of the total U.S. population have some communicative disorder. About 11 percent have a hearing loss, and approximately 6 percent have a speech, voice, or language disorder. Many of those with hearing losses also have speech, voice, or language disorders. Six to ten million Americans (about .03% of the population) have a disorder of swallowing (Castrogiovanni, 1999b, c), and many of these individuals also have a communicative impairment. While these figures are relatively low, it is likely that more, generally mild, cases are not reported (Tierney, McPhee, & Papadakis, 2000).

T H O U G H T Q U E S T I O N S

What is the prevalence of communication disorders in your Communication Disorders class? How does it compare with national figures? What could explain any differences?

Several theories attempt to explain sex differences in communication disorders. Certain disorders, such as autism spectrum disorder, are four times as prevalent in males. Some disorders may be related to a weak X or female chromosome, which can be contributed by either parent. Girls have two X chromosomes and may inherit a "protective gene" on the X contributed by the father that can override a weak X from the mother (Skuse, 2000). With only one X, boys have no such protection.

The percentage of people with hearing loss increases with age. Between 1 percent and 2 percent of people under 18 years of age have a chronic hearing loss, compared with approximately 32 percent of those over age 75. Exposure to noise has contributed to the hearing loss in about one-third of those affected (Castrogiovanni, 1999a).

Impairments of speech-sound production and fluency are more common in children than adults and more common among males than females. Speech disorders due to neurological disorders or brain and spinal cord injury occur more often among adults. It has been estimated that anywhere between 3 percent and 10 percent of Americans have voice disorders; this percentage is greater among school-age children and people over age 65 (Castrogiovanni, 1999b).

Language disorders occur in 8 to 12 percent of the preschool population; the prevalence decreases through the school years. Language deficits in older adults may be associated with stroke or dementia. It is likely that 5 to 10 percent of people over age 65 experience language disabilities related to these disorders (Bello, 1994; Castrogiovanni, 1999b). Table 2.4 highlights some communication disorders that may appear at different life stages.

SUMMARY

Communication is an exchange of ideas; it involves message transmission and response. Human communication is remarkable and may take many forms. It is strongly influenced by culture and environment. Not only do people speak different languages, but within language groups, age, gender, socioeconomic status, geographical background, ethnicity, and other factors influence our communication.

The primary vehicle of human communication is language. It may be spoken, written, or signed. Speech communication has been described in terms of form, content, and use. Form refers to the sound system, or phonology; word structure, or morphology; and syntax, or how the words are arranged in sentences. Content is semantics or meaning, and use is the purpose or pragmatics of the communication. Communication is also transmitted by nonverbal behaviors and characteristics.

A breakdown can occur in any aspect of communication. When communication is unimpaired, we tend to take it for granted, but when it fails us, we may feel frustrated and isolated. About 17 percent of the U.S. population currently experience some limitation of hearing, speech, and/or language.

TABLE 2.4

Communication disorders that may manifest themselves at different life stages

Age Range	Disorders	Receptive Communication	Expressive Communication	Swallowing
Infancy	Hearing impairment Fetal alcohol or drug-exposure syndrome Parental neglect/abuse Cerebral palsy	Limited response to sound/speech Limited response to others Atypical physical postures and movement	Atypical birth and other early cries Deaf infants vocalize normally for first 6 mos. Others may have little vocalization Passivity	May have difficulties with breast or bottle; later problems with solid foods
Toddler	Autism/Pervasive developmental disorder may be identified (hyper-sensitive to stimuli) Mental retardation not suspected earlier may now become apparent Brain injury due to falls	Comprehension of spoken language limited	Delay in first spoken word Utterances limited May use objects ritualistically	Rigid food preferences/dislikes Caution needs to be taken to prevent putting small objects in mouth that may be swallowed/choked on
Preschool	Delays that were suspected earlier may become more pronounced Fluency difficulties may emerge Specific language disabilities Middle ear problems common	Interactions with peers and others may be difficult	Inappropriate use of toys/objects Vocabulary may be limited, utterances short Alternative/augmentative communication may be recommended; Excessive dysfluency; delayed phonology and grammatical development	Food preferences may be more entrenched
School-Age	Language learning problems Hyperactivity/Attention deficit disorder Brain injury due to falls and other accidents	Difficulties attending, following directions, speech and reading comprehension	Narrative and other pragmatic skills may be affected	Inappropriate eating habits may become established

continued

TABLE 2.4 continued

Communication disorders that may manifest themselves at different life stages

Age Range	Disorders	Receptive Communication	Expressive Communication	Swallowing
Young Adulthood	Brain injury due to bike, motorcycle, car, and other accidents most prevalent in these years	Comprehension affected, generalized confusion, abstract thinking impaired	Pragmatic skills affected Life plans altered Dysarthria and apraxia may affect speech intelligibility	Neuromotor injury may impact on swallowing
Middle Adulthood	Hearing often starts to decline Life-threatning illnesses such as cancer may be diagnosed Neurogenic problems may appear; multiple sclerosis, ALS, Parkinson's, and Alzheimer's diseases; stroke (aphasia)	Speech in noise may be hard to comprehend Aphasia and Alzheimer's may result in comprehension difficulties	Illness-related depression may affect expressive communication Dysarthria and apraxia may impair speech intelligibility Alzheimer's and aphasia cause language impairments	Eating/swallowing not usually impaired in early stages
Old Age	Hearing deficits common Neurogenic problems become progressively worse	Difficulty understanding speech may cause "tuning out"	Voice may be weak Word finding problems Inappropriate speech Perseveration	Disinterest in food; swallowing impairments may lead to aspiration pneumonia

Sources: Owens (1999); Shadden & Toner (1997).
Note: This is a sampling of problems that may be seen. Variability within each age group is the norm.

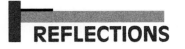

REFLECTIONS

- How do social and cultural aspects of human beings influence communication?
- In what ways can disorders of communication be described and classified?

- What communication disorders are likely to be diagnosed in different age groups?
- How are estimates made regarding the number of people with communication disorders?

SUGGESTED READINGS

Axtell, R. E., & Fornwald, M. (Illustrator). (1998) *Gestures: The do's and taboos of body language around the world.* New York: John Wiley & Sons.

Hamaguchi, M. P. (1995). *Childhood speech, language, and listening problems: What every parent should know.* New York: John Wiley & Sons.

Hirsh-Pasek, K., & Golinkoff, R. M. (1999). *The origins of grammar: Evidence from early language.* Cambridge, MA: MIT Press.

Morrison, T., Conaway, W. A., et al. (1995). *Kiss, bow, or shake hands: How to do business in 60 countries.* Avon, MA: Adams Media Corp.

Ruben, B. D., & Stewart, L. P. (1998). *Communication and human behavior* (4th ed.). Boston: Allyn and Bacon.

Winner, E. (1997). *The point of words: Children's understanding of metaphor and irony.* Boston: Harvard University Press.

ON-LINE RESOURCES

http://asha.org   American Speech-Language-Hearing Association.

Information for the general public concerning communication disorders.

http://www.nonoise.org   The Noise Pollution Clearinghouse.

A national nonprofit organization with extensive on-line noise-related resources. Its goal is to raise awareness about and combat noise pollution.

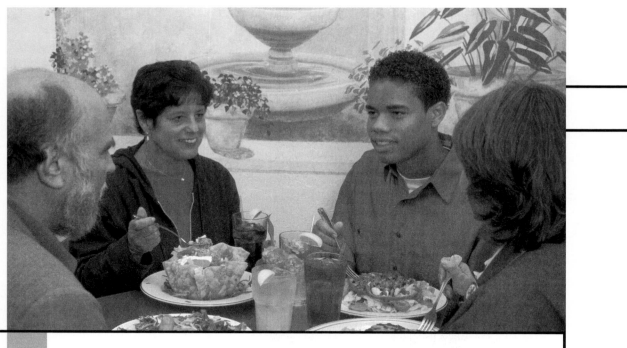

When you finish this chapter, you should be able to:

- Describe the respiratory/pulmonary system

- Explain the respiratory processes for quiet breathing and for speech breathing

- Describe the laryngeal system

- Explain the phonation process

- Describe the structures of the central nervous system involved in speech production

- Explain the general aspects of speech motor control and language processing

- Describe the articulation/resonance system

- Explain the articulatory and resonating processes for human speech

Anatomy and Physiology Related to Speech, Hearing, and Language

Speech production is generally taken for granted as a biological function that takes care of itself; thoughts and ideas are expressed with little or no apparent effort. But for all its apparent simplicity, the production of speech requires an incredibly complex coordination of biophysical events involving hundreds of muscles and millions of nerves. It is paradoxical that such complex physiological behavior appears to be so effortless. This natural paradox, however, is probably necessary. If we had full conscious comprehension of what we are doing when we speak, we would probably be unable to utter a single word. Monitoring all the nerves and muscles, the tone of the voice, facial expression, and word order would be an impossible intellectual feat (Thomas, 1979).

For many individuals, however, speech production is anything but effortless. Sometimes abnormalities of anatomical structures and physiological systems that support speech interfere greatly with speech production. As such, knowledge of the anatomy and physiology of the speech mechanism is fundamental to understanding many different communication disorders that are evaluated and treated by speech-language pathologists. Successful treatment of voice and swallowing disorders, laryngectomy (the surgical removal of the larynx), and cleft palate requires a thorough understanding of the anatomy and physiology of the speech mechanism.

Anatomy is the study of the structures of the body and the relationship of these structures to one another. **Physiology** is a branch of biology and is defined as a science concerned with the functions of organisms and bodily structures. This chapter will present an overview of the anatomy of the speech mechanism and the physiology of the systems that support speech production. The systems that support the production of speech include the **respiratory, laryngeal,** and **articulatory/resonating systems.** The structural support, some of the muscles, and the way these three systems are used for speech production will be discussed in this chapter. Consideration is also given to parts of the human nervous system that regulate the physiological systems underlying speech, language, and hearing.

THE RESPIRATORY SYSTEM

The primary biological functions of the respiratory system are to supply oxygen to the blood and to remove excess carbon dioxide from the body. This process is automatic and controlled by the respiratory centers located within the brain stem of the central nervous system. Although the primary function of respiration is to sustain life, it also serves as the generating source for speech production. Through the respiratory system, air is inhaled into the lungs to become the potential energy source for sound production. The air is then expelled in a controlled manner, to be modified by the vocal folds and/or articulators to generate speech sounds. We will consider the skeletal framework that supports the respiratory system, the major components of the pulmonary system, some of the muscles that are involved in inhalation and exhalation, the physiology of quiet breathing, and the physiology of speech breathing.

STRUCTURAL FRAMEWORK OF THE RESPIRATORY SYSTEM

The structural framework of the respiratory system, presented in Figure 3.1a, consists of the **vertebral column,** the **rib cage** or **thorax,** the **pectoral girdle,** and the **pelvic girdle.** The vertebral column comprises thirty-two bony vertebrae joined together by ligaments or fibrous connective tissue; some are separated from one another by cartilages called disks. Vertebrae are arranged in five different regions as shown in Figure 3.1b. The uppermost vertebrae are called the **cervical** vertebrae. There are seven cervical vertebrae. Immediately below the cervical vertebrae are twelve **thoracic** vertebrae, followed by five **lumbar,** five **sacral,** and three **coccygeal** vertebrae. Sacral and coccygeal vertebrae are fused and are often referred to as structures named the **sacrum** and **coccyx,** respectively.

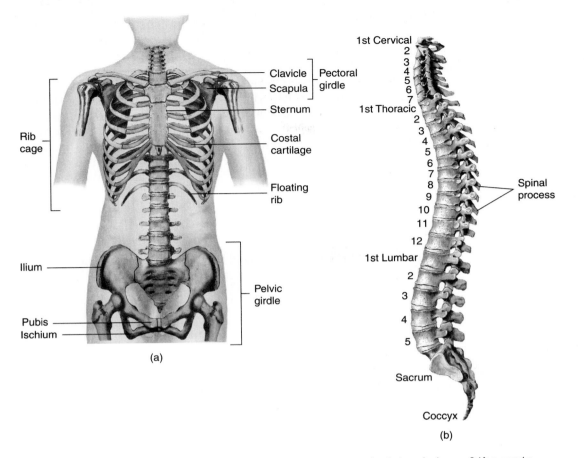

FIGURE 3.1   Anterior view of the thorax and pelvis (a) and a lateral view of the vertebral column (b)

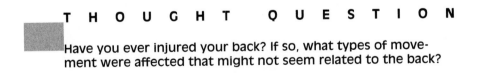

T H O U G H T   Q U E S T I O N

Have you ever injured your back? If so, what types of movement were affected that might not seem related to the back?

THE PULMONARY SYSTEM

The pulmonary system consists principally of the **trachea** and **lungs**, shown in Figure 3.2. The trachea is a cartilaginous and membraneous tube that extends downward from the larynx and divides into two bronchi. The trachea consists of sixteen to twenty horseshoe-shaped

The lungs are held in tight contact to the inner walls of the thorax and diaphragm by two layers of tissue called pleura. A painful condition, pleurisy, results when the pleura becomes inflamed.

rings of cartilage, placed one above the other and separated by fibroelastic tissue. The open portion of the horseshoe is posterior and lies in direct contact with the esophagus. At its inferior border, the trachea bifurcates or divides into two bronchial tubes that supply the lungs.

The bronchi are similar to the trachea in composition, but their diameter is approximately half that of the trachea. These two bronchi continue dividing into smaller and smaller tubes within the lungs until they become microscopic bronchioles. Bronchioles open into minute air sacs that are covered with millions of small depressions called alveoli. The exchange of carbon dioxide for oxygen occurs in capillaries that cover the alveoli. We will have more to say about the process of breathing later in this chapter.

MUSCULATURE OF THE RESPIRATORY SYSTEM

Respiratory musculature is divided functionally into muscles of inhalation and muscles of exhalation. In general, muscles of inhalation

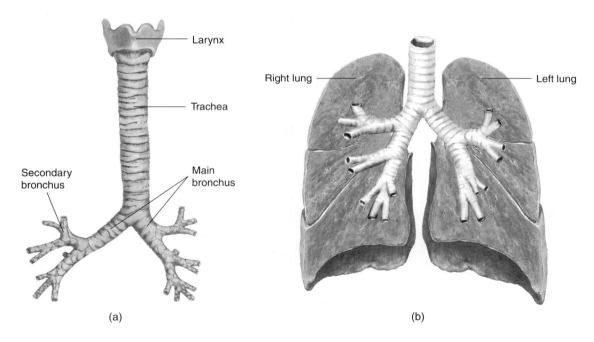

(a)

(b)

FIGURE 3.2 Anterior view of the trachea and bronchi (a) and an anterior view of the bronchi entering the right and left lungs (b)

are found above the diaphragm, and muscles of exhalation are found below the diaphragm. With the exception of the diaphragm, all respiratory muscles are paired or found on both the right and left sides of the body.

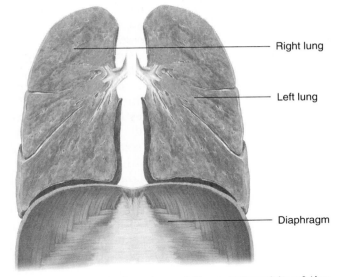

Right lung

Left lung

Diaphragm

FIGURE 3.3 Anterior view of the relationship of the diaphragm to the lungs; the lungs and diaphragm have been cut in half

MUSCLES OF INHALATION

Inhalation is part of the respiratory process that allows oxygen to be taken into the lungs. The **diaphragm** is the most important single muscle of respiration. It is a thin, dome-shaped structure composed of muscle fibers and a broad tendon on its superior surface. The diaphragm separates the thoracic and abdominal cavities. Figure 3.3 shows the relative position of the diaphragm at rest. In addition to the diaphragm, numerous thoracic and neck muscles contribute to the inhalation process.

MUSCLES OF EXHALATION

Exhalation is the part of the respiratory process that allows carbon dioxide to be expelled from the body via the lungs and speech to be produced. Some muscles in the thoracic cavity and some muscles of the back can assist in exhalation, but the primary muscles of exhalation are located in the anterior and lateral aspects of the abdomen.

T H O U G H T   Q U E S T I O N

Why do bodybuilders have stomachs that look like a washboard? What causes this appearance?

THE PHYSIOLOGY OF QUIET BREATHING AND SPEECH BREATHING

Quiet breathing is breathing to sustain life. As you are reading this chapter, you are using quiet breathing. The rate and depth of breaths taken during quiet breathing are determined by the body's oxygen needs and the amount of carbon dioxide in the blood. Contraction of inhalation muscles causes the thorax, and in turn the lungs, to expand. Expansion of the lungs results in an increase of lung volume and air pressure within the lungs drops below atmospheric pressure. Air rushes into the lungs, equalizing lung pressure with atmospheric pressure. Approximately one-half liter of air is inhaled when you are sitting and breathing quietly. Such breathing is also called **tidal breathing.**

Muscles of inhalation cease contracting at the end of an inhalation, the rib cage is elevated, and the lungs expand. As exhalation begins, the size of the thorax decreases, reducing lung volume. Air pressure within the lungs elevates to levels that are above atmospheric pressure and air rushes out of the lungs.

Exhalation during quiet breathing does not require active contraction of expiratory muscles. Gravity acting on the elevated rib cage and the elasticity of lung tissue help to return the thorax and lungs to their relaxed state, ready to begin the next respiratory cycle. Nonmuscular forces that return the respiratory system to its rest position are called **passive recoil forces.** A respiratory cycle is defined as one inhalation followed by one exhalation. During quiet breathing, inhalation and exhalation are approximately equal in duration.

Speech breathing is the kind of breathing you do when speaking aloud, and it differs from quiet breathing in a number of ways. First, during speech breathing, inhalations occur only at major linguistic boundaries such as the end of phrases or sentences. One would never inhale in the middle of a word or phrase.

T H O U G H T   Q U E S T I O N

Say the word "baseball" normally. Now say it again, but take a breath between "base" and "ball." What happened to the normal flow of your speech?

Speech breathing differs from quiet breathing in many ways, but the oxygen and carbon dioxide ratio in the blood is the same for both types of breathing.

During speech breathing, the time spent inhaling is shortened greatly, and the time spent exhaling is increased greatly. Additionally, one may inhale as much as 2 liters of air during speech breathing, depending on the specific demands of the utterance. Speaking is usually begun at lung levels above tidal breathing. In contrast to quiet breathing, speech breathing frequently requires active muscle contraction during exhalation. At the beginning of an utterance, muscles of inhalation may be active, controlling the descent of the rib cage, whereas at the end of an utterance, muscles of exhalation may be active to sustain lung pressure for longer utterances.

The respiratory system's primary role during speech breathing is to control vocal intensity. The loudness of one's voice is directly proportional to the amount of air pressure the lungs apply to the inferior aspects of the vocal folds. This air pressure, called **subglottal** pressure, will be discussed in more detail later in this chapter.

LIFE SPAN ISSUES OF THE RESPIRATORY SYSTEM

At birth, the newborn infant has a tidal breathing rate at rest between thirty and eighty breaths per minute. By 3 years of age, this tidal breathing decreases to between twenty and thirty breaths per minute. The newborn has very few alveoli, but adults have several million (Zemlin, 1998). Watch a preschool child speak. Note the more frequent and deeper inhalations compared to adult speakers.

As a child develops, the respiratory system's structures increase in size, and lung capacities increase. Maximum lung capacities are reached

This client is using biofeedback to monitor speech production.

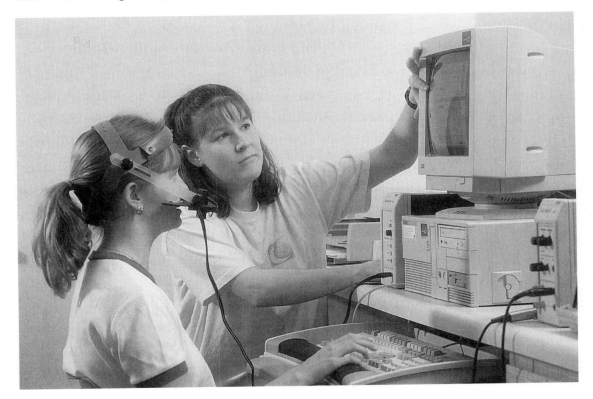

in early adulthood and remain fairly constant until middle age. Respiratory function is affected by exercise, health, gender, age, and smoking. It is estimated that smoking in older people could result in a 500 milliliter (approximately 1 pint) cumulative loss in pulmonary function every ten years (Kent, 1997).

THOUGHT QUESTIONS

Have you ever heard a heavy smoker complain of shortness of breath? How does the shortness of breath affect speech breathing patterns?

THE LARYNGEAL SYSTEM

The **larynx** is the organ of the laryngeal system. Although the larynx is the principal sound generator for speech production, it has several important primary biological functions. As the superior termination of the trachea, the larynx is a protective organ that prevents foreign objects from entering the trachea and lungs. Additionally, the larynx can impound air for forceful expulsions of foreign objects or coughing if those objects threaten the lower airways. We will discuss the structural support of the larynx, laryngeal musculature, and how the larynx is used during the production of speech.

STRUCTURAL SUPPORT OF THE LARYNGEAL SYSTEM

The **hyoid bone** is the point of attachment for both laryngeal and tongue musculature. Horseshoe shaped and not connected to any other bones of the body, the hyoid bone lies horizontally in the neck at the level of the third cervical vertebra. The larynx appears to be suspended from the hyoid bone by the **thyrohyoid membrane.** You can locate the two posterior ends of the major horns of your hyoid bone. Place your thumb and middle finger on the lower angle of the mandible, or lower jaw. Slide your fingers down about 1 inch and push in. You will feel two prominences that you can move from side to side. These prominences are the posterior projections of your hyoid bone.

The larynx consists of several cartilages connected to one another by ligaments and membranes. The primary cartilages of the larynx are shown in Figure 3.4. The **thyroid cartilage** is the largest laryngeal cartilage, and it forms the anterior and lateral walls of the larynx. The anterior aspect of this cartilage forms a V-shaped protrusion known as the **laryngeal prominence,** or Adam's apple, which is very prominent in some adult males.

The thyroid gland that helps to control aspects of growth and metabolism is located on the lateral aspects of the thyroid cartilage.

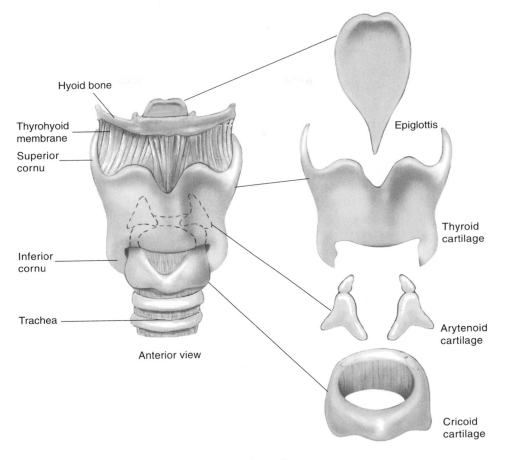

Hyoid bone

Thyrohyoid
membrane

Superior
cornu

Inferior
cornu

Trachea

Anterior view

Epiglottis

Thyroid
cartilage

Arytenoid
cartilage

Cricoid
cartilage

FIGURE 3.4 Anterior view of laryngeal cartilages

The posterior borders of the thyroid cartilage are upper and lower projections known as the superior and inferior thyroid cornu, respectively. The upper cornu connect the thyroid cartilage with the hyoid bone and the posterior cornu connect the thyroid and **cricoid cartilages.**

The cricoid cartilage sits immediately above the first tracheal ring and directly below the thyroid cartilage. It is a single structure in the shape of a signet ring consisting of an anterior arch or ring portion and a posterior signet portion. On the posterior and superior border of the cricoid cartilage are the paired **arytenoid cartilages.**

The **epiglottis** is a large leaf-shaped cartilage that is attached to the thyroid cartilage just below the laryngeal prominence. Its midportion is attached to the body of the hyoid bone, whereas the superior aspect of the epiglottis is free, extending to the root of the tongue. The epiglottis assists in preventing food from entering the larynx and lower airways during swallowing but has no function during speech production.

LARYNGEAL MUSCULATURE

Muscles of the larynx and its supporting structure are divided into three groups: **extrinsic, supplemental,** and **intrinsic muscles** (Zemlin, 1998). Extrinsic and supplemental laryngeal muscles serve to move the larynx up and down during swallowing. Put your index finger on your larynx and swallow; your larynx will be elevated by these muscles. Intrinsic laryngeal muscles are associated with voice production. They are responsible for changing the pitch of the voice and opening and closing the vocal folds.

THE VOCAL FOLDS

When viewed from above, the paired vocal folds appear to be ivory-colored bands of tissue. Vocal fold vibration produces the human voice, and voice production will be discussed later in this chapter. Figure 3.5 pictures the human vocal folds during a single vibratory cycle. Sustained vocal fold vibration is shown on the book's CD-ROM.

Some of the significant developmental changes that affect the larynx and the vocal folds over the life span are discussed in "The Voice and Voice Disorders" (Chapter 9).

THE ARTICULATORY/ RESONATING SYSTEM

The articulatory/resonating system comprises the **pharyngeal cavity** or neck, the **oral cavity,** and the **nasal cavity.** Collectively, these three cavities form the vocal tract, which is a resonant acoustic tube where all the sounds of spoken English are formed. Structures important for speech production such as the teeth, tongue, and soft palate are housed within these three cavities. Figure 3.6 illustrates the relationship of these three cavities.

STRUCTURAL SUPPORT OF THE ARTICULATORY/RESONATING SYSTEM

The supportive framework for the articulatory/resonating system consists largely of the twenty-two bones that make up the face and cra-

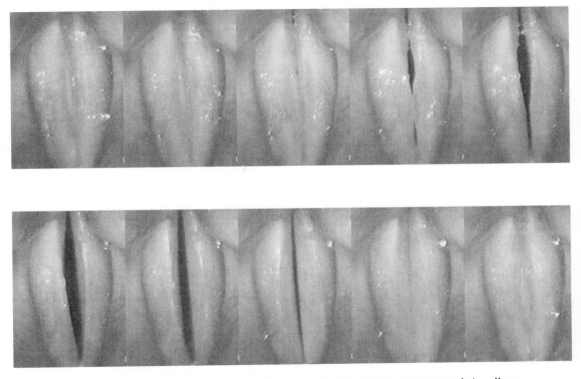

FIGURE 3.5 Stroboscopic film images of the vocal folds during one complete vibratory cycle. (Photograph courtesy of Robert Orlikoff, Ph.D., Memorial Sloan-Kettering Cancer Center, New York, NY)

nium. Some of the bones of the face and cranium are shown in Figure 3.7. With the exception of the lower jaw or **mandible,** facial and cranial bones are interlocked tightly with one another by mean of sutures. The mandible articulates with the temporal bone by means of a complex joint known as the **temporomandibular joint (TMJ).** This joint allows the mandible to move up and down and from side to side, as occurs during chewing.

Temporomandibular joint syndrome (TMS) is a painful condition that is associated with a partial dislocation of the joint.

THE TONGUE

An important structure for speech production within the oral cavity is the tongue. Tongue musculature is complex, comprising intrinsic and extrinsic muscles. Extrinsic tongue muscles serve to move the tongue's position in the mouth and intrinsic tongue muscles serve to change the shape of the tongue.

The primary biological function of the tongue is to move food in the mouth while chewing and direct it posteriorly for swallowing.

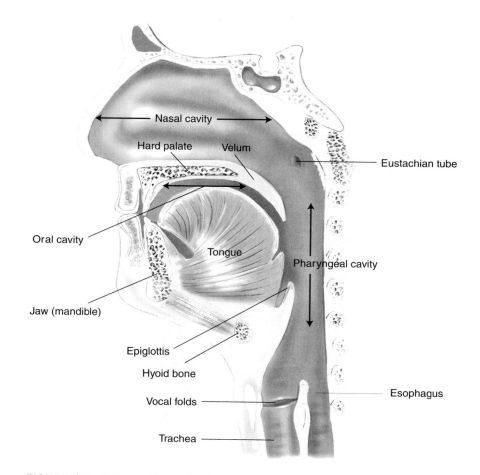

FIGURE 3.6 Schematic of the human vocal tract

TEETH

Adults have a total of thirty-two teeth that are held within the **alveo-lar processes** of the mandible and the **maxilla,** or upper jaw. Figure 3.8 shows structures of the **bony hard palate,** or roof of the mouth and the relationship of maxillary teeth. The obvious biological function of teeth is chewing food, but the teeth are also important for the proper production of a number of English speech sounds. Try, for example, to say the "th" sound in "think" without your tongue contacting your teeth. It can't be done.

Horizontal bones of the maxilla form the bony hard palate, which comprises the anterior two-thirds of the roof of the mouth. The soft palate, or **velum,** is attached to the posterior aspect of the hard palate.

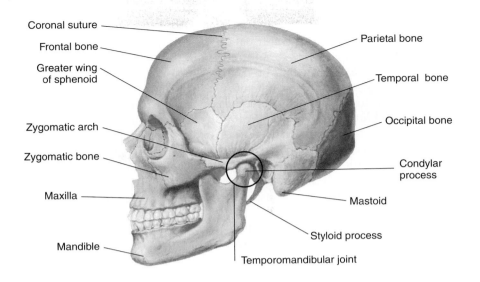

FIGURE 3.7 Lateral view of skull bones

Coronal suture
Frontal bone
Greater wing of sphenoid
Zygomatic arch
Zygomatic bone
Maxilla
Mandible
Parietal bone
Temporal bone
Occipital bone
Condylar process
Mastoid
Styloid process
Temporomandibular joint

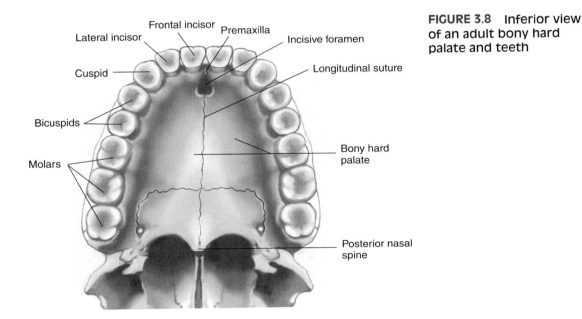

FIGURE 3.8 Inferior view of an adult bony hard palate and teeth

Lateral incisor
Frontal incisor
Premaxilla
Cuspid
Incisive foramen
Bicuspids
Longitudinal suture
Molars
Bony hard palate
Posterior nasal spine

THE VELUM

Located in the pharynx, the soft palate, or velum, hangs like a curtain in the posterior aspect of the oral cavity, coupling the nasal cavity with the pharyngeal cavity during breathing. Separation of the pharyngeal and nasal cavities is accomplished by a posterior and superior movement of the velum. When the velum is elevated, it is in contact with the posterior and lateral walls of the pharynx. Separation of the nasal and pharyngeal cavities is essential during swallowing and for the production of most speech sounds. Failure to separate these cavities during swallowing would result in food passing into the nasal cavity rather than the esophagus. Failure to separate these cavities during speech production would result in air escaping through the nose and excessively nasal-sounding speech. There are, however, three sounds in the English language—/m/, /n/, and /ng/—that require lowering the velum during their production. The velum's role in speech production is discussed extensively in Chapter 11.

Soft palate and pharyngeal musculature make up the velopharyngeal mechanism. Separation of the nasal and oral cavities is achieved through elevation of the soft palate itself and medial motion of pharyngeal walls.

LIFE SPAN ISSUES OF THE ARTICULATORY/RESONATING SYSTEM

The bones of the skull grow rapidly during the first years of life and reach the size of an adult at about 8 years of age. At birth, the newborn has forty-five separate skull bones, which ultimately fuse into twenty-two bones by adulthood. When they are fused together, as in adulthood, the cranium appears to be one solid bone.

The bones of the lower portion of the face grow at a much slower rate than the bones of the skull. These lower facial bones do not reach their maximum adult size until about 18 years of age. Because of the different growth patterns of the skull bones and the facial bones, the face is allowed to grow downward and forward relative to the cranium (Kent, 1997).

Dentition in the infant begins to emerge at about 6 months of age. First teeth are temporary and are usually referred to as primary or deciduous dentition. Emergence of the primary dentition is usually complete by 3 years of age. At approximately 5 years of age, children begin losing their primary teeth, and their permanent or secondary teeth begin to appear. The emergence of the secondary teeth is usually complete by 18 years of age.

The tongue of the newborn is large enough to occupy most of the oral cavity (Kent, 1997). As the infant grows during the first several years, the posterior portion of the tongue descends into the pharyngeal cavity, and the tongue reaches its mature size at about 16 years of age. In general, the growth of the tongue is similar to the growth of the mandible and the lips (Kent, 1997).

The lips experience two major growth spurts. The first occurs during the first two years of life, and the second occurs during the early and middle teenage years. During these growth spurts, the lips increase in width, height, and convexity.

THE NERVOUS SYSTEM

The nervous system consists of the brain, spinal cord, and all associated nerves and sense organs. The **neuron** is the basic unit of the nervous system. Each neuron consists of three parts: the cell body, a single long *axon* that transmits impulses away from the cell body, and several branching *dendrites* that receive impulses from other cells and transmit them toward the cell body. A nerve is a collection of neurons. Neurons do not actually touch but are close enough that electrochemical impulses can "jump" the minuscule space, or **synapse,** between the axon of one neuron and the dendrites of the next.

CENTRAL NERVOUS SYSTEM

The brain and spinal cord make up the **central nervous system (CNS).** The CNS communicates with the rest of the body through the nerves. All incoming stimuli and outgoing signals are processed through the CNS.

The brain consists of the brain stem, the cerebellum, and the **cerebrum** or upper brain. The cerebrum is divided into two halves, designated the left and right hemispheres. The sensory and motor functions of the cerebrum are **contralateral,** which means that each hemisphere is concerned with the body's opposite side. With the exception of hearing and vision, the nerves from each side of the body cross to the opposite hemisphere somewhere along their course.

Hearing is predominantly contralateral, but not exclusively. Approximately 60 percent of the signal from each ear crosses to the other hemisphere; 40 percent remains on the same side.

Each hemisphere consists of white fibrous connective tracts covered by a gray **cortex** of cell bodies approximately one-fourth inch in thickness. The cortex has a wrinkled appearance caused by little hills called **gyri** and valleys called **fissures,** or **sulci.** Each hemisphere is divided into four lobes, which are labeled frontal, parietal, occipital, and temporal (Figure 3.9).

The frontal and temporal lobes are separated by the deep **lateral sulcus,** or *fissure of Sylvius.* The **central sulcus,** or *fissure of Rolando,* separates the frontal lobe from the parietal. Immediately in front of the central sulcus is the **primary motor cortex,** a 2-centimeter-wide strip

The modified contralateral nature of hearing has survival value. If one ear is damaged, both sides of the brain still receive information. If one hemisphere is damaged, information from both ears is still reaching the brain.

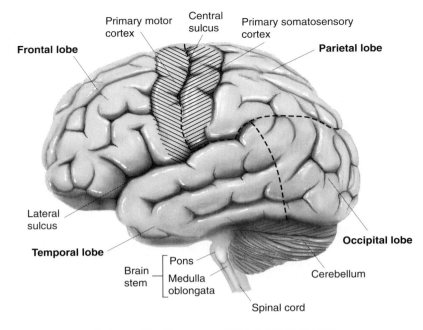

FIGURE 3.9 Schematic diagram of the human brain

that controls motor movements. Behind and parallel to the motor cortex is the somatosensory cortex, which receives sensory input from the muscles, joints, bones, and skin. Other motor and sensory functions are found in specialized regions of the cortex. It is too simplistic to conceive of the brain as merely consisting of localized sensory and motor mechanisms. The integration of sensory and motor information is required for the body to respond. Below the level of the cortex, the brain is crisscrossed with bands of neural fibers that link the hemispheres, coordinate motor and sensory areas, integrate sensory information, and aid recall from scattered storage areas.

HEMISPHERIC ASYMMETRY

Although the cerebral hemispheres are roughly symmetrical, for specialized functions such as language, they are asymmetrical, and processing is the primary responsibility of one hemisphere. Still, the hemispheres are complementary, and information passes readily between them via subcortical bodies. Overall, neither hemisphere is dominant, since each possesses specialized talents and different skills. Neither hemisphere is competent to analyze data and program a response alone.

The right hemisphere in humans is specialized for holistic processing through the simultaneous integration of information. It is dominant in visuospatial processing such as depth and orientation in space and perception and recognition of faces, pictures, and photographs. In addition, the right hemisphere is capable of holistic or simultaneous recognition of printed words but has difficulty decoding information using phonic or printed symbol-phoneme decoding. Other language-related skills include comprehension and production of speech prosody and affect; metaphorical language and semantics; and comprehension of complex linguistic and ideational material and of environmental sounds, such as nonspeech sounds, music, melodies, tones, laughter, clicks, and buzzes (Millar & Whitaker, 1983; Shapiro & Danley, 1985).

In nearly all humans, the left hemisphere is specialized for most aspects of receptive and expressive language, temporal or linear order perception, arithmetic calculations, and logical reasoning. Unlike the right hemisphere, which engages in holistic interpretation, the left is best at step-by-step processing. The left hemisphere is adept at perceiving rapidly changing sequential information, such as the acoustic characteristics of phonemes in speech. Processing these phonemes for meaning, however, involves representation in both hemispheres (Molfese, Molfese, & Parsons, 1983). The left hemisphere is also dominant for control of speech- and nonspeech-related oral movements.

When you recognize a face but can't recall a name, is it possible that two parts of the brain are not working together?

Not all human brains are organized as described, although approximately 98 percent of humans are left hemisphere-dominant for language. In general, all right-handers and approximately 60 percent of left-handers are left-dominant for language. The remainder of left-handers are right-dominant. A minuscule percentage of humans display bilateral linguistic performance with no apparent dominant hemisphere. Most likely, lateralization is a matter of degree for each human; some have more, others less.

The primary anatomical asymmetry in the brain is found in the left temporal lobe. This enlarged area, found even in the fetal brain, may account for the dominance of the left hemisphere in speech and language reception and production. In addition, this area continues to grow even larger in the mature brain and to mature at a slower rate than corresponding areas on the right (Geschwind & Galaburda, 1985).

SUBCORTICAL AND LOWER BRAIN STRUCTURES

The **thalamus** consists of a pair of spherical structures divided into neuron cell body clusters. Each sphere acts as a receiving station for relaying information. The thalamus transmits motor information to the muscles and receives sensory information for higher processing in the brain. In addition, the thalamus may set the tone for the brain, alerting it to prepare to receive or to transmit information.

The **basal nuclei,** a cluster of neuron cell bodies sometimes referred to as the **basal ganglia,** regulate motor functioning and maintain posture and muscle tone. The basal nuclei also send information on motor movement to the motor cortex to modify neural impulses. Damage to the basal nuclei can result in involuntary movements called **tremors** and abnormal posture and muscle tone.

Located below the cerebrum, the **brain stem** is important for regulating respiration, chewing, swallowing, and automatic, or *autonomic,* activities of the body. In addition the brain stem carries messages between the brain and the rest of the body.

Consisting of two hemispheres, the **cerebellum** is connected to many other parts of the brain and has access to much of the brain's information. Although the cerebellum generates no nerve impulses itself, it smoothly regulates and coordinates the control of purposeful muscle movement, including very complex and fine motor activities. The cerebellum revises the transmission from the cortex's motor strip to produce accurate, precise movements. For example, the cerebellum may inhibit excessively strong impulses from the motor cortex to achieve smoother, less jerky movements. In addition, the cerebellum helps to maintain balance on the basis of information from the inner ear. The general location of the subcortical and lower brain structures is shown in Figure 3.10.

Subcortical structures modify the brain signals to the muscles and maintain muscle tone and readiness.

FIGURE 3.10 Subcortical and lower brain structures

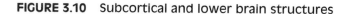

Basal nuclei

Thalamus

Brain stem — Midbrain
Pons
Medulla

Cerebellum

Spinal cord

How important is the cerebellum? If the motor cortex can only send the signal to muscles or muscle fiber groups for contraction, how do we make very precise movements necessary for drawing or painting or for playing musical instruments?

The **spinal cord,** located within the bony spinal column, is a collection of neuron cell bodies protected within a fatty myelin sheath. The spinal cord approximates (comes close but does not connect) with thirty-one pairs of peripheral nerves.

PERIPHERAL NERVOUS SYSTEM

Located outside the CNS, the **peripheral nervous system (PNS)** consists of twelve pairs of cranial nerves, thirty-one pairs of spinal nerves, and portions of the autonomic nerves that regulate smooth muscles and glands. By transmitting messages to muscles and glands and receiving sensory messages, the PNS helps the CNS to communicate with the body. For these functions, the PNS is generally divided into motor or efferent and sensory or afferent nerves.

The **cranial nerves** (Figure 3.11) are especially important for the control of motor speech. Having motor, sensory, and mixed functions, cranial nerves approximate the base of the brain at the brain stem and run to the structures they innervate. Because cranial nerves are arranged vertically along the brain stem, they are referred to by Roman numerals corresponding to their vertical order. Thus, number VII, the facial nerve, is seventh from the top.

Spinal nerves exit and enter through the bony spinal column. Many are important for innervating the muscles necessary for breathing, the foundation of speech production.

MUSCLE CONTROL

The muscles of speech are activated by the cranial nerves, which cause them to contract. Muscles are told when, how much, and for how long to contract. Three factors—the timing of muscle movements, muscle strength, and muscle tone—are important for correct speech production (Netsell, 1986).

Timing of the beginning and ending of muscle contraction and the duration of that contraction is essential to accuracy of movement. Bundles of muscle tissue must be coordinated to activate each muscle, and in turn, muscles must be synchronized to achieve movement. For example, no movement would result if two opposing muscles contracted simultaneously. Try this yourself by attempting to raise your

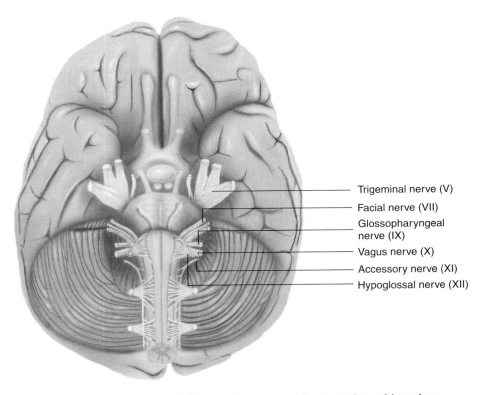

Trigeminal nerve (V)

Facial nerve (VII)

Glossopharyngeal nerve (IX)

Vagus nerve (X)

Accessory nerve (XI)

Hypoglossal nerve (XII)

FIGURE 3.11 Cranial nerves that are important in speech and hearing

Trigeminal (V): A mixed nerve with both sensory and motor functions for the jaw and tongue for speech and chewing.

Facial (VII): A mixed nerve for sensation of taste and motor control of the facial muscles important in facial expression, such as smiling, tearing, and salivation.

Glossopharyngeal (IX): A mixed nerve with sensory input from the tongue for taste and motor control of the pharynx for salivation and swallowing.

Vagus (X): A mixed nerve serving the heart, lungs, and digestive system. A sensory nerve to the larynx and throat. A motor nerve for the larynx for phonation, the soft palate for lifting, and the pharynx for swallowing.

Accessory (XI): A motor nerve controlling the muscles of the pharynx, soft palate, head, and shoulders.

Hypoglossal (XII): A motor nerve controlling the muscles of tongue movement.

arm while simultaneously attempting to lower it. The result is no movement. This is the principle that is used in isometric exercises, in which one muscle group is pitted against another, negating the need for weights.

Some muscle responses to stimuli, called **reflexes,** are automatic, seemingly instantaneous motor movements. Reflexes are processed at the level of either the spinal cord or the brain stem rather than at the cortex, accounting for the rapid response time.

Strength is the power or force of muscle contraction and the accompanying amount of work a muscle can accomplish. All of us occasionally have to ask for assistance when something turns out to be heavier than it looks. Remember the last time you asked for or provided help opening a particularly sticky jar lid?

Tone, or resistance to stretch, is the near constant state of a muscle. Tone can be increased or decreased with contraction and the activities required of the muscle. Overall tone also may vary over time. Muscles may become either more flaccid or more rigid. The tone of opposing muscle groups, such as biceps and triceps in the upper arm, ensures smooth, controlled movement.

Neurogenic speech impairments are a disturbance in the control of motor movement. Timing, strength, and/or tone may be affected.

THE PROCESS OF MOTOR SPEECH

Every language message relies on some motor system for transmission. Once a message is formulated, it is transmitted to another person via speech, writing, gesture, manual signs, some communication device, or a combination of these. Different output systems have different processes of motor control and coordination. We'll concentrate on speech.

The process of coordinating speech is complicated. Figure 3.12 presents a simplified schematic of the process. Nerve impulses generated in the motor cortex are sent to the muscles by two cooperating systems to control motor movement. These are the pyramidal and the extrapyramidal pathways, which can be thought of as complementary, each reinforcing the task of the other and resulting in a coordinated whole.

Usually described as the primary voluntary motor control system, the **pyramidal tract** is a bundle of nerves that originates in the primary motor cortex and travels uninterrupted to the spinal cord, crossing to the other side of the body in the brain stem. Within the pyramidal pathway are different tracts for specific areas of the body, including the structures that are important for speech. After crossing over, these **upper motor neurons** contact a second set of **lower motor neurons,** consisting of the cranial and spinal nerves of the peripheral nervous system, that innervate the muscle.

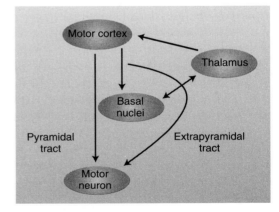

FIGURE 3.12 Schematic of the speech coordination process

A lesion in either the upper or lower motor neurons can result in **paralysis,** or an inability to move typically. Damage to the *upper* motor neurons causes rigidity, or increased tone in the muscles, while damage to the *lower* results in flaccidity, or softness and weakness in muscle tone.

The complex stimulation of a nerve can be imagined by forming the entire population of the earth into millions of human chains linked by hand. Each person is a neuron, and hands are actually held a short distance apart to simulate a synapse. Chains are intertwined to form a few hundred strands, called nerves. A nerve impulse would begin with squeezing of the hands that are closest to the brain and would progress through each chain with hand squeezes at each "synapse." Stronger impulses would involve stronger squeezing, more hands, and more chains.

The cooperating **extrapyramidal tract,** a more indirect system, involves the brain stem, cerebellum, and basal nuclei and complements the pyramidal tract by smoothing and coordinating movement. Unlike the pyramidal tract, the extrapyramidal has a more diffuse origin and several synaptic "stations" along its path.

The distinction between the two tracts may help you to understand some of the disorders that we will be discussing. As with language disorders, however, the location of the lesion does not directly correlate to the resulting type of disorder.

LANGUAGE PROCESSING

Linking language processing with specific cortical location is difficult because these processes are often not localized. The processes often overlap, and a particular region of the brain may be responsible for both incoming and outgoing information. In addition, language processing is extremely complex, requiring a broad range of functions. We will consider the parallel but opposite processes of comprehension and production.

Comprehension consists of linguistic auditory processing and language symbol decoding. We will concentrate on auditory processing because it is the primary sense used in conversation. Auditory processing is concerned with the nature of the incoming auditory signal. Symbol decoding considers the representational meaning and underlying ideational concepts of the auditory signals. Processing begins with attending to incoming auditory stimuli. Since it has a limited capacity to process incoming data, the brain must allocate this capacity by focusing its attention on certain stimuli while ignoring or inhibiting others.

Auditory signals are relayed to an area in each hemisphere called **Heschl's gyrus** (Figure 3.13). Heschl's gyrus and the surrounding auditory association areas separate the incoming information, differentiating significant linguistic and paralinguistic information from nonsignificant background noise. Linguistic information is sent to the

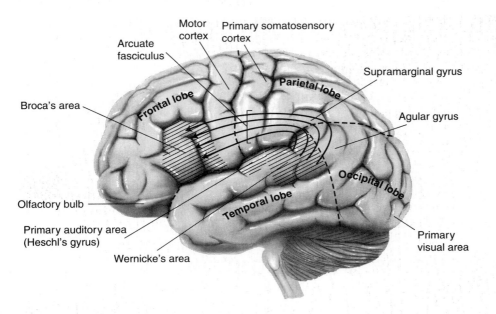

Labels on figure:
- Motor cortex
- Primary somatosensory cortex
- Arcuate fasciculus
- Supramarginal gyrus
- Parietal lobe
- Broca's area
- Agular gyrus
- Frontal lobe
- Olfactory bulb
- Occipital lobe
- Primary auditory area (Heschl's gyrus)
- Temporal lobe
- Primary visual area
- Wernicke's area

FIGURE 3.13 Linguistic processing and the brain

left temporal lobe for processing, while paralinguistic input (intonation, stress, rhythm, rate) is directed to the right temporal lobe.

Linguistic analysis is accomplished in **Wernicke's area,** located in the left temporal lobe (Figure 3.13). The **angular gyrus** and the **supramarginal gyrus** assist in this process by integrating visual, auditory, and tactile information and linguistic representation. Damage to these areas disrupts the connection between oral and visual language and may necessitate the use of reading aloud for comprehension. Although their functioning is not totally understood, the angular gyrus aids in word recall, and the supramarginal gyrus is involved in processing longer syntactic units, such as sentences. Written input is received in the visual cortex and transferred to the angular gyrus, where it may be integrated with auditory input. This information is then transmitted to Wernicke's area for analysis.

Obviously, analysis for comprehension depends on memory storage of both words and concepts. The store of word meanings is diffusely located, centered primarily in the temporal lobe, although the exact location is unknown. Incoming information is transmitted to the *hippocampus* on the underside of the temporal lobe and to related areas for consolidation before storage.

Production processes are located in the same general area of the brain as comprehension. The conceptual basis of a message to be produced

> Wernicke's area is central to both incoming and outgoing linguistic processing.

forms in one of the many memory areas of the cortex. The underlying structure of the message is organized in Wernicke's area; then the message is transmitted through the **arcuate fasciculus,** a white fibrous tract underlying the angular gyrus, to **Broca's area,** in the frontal lobe (Figure 3.13). Broca's area is responsible for detailing and coordinating the programming for verbalizing the message. Signals are then passed to the regions of the motor cortex that activate the muscles that are responsible for respiration, phonation, resonation, and articulation. The outgoing message is conceived abstractly and given specific form as it passes from the posterior ideational areas to anterior motor execution areas.

The actual processes are much more complex than our brief description suggests. Many areas of the brain have multiple or as yet unknown functions. In addition, describing the location of a function does not explain how that function is performed.

MOTOR SPEECH CONTROL

In the process of producing motor speech, first the movement plan is conceived, detailed, and programmed in the cortex; next it is sent to the motor control areas; then it is transmitted with precise timing along the nerves to the muscles and structures of the speech mechanism, resulting in sequences of acoustic signals recognizable as speech sounds. Along the way, these nerve impulses are modified to ensure precise, smooth muscle movement.

Typical movement patterns are purposeful and efficient and are under the control of the individual, thus enabling her or him to change or modify the movement. The tennis player who is ready for one type of serve must change her response quickly if another type of serve occurs instead. Reach for your pen, then change and scratch your nose instead. Do it again and notice how smoothly the action is executed.

If feedback is disordered in some way, movement will also be affected.

Motor responses are initiated, changed, and coordinated on the basis of both external and internal sensory information. External sensory mechanisms detect and analyze the external environment. Internal proprioceptive or movement feedback from the muscles and nerves helps us to know the position and movement of body structures in space. In speech, additional auditory feedback is a further check on the correct coordination of the speech mechanism.

SPEECH PRODUCTION PROCESS

The production of speech begins with the sound produced by vocal fold vibration, or **phonation.** Phonation is initiated by approximating or adducting the vocal folds and closing the glottis through active contraction of intrinsic laryngeal adductor muscles. Once the vocal folds are closed, air pressure generated by the respiratory system increases beneath the vocal folds. The air pressure that builds beneath the vocal folds is called subglottic pressure.

As subglottic air pressure increases, vocal fold tissue is displaced in a lateral or sideward and superior or upward direction (frames 1, 2, and 3 of Figure 3.14), and the vocal folds are literally blown apart once the subglottic pressure reaches a critical value, as illustrated in frame 4. Air rushing through the glottis increases in velocity. This increase in velocity produces a negative pressure (partial vacuum) between the medial edges of the vocal folds, which tends to pull the vocal folds toward one another, closing the glottis (frames 5, 6, and 7).

This phenomenon is called the **Bernoulli effect.** In addition to the Bernoulli effect, two other forces bring the vocal folds back to an adducted state during phonation. The first force is the natural elasticity of the vocal folds, which acts to restore them to their original adducted state. The second force is the contraction of adductory intrinsic laryngeal muscles. It is important to realize that the opening of the vocal folds during phonation results solely from subglottic air pressure blowing the folds apart. No abductory muscle activity is associated with vocal fold opening during phonation.

Each time the vocal folds open and close, one complete vibratory cycle, the air in the vocal tract is set into vibration, producing sound. The sound that results from vocal fold vibration is complex, containing a **fundamental frequency,** or the lowest frequency component that is directly related to how fast the vocal folds are opening and closing, and approximately forty additional higher frequencies called **harmonics.** Figure 3.15 is a stylized spectrum of the complex sound that is produced by vocal fold vibration. A spectrum represents the frequencies of a complex sound along the horizontal axis, and their relative intensity is represented on the vertical axis. Note the relationship of the harmonic

FIGURE 3.14 Anterior view of the voice folds during one cycle of vibration. Air from the lungs creates a pressure beneath the vocal folds (1, 2, and 3). This pressure causes the vocal folds to separate (4). Decreased pressure in the glottis and elastic recoiling of vocal fold tissue cause the vocal folds to begin to close (5 and 6). The vocal folds close the glottis to end the cycle, and the next cycle begins (7)

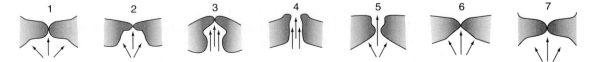

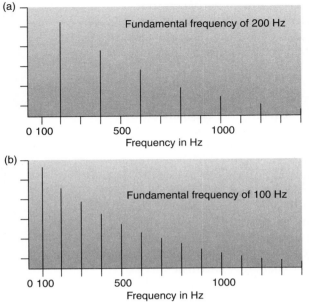

(a)

Fundamental frequency of 200 Hz

0 100   500   1000
        Frequency in Hz

(b)

Fundamental frequency of 100 Hz

0 100   500   1000
        Frequency in Hz

FIGURE 3.15 Spectrum illustrating a fundamental frequency of 200 Hz and related harmonics (a) and a spectrum of a fundamental frequency of 100 Hz and related harmonics (b)

frequencies to the fundamental frequency. The harmonic frequencies are whole-number multiples of the fundamental frequency. For example, when the fundamental frequency is 100 Hz, the second harmonic is 200 Hz, the third is 300 Hz, and so on. Note that the relative intensity decreases systematically with increases in harmonic frequency. Observe these relationships in the spectra shown in Figure 3.15.

The vocal tract is an acoustic resonator that will modify the quality of the sound produced by the larynx. In any acoustic resonator, some frequencies in a complex sound are reduced or attenuated and other frequencies are enhanced. Certain physical aspects (for example, the volume) of the resonator will determine which frequencies are attenuated and which frequencies are enhanced.

Air-filled cavities are acoustic resonators. The frequency or frequencies at which a filled cavity will resonate are determined by the volume of the cavity, the area of the opening of the cavity, and the length of the opening of the cavity.

THOUGHT QUESTION

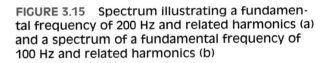

You are drinking soda from a bottle. After you have taken a few sips, you blow air across the opening on the top of the bottle, and a sound is produced. After taking a few more sips, you again blow across the opening. Was the sound different the second time you blew across the top of the bottle? The bottle is a resonator. What characteristics of the resonator changed and how did those changes influence the sound that was produced?

Movement of the tongue, lips, and larynx will change the shape of the vocal tract and in turn modify the sound emanating from the larynx. Produce the vowels /i/ (as in the word "bee") and /u/ (as in the word "boot"). Try to sense how your tongue and lips change position for the production of these two vowels. Changes in the position of your lips and tongue in turn change certain physical characteristics of the vocal tract that directly affect the quality of the sound that emanates from your mouth.

Figure 3.16 represents how changes of vocal tract shape influence which frequencies are enhanced and which are attenuated. A complex sound is produced by vocal fold vibration (a), and the vocal tract acts as a filter attenuating some frequencies and enhancing others (b). The sound that emanates from the mouth during vowel production (c) is

FIGURE 3.16   Spectra of glottal sound source (a) that sets the air in the vocal tract (b) into vibration. The vocal tract filters the glottal sound source differently for the vowels /i/ and /u/ as seen in the radiated spectra (c)

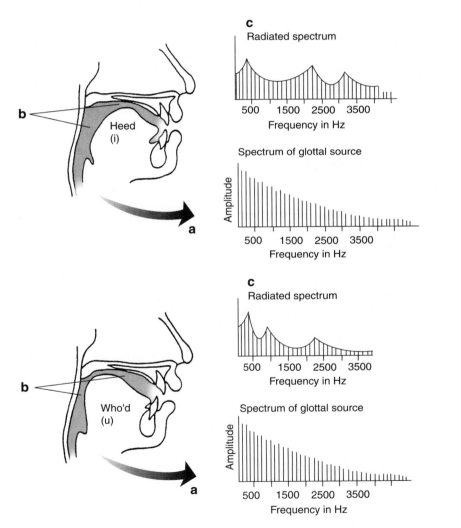

related directly to the general shape of the vocal tract determined largely by tongue position. Note that for the /u/ vowel, low frequencies are enhanced, whereas high frequencies are somewhat attenuated. For the /i/ vowel, low frequencies are somewhat attenuated, whereas high frequencies are enhanced.

During consonant production, the tongue is sometimes used to momentarily occlude the vocal tract for the production of stop sounds such as /t/, /d/, /k/, and /g/. Production of sounds such as /s/ and /sh/ require the tongue to form a constriction in the vocal tract that will produce frication noise when air is passed through the constriction.

Consonants are classified broadly as **voiced** and **voiceless.** Voiced consonants require vocal fold vibration, whereas voiceless consonants do not. When you produce the /s/ sound, as in the word "seal," you momentarily abduct the vocal folds, ceasing vocal fold vibration. The /s/ sound is a voiceless consonant. In contrast, when you produce the /z/ sound, as in the word "zeal," vocal fold vibration is required. The /z/ sound is a voiced consonant.

SUMMARY

This chapter has been a brief overview of the anatomy and physiology of the speech and voice mechanism. The study of the structures that are used to produce speech and their function is extensive and complex. It is important to remember that although anatomy is static, these structures are capable of dynamic movement that can result in the unique human processes of speech.

The study of anatomy and physiology is essential for the speech-language pathologist. Knowledge and understanding of this topic will assist in the evaluation and treatment of clients whose communication disorder is the direct or indirect result of a breakdown within these systems.

REFLECTIONS

- Describe the skeletal framework for respiration.
- Describe the components of the pulmonary system.

- Explain the respiratory processes for quiet breathing and for speech breathing.
- Describe the framework of the larynx.
- Explain the phonation process.
- Describe the skeletal framework of articulation and resonance.
- Describe the vocal tract cavities.
- Explain the articulatory and resonating process for human speech.
- Describe the components of the central nervous system.
- Explain the process of speech production.

SUGGESTED READINGS

A.D.A.M.®Animated Dissection of Anatomy for Medicine. Atlanta, GA: A.D.A.M. Software, Inc.

Kent, R. D. (1997). *The speech sciences.* San Diego, CA: Singular Publishing Group.

The Respiratory System (CD-ROM). New York: Insight Media.

Thomas, L. (1979). *The medusa and the snail: More notes of a biology watcher.* New York: Viking.

Zemlin, W. R. (1998). *Speech and hearing science anatomy and physiology* (4th ed.). Boston: Allyn and Bacon.

ON-LINE RESOURCES

http://www.madsci.org/~lynn/VH/   Animated anatomical images of the three major body planes and more.

http://www.uchsc.edu/sm/chs/   Anatomical views of various body structures.

http://faculty.washington.edu/chudler/introb.html   Excellent information about the nervous system.

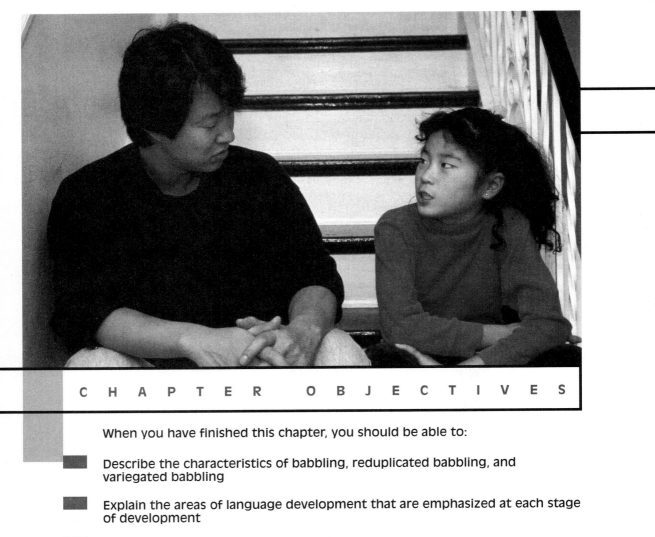

C H A P T E R   O B J E C T I V E S

When you have finished this chapter, you should be able to:

◼ Describe the characteristics of babbling, reduplicated babbling, and variegated babbling

◼ Explain the areas of language development that are emphasized at each stage of development

◼ Describe the major difficulties that individuals may encounter in speech, language, and communication throughout the life span

4

Communication Development

In any area of development, compare the somewhat limited abilities of infants with your own abilities. For example, in terms of locomotion, how did you go from being a newborn who was unable even to roll over to an adult who may be able to rollerblade, snowboard, swim, run, bicycle, and/or drive a car? Yet, the infant is a complete being and contains all the potential to develop into a competent adult.

The most complex and challenging task newborns face is learning the abstract code called language that those around them use to communicate. To do this, infants must first learn the rudiments of communication and begin to master the primary means of language transmission, called speech. As you know

from Chapter 1, speech, language, and communication are all different but interdependent, and their development is similarly separate but intertwined. The early establishment of communication between children and their caregivers fosters the development of speech and language, which in turn influences the quality of communication. This intricate pattern is further complicated by physical, cognitive, and social development as children mature. We can go even further to suggest studies in several languages that reveal that language proficiency is critical to development of higher cognitive skills, even nonverbal ones (Oller, Kim, Kunok, & Choe, 2001).

Communication is established very early between the child and caregiver.

Are newborns totally helpless? Next time you're with one, observe the things the child can do and try to make a mental list of the abilities of a newborn.

Every person's speech and language continue to change until the end of life. Communication reflects the changes occurring in us and around us. Even the means of communication can change. Your great-grandparents might have begun life without a telephone and had to learn this new means of communication. Your grandparents probably began life without television. We, the authors, had to learn to use computers to communicate when we were well into our adult lives. You, on the other hand, grew up with the Internet.

Languages change too. New words and phrases have entered American English within your lifetime, such as *Internet, compact disc, disco, rollerblade, clap skate, rap,* and *European Union.* Other cultures and languages have contributed *mullah, sushi, mensch, tortilla,* and *salsa.* The competent communicator continues to adapt to changes in the language and in the communication process.

T H O U G H T   Q U E S T I O N S

Have you become dependent on e-mail to communicate with your friends? Do you routinely use the Internet to chat or explore areas of interest? Only a few years ago, neither was available to college students. (How did they survive?)

Children become communicators because we treat them as if they already are.

The key to becoming a communicator is being treated as one. While both speech and language are dependent on physical and cognitive maturation, neither is sufficient to account for the rapid developments in children's communication. Most linguists would also agree that language has strong biological underpinnings, although this too is an insufficient explanation in itself of the language learning process.

The process of learning speech and language is a social one that occurs through interactions of children and the people in their environment. Speech and language are learned within routines and familiar activities that shape children's days and within conversations about food, toys, and pets and later about school, social life, and the like. As listeners, we use a variety of lexical, syntactic, and stress-pattern cues flexibly to break continuous speech into more readily interpretable chunks (Sanders & Neville, 2000).

In different cultures, the type of child-caregiver interaction, the model of language presented to the child, and the expectations for the child differ, but each is sufficient for the learning of language. Learning to become an effective communicator is a dynamic and active process in which children in our culture become involved in the give-and-take of conversations. Even the more formal educational processes of learning to read and write are initially social and occur within book-reading activities in the home involving children and caregivers.

In the remainder of this chapter, we'll describe speech, language, and communication development as we move through the life span.

A CHRONOLOGY

We'll begin our study of communication development with the newborn and trace changes through to the elderly communicator. Highlights are presented in Table 4.1. At each level of development, we'll examine important changes in speech, language, and communication. As you might guess, the relative importance of each will vary with maturational level. For example, speech development, while rapid in preschool and early elementary school, is unremarkable in later life. As we progress through the life span, we will stop periodically to note possible problems that might impair development. These impairments will be examined in more detail in later chapters. We also quickly discuss physical, social, and intellectual maturation because these are closely related to communication.

INFANTS AND TODDLERS

Newborns, or **neonates,** are oddly proportioned little creatures when compared to adults. Figure 4.1 presents a comparison. Their heads are approximately a quarter of their total body length, and their torso and limbs are small by comparison. The head is large to accommodate the brain, which grows rapidly during gestation and infancy. The skull must solidify early to protect the delicate brain, but not before the brain has had time to reach sufficient size.

Unable to control their motor behavior smoothly and voluntarily, newborns are all twitches, jerks, and seemingly random movements. These automatic, involuntary motor patterns, called *reflexes*, allow newborns to react to things in the world while learning to control their bodies. Most reflexes, such as sucking in response to oral stimulation, disappear, but some, such as the gag reflex, remain with us for life.

Although unable to respond with specific, volitional movements, newborns are nonetheless able to perceive stimuli in the environment, especially sights and sounds. Although nearsighted at birth, newborns are sensitive to both brightness and color. Short-term visual memory

TABLE 4.1

Development of speech, language, and communication

Age	Accomplishments
Newborn	Prefers human face and voice. Able to discriminate loudness, intonation, and phonemes.
3 months	Begins babbling. Responds vocally to partner.
6 months	Begins reduplicated babbling "Ba-ba-ba."
8 months	Begins gesturing. Begins variegated babbling. Imitates tonal quality of adult speech, called jargon.
10 months	Adds phonetically consistent forms.
12 months	First word spoken. Words fill intentions previously signaled by gestures.
18 months	Begins combining words on the basis of word-order rules.
2 years	Begins adding bound morphemes. Average length or mean length of utterance (MLU) is 1.6–2.2 morphemes.
3 years	More adultlike sentence structure. Mean length of utterance (MLU) is 3.0–3.3 morphemes.
4 years	Begins to change style of talking to fit conversational partner. Mean length of utterance (MLU) is 3.6–4.7 morphemes.
5 years	Ninety percent of language form learned.
6 years	Begins to learn visual mode of communication with writing and reading.
8 years	All American English speech sounds acquired.
Adolescence	Able to competently participate in conversations and telling of narratives. Knows multiple meanings of words and figurative language. Uses a gender style, or genderlect, when talking.
Adult	Vocabulary has expanded to 30,000–60,000 words. Specialized styles of communicating with different audiences and for diverse purposes.

Sources: Klee, Schaffer, May, Membrino, & Mougey, 1989; Miller, 1981; Scarborough, Wyckoff, & Davidson, 1986; Wells, 1985.

is limited to recognition when an object reappears within 2 ½ seconds. Within limits, newborns learn to distinguish some people and objects. By 2 months of age, infants have some short-term mental images for common objects and people in their environment.

Newborns possess good auditory abilities, although their middle ears are filled with fluid and the portion of the brain that integrates sounds is still immature. Despite these limitations, newborns are able to distinguish loudness or intensity and duration of sound. Within two weeks after birth, the middle ear becomes more sensitive to sound as fluid is absorbed and drained.

Possibly before birth and most certainly within the first few days after birth, infants can discriminate between different meaningful speech sounds or *phonemes*. This is not the same as comprehending words. The human voice often causes an infant to stop sucking and can usually soothe a crying baby.

During the first few weeks, infants learn to coordinate vision and hearing and to use these to examine nearby objects, people, and events by turning their heads toward sound sources. Within a few months, vision and reach become coordinated, and the infant is able to reach and grasp.

The downward progression of large muscle control enables infants to gain control of their heads and neck followed by trunk control and unsupported sitting by about 6 months. In this upright position, infants' hands are free to explore and examine objects. Knowledge of object functions and characteristics thus gained form early concepts that will become the bases for word definitions later.

By age 1, infants have progressed from sitting through crawling and cruising, or holding onto furniture while moving, to independent walking. Much of the second year is spent in perfecting the latter.

During the second year, toddlers seem absorbed in speech and language play. They like rhymes, songs, and stories, and much of their activity, such as playing and eating, is accompanied by speech.

Two-year-olds are relatively independent, though still very dependent on adults for protection and well-being. They have a good concept of the immediate environment and an expectation of daily routines. They have the social skills to gain and hold the attention of others and to express some emotions. Increased mobility enables them to explore the environment and to modify it, in part by using their linguistic skills to influence others.

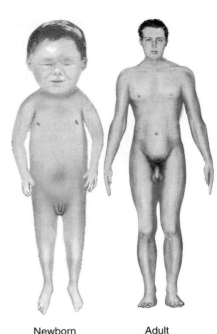

Newborn   Adult

FIGURE 4.1 Comparison of newborn and adult bodies

Control of large muscles moves progressively downward. First, the child gains some ability to lift and turn the head, then to control the shoulders, and finally to control down to the back. Soon he or she will be able to sit unsupported, then stand, and finally walk.

Children become communicators because they are treated as if they are communicators.

COMMUNICATION

Much of the first year of life is spent learning to be a communicator. Caregivers treat infants as if they are communicators. Caregivers talk to newborns as if these children understand what the adults are saying. For example, adults ask questions, then pause for a response. Later on, as children begin to comprehend language in limited ways, caregivers will modify their style of talking to maximize comprehension and participation by the child. Listen to the caregiver-child conversations on the accompanying CD-ROM.

T H O U G H T   Q U E S T I O N

As a speech-language pathologist, should you treat your clients as you treat infants even if they are adults but are unable to speak or to use language?

Shortly after birth, infants become actively involved in a reciprocal process with caregivers. By 1 month of age, infants initiate interactional sequences by gazing at their caregivers' faces and vocalizing. Infants also respond to their caregivers' vocalizations and movements.

Infants are especially responsive to their caregivers' voices and faces. By as early as two weeks, infants are able to distinguish their caregivers from strangers. Infant cooing increases and is easily stimulated by attention and speech and by toys that are moved before the baby.

To maintain attention, caregivers must provide the appropriate level of stimulation. They exaggerate their facial expressions and voice and vocalize more often. In turn, infants respond. Both partners affect their mutual interaction. Developmental changes affect the dynamic relationship between child and caregiver behaviors and the context (Sameroff & Fiese, 1990).

For some children with communicative impairment, the caregiver-child interaction is disrupted. For example, a child with either mental retardation or autism might not respond in the expected manner. Children with autism may ignore their parents' behaviors or actually turn away. To their credit, parents of children with autism continue to try to engage their children in interactions with patience and perseverance.

T H O U G H T   Q U E S T I O N

How would you respond to a child who went limp or stiff when held and would not make eye contact? Or a child who was more interested in objects than in people?

Dialogues become more important as handling decreases with increased age. Infants are full partners and their behavior is influenced by the communication behavior of their caregivers, whether mother, father, sibling, or daycare worker. For example, the 12-week-old is twice as likely to revocalize if his or her caregiver responds verbally to the infant's initial vocalization rather than responding with a touch, look, or smile.

This "conversational" turn taking by adults benefits infant babbling and turn taking. Infant babbling becomes more speechlike and mature, containing syllables rather than individual sounds.

A shift in infant-caregiver vocalization begins at about 12 weeks. From the predominantly simultaneous vocalization pattern, more conversational turn taking gradually begins to emerge. One partner begins, the other responds, followed by the first revocalizing, and so on.

Eye gaze is very important in these early dialogues. By 6 weeks of age, infants are able to fix visually on their caregiver's eyes and hold the fixation, with eye widening and brightening. Infants are more likely to begin and to continue looking if their caregivers are looking at them. In return, the caregivers' behavior becomes more social, and play interactions begin.

During the first three months, caregivers' responses teach children the "signal" value of specific behaviors. Infants learn the stimulus-response sequence. If they signal, caregivers will respond. Thus, they develop an expectation that they can change or control the environment. In addition, they learn that a relatively constant stimulus or signal results in a predictable response.

By 3 to 4 months, two additional joint action patterns have emerged: rituals and game playing. Rituals, such as feeding and diaper changing, provide children with predictable patterns of behavior and speech. They learn that interactions and communication can unfold in predictable ways; they begin to form expectations of events. Games such as "peekaboo," "this little piggy," and "I'm gonna get you" have many of the aspects of communication. There is an exchange of turns, rules for each turn, and particular slots for words and actions. Games, like communication, are also predictable.

Games and rituals share many characteristics with conversations.

As infants approach 6 months of age, interest in toys and objects increases. From this point on, interactions often include the infant, the caregiver, and some object. In recognition of their infants' interest in objects and increasing ability to follow conversational cues, caregivers make increasing reference to objects, events, and people outside of the immediate context.

Nine-month-olds can follow caregivers' pointing and glancing or regard. Visual orientation of both infants and their caregivers is usually accompanied by caregiver naming. Infant gazing is more likely to be initiated and maintained when caregivers are vocalizing and/or gazing back, and in turn, caregivers are more likely to initiate and maintain vocalization when infants are looking at them.

At about 8 to 9 months, infants also develop **intentionality,** or goal directedness, in their interactions with their caregivers and the ability to share goals with others primarily through gestures. Even children who are deaf will begin to gesture and to communicate meaningfully with immature signs at about this age. For the first time, a child considers the audience or other person when attempting a potentially communicative act. In this way, communicative behaviors, such as requesting, interacting, and attracting attention, are first fulfilled by prelinguistic communicative means and only later by language.

From birth to 7 or 8 months, infants have failed to signal specific intentions beyond those behaviors that will sustain an interaction. Toward the end of this period, as infants become more interested in manipulating objects, they begin to use gestures that demonstrate an understanding of object purpose or function, such as bringing a cup to the lips or a telephone receiver to the ear. Infants also begin reaching for objects they desire.

Functional communication development or intentional communication begins at 8 to 9 months when infants begin to use conventional gestures and/or vocalizations to communicate their intentions. Different behaviors signal different intentions. An intention to communicate is noted in gestures accompanied by eye contact with the child's communication partner, the use of consistent sound and intonational patterns for specific intentions, and persistent attempts to communicate. Children with autism may be so seemingly uninterested in communication that they do not even communicate with gestures. This lack affects the development of first words.

Initially, gestures appear without vocalizations, but the two are gradually paired. Consistent vocal patterns, dubbed **phonetically consistent forms (PCFs),** accompany many gestures. To be discussed in the following section, PCFs are a transition to words in a highly creative developmental period when the child is also adept at employing gestures and intonation.

Around 12 months, children use their first meaningful word. Children's intentions become encoded in a language symbol or word. Real words are used with or without gestures to accomplish the functions previously filled by gestures. The gesture, which initially stands for the entire message, gradually becomes the context for the word.

Early intentions, such as attracting attention, are established in gestures and first words fill these same functions, often with the accompanying gesture.

SPEECH

Newborns produce predominantly reflexive sounds, such as fussing and crying, and vegetative sounds, such as burping and swallowing. Production of both decreases with maturation.

Although some oral reflexes, such as gagging, coughing, yawning, and sneezing, remain for life, most disappear or are modified by 6 months of age. This disappearance is related to the rapid rate of brain growth and to myelination. **Myelination** is the development of a protective myelin sheath or sleeve around the cranial nerves. When myelination is completed in adulthood, the organism has the capacity for full neural functioning.

The rate of myelination may be affected by overall health. Children who are exposed to toxins or poor diet may experience delayed myelination or brain damage that retards or alters development.

Initially, newborns cry on both inhalation and exhalation. The expiration phase—a more efficient sound production source—gradually increases. By the end of the first month, primary caregivers can usually tell the reason for crying by its differing sound patterns.

T H O U G H T   Q U E S T I O N

Try saying "Ah-h-h" on inhalation and on exhalation. Inhalation vocalization is very inefficient and may even hurt a little. Although some languages have a few sounds that are produced on inhalation, excessive vocalization in this way may harm the vocal folds.

Crying helps children to become accustomed to air flow across the vocal folds and to modifying their breathing patterns. Since speech sounds originate at the level of the larynx, this early stimulation is necessary. However, noncrying vocalizations are far more important in the development of speech.

Noncrying sounds usually accompany feeding or are produced in response to smiling or talking by the caregivers. These noncrying vowel-like sounds contain some **phonation** or vibration at the larynx, but the child has insufficient ability to produce fully resonated and articulated speech sounds. **Resonation** is a modification of the vibratory pattern of the laryngeal tone through changes in the size and configuration of the vocal tract, which consists of the nasal cavity, the oral cavity or mouth, and the pharynx or throat. **Articulation** is rapid and coordinated movement of the tongue, teeth, lips, and palate to produce speech sounds. Initially, production of sounds is by chance.

By 2 months of age, infants develop nondistress sounds called either "gooing" or "cooing" and consisting of vocalizations with a velar to uvular closure or near closure. The velum, you will recall, is the soft and somewhat mobile portion of the palate. During gooing, infants produce back consonant sounds similar to /g/ and /k/ and middle and back vowel sounds, such as /ʌ/ and /ʊ/, with incomplete resonance.

By 3 months of age, infants vocalize in response to the speech of others as noted earlier. Infants are most responsive if their caregivers respond to them. The amount of crying and vegetative sounds decreases.

At 5 months, infants are able to imitate the tone and pitch signals of their caregivers. Most infant imitative and nonimitative vocalizations are single-syllable units of consonant-vowel (CV) or vowel-consonant (VC) construction. These sound units that begin at 4 months are called **babbling.**

With maturity, longer sequences and prolonged individual sounds evolve. Children produce increasingly more complex combinations. Sounds are now more fully resonated and more like adult speech. Muscle control moves forward from the back of the oral cavity. Thus, we see strong tongue projection in 4- to 6-month-olds. Initially, back consonants predominate in babbling, but by 6 months, labial or lip sounds, such as /m/ and /p/, are produced more frequently.

Babbling is random sound play, and even deaf infants babble. During babbling, infants experiment with sound production. Often the sounds that are produced do not appear in the native language. Because babbling is random, children may produce sounds that they will be unable to produce later when they attempt words containing that sound. With age, children's babbling increasingly reflects the syllable structure and intonation of the caregivers' speech.

The consonant-vowel (CV) syllable becomes one of the predominant building blocks in first words.

At about 6 or 7 months, infants' babbling begins to change to **reduplicated babbling,** which contains long strings of consonant-vowel syllable repetitions or self-imitations (CV-CV-CV), such as "ma-ma-ma-ma-ma." Hearing ability appears to be very important. Children with deafness continue to babble, but the range of consonants decreases, and few reduplicated strings are produced.

Hearing children practice speech sounds for long periods each day. They may even repeat at a caregiver's urging. Although babbling may have been slow and somewhat restricted, reduplicated babbling more closely approximates mature speech in its resonant quality and timing. The child is beginning to adapt the speech patterns of the environment. Regardless of the language modeled for infants, their vocalizations and later first words have similar phonological patterns. For example, stops (/p, b, t, d, k, g/), nasals (/m, n, ŋ/), and approximants (/w, j/) constitute approximately 80 percent of the consonants in infant vocalizations and in the first fifty words of Spanish-, Korean-, and English-speaking children.

The period from 8 to 12 months has been called the *echolalic* stage. **Echolalia** is speech that is an immediate imitation of some other speaker rather than a spontaneous production by the child. At first, children imitate only those sounds that they have produced spontaneously on their own.

Gradually, infants begin to use imitation to expand and modify their repertoire of speech sounds. Babbled speech sounds that are not in the native language decrease and gradually drop out. Although children at this stage may echo or repeat "ma-ma" when an adult says "Mama," the child will probably not yet associate the sound with the actual referent or entity, although some associations are made.

At about the same time, infants begin using gestures, with or without vocalizations, to communicate. They may point, show and give objects, request, signal "no" or noncompliance, show off for attention, wave bye-bye, and give kisses. Speech during this period is characterized by **variegated babbling,** in which adjacent and successive syllables in the string are not identical.

In the second half of the first year, children begin to notice contrasts in pitch, in vowels, and in consonants in CV syllables. They begin to recognize recurring patterns of sounds within specific situations. The child may even produce sounds in these situations. For example, the child might begin to say "M-m-m" during feeding if this sound is modeled for him or her.

In response to caregiver conversations, infants may begin to experiment with **jargon,** long strings of unintelligible sounds with adultlike intonation. Gradually, children's babbling begins to resemble the intonational pattern of the language to which the child is exposed. Jargon may sound like questions, commands, and statements.

T H O U G H T   Q U E S T I O N

Try to produce jargon yourself. Say the sentence "How are you today?" with exaggerated intonation as if talking to an infant. Now do it again but substitute "la" for each syllable. Congratulations, you're jargonning with the best of 'em!

Many speech sounds will develop sound-meaning relationships. Called phonetically consistent forms (PCFs), mentioned earlier, these sound patterns function as "words" for the infant (Dore, Franklin, Miller, & Ramer, 1976). Children may develop several PCFs before they speak their first adult-type words. By establishing sound-meaning relationships, children demonstrate a recognition of linguistic regularities. In short, infants have noticed that adults consistently use certain sound patterns to refer to the same things in the environment.

PCFs are the child's first attempt at consistent use of a sound to represent or "stand for" something else.

Word production depends upon sound grouping and sound variation. Children adopt a problem-solving or trial-and-error approach to word production. The resultant speech is a complex interaction of the ease of production and perception of the target syllable and its member sounds.

Phonetic production is essential for the establishment of first words. The number of consonants produced at 9 months is positively correlated with the size of the child's lexicon at 16 months (McCune & Vihman, 2001).

Any perceptual difficulty such as learning disability (LD), sensory deficit such as deafness, neuromuscular problem as in cerebral palsy (CP), or structural abnormality such as cleft palate may result in speech production problems. For example, children with CP or with clefts of the palate or palate and lip may have great difficulty with control of the soft palate or velum. In addition, children with cerebral palsy may have tongue movement deficits, resulting in feeding and babbling difficulties.

LANGUAGE

To develop spoken language, children must be able to store sounds, use this information for later comparison and identification, and relate these sounds to meaning. By 6 months of age, children have some limited knowledge of speech. They know that

1. Speech predicts the presence of humans.
2. Speech affects listeners.
3. Speech can fill a conversational turn.

Now children must discover what it all means.

The task of learning language is one of learning to represent and to symbolize and is strongly related to cognitive abilities. Children with cognitive processing difficulties, such as LD, or limited cognitive abilities, such as mental retardation (MR), may have problems breaking the language code. **Representation** is the process of having one thing stand for another. For example, in play, a piece of paper might be used as a blanket for a doll.

After repeated exposure to mom's face, an infant will smile in recognition upon reexposure. Soon, the mother's voice alone will be enough to recall her image. Her voice *represents*, or stands for, her image. Other entities associated with mom, such as her shoes, hat, or dress, may also represent her. In like fashion, noises and objects will come to represent events and other objects in the environment.

Later, an arbitrary symbol or word, such as *mama* or *mommy*, will be enough to recall the image or concept of mom. The symbol comes from the linguistic code that is used in the child's environment by caregivers. The image has also undergone subtle change to a concept that includes mother's characteristics and her past experiences with the child. Still later, the concept will be expanded to include a definition of mother. In this very simplified explanation, the symbol has come to represent the referent or to symbolize it. At about 18 months of age, by using the word, the child will be able to refer to mom even though she is not present.

By the second half of the first year, infants respond consistently to a few frequently used symbols. For example, the infant may look at a few very familiar objects, such as *doggie,* that are named. By 10 months, he or she can recognize a familiar word within a short sentence.

Children "understand" or comprehend in a limited way on the basis of word sounds, nonlinguistic and paralinguistic cues, and context. Words are probably not comprehended by sound alone. The exceptions may be the child's name and *no,* which children seem to recognize out of context. As a result of continued exposure, children learn to reproduce aspects of these sound patterns in contexts in which they occur.

Around the first birthday, children produce their first meaningful word in the presence of the referent or the thing to which the word refers. Generally, first words name favorite toys or foods, family members, or pets. Common first words are *mama, dada, no, bye-bye, cookie,* and *juice.* To learn words, children must make some assumptions, among them that each word refers to a specific referent but can be used with similar referents, that use is consistent and predictable, and that different referents have different names.

By 18 months, children usually can produce approximately fifty single words and begin to combine two words in predictable ways. Within a few short months, three- and four-word combinations appear. Accompanying the increases in utterance length and vocabulary is a decrease in the use of jargon and babbling, although the child continues to use both.

USE   People who are unfamiliar with young children's language often think that children either imitate all first words or use them only to name. In fact, single words are used to make requests, comments, and inquiries. A child may use a single word to signal a variety of purposes by altering the word's pitch contour or accompanying it with a gesture.

Words are acquired first within the intentions that the child is able to express in previously acquired gestures. Several early intentions are presented in Table 4.2. Note all the uses or intentions expressed in the conversation presented in Box 4.1 on page 99.

T H O U G H T   Q U E S T I O N

Try altering a word's purpose or intention by changing the pitch contour and the gesture. Say the word "cookie" as a statement, as a question, and as a demand. A question has a rising intonation, implying "Is this a cookie?" A demand might employ a reach and a whining or insistent intonation. Intent can easily be inferred from these behaviors.

CONTENT AND FORM   The second year is one of vocabulary growth and word combinations. Vocabulary growth is slow for the first few months,

TABLE 4.2

Examples of early intentions of children

Intention	Example
Wanting demand	Says the name of the desired item with an insistent voice. Often accompanied by a reaching gesture.
Protesting	Says "No" or the name of the item while pushing it away, turning away, and/or making a frowning face.
Content questioning	Asks "What?," "That?," or "Wassat?" while pointing and/or looking at an item.
Verbal accompaniment	Speech accompanies some action, such as "whee-e-e" when swung or "Uh-oh" when something spills.
Greeting/farewell	Waves hi or bye with accompanying words.

Note: A fuller list can be found in Owens (2001).

when toddlers may be concentrating on refining their walking. After that, vocabulary increases rapidly. By age 2, the toddler has an expressive vocabulary of about 150–300 words.

Adult and toddler definitions are very different, toddler definitions being based almost exclusively on experience while adult ones are based more on meanings shared with others.

Each toddler has his or her own **lexicon,** or personal dictionary, with words that reflect that child's environment. In general, toddlers' definitions, based on each child's limited experience, are not the same as those of adults. Much toddler speech consists of single words, jargon, or a combination of the two. Phrases that adults frequently use in the child's environment may be repeated as single words. For example, many children say "Wassat?" and "Go-bye" as some of their first "words."

Early word combinations follow predictable word-order patterns based on semantic categories into which words are placed. For example, *agents,* which cause action, are placed before the *action,* which in turn precedes *objects,* which receive action. As a result, we hear *Daddy eat* and *Mommy throw,* plus *Eat cookie* and *Throw ball,* but only rarely the reverse, such as *Cookie eat.* Other common utterances are *More cookie, Big doggie, No night-night,* and so on. Within a few months, short-term memory has increased, so the child can attempt a few longer constructions such as *Daddy eat cookie* or *Throw ball me.* Children

BOX 4.1

Example of Toddler Language

Stacy and her mother are coloring and talking while they do. Note that the language concerns the task. Stacy's mom keeps her utterances short and cues Stacy to respond by asking questions. Stacy participates by talking about the task, often incorporating part of the previous utterance into her own.

Mom: What are you making?
Stacy: Doggie.
Mom: Are you making a doggie? Oh, that's nice, Stacy.
Stacy: Where more doggie?
Mom: Is there another doggie underneath?
Stacy: Yeah.
Mom: Where? Can you find the picture? Is that what you're looking for, the picture of the doggie? Where's a doggie?
Stacy: A doggie. Color a doggie.

Mom: Okay, you color the doggie.
Stacy: Mommy color crayon.
Mom: Mommy has crayons. Mommy's coloring. What's mommy making?
Stacy: Doggie.
Mom: A doggie.
Stacy: Okay.
Mom: All right, I'll make a doggie. Is this the doggie's tail?
Stacy: Doggie's tail. More.
Mom: More doggie?
Stacy: Okay.
Mom: Can Stacy color? Hum?
Stacy: More doggie there. More doggie daddy.
Mom: More doggie daddy?
Stacy: Want a more doggie. More doggie. Put more doggie there.
Mom: Okay, you color the doggie on this page. What color's your doggie?
Stacy: Blue. Color this page, mommy.

use strategies that simplify adult forms into the more truncated forms just described.

Caregivers can have a direct effect on the amount of toddler talking. Behavior control strategies, commands, and directives are associated with low toddler productivity, while conversational strategies, such as asking questions and asking for clarification, are associated with more toddler talking and more complex child utterances (Girolametto, Weitzman, van Lieshout, & Duff, 2000).

When faced with a difficult word, children adopt similar strategies. Armed with the consonant-vowel (CV) structures of babbling and the CV-CV-CV strings of reduplicated babbling, children attempt to pronounce the adult words they encounter. It is not surprising, therefore, that many words are reduced to variations of a CV structure or other simplification. These adaptations, called phonological processes, are presented in Table 4.3.

TABLE 4.3

Phonological processes of young children

Process	Explanation	Example
Deletion of final consonant	Reduces CVC structure to more familiar CV	*Cat* becomes *ca* (/ka/) *Carrot* becomes *cara* (/kara/) CVCVC → CVCV
Deletion of unstressed syllable	Reduces number of syllables to conform to the child's ability to produce multisyllable words	*Telephone* becomes *tephone* (/tefon/) *Vacation* becomes *cation* (/kaʃən/)
Reduplication	Syllables in multisyllable words repeat	*Baby* becomes *bebe* (/bibi/) *Mommy* becomes *mama*
Reduction of consonant clusters	Reduces CCV+ structures to the more familiar CV	*Tree* becomes *te* *Stay* becomes *tay*
Assimilation	One consonant becomes like another, although the vowel is usually not affected	*Doggie* becomes *goggie* /gɔgi/
Substitution	One group of difficult sounds, such as fricatives (/f/, /v/, /s/, /z/, and others) are replaced by easier sounds, such as stops (/b/, /p/, /d/, /t/, /g/, /k/)	*Face* becomes *pace* *This* becomes *dis*

Toddlers often omit final consonants, resulting in a CVC word being produced as CV, as in *cake* pronounced as *ca*. It is also possible that children will add an additional vowel to form the CV-CV *cake-a*. Multisyllable words may be reduced to one or two syllables, or the syllables may be repeated. For example, *telephone* might become *tephone*, and *baby* might be modified to *beebee*. If the syllables are not duplicated, only the consonants may be, as in *doggie* becoming *goggie*. Consonant blends might be shortened to single consonants, as in *stop* becoming *top*. Finally, one type of sound might be substituted for another. For example, all initial consonants in words might be pronounced as the same consonant, as in, *Go bye-bye* becoming *Bo bye-bye.*

Not all children will demonstrate all of these phonological patterns. The number and length of time each is used will vary greatly. Children with chronic ear infections or those with perceptual difficulties, such as LD, may experience problems when attempting to reproduce the sound patterns in words heard in the environment. They may develop multiple phonological processes that they continue to use into the preschool years. This is described further in Chapter 10, "Disorders of Articulation and Phonology."

T H O U G H T   Q U E S T I O N

Take a three- or four-syllable word and apply several phonological patterns. Note how the word may be altered beyond recognition. Is it any wonder that you might have some difficulty understanding some young speakers?

PRESCHOOLERS

Three-year-olds are relatively independent and capable of many self-help skills, such as dressing themselves. They love to explore and to take things apart.

Very social beings, 4-year-olds have the linguistic skills and the short-term memory to be good, albeit limited, conversationalists. Four-year-olds are curious and very anxious to exhibit their knowledge and abilities. Socially, most 4-year-olds play well in groups and cooperate effectively with others. Although there is still a lot of object play, role play becomes increasingly frequent.

COMMUNICATION

Preschool children's primary means of communication are speech and language. Most communication still occurs within the framework of conversations with caregivers. With increased memory, children expand their conversational skills to include recounting the past and remembering short stories. This memory and recall are aided by the child's increased language skills. Preschool children communicate well within and about familiar environments.

LANGUAGE

Preschool language learning is not a passive process. From interaction with others, children form hypotheses about the rules of language and use these hypotheses to produce ever more complex language. Caregivers in each child's environment provide feedback on the child's

Language rule learning is a lengthy process that involves hypothesis testing and refinement.

attempts and models for further growth. Through this process of further and further refinement, children's language increasingly reflects that used in their environment.

Many interrelated variables, such as maternal education level and socioeconomic status (SES) affect the child's language development. Maternal education is positively correlated with longer, more complex child speech and the production of more and different words (Dollaghan, Campbell, et al., 1999). Within African American families, middle-class mothers include more language in their play with the child and use a wider range of words than do lower-class mothers (Scheffner Hammer & Weiss, 1999).

The process of language rule hypothesis building is evident in constructions such as *eated* and *goed* that are not found in adult speech but represent a rule in English: Verbs are made past tense by adding *-ed.* Some children and adults with severe MR may have very limited ability to hypothesize about language rules inferred from the language they hear. Children with LD may be unable to perceive the subtle difference of adding a bound morpheme, such as *-ed,* to change word meaning.

Language becomes a tool for exploring the world much as physical exploration was used previously. As a result, the typical 4-year-old is full of questions. In the process of exploration, each child's language is refined and modified.

USE   Within conversations with caregivers, preschool children introduce topics and maintain these topics for an average of two to three turns before introducing another one. On-topic turn taking is complex and requires speakers to consider the other speaker's turn while formulating a relevant comment on the same topic. It is often easier for preschool children to introduce a new topic, as in the following example:

> *Child:* I got a new bike.
> *Partner:* What color is it?
> *Child:* Red.
> *Partner:* Was the weather nice enough to ride it on your birthday?
> *Child:* Mommy saw a spider.

Within conversations, maturing preschool children begin to consider the speaker's perspective in the use of words such as *here, there, this,* and *that;* the listener's need to know certain information and the amount of information needed; and the need to change conversational style when speaking to younger children. A typical preschool conversation is presented in Box 4.2. Another example is presented on the accompanying CD-ROM.

Style of talking is also reflected in role playing and narration or storytelling. The ability to carry a role through story play is reflected in the narratives of 4-year-olds. These children can tell simple sequential stories of their own or others' authorship.

BOX 4.2

Example of Preschool Language

G and B are young 4-year-olds. They are playing with firefighter hats, dishes, and dolls. Notice how different this sample is from the toddler language in Box 4.1. Each child supports her portion of the conversation. The syntax seems adultlike, but the content is pure preschool. The rapid change of topics gives this sample a nonsensical quality. With no adult to maintain a cohesive topic structure, this is a free-for-all with only one or two turns on each topic before it shifts.

G: And I gonna wear both of these.
B: At the same time? No, I'm wearing this one.
G: I'm wearing this one.
B: And then I do this.
G: You wear this and I'll wear this.
B: Two colored cups. You drink out of this one. I drink out of the big one. I'm putting the box up there.
G: Okay, I will. I have this and you have this.
B: Stay up there.
G: She doesn't look too happy.

B: Uh-oh. Why did I spill it?
G: Mine will only stand.
B: Mine sat.
G: All done with supper. What kind of spoon is this?
B: A plastic one, what else? Now it's time for me to make my own dinner.
G: Time for me too. I have to use this. My baby has to go to bed now. We have to first change their diapers.
B: No we don't.
G: Come here, look.
B: There's a button. I want something to drink.
G: Okay, I'll give you some. Look at this. Watch this. I'm gonna try and make this stand. Do you think this is a girl or a boy?
B: A boy.
G: Oh, cause the boy has the pants on and the girl has the dress on.
B: Happy birthday to you.
G: Grab everythin' up. I'm grabbing most of the doll stuff.

CONTENT   From a few words at age 1, children's expressive vocabularies grow to approximately 300 words by age 2, then mushroom to 900 and 1,500 at ages 3 and 4, respectively. Children may comprehend two or three times that many words in context.

Words are learned quickly through a process called **fast mapping** in which the child infers the meaning from context and uses the word in a similar manner. Fuller definitions evolve over time. It is easier to fast map words with fewer morphological variations (Bedore & Leonard, 2000).

In addition to single words, preschool children acquire some relational words and phrases that are used to join other words and create longer units of language. Categories of relational words include locational terms such as *in*, *on*, and *under*; temporal terms such as *first* and *last*; quantitative terms such as *more than*; qualitative terms such as *bigger than*; and familial terms such as *brother*.

Word order is still the predominant strategy for determining meaning. Even 4-year-olds ignore words such as *before* and *after*, instead relying on word order for interpretation of temporal information. For example, the 4-year-old interprets the following sentences to mean the same:

Go home after you eat.

Go home before you eat.

The order-of-mention strategy results in the interpretation *Go home, then eat* for both.

Conjunctions such as *and* and *then* may be used to join whole sentences together, resulting in those long run-on sentences that only a preschooler could love:

We saw a Grinch movie on television and he made his dog pull the sled and he stoled all the toys and he took the little—What was her name, mom?—yeah, little Who girl's candy cane, and then he went up the mountain again and the people started singing and his heart got exploded and he brought back all the toys and he was nice.

Other conjunctions used by the end of preschool but only rarely to join sentences are *if*, *so*, *but*, and *because*. These words may be used alone or to begin an utterance, as in the following:

Partner: Why are you doing that?
Child: 'Cause I want to.
Partner: You'll get into trouble.
Child: So?

In part, semantic development reflects cognitive development. Four-year-olds demonstrate categorization skills that seem to indicate more advanced procedures for storage of learned information than are seen in younger children. They can name the primary colors and label some coins. Although they can count to five by rote, 4-year-olds have no notion of quantity beyond three.

FORM During the preschool years, the emphasis in language development shifts from semantics and pragmatics, or development of intentions, to language form. The resultant changes in language form are very dramatic.

Syntax and Morphology. Beginning with short, two- to four-word sentences at age 2, children acquire 90 percent of adult syntax by age 5. For the English-speaking preschooler, language becomes more complex as it becomes longer. This relationship can be measured, and we can describe children's language development by calculating the average or **mean length of utterance (MLU)** in morphemes. The calculation of MLU will be discussed in Chapter 6, "Childhood Language Impairments." Some MLU values are presented in Table 4.1.

The simple word-order rules found in the utterances of 18- to 24-month-olds form the basis for a more elaborate grammar, and by age 3, most children's utterances contain both a subject and a verb. This basic structure is elaborated with the addition of articles, adjectives, auxiliary verbs, prepositions, pronouns, and adverbs. Nouns usually have no more than an article and one preceding element, as in *the big doggie.*

In addition, adultlike negative, interrogative, and imperative sentence forms evolve. For example, the toddler negative consisting of a Negative + X form, as in *No cookie, No ni-night,* and *No daddy go bye-bye,* is modified by words such as *no, not, can't, don't,* and *won't* being placed between the subject and verb, as in *Doggie no eat* and *Mommy can't catch me,* to which other negatives such as *wouldn't, couldn't, is not,* and *isn't* are added later.

Similarly, interrogatives or questions go from single words, such as *Doggie?* and *What?* or *Wassat?,* to more complex questions that ask *what* and *where,* followed developmentally by *who, which* and *whose,* and finally *when, why* and *how,* and a more mature form in which the verb and subject or the auxiliary verb and subject are reversed, as in *Are you happy?* and *When are we going to go?,* respectively.

By the end of preschool, children are joining two or more sentences or independent clauses together to form compound sentences, such as the run-on sentence example above. Late preschoolers can also attach dependent clauses to independent clauses to form complex sentences such as *I didn't liked the big dog that barked at grandpa last night.* These structures appear infrequently and will develop slowly and be refined throughout the school-age years.

Several bound morphemes are added during the preschool years. These include the present progressive verb ending *-ing,* as in *running* and *jumping;* plural *-s,* as in *dogs* and *cats;* possessive *-'s* (or *-s'*), as in *mommy's* and *babies';* and the past tense verb ending *-ed,* as in *walked* and *talked.* Often a more obvious or simpler form such as word order is used before mastery of the morphological ending. For example, children may use word order to mark possession, as in *Mommy sock* before children develop the possessive *-'s* to form *Mommy's sock.*

As might be expected, it takes children some time to acquire the use of these morphemes, and it is not uncommon to hear words such

Adultlike forms of many sentences evolve during the preschool years.

as *eated*, *goed*, *sheeps*, and *foots*. Some morphological development is complicated by phonological rule acquisition. For example, we say *dogs* (/z/), *cats* (/s/), and *bridges* (/ɪz/). The concept of plural is simple, but the phonological rule is somewhat more complicated. Two samples of the speech and language of 3-year-olds is presented on the accompanying CD-ROM.

T H O U G H T   Q U E S T I O N

Let's be fair about this. You're a mature speaker, and you don't make mistakes with the plural ending. Can you figure out the three rules for the plural ending well enough to state them? It's not easy.

Phonology Most of the phonological processes described for toddlers have disappeared by age 4. Consonant blends consisting of two or more adjacent consonants, as in *strong*, continue to be difficult for some children, and simplification strategies, resulting in *tong*, may continue into early elementary school. Children who experience continuing phonological difficulties may persist in the use of more immature phonological processes. These are discussed in Chapter 10.

SPEECH

Development of individual sounds is dependent on the location in words, frequency of use, and the influence of other speech sounds.

Children continue to master new speech sounds throughout the preschool period. The acquisition process is a gradual one and depends on the individual sound, its location in words, its frequency of use, and its proximity to other speech sounds. A sound may be produced correctly in single words but not in connected speech. Mastery is considered to be the point at which 90 percent of children are producing the sound correctly 90 percent of the time.

We can make a few generalizations about the speech sound acquisition by young children:

1. Phoneme acquisition is a gradual process.
2. Vowels are easier to master than consonants. Usually, English vowels are acquired by age 3, while some consonants may not be mastered until age 7 or 8.
3. Many sounds are first acquired in the initial position in words.
4. Consonant clusters (*cons*ider) and blends (*str*eet) are not mastered until age 7 or 8, although some clusters appear as early as age 4.
5. Some sounds are easier than others and are acquired first by most children. As a group, stops (/p, b, t, d, g, k/) and nasals (/m, n, ŋ/) are acquired first.
6. Much individual difference exists.

By age 3, most children have mastered vowel sounds and the consonants /p/, /m/, /h/, /n/, /w/, /b/, /k/, /g/, and /d/. Most 4-year-olds have added /t/, /f/, and /j/. In addition, at least 50 percent of all 4-year-olds can produce /r/, /l/, /s/, /tʃ/, /ʃ/, and /z/. This information is presented visually in Table 4.4. Children with neuromuscular problems, sensory deficits, perceptual problems, or poor learning skills are going to have difficulty acquiring all the sounds of the language.

SCHOOL-AGE CHILDREN AND ADOLESCENTS

When children begin to attend school, they start the long process of establishing their identity independent of their family. New friendships and social groupings are found, and most communication occurs in conversations outside the home. In part, the status of adolescents within their own social grouping is determined by communication skills. The child with a language problem, an inappropriate voice pitch, or disfluent speech may be unpopular and unhappy.

Brain maturation slows but continues and with it the child's ability to think, adapt, and solve problems. Concrete thought gives way to abstract thinking. Even so, some anatomical areas of higher brain function, such as the left temporal cortex used in language encoding and decoding, must wait until early adulthood before they are finally mature.

TABLE 4.4

Mastery of English speech sounds

Ages by which most children have acquired speech sounds in all positions. Vowels are not included because they are usually mastered by age 2–3 years.

Age 2	p, h, n, b, k
Age 3	m, w, g, f, d
Age 4	t, ʃ ("sh"), j ("y")
Age 5	s, v, ŋ("ng"), r, l, tʃ ("ch"), z, dʒ ("j")
Age 6	θ ("th" in "thin"), ð ("th" in "the"), ʒ ("zh" in "measure")
Age 8	Consonant blends and clusters

Sources: Compiled from Olmsted (1971); Prather, Hedrick, & Kern (1975); and Sanders (1972).

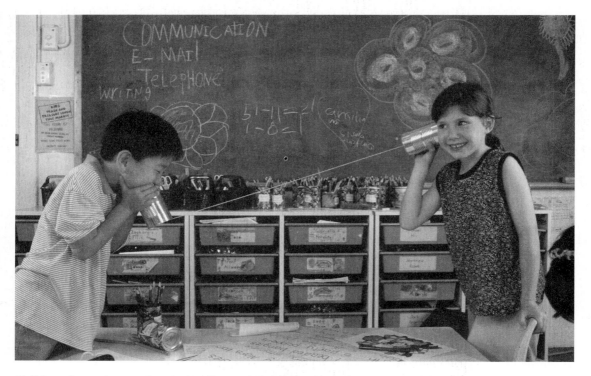

Children learn to use language through interactions
with many individuals and in varying situations.

Physical development finalizes in the adult as trunk and limbs
lengthen. Some final fine motor skills, such as finger movement, continue to improve.

COMMUNICATION

The means of communication change in school as children learn to read
and write. In turn, this skill enables children to use computers and
opens a whole new world of information. Reading and writing are first
introduced within interactions of children and caregivers. Gradually,
children come to realize that it is the written symbols on the page, not
the pictures, that contain the verbal information. This realization is
reflected in their own drawing, to which they may begin to add words
following their own creative spelling of those words. See samples of
early "writing" on the website.

Formal school-based reading and writing training removes language
from the conversational context and thus requires the child to consider

language in the abstract. It is not surprising, therefore, that reading, writing, and metalinguistic skills seem to be related. **Metalinguistic skills** enable the child to consider language in the abstract, to make judgments about its correctness, and to create verbal contexts, such as in writing. Younger children are unable to make such judgments, especially without a supporting nonlinguistic context.

Children with poor oral language skills will most likely have difficulty with visual language. Five kindergarten variables predict reading success by second grade: letter identification, oral sentence imitation, phonological awareness, rapid oral naming, and the mother's education level (Catts, Fey, Zhang, & Tomblin, 2001).

T H O U G H T   Q U E S T I O N

Does the possibility of difficulty reading in school justify early intervention with preschool children who have slow language development? When should we become concerned?

Conversation continues to be the primary locus of communication. Through interactions with many different conversational partners, children and adolescents learn to be more effective and efficient communicators.

Adolescents consolidate their self and personal identity through multi-tiered peer relationships and restructured family interactions. Slang is used within the peer group to distinguish adolescents from both children and adults. Communication is important as adolescents attempt to gain more freedom from and more equality within the family. The equality of the peer group aids in this transition at the same time that the lessons of family relationships form a basis for the deepening relationships with peers (Whitmire, 2000).

LANGUAGE

Five-year-olds use very adultlike language form, although many of the more subtle syntactic structures are missing. In addition, these children have not acquired some of the pragmatic skills that are needed to be truly effective communicators. Still, their language abilities are formidable. They can use language to converse and to entertain, to tell stories, to demonstrate their budding sense of humor, to tease, and to discuss emotions.

Over the next few years, language development slows and begins to stabilize, but it will be nonetheless significant. By age 12, children have many of the cognitive and linguistic skills of adults. Language development does not stop, however, and many complex forms and subtle linguistic uses are learned in the adolescent period. The preschool emphasis on development of language form becomes less prominent, and semantic and pragmatic development blossoms.

Even with the development of writing, conversation is still the predominant use for language.

USE During the early school-age years, children's language use changes in two ways: Conversational skills continue to develop, and narratives expand and gain all the elements of mature storytelling. Children refine their conversational skills to become truly effective communicators. They learn effective ways to introduce new topics and, once begun, to continue and to end conversations smoothly and appropriately. By age 9, the number of turns on a topic expands beyond the two or three seen in preschool conversation. While in a conversation, they make relevant comments and adapt their roles and moods to fit the situation. In addition, school-age children learn to make even more and increasingly subtle assumptions about the level of knowledge of their listeners and to adjust their conversations accordingly. This communication development reflects children's growing appreciation for the perspectives of others.

Adolescents spend increasing amounts of time socializing with peers (Raffaelli & Duckett, 1989). Peer support is an important source of information, emotional support, and personal well-being. Within these conversation, teens demonstrate more affect and discuss topics infrequently mentioned at home. The number of turns on a topic increases greatly and topic shifts become less abrupt. Although interrupting increases, it has evolved into behaviors, such as asking pertinent questions, that serve to move the topic along (Larson & McKinley, 1998).

Narratives, both in conversation and in writing, gain the elements needed in our culture to be considered satisfying. English literate narratives contain an introductory setting statement and a challenge or challenges that the characters overcome after their initial reaction by planning a course of action and acting upon that plan to some conclusion. Events are organized both sequentially and by cause and effect. Compare this organization to the Grinch narrative of the 4-year-old mentioned previously.

CONTENT Vocabulary continues to grow but number of words is only the most superficial measure of semantic change. The vocabulary of 5-year-olds grows to about 2,200 words, although word definitions still lack the fullness of adult meanings. First graders have an expressive vocabulary of approximately 2,600 words but may understand as many as 8,000 root English words and possibly 14,000 when various derivations are included. Aided in school, this receptive vocabulary expands to approximately 50,000 words by sixth grade and to 80,000 words by high school. Multiple word meanings are also acquired.

Definitions become more dictionary-like, which means that they become less experiential or less based on individual experience, more shared, categorical, as in *An apple is a kind of fruit*, and more precise. The increasing size of children's vocabularies requires more precision and an organization into categories for easy retrieval.

Categorical organization enables language users to be more efficient and more flexible as demonstrated by the development of divergent and convergent language abilities. *Divergent semantic abilities* enable the production of a great variety of words, word associations, phrases, and sentences from a given topic. For example, the words *dog* and *cat* are associated as house pets and mammals but also figuratively, as in *raining cats and dogs*. In addition, *dog* can be an adjective, as in *dog days of summer* or *dog tired*, or a verb, as in *he dogged my footsteps*. Divergent abilities add originality, flexibility, and creativity to language. *Convergent semantic abilities* enable selection of a unique semantic unit given specific linguistic restrictions. For example, there are only a few words that can complete the sentence "The opposite of *large* is _____."

Finally, school-age children also learn to understand and use **figurative language** consisting of idioms, metaphors, similes, and proverbs. Unlike literal meanings, figurative language does not always mean what it seems to mean. *Idioms* are expressions that often cannot be justified literally, such as "hit the road" or "off the wall." *Metaphors* and *similes* offer implied comparisons, such as "I have butterflies in my stomach" and "That elephant is as big as a house," respectively. *Proverbs* offer advice that is not intended to be taken literally. For example, "Don't put all your eggs in one basket" concerns caution in planning for the future, not advice for chicken farmers. Figurative language enriches communication but requires higher language functions of interpretion. Use of figurative language generally does not begin until the child attends school. Some forms are not comprehended until adulthood. Learning appears to be related to familiarity and to reading and listening comprehension (Nippold, Moran, & Schwarz, 2001). Children with MR, LD, or traumatic brain injury may be very concrete in their interpretation and have great difficulty with figurative language.

FORM   Following the rapid development of language form in preschool, there is a gradual slowing, although development continues at this lesser pace. Many forms will continue to develop into adolescence. Oral language and written language forms differ somewhat, and forms that are used in one, such as the use of fillers—*ah-h, um-m, ya know*—and the substitution of /n/ for /ŋ/ in speech, as in *runnin'*, are used orally but not in writing. Initially, children's speech is much more complex than their writing, but the relationship reverses permanently for most of us in late elementary school.

If mastery of language form is a slow process during the school years, when do we decide that a child is having enough difficulty to require therapeutic intervention?

Syntax and morphology. By age 5, children use most verb tenses, such as regular and irregular past tenses of common verbs, the future tense *will*, and other auxiliary verbs, such as *would, should, must,* and *might,* although they still have some difficulty with multiple auxiliary verbs, as in *should have been;* possessive pronouns (*his, her, your*); the conjunctions *and, but, if, because, when,* and *so;* and the past tense of the verb *to be* (*was* and *were*). Five-year-old children also have limited use of the comparative *-er,* as in *bigger,* and superlative *-est,* as in *biggest;* relative pronouns used in complex sentences (I know *who* lives next door); gerunds (We go *fishing*); and infinitives (I want *to eat* now).

Many syntactic structures appear slowly, and many children struggle with acquisition well into the school years. During the school years, children gradually add passive sentences, such as *The cat is chased by the dog,* in which the entity performing the action is placed at the end rather than the beginning of the sentence; reflexive pronouns, such as *myself, yourself, himself,* and *themselves;* conjunctions, such as *although* and *however;* variations of compound and complex sentences; and conversational devices, such as *on the other hand, in contrast, well,* and *relative to that,* that are used to tie utterances together. Gradually, school-age children begin to comprehend sentences as a whole and no longer depend solely on word order for interpretation.

It frequently takes the child several years of practice to gain complete control of these linguistic structures. Children from stimulation-poor environments may take even longer.

As might be expected, children with perceptual problems, as in LD, frequently miss subtle differences of meaning. Children with neuromuscular difficulties may have difficulties making the oral movements to produce the *bigger-biggest* contrast.

Morphological development focuses on derivational suffixes—word endings that change the word class, such as adding *-er* to a verb to make a noun, as in *paint/painter*—and prefixes. By second and third grades, children attain accurate use of the rules for noun (*-er*) and adverb derivation (*-ly*). Other derivational morphemes include *-ist,* used to change the verb *cycle* to the noun *cyclist; -ful,* used to change the noun *joy* to the adjective *joyful;* and *-able,* used to change the verb *rely* to the adjective *reliable.* Development of prefixes, such as *un-, ir-,* and *dis-* will continue into adulthood.

Phonology By early elementary school, most children's phonological system resembles that of adults. A few children will still have difficulty with multiple consonant blends, such as *str* and *sts*, as in *str*eet and bea*sts*, respectively.

Other developments such as **morphophonemic** contrasts—changes in pronunciation as a result of morphological changes—will take several years to master, some extending into adulthood. For example, in the verb *derive*, the second vowel is a long "i," transcribed phonetically as /aɪ/. When we change *derive* to the noun *derivative*, the second vowel is changed to sound like the "i" in *give*, transcribed as /ɪ/. Other contrasts, mentioned in Chapter 2, include changes in emphasis and more subtle changes in pronunciation, as in the verb re*cord* and the noun *rec*ord. Although there are phonological rules to be derived from speech, many of these contrasts are learned word by word.

SPEECH

Most 5-year-olds can correctly articulate the /p/, /m/, /ŋ/, /n/, /w/, /b/, /k/, /g/, /d/, /t/, /h/, /f/, /j/, /r/, /l/, /s/, /ʧ/, /ʃ/, /z/, /dʒ/, and /v/ consonant sounds. At least 50 percent can produce the "th" in "*th*ere" sound /ð/ correctly (Table 4.4). Five-year-olds still have difficulty with a few consonant sounds and with consonant blends. Six-year-olds have acquired most English speech sounds, adding the /θ/ and /ʒ/ sounds, as in *th*in and trea*s*ure. By age 8, children have acquired consonant blends, such as *str*, *sl*, and *dr*.

ADULTS

By adulthood, speech and language have matured and adults are able to communicate in a variety of modes, using not only speech and language, but paralinguistic and nonlinguistic signals effectively. A subtle pause or shift in word emphasis can signal vast differences of meaning in speech. With the advent of computers, reading and writing have been re-established as essential communication tools.

COMMUNICATION

Unless debilitated in some way through accident, disease, or disorder, adults continue to refine their communication abilities throughout their lives. Writing and speaking abilities continue to improve with use, new words are added to vocabularies, and new styles of talking are acquired. Some communication disorders of childhood, such as those from cleft palate, cerebral palsy, and stuttering, may persist into adulthood and require continuing intervention services.

Language and communication should continue to develop throughout one's life.

LANGUAGE

Language development proceeds slowly throughout adulthood. Even people with delayed development, such as individuals with MR experience continued but slowed language growth.

USE   Through the use of various communication techniques, competent adults can influence others, impart information, and make their needs known. Some adults are even capable of oratory on a par with that of a Winston Churchill or a Martin Luther King that can call up the heroic and the unselfish in others.

Compared to children, adults are very effective communicators and skilled conversationalists who have a variety of styles of talking from formal to casual adapted from their many roles at work and home. Styles require modification not only in the manner of talking, but also in the topics introduced and the vocabulary used. As the Little Prince noted when talking with adults (Saint-Exupéry, 1968):

> I would never talk . . . about boa constrictors, or primeval forests, or stars. I would bring myself down to his level. I would talk . . . about bridge, and golf, and politics, and neckties. And the grown-up would be greatly pleased to have met such a sensible man.

Competent adult communicators quickly sense their role in an interaction and adjust their language and speech accordingly. For example, some people are addressed as *sir* and some as *honey*, and adults do well not to confuse the two. It might be inappropriate to address even a loved one as *honey* in certain formal situations. Communication may vary from direct, as in *Turn up the heat*, to indirect, as in *Do you feel a chill?* The goal is the same, but the linguistic methodology is very different.

The number of communicative intentions increases gradually so that adults are able to hypothesize, to cajole, to inspire, to entice, to pun, and so on. The skilled speaker knows how to fulfill these intentions and when to use them. For example, puns and jokes are inappropriate at a funeral. Likewise, analyzing and reanalyzing a decision long after it has been made is annoying to others.

Adult language use is extremely flexible because of the variety of language forms, the large size of the vocabulary, and the breadth of language uses.

CONTENT   Adults continue to add to their personal vocabularies and most use between 30,000 and 60,000 words expressively. Receptive vocabularies are even larger. Specialized vocabularies develop for work, religion, hobbies, and social and interest groups. Some words fade from the language and are used less frequently while new words are added. For example, you no longer *dial* a telephone number. Multiple definitions and figurative meanings are also expanded.

FORM   Within language form, adults continue to acquire prefixes, morphophonemic contrasts, and infrequently used irregular verbs. Language units become more cohesive through more effective use of linguistic devices, such as pronouns, articles, verb tenses, and aspect (which, for example, allows us to talk about the past from the vantage point of the future, as in *Tomorrow, I'll look back and say "That was a great picnic"*). In general, written language continues to be more complex than spoken language.

T H O U G H T   Q U E S T I O N S

Are there more things to learn about language form as an adult? Try some of these. Can you state the past tense of the verbs "lay" and "lie"? What is the difference between "effect" and "affect"? Do "uninterested" and "disinterested" mean the same thing?

SPEECH

Speech sound acquisition is completed long before adulthood, and efficient speech sound production should continue throughout life. However, cerebrovascular accident or stroke, uncontrollable voice, pitch, or rate changes as a result of illness, or a brain trauma from a motorcycle accident may result in a loss of efficient speaking ability.

SUMMARY

The development of speech, language, and communication is very complex. Together, they pose the most difficult learning task faced by humans. Nevertheless, most of us become effective in all three. Initial sounds, nurtured by the environment, mature into words and sentences. The early expression of intent through gestures matures into the subtle intentions expressed through sentences. As we mature, grammar becomes more complex and conversations more cohesive. Intonational patterns help mature speakers to convey and interpret meaning.

Newborns are treated as communication partners by their caregivers. Gradually, the child learns to attract attention and begins to realize that he or she can influence others by making sounds or movements. At around 8 months, the child begins to use gestures to signal his or her intent and to look to the communication partner to ensure that he or she is paying attention.

Meanwhile the production of speech sounds is maturing from individual syllables through repetitive syllables to strings of different syllables. As the child gains a realization that adults use consistent sounds to refer to entities, she or he begins to use consistent sound sequences to also refer.

At around age 1, the infant's comprehension, gestural intentions, and consistent speech sound use come together in the production of the first true word recognizable by adults. Within a few months, the child has begun to join words together following simple word-order rules based on semantic categories.

During preschool, language development concentrates on language form. By kindergarten, the child has acquired 90 percent of adult syntax, many morphological endings, and most speech sounds. Language is used in conversations and narration, and the child is capable of initiating, maintaining, and terminating conversations and topics and changing the style of talking for the listener.

School-age and adult years are spent perfecting language form, expanding semantics and pragmatics, and learning and perfecting a new mode of communication: reading and writing. With maturity, the child becomes increasingly flexible in his or her use of language for a variety of communication uses. Vocabulary growth reflects these many uses and the interests, education, and employment of the speaker.

Some of us, because of cognitive, sensory, perceptual, neuromuscular, anatomical and physiological, environmental, and personal difficulties or faulty learning, find language learning and use difficult. You will meet some of these people as we progress through the rest of this book. You are about to enter the fascinating world of communication disorders.

REFLECTIONS

- Can you describe babbling, reduplicated babbling, and variegated babbling?
- What are the major differences between the language of toddlers and preschoolers?
- What generalizations can we make about speech sound development?

- What areas of language development are emphasized in each stage of development? Toddler? Preschooler? School age?
- State some of the major difficulties that individuals may encounter in speech, language, and communication throughout the life span.
- What are some of the changes in language that adults experience?

SUGGESTED READINGS

Hulit, L. M., & Howard, M. R. (1997) *Born to talk: An introduction to speech and language development* (2nd ed.). Boston: Allyn and Bacon.

Nippold, M. A. (Ed.). (1998). *Later language development: The school-age and adolescent years* (2nd ed.). Austin, TX: Pro-Ed.

Owens, R. E. (2001) *Language development: An introduction* (5th ed.). Boston: Allyn and Bacon.

ON-LINE RESOURCES

http://poppy.psy.cmu.edu/childes/   International Child Language Data Exchange System.

http://atila-www.uia.ac.be/IASCL/Inhoud.html   Association for the Study of Child Languages.

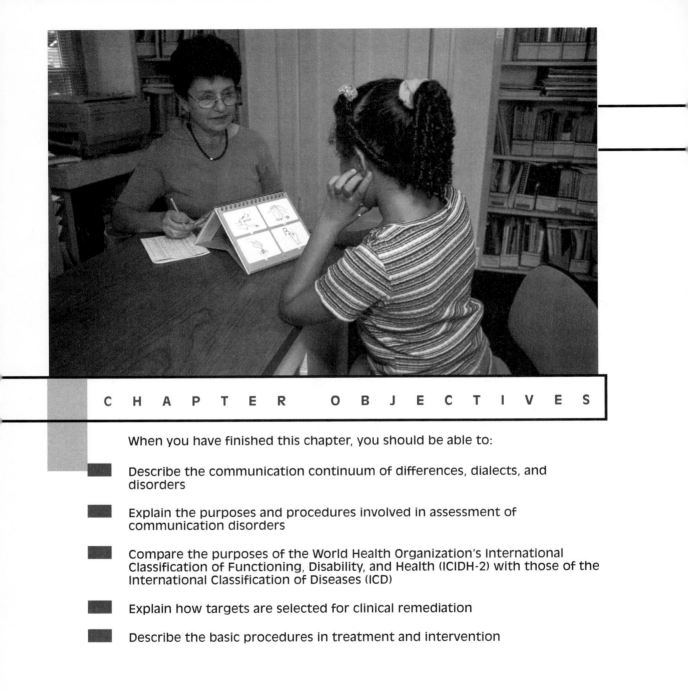

When you have finished this chapter, you should be able to:

Describe the communication continuum of differences, dialects, and disorders

Explain the purposes and procedures involved in assessment of communication disorders

Compare the purposes of the World Health Organization's International Classification of Functioning, Disability, and Health (ICIDH-2) with those of the International Classification of Diseases (ICD)

Explain how targets are selected for clinical remediation

Describe the basic procedures in treatment and intervention

Assessment and Intervention

The human communication process is remarkable but not flawless. Each of us has experienced frustration at not remembering someone's name or faltering when trying to express ourselves clearly. We also know that sometimes a friend speaks to us, and we don't fully understand what she or he is trying to say. The reverse happens, too, when we know that someone else misinterprets what we say. But when do these often minor annoyances constitute a problem? How do we determine that a communication disorder exists? And how do we categorize its nature?

In this chapter, we provide an overview of assessment procedures. We also examine principles and techniques for assisting people who have communication disorders.

DIFFERENCES, DIALECTS, DISORDERS

Age influences all aspects of communication; however, considerable variation exists within each age group.

We learned in Chapter 2 that communication takes place within a social context. We communicate with other people. Our own culture and that of others influence the nature and success of this interaction. Ordered and disordered communication can be described only within cultural standards. It is obvious that the communication skills of a 4-year-old generally will be less sophisticated than those of a 12-year-old. Age, therefore, is one determiner of communicative proficiency. But factors such as gender, ethnicity, geographical region, language background, and socioeconomic status also contribute to the ways in which we communicate. The speech-language pathologist must recognize that variety is typical, and she or he must be able to distinguish differences from disorders.

A COMMUNICATION CONTINUUM

Everyone in Carol's family, including Carol, speaks rapidly; sometimes their words come out so fast they are hard to understand. Peter comes from a family of slow and deliberate speakers; occasionally, such a long lag time appears between Peter's words that one wonders whether he's going to complete his sentence. Carol and Peter represent different ends of the speech rate continuum. While they are clearly not speakers you might encounter every day, you might wonder whether they are different enough to have disordered speech. To make this determination, consider the following:

1. Does the speaker feel embarrassed or uncomfortable?
2. Do listeners react negatively?
3. Is the intent of the speaker communicated?

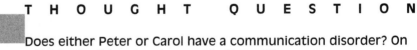

T H O U G H T   Q U E S T I O N

Does either Peter or Carol have a communication disorder? On what basis did you make your judgment?

The World Health Organization developed the International Classification of Impairments, Disabilities, and Handicaps (ICIDH) in 1980. Although the term *Functioning* is now used rather than *Impairments*, the original letters (ICIDH) have been kept. The ICIDH-2 is appropriate not only for individuals with impairments, but also for those who are functioning well.

Even experts do not always agree on what is an acceptable variation and what constitutes a disorder (Yairi & Ambrose, 2001). The World Health Organization (WHO) has developed a health classification system that describes individuals within an array of health and health-related domains. Items are rated on a continuum: no problem, mild problem, moderate problem, severe problem, or complete problem. WHO's International Classification of Functioning, Disability, and Health (ICIDH-2) describes two broad components: (1) body functions and structures and (2) activities and participation. In addition, environmental and personal factors are included because they provide a context for an individual's health status. Figure 5.1 shows an overview of the ICIDH-2 with an example that relates to communication. Unlike the International Classification of Diseases, Tenth Revision (ICD-10),

FIGURE 5.1 An overview of ICIDH-2 (with a communication example).
Adapted from World Health Organization (2001).

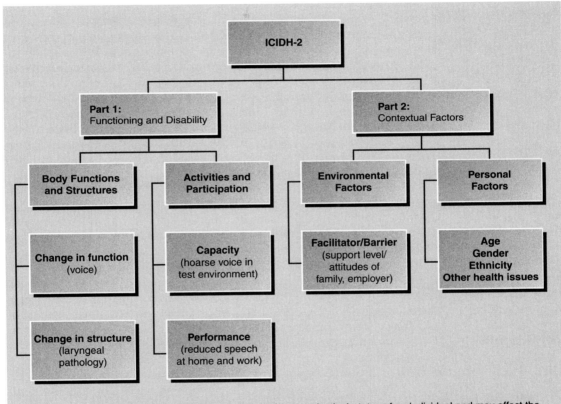

Note 1: All factors interact in determining the health (communication) status of an individual and may affect the outcome of different interventions.

Note 2: All components are quantified using the same scale:

0	NO problem	(none, absent, negligible . . .)
1	MILD problem	(slight, low . . .)
2	MODERATE problem	(medium, fair . . .)
3	SEVERE problem	(high, extreme . . .)
4	COMPLETE problem	(total . . .)

to be discussed a little later in this chapter, the ICIDH-2 does not provide a diagnosis of diseases, disorders, or other health conditions (World Health Organization, 2001).

DIALECTS

Dialects are variations of a language. Whereas languages typically, but not always, represent the political boundaries of a country, dialects usually represent less formal geographical distinctions. We can usually distinguish people from Boston and Dallas by their distinctive ways of speaking. Ethnicity may also result in a dialect. Ebonics, also called African American English or Black English, is an example of this. Foreign language background contributes to dialect, too. Within each region, ethnicity, and language background, additional variations exist. Not all Bostonians or African Americans share a common dialect. Similarly, speakers of Spanish (or French or any language) from different countries and regions are not identical in their communicative patterns. For example, the speech of a person from Quebec is distinct from that of someone from Haiti, which is different from that of a Parisian. Women and men, too, often differ in their manner of communication, giving rise to **genderlect,** or gender-based dialect.

Everyone uses a dialect. People with a dialect that differs from yours do not have a disorder of communication. It is important to recognize that dialects are normal variations; they are not pathological.

Individuals who use a particular dialect belong to the same **speech community** and "share knowledge of the communicative constraints and options governing a significant number of social situations" (Gumperz, 1972, p. 16). Speech communities may differ from one another in specifics of vocabulary, grammar, pronunciation, rate and rhythm of speech, topics of communication, body language, and pragmatic rules.

Pragmatic dialect differences are not always obvious. For example, narrative or storytelling styles of schoolchildren may reflect their ethnic background. If this is not recognized, those who tell stories in a manner that differs from that of the teacher may be considered deficient. European American youngsters, like their elders, tend to build a story to its climax and then provide a resolution. Algonquin and Chinese American children typically develop a story to its high point and then stop. From the European American viewpoint, the Algonquin and Chinese tales may appear incomplete, but to someone from these cultures, this might be seen as a positive technique for leaving the listener in the midst of the story (Crago, Eriks-Brophy, Pesco, & McAlpine, 1997).

T H O U G H T   Q U E S T I O N

What pragmatic differences can you think of that distinguish female genderlect from male genderlect?

In summary, dialects are variations of Standard American English. Although they are not "standard," they should not be considered "substandard" or "wrong." The ICIDH-2 designation for someone with a dialect that differs from the local community would reflect a problem only if this speech pattern impaired participation in this individual's daily life. Table 5.1 highlights a few dialect differences.

TABLE 5.1

A few examples of possible dialect differences

Although features can be identified as characteristic of a particular dialect, you should recognize that each dialect contains variations. For example, Latino English is spoken by people from Spain, Mexico, Puerto Rico, and many parts of South and Central America, and their linguistic patterns are not identical. In addition, individual speakers may use some or none of the features listed below. It must be emphasized that dialects are not "wrong," they are rule-based modifications of the standard. The examples that follow are a small sample of differences based on ethnicity and language background.

SAE = Standard American English, BE = Ebonics, ME = Mandarin English, LE = Latino English.

Grammar

Past tense

(SAE) I talked to her yesterday.
(BE) I talk to her yesterday.
(ME) I talk to her yesterday.
(LE) I talk to her yesterday.

Possession

(SAE) That is Mary's dress.
(BE) That is Mary dress
(ME) That is dress of Mary.
(LE) That is dress of Mary.

Negation

(SAE) She doesn't like him.
(BE) She don't like him.
(ME) She don't no like him.
(LE) She no like him.

Phonology

Substitutions, Omissions

(SAE) "feet" "it"
(BE) "fee-" "i-"
(ME) "fit" "eat"
(LE) "fit" "eat"

Pragmatics

Direct eye contact

(SAE) Sign of respect and that attention is being paid
(BE) Used by speaker but may be considered disrespectful when used by listener
(ME) Generally avoided
(LE) Generally avoided

Laughter/giggling

(SAE) Response to humor
(BE) Sign of friendliness
(ME) Indication of shyness
(LE) Response to humor

Source: Adapted from Owens (2001) and Paul (1995).

In addition to dialect, we must consider **idiolect,** which is an individual's unique way of speaking. Idiolect is based on an interaction of such things as age, education, personality, family, geographical background, and linguistic background. Not everyone in your hometown sounds the same. Some Iowans might "sound" Californian, while others demonstrate a Japanese influence when they speak English. What is more, some people will use one or two aspects of a dialect, such as vocabulary (even just a few words) or grammar, and others will use different aspects such as pronunciation. Many people are bidialectical or multidialectal; they are competent in more than one dialect. They will choose the dialect that is appropriate to the setting and conversational partners.

T H O U G H T   Q U E S T I O N

Do you think someone who speaks with a foreign dialect has a communication disorder? Why? Why not?

DISORDERS

Communication disorders may affect language processing and/or transmission, that is, any aspect of speech, hearing, listening, reading, or writing. The American Speech-Language-Hearing Association (ASHA) defines a communication disorder as "an impairment in the ability to receive, send, process, and comprehend concepts or verbal, nonverbal and graphic symbol systems" (ASHA, 1993, p. 40). The exact nature and degree of impairment will vary from individual to individual. It is the task of the speech-language pathologist or audiologist to describe the problem clearly and identify its extent.

Some clinicians object to the term "disorder," especially when it is used simply to report test results that are below average. They suggest that differences make us distinct as human beings and that we should redirect our attention toward people's strengths (Miller, 1993). While we agree, we also recognize, as do other specialists, that terminology is needed to identify people who are in need of speech, language, or hearing services, and to state that a person has an impairment, disability, or disorder should not carry with it negative stigma. It is important to recognize that an individual with a communication disorder is not a disordered person. We do not label a person as a "stutterer" or a "lisper" but rather "a person who stutters or lisps." The person is primary; the disorder is simply one aspect of the individual.

How do you react to the words "disability," "disorder," "handicap," "impairment," "atypical," and "abnormal"? Are the words loaded? Can you propose a solution to this dilemma? What is your opinion of the concept of so-called politically correct terms such as "communicatively challenged"?

IS THERE A PROBLEM?

Not everyone is assessed for communication disorders. When there is a possibility of a problem, recognition of this precedes formal assessment. Selection for assessment may come from either referral or screening.

REFERRALS

Individuals at any age may be referred from various sources for an evaluation for a communication disorder. An infant in a hospital neonatal intensive care unit who has feeding or other oral difficulties may be referred to the speech-language pathologist (SLP) for evaluation and management of these problems.

A pediatrician may refer a toddler. Sometimes a parent, grandparent, neighbor, or friend observes that a young child is not communicating as well as others of the same age. This person might take appropriate steps so that an assessment will occur. A phone call to an area speech and hearing center, school system, rehabilitation program, or to a clinician in private practice might lead to a formal evaluation of the youngster's hearing and speech.

For children enrolled in a preschool or regular school, it is common for a teacher to express a concern about a child's speech and recommend an assessment by an SLP or audiologist. When a speech-language pathologist is employed by a school system, this person may send an annual notice to teachers asking them to refer youngsters who appear to have communication problems. Often a checksheet helps teachers in making these identifications. Table 5.2 contains a range of behaviors to look for, including aspects of form (e.g., "Difficult to understand"), content (e.g., "Nonspecific vocabulary"), and use (e.g., "Inappropriate responses"). The pioneering work with bilingual children of Damico, Oller, and Storey (1983) contributed guidelines for considering diverse aspects of children's speech.

Specialists in communication disorders may encourage referrals from other professionals and concerned individuals by publicizing the nature of the services that they provide.

TABLE 5.2

Sample teacher checksheet for possible signs of communication problems in preschool and kindergarten children

Dear Teacher,

Your help is requested in identifying children who are at risk for language disorders. Please observe the children in your class and indicate by a check the symptoms noted below. Few children are expected to show *all* of these symptoms. Return forms to me by _____ for those children for whom you are concerned. I will contact parents and the Committee on Special Education to schedule evaluations for those children referred to me.

Thank you.

Jane Jones, M.S., SLP-CCC
Speech-Language Pathologist

Student's Name _____ Date _____ Class _____ Teacher _____

_____ *Short attention span for language-related activities.* Does not sit still to look at a book or listen to a story.

_____ *Relies heavily on imitation.* Creates few original utterances. Basically just repeats what others say.

_____ *Difficult to understand.* Child's speech is not easily intelligible to unfamiliar adults. *Many* sounds are misarticulated/mispronounced.

_____ *Limited social interaction.* Shows little interest in engaging with other children or adults.

_____ *Little interest in using language to learn more about language and the world.* Does not ask "What's that?" or "Why?" questions.

_____ *Limited play.* Does not engage in imaginative symbolic play with other children.

_____ *Problems understanding speech.* Shows difficulty understanding language that is not supported by nonverbal cues.

_____ *Limited expressive language.* Produces few nonimitated or rote utterances that are three words or more in length.

_____ *Linguistic nonfluency.* Disruption of speech production by a high number of repetitions, unusual pauses, and excessive use of fillers such as "um," "er," "uh."

_____ *Nonspecific vocabulary.* Use of expressions such as *this, that, then, he,* or *over there,* without making the referents clear to the listener; also the overuse of all-purpose words such as *thing, stuff, these,* and *those.*

_____ *Delays before responding.* Inordinate pauses following communication attempts initiated by others.

_____ *Poor topic maintenance.* Rapid and inappropriate changes in the topic without providing transitional clues to the listener.

_____ *Revisions.* Breakup of speech production by numerous false starts or self-interruptions; multiple revisions are made as if the child keeps coming to a dead end in a maze.

_____ *Inappropriate responses.* The child's utterances appear to indicate that the child is operating on an independent discourse agenda—not attending to the prompts or probes of the adult or others.

_____ *Voice is harsh or inappropriate.* Speech is too loud or too soft. Voice quality sounds hoarse, strained, or unpleasant.

Source: Adapted from Damico, J.S., Oller, J.W., & Storey, M.E. (1983). The diagnosis of language disorders in bilingual children: Surface-oriented and pragmatic criteria. *Journal of Speech and Hearing Disorders, 48,* 388, and Nelson, N.W. (1998). *Childhood language disorders in context: Infancy through adolescence* (2nd ed.). Boston: Allyn and Bacon, p. 290. Used with permission.

In many schools, the teacher must first notify the Child Study Team (CST), which is usually composed of teachers, the school principal, a reading specialist, a psychologist, and an SLP. If the CST believes that an evaluation is appropriate, it informs the Committee on Special Education (CSE), which then sends a letter to the parents requesting permission to test the child. This procedure can sometimes be shortened if the teacher speaks directly to the SLP, who can then contact the parents and suggest that they write a letter to the CSE requesting testing for their child.

Adults may refer themselves if they feel they have a communication disorder. Sometimes a person might feel handicapped professionally and/or socially because of hearing or speech limitations. Often a family member takes the initiative in seeking help. Frequently, a physician refers an individual who has had an accident or a medical problem such as a stroke.

SCREENING

The legislation in IDEA (see Chapter 1) mandates that *all* children from birth to age 20 be given the opportunity to receive special services if needed. To ensure this, departments of health and welfare and departments of education throughout the country must provide a system for identifying at-risk individuals at no personal expense. Children between the ages of birth and 36 months may be brought to special centers for screening for speech, language, hearing, motor, and other functions. Older children are screened in preschools and schools.

Several states in the United States have passed legislation requiring that hearing screening tests be given to infants at their birthing facility or as soon after birth as possible. Babies who are identified as being at risk for hearing loss are then assessed more fully, and steps toward appropriate intervention are initiated. It is likely that universal infant hearing screening will be soon mandated throughout the United States.

For individuals who are able to respond to simple directions, hearing is usually screened with **pure tones.** The client is presented with tones in the speech frequency range at what is normally a just audible sound level. If the client does not respond to any tone in either ear, more complete testing is recommended. The integrity and health of the tympanic membrane (eardrum), middle ear, and auditory and facial nerves are often screened with **acoustic immittance** testing using a **tympanometer.** A probe tip is held in place in the ear canal, the **compliance,** or mobility, of the membrane is measured, and an ipsilateral acoustic reflex is elicited. These techniques are described in more detail in Chapter 14, "Audiology and Hearing Loss."

Some SLPs devise and use their own speech and language screening test; others use commercially available ones such as the *Fluharty*

Speech and Language Screening Test-2 (Fluharty, 2002) or the *Adolescent Language Screening Test* (Morgan & Guilford, 1984). Table 5.3 is an example of a screening test developed by SLPs who work together in the same school district.

Preschool children, especially those from nonwhite, non-middle-class backgrounds, often do not respond well to formal tests. Test results may not accurately reflect communication ability in real-life situations (see Issues in Screening in the next section of this chapter). To solve this problem, some researchers developed an "authentic assessment approach" to preschool speech-language screening (Schraeder, Quinn, Stockman, & Miller, 1999). Three-year-olds who are determined to be at-risk for communication disorders based on parent interviews, hearing screening, physical evaluation, and other parameters are observed for 45 to 60 minutes during regular preschool activities or during interaction using familiar materials. The clinician uses a checksheet to record the presence of specific language behaviors. Those children who exhibit fewer than 80 percent of the items fail the screening and are referred for a comprehensive evaluation. Although this screening procedure appears to require more time than a formal test, it is considered more accurate and may actually reduce time for the SLP by limiting the number of children who require complete assessments.

ISSUES IN SCREENING

When individuals are screened for any type of problem, four outcomes are possible (see Figure 5.2):

1. Test results suggest a problem, but the person in truth does not have a problem.
2. Test results suggest a problem, and the person actually has one.
3. Test results show no problem, and none exists.
4. Test results show no problem, but the person in truth does have a problem.

Outcome "1" (fails test but has no problem) is called a **false positive** or a **Type 1 error.** Outcome "4"

FIGURE 5.2 Possible outcomes of screening tests

ACTUAL CONDITION

	No Problem	Problem
Fail (problem)	False positive (Type 1 error) *Outcome* 1	True positive *Outcome* 2
Pass (no problem)	True negative *Outcome* 3	False negative (Type 2 error) *Outcome* 4

TEST RESULTS

TABLE 5.3

Clinician-developed speech and language screening test

Student's Name _____   Date _____

Age _____   Grade _____   Pass _____   Refer _____

Comments: _____
_____

Articulation
Errors: _____
Oral-motor: _____
WNL: _____

Auditory Skills
Digit Memory: 4-3-3 _____   5-4-2 _____   7-1-6 _____
                     2-7-3-3 _____   6-3-5-1 _____   8-2-9-3 _____

Wh- Questions: "One night Sally brought pizza to John's house. Sally and John ate the pizza and drank orange soda. They were so full that they couldn't eat the last piece."

Who ate pizza? _____   What did they drink? _____
Where did they eat the pizza? _____
How many pieces were left? _____

Definitions
bird   _____
apple   _____
brown   _____
ice   _____
bed   _____
cow   _____

Informal Language Sample (+ –)

	Simple	Compound
MLU _____	sentences _____	sentences _____
Pragmatics:		
Use _____	Topic maintenance _____	Turn taking _____
Syntax _____		
Semantics: Expressive vocabulary _____		Word finding _____

continued

TABLE 5.3

Clinician-developed speech and language screening test
continued

Concepts (_____ /20 correct)

top	_____	over	_____	side	_____	through	_____
bottom	_____	nearest	_____	first	_____	right	_____
inside	_____	farthest	_____	last	_____	left	_____
around	_____	next to	_____	same	_____	front	_____
under	_____	middle	_____	different	_____	back	_____

Voice
WNL* _____   Questionable _____

Fluency
WNL* _____   Questionable _____

Grammar: Evoked Sentences   **Articulation**
                                                          circle if incorrect

1. Susan saw a mouse and a lizard.	s z
2. They thanked her mother for the cloth.	θ ð
3. The little boy wants a yellow balloon.	l
4. The treasure chest was not in the usually place.	ʒ
5. Karl had a cookie and some cake after school.	k
6. He was wearing his red suspenders.	r
7. Biff laughed when he caught the fish.	f
8. She wished for a dish of ice cream with syrup.	ʃ
9. John couldn't budge the heavy chair, could he?	dʒ
10. Charlie didn't watch television because he wanted to play checkers.	tʃ

Error score _____

Suggested cut-offs: Kindergarten—12 errors; Second Grade—5 errors;
Fifth Grade—4 errors

*Within Normal Limits

Source: Adapted from Speech & Language Department, Marlboro Central School, NY.
Used with permission.

(passes test but has a problem) is called a **false negative** or a **Type 2 error.** No screening tool is perfectly accurate, and both false positives and false negatives occur. Both of these errors might be caught at a later time, and appropriate in-depth assessment and treatment, when warranted, may follow. However, children who pass screening tests but are in need of services can lose important time in developing speech, language, and academic skills. Those who are incorrectly identified as having a disability can become stigmatized, lose self-confidence, and perform below their capability.

A person who has been identified during screening as having a communication disorder is likely to have a problem. However, a screening is not a diagnostic evaluation. Screenings simply suggest which individuals should receive further evaluation.

T H O U G H T   Q U E S T I O N S

Imagine a ten-minute preschool communication screening. What difficulties might be encountered by someone with outcome "1" (fails test but has no problem)? What difficulties might be encountered by someone with outcome "4" (passes test but has a problem)? Which situation do you think is worse? Why do you think a ten-minute communication screening might not always yield accurate results?

DEFINING THE PROBLEM

Assessment of communication disorders is the systematic process of obtaining information from many sources, through various means, and in different settings to verify and specify communication strengths and weaknesses, identify possible causes of problems, and make plans to address them. Once an individual has been selected for evaluation, assessment may begin. If a problem is identified, speech-language pathologists may make a **diagnosis,** which distinguishes an individual's difficulties from the broad range of possible problems. Although a diagnosis includes a label such as "harsh voice," it should also contain a more complete understanding of this disorder that reflects the person's ability to communicate, variability of symptoms, severity, and possible causes (Haynes & Pindzola, 1998). (See Figure 5.1 and Table 5.7.)

ASSESSMENT GOALS

The goals of assessment are listed in Table 5.4 and explained in the paragraphs that follow. The procedures that are used in meeting these objectives are described later in this chapter.

VERIFICATION OF COMMUNICATION PROBLEMS

Pretend that your grandmother just had a stroke. The speech-language pathologist in the hospital reported that she did not pass some

TABLE 5.4

Goals of assessment

The communication disorders specialist is charged with answering the following questions when assessing an individual:

1. Does a communication problem exist?
2. What is the diagnosis?
3. What are the deficit areas? How consistent are they?
4. What are the individual's strengths?
5. How severe is the problem?
6. What are the probable causes of the problem?
7. What recommendations should be made?
8. What is the prognosis (likely outcome) without and with intervention?

Source: Adapted from Lund & Duchan (1993).

preliminary tests regarding both language function and swallowing. You want to know exactly what is wrong. You are concerned whether this is a temporary situation or whether the problems will persist. You also want to know the severity of these deficits. The SLP must probe in depth to provide answers by using a variety of tools and techniques, which are described a little later in this chapter and in subsequent chapters. Simple answers might not be possible immediately. Sometimes **diagnostic therapy** is suggested. This means that the clinician will work with the client for a time and will obtain a clearer picture of the person's communication abilities and limitations in the process.

DESCRIPTION AND QUANTIFICATION OF DEFICITS AND STRENGTHS

We learned in Chapter 2 that communication impairments may involve hearing, speech, language, and/or processing or, more likely, some combination of these. During assessment, specifics of all of these are probed. Both the client's communicative strengths and limitations are noted. Techniques that the client uses for overcoming difficulties are observed. The SLP provides data reporting the consistency of behaviors and indicates how the client compares with peers. In short, assessment must provide detailed information about all aspects of the client's communicative disabilities and abilities, recognizing the interrelatedness of speech, language, and hearing. Oral, written, signed, or other modes of communication may be affected.

What are the differences between screening, evaluation, and diagnosis?

STATEMENT OF SEVERITY

If a problem exists, you will want to know how serious it is. At a general level, the clinician will determine whether the disorder is profound, severe, moderate, mild, or borderline. Individuals with a profound impairment have very little functional speech communication. A person with a severe disorder would require a great deal of intervention and support. Moderate disorders also require significant treatment and accommodation. A mild or borderline communication problem might not be readily apparent to the individual himself or herself or to others. However, even subtle communication problems can have a negative impact on social, academic, and professional success.

Exactly what determines a particular severity rating varies with each disorder. For example, an individual whose articulation is so poor that less than 5 percent of the person's words can be understood would likely have a severe impairment (see Chapter 10, "Disorders of Articulation and Phonology"). Stuttering severity may be assessed by the number of stuttered words, their duration, and additional related behaviors and attitudes (see Chapter 8, "Fluency Disorders"). Moderate ratings in more than one aspect of communication would combine to produce a more severe problem.

Beginning and experienced clinicians often differ in their judgments of the severity of a disorder. Objective criteria are needed to ensure consistency in this determination.

Published tests often suggest severity ratings depending on a client's performance scores. These must be used with caution. The clinician must be aware that there is always a range of typical communication behavior and also that a single test should not be overly relied upon.

How would you feel if your ability were determined on the basis of a single test such as the SAT or GRE? What information is missing from this measure?

ETIOLOGY

Etiology is the study of cause. The SLP must try to ascertain the reason(s) for the presenting problem. Three categories of cause may be identified. A **predisposing cause** describes the underlying factor that led to the problem, for example something genetic. A **precipitating**

cause is a factor that triggered the disorder, such as a stroke. A **maintaining** or **perpetuating cause** is something that keeps the problem going. In the case of Sally M. that follows, the SLP formed hypotheses concerning all three categories of etiology.

Sally M., age 7, had multiple articulation, phonological, and morphological errors in her speech. The SLP learned that Sally had frequent ear infections during her second and third years of life. The SLP hypothesized that inability to hear adequately during this period may have interfered with mastery of the sound system of English. Sally was ill so much that she may not have had the energy to focus on learning speech. The SLP observed that Sally's mother laughed good-naturedly at Sally's way of speaking. The SLP reported that the likely predisposing cause of Sally's communication difficulties was a tendency toward ear infections. The precipitating cause may have been the history of middle ear infections (otitis media). Possible maintaining factors were the attention and "rewards" Sally received from her immature speech.

Causality is sometimes viewed from another perspective. The terms **organic/somatogenic** and **functional/psychogenic** may also be used in describing etiology. An organic disorder has an identifiable physical cause; for example, cleft palate, cerebral palsy, and cancer of the larynx all are likely to result in communicative difficulties. The term "somatogenic" means coming from the body, and it therefore indicates a physical basis.

When no physical cause can be identified, the disorder is considered functional. Functional disorders may be due to psychogenic (psychological) factors; for example, in elective mutism, an individual has no physiological reason for not being able to speak but decides not to talk, perhaps as retaliation toward an abusive parent (Haynes & Pindzola, 1998).

It is helpful to remember that the causes of communication problems are often elusive; sometimes we simply cannot figure out what they are. In these cases, clinicians report that the etiology is unknown. The mystery may be partly because original causes do not always persist; for example, Sally M.'s ear infections are no longer apparent at age 7. Furthermore, we have no way of knowing why Sally was especially vulnerable to getting ear infections in the first place. Finally, causality is often complex, with many factors coming together to result in the development of a particular disorder.

T H O U G H T   Q U E S T I O N S

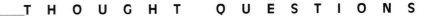

Do you think the etiology of Sally's communication problems is organic/somatogenic or functional/psychogenic? Could it be a combination? What are the limitations of this terminology? Why is it important to attempt to determine the cause(s) of communication problems?

THE TREATMENT PLAN

The **treatment plan** contains recommendations for addressing the client's communicative deficiencies. It is often the most read portion of an assessment report. In making a plan, the first decision is whether any intervention at all is warranted. If it is, then its nature must be described. Should the client be enrolled in speech and language therapy? Where? How frequent and how long should therapy sessions be? Would the client benefit more from individual or group work? What specific targets should be addressed initially? What style of therapy might be optimal? Some options include high or low structure, client or clinician directed, behavioral or cognitive, direct or indirect, pull-out or push-in. These are described later in this chapter in the section on treatment procedures. Recommendations for counseling are also noted. The plan should also indicate referrals for other services such as psychological or medical evaluation. The treatment plan is essentially a "working hypothesis" (Haynes & Pindzola, 1998, p. 11); the initial recommendations may need to be altered as intervention proceeds. Assessment continues throughout treatment, and one affects the other in a circular fashion (see Figure 5.3).

PROGNOSIS

A **prognosis** is an informed prediction of the outcome of a disorder. For example, a parent of a 5-year-old with very disfluent speech will want to know what will happen if this is left untreated and whether therapy will prevent the child from stuttering later in life.

In communication disorders, the SLP makes a prognosis regarding whether the problem will persist if no intervention occurs and what the likely outcome is if a course of therapy or other treatment plan is followed. The SLP must consider the nature and severity of the disorder; the client's responsiveness to trial therapy during assessment; and the client's overall communicative, intellectual, and personal strengths and weaknesses. The client's

FIGURE 5.3 The assessment/treatment cycle

Assessment is an ongoing process. The initial assessment determines the treatment plan. A thorough assessment includes trial therapy. As treatment proceeds, the client's functioning is monitored (assessed) and modifications in treatment are made.

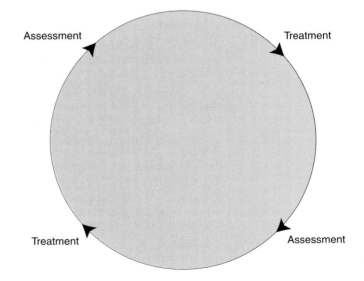

Assessment

Treatment

Treatment

Assessment

Family members and clients are often eager to know the prognosis. They will ask questions such as "Will my child outgrow this problem?" "How long will it take to correct this disorder?"

environment is also important. Are family members able and willing to help? Is support available within the school or through other agencies involved with the client?

ASSESSMENT PROCEDURES

Assessment may take many forms. Ideally, the clinician should sample a broad variety of communication skills through multiple procedures in several settings. The focus should be on the collection of **authentic data,** that is, actual real-life information, in sufficient quantity to be able to make meaningful and accurate decisions (Damico, 1997). Several aspects of a typical evaluation are presented on the accompanying CD-ROM.

Background information needs to be obtained from case histories and interviews. Hearing and oral-motor function should be screened. The client's communicative skills should be observed, preferably in more than one situation, and evaluated. Formal tests of areas of concern, such as articulation or expressive vocabulary, should be administered and scored. The client should be given more than one opportunity to demonstrate specific competencies. All the data obtained should be organized and synthesized. Sometimes a **portfolio** of information about the client is gathered that contains such items as audiotapes, videotapes, and written observations and comments by numerous people (Kratcoski, 1998). A report must be written that includes a summary of the assessment findings, including prognosis and recommendations. Provisions should be made for reevaluation.

CASE HISTORY

The written **case history** provides background information that helps the SLP to prepare for an evaluation. Most speech-language pathologists require that histories be completed before the client's first visit. Normally, one form is tailored for adult clients, and a comparable one is for a parent or other responsible person to use with regard to a child. These forms tend to be quite detailed. In addition to basic information such as name, address, and birth date, they include questions about languages spoken in the home, the nature and history of the problem, health, education, and occupation.

Although the written case history is a valuable tool, its reliability may be limited for various reasons. The respondent might not have understood all the questions. She or he might not know the answers to many questions and might guess or recall incorrectly. Cultural differences can influence the manner of response to some items (Shipley & McAfee, 1998, p. 5). Table 5.5 lists some possible limitations of written case histories.

TABLE 5.5

Possible limitations of written case histories

1. The respondent might not have understood all the questions.
2. The respondent might not know the answers to many questions and might guess or recall incorrectly.
3. Cultural differences might influence the manner of response to some items.
4. The respondent might be embarrassed about some aspects of the history and try to make a good impression.

T H O U G H T   Q U E S T I O N

Can you think of other factors in addition to those suggested in Table 5.5 that could interfere with the accuracy of a written case history?

OPENING INTERVIEW

Once the SLP has the completed case history form, additional background information is obtained through an interview. The basic purposes of the initial interview are (1) to learn more about the client that might be relevant to his or her communication and (2) to answer questions and provide reassurance and support for the client and/or family. Open-ended questions are used to encourage the respondent to provide adequate detail. In addition, the respondent must be given the opportunity to express concerns. The clinician must be sure to listen openly and nonjudgmentally. Experienced SLPs are able to guide the interview so that the objectives are met in a supportive, natural way within the allotted time frame.

The SLP obtains background information about a client from a written case history completed by the client, parent, or significant other; an interview; and reports from other professionals.

SYSTEMATIC OBSERVATION/SAMPLING

Watching the client in more than one setting and with different people can provide considerable insight into the individual's communicative skills. One 5-year-old client stuttered severely with his gruff 60-year-old father but very little with the SLP.

Clinicians often begin their observation when the client and a family member are in the waiting room. Some children are very talkative with a parent but become silent with a stranger. Classroom and recess or lunchtime observations for school-age children can be revealing.

Hospitalized clients could be observed with significant others when possible.

Most clinicians use a **speech** and/or **language sampling** technique when assessing the communication of both children and adults. Activities for obtaining this sample generally are planned beforehand on the basis of the age and interests of the client. The clinician records the interaction of the client with the clinician, a parent, and/or a similarly aged person. The sample is then transcribed and analyzed. Guidelines for sample collection and analysis are described in Chapter 6, "Childhood Language Disorders," and Chapter 10, "Disorders of Articulation and Phonology."

HEARING SCREENING

Hearing is routinely screened in most communication evaluations. Since hearing is so important to speech, the SLP needs to ascertain that the client's hearing is normal for speech purposes. The pure tone and

Trial therapy is an important part of the assessment procedure.

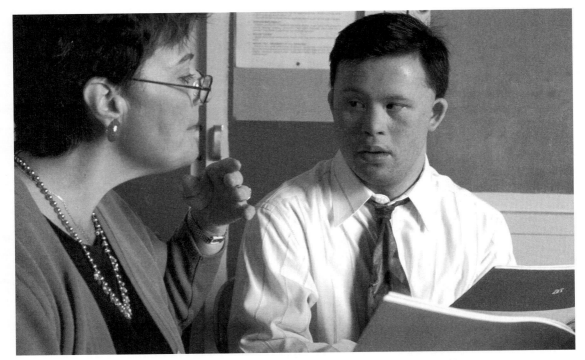

administered by different clinicians and at different times. When selecting a test for use with a particular client, in addition to selecting an instrument that is generally reliable and valid, the SLP must determine that others from the client's cultural background were included in the sample population.

Published norm-based tests generally provide several types of scores, including raw scores, standard scores, percentile ranks, and age equivalents. The **raw score** is usually simply the number correct and tells you little. **Derived scores** are based on the normal curve (see Chapter 2 and Figure 2.1). Derived scores include *percentile ranks, standard scores,* and *age equivalents*. **Percentile ranks** indicate the percentage of people who scored below a particular score. For example, someone with a percentile score of 40 scored better than 40 percent of those with whom she or he is being compared; conversely, this score is also lower than that received by 60 percent in the comparison group. If your percentile rank is 50; you are exactly in the middle. Several different types of **standard scores** are used. A common system, used in IQ tests and some communication scales, is to call the middle of the bell curve "100." In other words, the average score for the sample population would be converted to 100. With the use of statistical formulae, scores below the average would be assigned standard scores lower than 100, and those above the average would receive higher standard scores. Both percentile ranks and standard scores are useful in determining how one person performs relative to others.

Age-equivalent scores are the average score of people of a given age. For example, if the average raw score of 5-year-olds is 15 on a certain test, 15 would be an age-equivalent score of 5 years. A 10-year-old receiving a raw score of 15 would have an age-equivalency of 5 years based on this test. This may be misleading, since age-equivalent scores do not account for normal variability in a given age group. Furthermore, while a one-year age difference is usually quite significant in comparing a 1-year-old child and a 2-year-old child, a one-year difference means less and less with advancing age.

T H O U G H T   Q U E S T I O N S

Can different data be collected from systematic observation and formal testing? What are the relative advantages and disadvantages of each type of information gathering?

CONSOLIDATION OF FINDINGS: MAKING THE DIAGNOSIS

It is axiomatic to say that professionals must treat the "whole person" and not just the disorder. After the speech-language pathologist has

The SLP makes a determination about a client's current functioning and the nature of the problem from background information, careful observation, hearing screening, an examination of the peripheral speech mechanism, speech sampling, and formal and informal testing.

obtained information about the client from various sources, it is necessary to summarize the results and make connections between the findings. For example, background information may give insights into presenting behavior. Scores from norm-based tests need to be reconciled with observations by the SLP and other important people in the client's life. The client's communicative limitations must be viewed in the context of strengths, such as motivation and family or other support (see Figure 5.1). Often an individual is more capable in some aspects of communication, while other features are weak. For example, a child's speech might be easy to understand (readily intelligible), although he or she has a limited expressive vocabulary. The SLP must attempt to obtain a well-rounded picture of the person who is being assessed.

T H O U G H T   Q U E S T I O N

Can you think of a situation in which a parent, a teacher, and a speech-language pathologist would each have a different perception of a child's communicative competence? (Do you know the story of the four blind men and the elephant?)

Communication disorders specialists working in any environment typically are required to put a name to the presenting disorder. It is not sufficient to be general and state that the client has a "communication problem." A diagnostic label is needed for funding reimbursement by third party payers such as insurance companies, Medicare, and Medicaid. School systems also require a diagnosis before an Individual Education Plan (see Table 5.8) can be devised for a child. The International Classification of Diseases (ICD-10), available in 2002, is the standard universal coding system. Table 5.7 lists some of the codes most often used or encountered by speech-language pathologists and audiologists. Sometimes a medical or psychological diagnosis is made before the SLP or audiologist does her or his evaluation.

CLOSING INTERVIEW

The client and/or family will want to know the outcome of the evaluation as soon as possible. When and how this information is shared may depend on whether the setting is a hospital, private clinic, university center, or public school. In addition, each facility will establish its own set of policies.

In general a brief conference is held immediately after the formal assessment. The SLP will probably indicate that all of the information gathered about the client has not yet been analyzed, so more complete recommendations will appear in the diagnostic report. The SLP might suggest another meeting to discuss this report.

TABLE 5.7

International classification of diseases

Codes used in identification and billing related to some communication disorders

MALIGNANT NEOPLASM OF LIP, ORAL CAVITY, AND PHARYNX (140-149)
PSYCHOSES (290-299)

290	Senile and presenile organic psychotic conditions
299.0	Infantile autism

NONPSYCHOTIC MENTAL DISORDERS (300-316)

307.0	Stammering and stuttering
307.23	Gilles de la Tourette's disorder
307.9	Developmental articulation disorder
309.83	Elective mutism
310.1	Mild memory disturbances associated with senile brain disease
313.2	Sensitivity, shyness, and social withdrawal disorder
314.0	Attention deficit disorder
315	Specific delays in development
315.3	Developmental speech or language disorder

MENTAL RETARDATION (317-319)

317	Mild mental retardation
318.0	Moderate mental retardation
318.1	Severe mental retardation
318.2	Profound mental retardation

HEREDITARY AND DEGENERATIVE DISEASES OF THE CENTRAL NERVOUS SYSTEM (330-337)

331.0	Alzheimer's disease
331.1	Pick's disease of the brain
332	Parkinson's disease
333.4	Huntington's disease
333.82	Orofacial dyskinesia
334	Spinocerebellar disease
335.20	Amyotrophic lateral sclerosis

OTHER DISORDERS OF THE CENTRAL NERVOUS SYSTEM (340-349)

340	Multiple sclerosis
342	Hemiplegia and hemiparesis
343	Infantile cerebral palsy
344.1	Paraplegia: Paralysis of both lower limbs
344.2	Diplegia of upper limbs: Paralysis of both upper limbs

345.1	Generalized convulsive epilepsy
345.2	Petit mal status
345.3	Grand mal status

DISORDERS OF THE PERIPHERAL NERVOUS SYSTEM (350-359)

351.0	Bell's palsy: Facial palsy
359	Muscular dystrophies and other myopathies

DISEASES OF THE EAR AND MASTOID PROCESS (380-389)

380	Disorders of external ear
380.1	Infective otitis externa
380.4	Impacted cerumen: Wax in ear
380.5	Acquired stenosis of external ear canal: Collapse of external ear canal
381	Nonsuppurative otitis media and Eustachian tube disorders
381.01	Acute serous otitis media
381.6	Obstruction of Eustachian tube
384.2	Perforation of tympanic membrane
385.0	Tympanosclerosis
385.21	Impaired mobility of malleus
386.0	Meniere's disease
387	Otosclerosis
388.01	Presbyacusis
388.12	Noise-induced hearing loss
388.3	Tinnitus
388.41	Diplacusis
388.43	Impairment of auditory discrimination
388.44	Recruitment
388.5	Disorders of acoustic nerve
389.0	Conductive hearing loss
389.1	Sensorineural hearing loss
389.14	Central hearing loss
389.2	Mixed conductive and sensorineural hearing loss

DISEASES OF THE RESPIRATORY SYSTEM (460-519)

464.0	Acute laryngitis
470	Deviated nasal septum
474.1	Hypertrophy of tonsils and adenoids
478.3	Paralysis of vocal cords or larynx
478.4	Polyp of vocal cord or larynx

continued

TABLE 5.7

International classification of diseases continued

DISEASES OF THE RESPIRATORY
SYSTEM (460-519) (continued)
478.6   Edema of larynx
518.0   Pulmonary collapse
519.4   Disorders of the diaphragm

DISEASES OF THE DIGESTIVE
SYSTEM (520-579)
520   Disorders of tooth development and
         eruption
524.7   Dental alveolar anomalies
526   Diseases of the jaws
529   Diseases and other conditions of the
         tongue

CONGENITAL ANOMALIES (740-759)
748.2   Web of larynx
749   Cleft palate and cleft lip
749.0   Cleft palate
749.1   Cleft lip
750.0   Tongue tie (Ankyloglossia)
756.0   Anomalies of skull and facial bones
759.81   Prader-Willis syndrome
759.82   Marfan syndrome
759.83   Fragile X syndrome

MATERNAL CAUSES OF PERINATAL
MORBIDITY AND MORTALITY (760-763)
760.71   Alcohol (fetal alcohol syndrome)
760.72   Narcotics
761   Fetus or newborn affected by maternal
         complications of pregnancy

OTHER CONDITIONS ORIGINATING IN
THE PERINATAL PERIOD (764-779)
764   Low birthweight due to slow fetal
         growth and fetal malnutrition
779.3   Feeding problems in newborn

SYMPTOMS, SIGNS, AND ILL-DEFINED
CONDITIONS (780-799)
781.3   Lack of coordination
784.3   Aphasia
784.4   Voice disturbance

784.41   Aphonia (Loss of voice)
784.49   Other change in voice (Dysphonia,
         Hoarseness, Hypernasality,
         Hyponasality)
784.5   Other speech disturbance (Dysarthria,
         Dysphasia, Slurred speech)
784.61   Alexia and dyslexia
797   Senility without mention of psychosis

INJURY AND POISONING (800-999)
931   Foreign body in ear
933   Foreign body in pharynx and larynx
934   Foreign body in trachea, bronchus, and
         lung

PERSONS WITH POTENTIAL HEALTH
HAZARDS RELATED TO COMMUNICABLE
DISEASES (V01-V09)
V08   Asymptomatic human immuno-
         deficiency virus [HIV] infection status

PERSONS WITH A CONDITION
INFLUENCING THEIR HEALTH STATUS
(V40-V49)
V40   Mental and behavioral problems
V40.0   Problems with learning
V40.1   Problems with communication
         [including speech]
V41.0   Problems with sight
V41.2   Problems with hearing
V41.4   Problems with voice production
V41.5   Problems with smell and taste
V41.6   Problems with swallowing and
         mastication
V53.2   Hearing aid

PERSONS ENCOUNTERING HEALTH
SERVICES IN OTHER CIRCUMSTANCES
(V60-V68)
V60.1   Inadequate housing
V60.2   Inadequate material resources
         (Economic problem, Poverty)
V60.3   Person living alone
V61.21   Child abuse

Source: Adapted from U.S. Department of Health and Human Services (1994).

REPORT WRITING

The diagnostic report is a summary of the client's history and a record of what transpired during the assessment. The implications of the findings should be clearly stated and thoughtfully justified. The report is normally the springboard for intervention and treatment. It may be sent to other professionals who will be working with the client. It is also available to the client or client's parents. The report must be carefully written. If technical terms are used, they should be explained. Speech-language pathologists may develop individual styles of writing, but most reports follow a similar format and contain comparable information. For children within a school system, information from the diagnostic report may be used in the development of Individual Education Plans (IEPs), which are mandated by federal law (see Chapter 1). The IEP will contain long-term goals and short-term objectives for the individual child. Table 5.8 on page 146 is an example of an IEP.

Effective writing skills are required to accurately convey assessment information to the client, the client's family, and other professionals.

INTERVENTION WITH COMMUNICATION DISORDERS

Intervention for individuals with communication disorders is influenced by the nature and severity of the disorder, the age and status of the client, and environmental considerations, as well as personal and cultural characteristics of both client and clinician. Despite this, some general principles and procedures can be identified.

OBJECTIVES OF INTERVENTION

Regardless of the specific nature of the problem, intervention in speech-language pathology has as its overriding goal the improvement of the client's communication skills.

1. The client should show improvement not just in a clinical setting; progress should generalize to his or her real-world environments, such as home, school, and work.
2. The client should not have to think about what has been learned; in large part, it should be **automatic.**
3. The client must be able to **self-monitor.** Although modifications should be automatic, they will still require monitoring. The client should be able to listen to and observe himself or herself and make corrections as needed without the therapist's being present.
4. The client should make optimum progress in the minimum amount of time.
5. Intervention should be sensitive to the personal and cultural characteristics of the client.

TABLE 5.8

A sample Individual Education Plan

Department of Communication Disorders
Preschool Program
Individual Education Plan

Name:	Matthew R.	*Date:*	September 1, 1999
Address:	123 Maple St.	*D.O.B.*	January 4, 1996
	Nice Town, AZ	*Age:*	3 yrs., 8 mos.
Phone:	123-321-1111	*Parents:*	Jack and Jill R.

Speech and Language Goals

Long-Term Goal 1: To develop presymbolic skills.

Short-term objective 1a: Matthew will localize to his name on 4 out of 5 occasions.

Short-term objective 1b: Matthew will imitate simple motor actions on 4 out of 5 occasions.

Short-term objective 1c: Matthew will maintain visual attention for the completion of a simple visual-motor task on 4 of 5 occasions.

Short-term objective 1d: Matthew will match 1–3 pictures or colored blocks from larger arrays as directed by an adult, with 80% accuracy.

Short-term objective 1e: Given verbal prompts, Matthew will utilize a pointing gesture to request a desired item on 4 of 5 occasions.

Long-Term Goal 2: To improve expressive language skills.

Short-term objective 2a: Matthew will develop functional use of the following words or signs: "more," "eat," "drink," "all gone."

Short-term objective 2b: With minimal cueing, Matthew will utilize an augmentative communication board/device for purposes of requesting and responding on 4 of 5 occasions.

Long-Term Goal 3: Improve receptive language skills.

Short-term objective 3a: Matthew will discriminate between two commonly used objects accurately in 80% of the opportunities presented.

TABLE 5.8

A sample Individual Education Plan (continued)

Long-Term Goal 3 (continued)

Short-term objective 3b: Matthew will follow one-step routinely used commands (e.g.: "sit down," "no," "come here,") given verbal and gestural cues in 80% of the opportunities presented.

Long-Term Goal 4:   To develop basic phonological skills.

Short-term objective 4a: Matthew will imitate vowel sounds as modeled by an adult in 80% of the opportunities presented.

Short-term objective 4b: Matthew will imitate early developing consonant sounds in CV structures 60% of the time.

Long-Term Goal 5:   To develop oral-motor skills.

Short-term objective 5a: Matthew will manipulate sensory materials without mouthing on 5 of 5 occasions.

Short-term objective 5b: Matthew will participate in oral-motor imitation tasks/exercises on 4 of 5 occasions.

Long-Term Goal 6:   To develop simple play behaviors.

Short-term objective 6a: Matthew will consistently use 20 objects for their intended purposes with a model provided during "active learning" times.

Short-term objective 6b: Matthew will engage in parallel play behaviors with peers for 5–10 minutes on 4 of 5 days.

Short-term objective 6c: Matthew will participate in reciprocal ball play for 3–5 turns on 4 of 5 days.

Long-Term Goal 7:   To develop self-feeding skills.

Short-term objective 7a: Matthew will drink from an open cup during meal times without spilling, dumping, or dunking foods on 4 of 5 occasions.

Short-term objective 7b: Matthew will utilize a spoon independently to eat soft-textured or semiliquid foods with minimal spilling on 4 of 5 occasions.

signed

Samuel Q. Brown, M.S., CCC-SLP
Arizona Licensed
Speech-Language Pathologist

Source: Adapted with permission from C. Augello, Speech-Language Pathologist.

TARGET SELECTION

The assessment report and/or IEP should provide long-term goals and short-term objectives for communication intervention. The clinician, however, will have to decide which specific targets should be addressed and in what sequence. The client's personal needs and the potential for generalization are most relevant in making meaningful choices. Likely success of mastery and typical behavior of others of the client's age and gender might provide additional insights.

CLIENT NEEDS

Each client has individual needs. The SLP must attempt to determine which are paramount at this time and then develop a plan to meet these needs.

The client's individual needs are paramount in target selection. For example, Johnny M. is a 6-year-old boy with numerous articulation and grammatical errors in his speech. When asked his name, he is reluctant to answer, but he may be coaxed to say, "Doddy." According to Mrs. M., people tease him about his pronunciation of his name, and this is a great source of anxiety for the child. Because of this, the phonemes /dʒ/ ("J" in Johnny) and /n/ are very important to this child and should be considered for early targeting.

HOW IT WILL GENERALIZE

Generalization refers to the use of the trained target with different people in varied environmental settings and linguistic contexts. If what has been learned in therapy is in conflict with patterns found in the home environment, generalization may be difficult. Going back to Johnny, let's assume that his major playing companion is a 5-year-old brother whose speech is even more difficult to understand. This situation may inhibit generalization. On the other hand, the phoneme /n/ is found in many common English words. Johnny will have ample opportunities to practice that sound not only in his name but also in many other words. Although /dʒ/ occurs less frequently in English, its prominence in this child's name and the frequency with which he may be expected to say it suggest an opportunity for it to generalize to many life situations.

Another type of generalization occurs when not only the targeted sound, word, or communicative behavior is modified. The SLP will anticipate that similar phonemes (see Chapter 10, "Disorders of Articulation and Phonology") and related linguistic skills also improve (Roth & Worthington, 1996).

EASE OF MASTERY

A careful assessment includes trial therapy. In the case of Johnny M., the clinician observed that he could correctly say /n/ and "knee" when these were modeled and he was asked to repeat what he heard; in other words, Johnny was stimulable for the /n/ sound. Johnny was not successful in producing /dʒ/ even though the clinician used a variety of techniques to elicit this sound; he was not stimulable for /dʒ/. On the basis of this information, Johnny will more quickly acquire /n/ than /dʒ/. However, recent research has concluded that once learned, nonstimulable phonemes prompt greater generalization than those that were stimulable (Gierut, 1998). For this reason, both /n/ and /dʒ/ are appropriate targets.

AGE APPROPRIATENESS

Knowledge of normal development and behaviors provides insights into which communication forms and functions are typical at different ages. For example, /n/ is generally mastered by age 2, and /dʒ/ is customarily correctly produced by age 4 (Stoel-Gammon & Dunn, 1985). This information confirms the decision to select the production of the phonemes /n/ and /dʒ/ as first objectives for Johnny.

In summary, target selection requires consideration of several variables. The clinician must make a decision that is appropriate for the particular client's needs. The selection of the targets /n/ and /dʒ/ for Johnny is a simplification. Children with multiple phonemic errors will likely be treated with a process approach, which is described in Chapter 10, "Disorders of Articulation and Phonology."

T H O U G H T   Q U E S T I O N

Mr. Brown had a stroke at age 75. He is able to say a few words, but these are often garbled, and the speech sounds are not correctly produced. He becomes frustrated when he tries to talk. He can accurately point to things around the room to express basic wants and needs. Using the criteria above, which is probably a better early communication target: (1) correctly pointing to pictures to express himself or (2) learning to produce the sounds (phonemes) of English?

BASELINE DATA

Before beginning a program of intervention, SLPs obtain **baseline data;** that is, they try to elicit the target behavior(s) multiple times and record the accuracy of the client's responses. This gives them information about the client's starting point. Baselines are essential to determine the client's progress and the success of the treatment program.

Unlike a language sample and standardized tests used in the initial assessment, baselines specifically probe the communication behavior that will be the focus of therapy. Let's return to Johnny M. The speech-language pathologist has decided that the phoneme /n/

Formal test results during assessment differ from baseline data. During formal testing, a wide range of communicative skills are evaluated. Baseline data reveal an individual's performance level with regard to a few selected potential targets.

is a first target. The child pronounces his name as "Doddy" and says "do" for "no" and "dife" for "knife." The SLP knows that Johnny can correctly imitate the sound /n/ and the word "knee." In baseline testing, the SLP may obtain ten pictures of objects beginning with /n/ and ten of objects ending with /n/. The SLP asks Johnny to name the objects. The percentage of correct /n/ productions in each of these positions is Johnny's baseline for the phoneme /n/. The SLP might record the following baselines: 20 percent success with /n/ at the beginning of words and 10 percent success with /n/ at the end of words in a nonmodeled condition. Johnny was accurate in 50 percent of the words presented when he was immediately imitating the clinician's speech. These data provide a starting point both for planning therapy and for measuring progress.

BEHAVIORAL OBJECTIVES

Notice the difference between long-term goals (see Table 5.8) and behavioral or short-term objectives. The former are somewhat general, while the latter are highly specific.

Once the clinician has obtained baseline data, short-term objectives are developed. These are the targets for each treatment session, but they may also serve for several sessions. A behavioral objective is a statement that specifies the target behavior in an observable and measurable way. To do this requires that the clinician identify what the client is expected to do, under what conditions, and with what degree of success. The letters ABCD might help you to remember the format for writing behavioral objectives:

A. Audience. Who is expected to do the behavior?
B. Behavior. What is the observable and measurable behavior?
C. Condition. What is the context or condition of the behavior?
D. Degree. What is the targeted degree of success?

Returning to Johnny M., the SLP has decided that she or he wants Johnny to experience early success and establishes the following as one behavioral objective for the first session:

A. Johnny
B. will produce the phoneme /n/ correctly
C. in the initial and final position of one-syllable words when modeled by the clinician
D. in 60 percent of the opportunities presented.

This seems a reasonable goal, since Johnny was accurate in this condition 50 percent of the time during baseline testing.

Behavioral objectives, sometimes called instructional objectives, may be used for a broad range of teaching targets. Table 5.9 lists ten objectives written by student clinicians. Read each one to see whether it

TABLE 5.9

Test yourself: Behavioral objectives

Which of the following is NOT a well-written behavioral objective and why? (Answers are at the bottom of the table, upside down.)

1. The client will understand the words "over" and "under" when they are said to him in 90 percent of the opportunities presented.
2. The client will answer "What" questions using sentences that are 5 words in length in response to 4 of 5 questions.
3. The client will use a rate of speech of no more than 150 wpm when reading aloud from the local newspaper for 5 minutes.
4. The client will correctly name 8 of 10 farm animals when shown cards with their pictures.
5. The client will correctly use the plural form.
6. The client will appropriately respond to the clinician's greeting at the beginning of the therapy session.
7. The client will follow two-part directions given by the clinician in 90% of the opportunities presented.
8. The client will improve vocal quality while reading sentences aloud.
9. The client will distinguish between the phonemes /s/ and /z/ when produced by the clinician.
10. The client will sustain the phoneme /a/ for 20 seconds at a loudness level of 50 decibels.

Answers: 1. No, can't observe or measure "understand." 2. Yes. 3. Yes. 4. Yes. 5. No, in what situation and how often? 6. No, how often? Just today? What is meant by "appropriate"? 7. Yes. 8. No, "improve" is not measurable, also no degree is given. 9. No, degree is not given. 10. Yes.

is a valid objective. Use the ABCD criteria. If the instructional objective for this task for readers of this text is 80 percent accuracy, did you meet it?

CLINICAL ELEMENTS

A TANDEM APPROACH: COGNITION AND TRAINING

Human beings possess an intellect that makes us able to think and understand things. This is known as our **cognitive ability.** Almost without exception, successful speech-language therapy depends upon the client's understanding what is to be learned and being motivated to do so. Most clinical sessions begin with the SLP explaining or reviewing the target.

TABLE 5.10

A possible format for a therapy session

A. Introduction
   Greetings
   Review previous sessions' targets and/or activities
   Summarize format for current session

B. Teach concept
   Explain
   Provide example
   Demonstrate (model)
   Provide strategy
   Define

C. Practice concept
   Game
   Worksheet
   Books/magazines
   Hands-on activity

D. Assess learning
   Ask specific questions
   Prompt problem solving
   Ask for paraphrasing

E. Summary/conclusion
   How does this skill affect daily life?

Notes

1. Steps A through E are appropriate for most individual or group sessions.
2. The specific techniques listed under each step are suggestions and will vary.
3. When possible, use more than one modality. For example, use visual, verbal, and tactile stimuli.
4. Use teachable moments to review previously learned skills unrelated to target concept.
5. In working with groups, recognize that there will be a variety of targets and skill levels.
6. Be sensitive to clients' cultural backgrounds.
7. Consider how to maintain high levels of motivation.
8. Recognize that details will need to be tailored to the needs of the individual client and will change as the client progresses in therapy.

Source: Adapted from scheme developed by D. Moneymaker, Beacon Central School System, NY. Used with permission.

The amount and complexity of the explanation vary with the training target and the client's age and cognitive ability. A behavior modification approach is widely used after the client has been prepared.

Behavior modification training programs have been shown to be successful for a broad variety of communication disorders (Hegde, 1993). Behavior modification is a systematic method of changing behavior. The speech-language pathologist typically proceeds as follows.

Before training, the SLP establishes a target and collects baseline data. During training, the SLP attempts to evoke the desired response from the client by providing a **stimulus.** The client is expected to *respond,* and the clinician **reinforces** this response. The SLP records the accuracy of the client's response on a tally sheet. For example, Johnny might be shown a picture of a "nest" (stimulus) and be asked to identify the picture (response); if his response is correct, the SLP may permit Johnny to move a peg up a "Good Speech" ladder (reinforcement). After training, the SLP counts the percentage of accurate responses and determines the next target response. Table 5.10 is a general format for a therapy session. It was developed by a school SLP to give to student clinicians to guide them in their preparation.

Even young and relatively low-functioning individuals are more responsive to therapy when they understand the goals.

HIGH AND LOW STRUCTURE

Behavior modification follows a highly structured format; it is directed by the speech-language pathologist. The SLP has a well-thought-out plan and works to guide the client through the stages required for mastery of the target.

Sometimes a low-structured or more client-led approach is used. The SLP follows the client's lead but teaches along the way. This is referred to as **incidental teaching.** For this to be effective, planning is also necessary so that targets are reached. The SLP provides an environment in which communication should occur naturally. For example, imaginary play with a young child or a cooking or art project with one who is older may serve as situations in which therapy occurs. The approach is described further in Chapter 6, "Childhood Language Impairments."

COUNSELING

In addition to direct work with the client on the communication problem, the SLP is a counselor for the client and other key people in the client's life. A person with a communication disorder may experience a host of feelings, including embarrassment, anger, depression, and inadequacy. Family members may have similar emotions regarding the client's communication and may also feel guilty, perhaps blaming themselves for the problem. Through counseling, the SLP tries to understand the client's motivations and to guide her or him toward mutually desirable outcomes.

Clients, family members, teachers, and others might not be completely open about their feelings. A skilled SLP knows how to listen empathetically, provide support, and guide the interaction toward a productive end. Some suggestions for effective counseling are found in Table 5.11.

PULL-OUT AND PUSH-IN

The traditional approach to speech and language therapy involves meeting with clients individually or in small groups in a clinical setting or

---

TABLE 5.11

Suggestions for effective counseling

1. *Empathize.* Speech-language pathologists should listen in an empathetic and nonjudgmental fashion. All clients must feel valued and respected.
2. *Be focused.* Speech-language pathologists should keep the interaction focused and minimize irrelevant, tangential conversation. While occasional side remarks are useful in building a rapport, the purpose of counseling should be paramount.
3. *Keep it simple.* Avoid jargon. Use language that the client is likely to understand. Give examples.
4. *Strive for cultural sensitivity.* Speech-language pathologists must be sensitive to the client's cultural background as it may pertain to personal values and verbal and nonverbal communication. For example, some cultural groups expect more mutual sharing and informal conversation, while others are more task oriented.
5. *Summarize.* Speech-language pathologists should review statements made periodically throughout the session and at the close of the session should provide a summary. This improves recall of the interaction as well an opportunity to revisit issues that may not be understood or resolved.
6. *Listen carefully and repeat.* Speech-language pathologists should paraphrase key points that the client makes to assure understanding.
7. *Avoid irrelevant revelations.* Speech-language pathologists should guard against probing or permitting too much personal disclosure early in the counseling relationship.
8. *Be in charge.* Speech-language pathologists should take the responsibility for moving the interview forward and bringing it to closure.

Source: Adapted from Shipley (1997).

---

therapy room. When this occurs within a school system, it is often referred to as **pull-out therapy,** because the child is pulled out of the classroom. Today, much communication treatment in schools occurs within the classroom, and it may be referred to as **push-in therapy.** A regular teacher, an aide, and a speech-language pathologist may jointly staff a preschool class for children with speech and language difficulties. The goal is for the three to work together to plan and implement a program that meets the special needs of each child.

In this **collaborative model** of intervention, the SLP may periodically go into a classroom and work with individuals and groups of children as the regular teacher conducts a lesson. The SLP provides special assistance as needed. She or he helps with vocabulary items, reading comprehension, and language processing and offers guidance in structuring and writing the reports. In the classroom setting, the teacher and the SLP reinforce speech and language targets that were developed for individual youngsters. Some of these children may also be seen by the SLP for pull-out therapy.

FAMILY AND ENVIRONMENTAL INVOLVEMENT

An individual might spend two hours a week with a speech-language pathologist and 110 awake hours alone and with other people. Very young language-delayed children are sometimes bombarded with questions at home. Others may have older siblings who do the talking for them. In Johnny's case, described earlier in this chapter, it might be recommended that the younger sibling with highly unintelligible speech receive therapy. This would benefit both youngsters.

The SLP needs to learn as much as possible about the home situation and provide guidance to optimize learning. He or she may show the parents such techniques as **incidental language teaching, modeling, expansion,** and **extension.** These are described in Chapter 6, "Childhood Language Impairments."

When children are seen for speech or language therapy, SLPs often ask that a parent observe the sessions on a regular basis. Depending on the family circumstances, family members may be asked to help the child with specific homework assignments. Some parents are overly eager to help and may correct the child continuously. The SLP needs to teach appropriate intervention techniques so that the client stays motivated and does not feel frustrated. Sometimes siblings or other peers may be taught how to assist in the progress of a child with a communicative disorder.

Classroom teachers are key figures in the lives of school-age children and must be involved in any communication intervention. For children with multiple handicaps, the speech-language pathologist must coordinate efforts with other specialists such as the physician, reading teacher, physical and occupational therapist, and psychologist. Teamwork is essential for the child to make optimum progress.

Families and friends may learn ways of helping adults with communicative impairments. A spouse may be critical in assisting therapy for an adult who had a stroke or has a voice problem due to recent accident or illness. The SLP must recognize the significant others in the client's life, from infancy through old age, and engage them in productive ways. **Support groups** consisting of individuals who have similar difficulties often provide an avenue to practice what has been learned in therapy, to share feelings related to the disability, and to maintain communication skills once formal treatment has been terminated.

Intervention for communication disorders occurs in many settings. Broadening the base for treatment helps to ensure that what is learned in a clinical setting is transferred to a variety of real-world contexts.

Whatever approaches are used, the client's interests and strengths should be utilized. For example, some individuals learn more easily when shown diagrams and pictures, whereas others profit more from a verbal approach. Some are quicker to grasp concepts; others learn more rapidly from drill. Some have families who can provide strong support; some must look elsewhere for this. Ongoing assessment helps the SLP to determine the most useful procedures for individual clients.

PROCEDURAL TERMINOLOGY

Clinicians need to document their activities with a client. Keeping accurate records of client progress and time spent in various activities is an important yet often overly time-consuming chore. Medicare, Medicaid, and many private insurance carriers require that speech-language pathology and audiology services be billed using the Current Procedural Terminology (American Medical Association Staff, 2001) system. However, despite this general agreement, considerable variability exists from state to state and from one insurance company to another so that service providers need to be well informed regarding the "business" of their professions as well as the theory and practice (Iskowitz, 1999).

MEASURING EFFECTIVENESS

The speech-language pathologist determines readiness for dismissal from therapy largely by assessing its effectiveness. Did the client meet the long-term goals and short-term objectives? SLP-designed **post-therapy tests** similar to those used to determine baselines are normally used to answer this question. In addition, it is essential that the client has gained a degree of *automaticity* in the use of the communication target. If he or she has to stop and think each time, overall communication will be impaired, and the targets will not have been fully mastered. Errors will occur, however, and the client should be able to *self-monitor* and self-correct when needed. If therapy has been effective, the client has been successful in *generalizing* learned skills to the out-of-clinic world. This might require the SLP to observe the client in different settings, such as home or school. More often, the SLP depends on reports from others to assess this type of generalization.

FOLLOW-UP AND MAINTENANCE

After a client has been dismissed from therapy, the SLP must take steps to ensure that the progress that was achieved is not lost. This is done in two ways: Upon dismissal, the client or family should be encouraged to return when anyone feels a need. More reliable is the establishment of a regular follow-up schedule. The client may be contacted by telephone or letter every six months for a period of two years or so after the termination of therapy. At this time, retesting may be suggested, and **booster treatment** may be provided if needed. In **follow-up testing,** the SLP evaluates the client's communication skills to see that they are at least at dismissal level. This usually consists of a combination of conversational interaction and systematic probing of therapy targets. During booster treatment, the SLP reintroduces the therapy targets and addresses them again. Often different and abbreviated procedures are used, and the client returns to the dismissal level of accomplishment relatively quickly.

SUMMARY

Assessment of communication disorders requires an understanding of communication in context. Dialects as a result of geography, ethnicity, foreign language background, and other factors contribute to our communicative individuality. The SLP recognizes that dialects and differences do not constitute disorders. Communication behaviors, as much of life, can be viewed as occurring on a continuum.

Referrals and screenings are the primary ways in which individuals are selected for assessment. During assessment, the SLP verifies and defines the client's problem, identifies deficits and strengths, probes causality, makes a treatment plan, and provides a prognosis for improvement. This is achieved through multiple techniques, including sampling of communicative behaviors in several settings.

Assessment and treatment function in a cyclical fashion, with one influencing the other. In many ways, an SLP is assessing the client each time the client is seen in therapy. Successful intervention often uses a team approach that involves family members as well as professionals.

Provisions for follow-up ensure that the gains made in therapy are maintained. In the chapters that follow, techniques for assessment and treatment of specific communication disorders will be described.

REFLECTIONS

- What is meant by the continuum connecting communication differences, dialects, and disorders?
- What are the basic goals of communicative assessment?
- Why is it important to obtain information about a client from several sources?
- What are some differences you might expect to find as a result of systematic observation and formal testing?
- What are the major components of the International Classification of Functioning, Disability, and Health framework?
- How does a speech-language pathologist decide what to target for intervention?
- How is the success of speech and language therapy determined?

SUGGESTED READINGS

Bliss, L. S. (2002). *Discourse impairments: Assessment and intervention applications.* Boston: Allyn and Bacon.

Coleman, T. J. (2000). *Clinical management of communication disorders in culturally diverse children.* Boston: Allyn and Bacon.

Hamayan, E. V., & Damico, J. S. (1991). *Limiting bias in the assessment of bilingual students.* Austin, TX: Pro-Ed.

Haynes, W. O., & Pindzola, R. H. (1998). *Diagnosis and evaluation in speech pathology* (5th ed.). Boston: Allyn and Bacon.

Klein, H. B., & Moses, N. (1999). *Intervention planning for adults with communication problems: A guide for clinical practicum and professional practice.* Boston: Allyn and Bacon.

Klein, H. B., & Moses, N. (1999). *Intervention planning for children with communication problems: A guide for clinical practicum and professional practice* (2nd ed.). Boston: Allyn and Bacon.

Roth, F. P., & Worthington, C. K. (1996). *Treatment resource manual for speech-language pathology.* San Diego, CA: Singular.

Shipley, K. G., & McAfee, J. G. (1999). *Assessment in speech-language pathology. A resource manual* (2nd ed.). San Diego, CA: Singular.

ON-LINE RESOURCES

http://professional.asha.org/resources/multcultural/reading_6.cfm

American Speech-Language Hearing Association Multicultural Issues Board: Service delivery with multicultural populations. Includes references to cross-cultural differences in beliefs about health and disorder, strategies for professionals, and relevant statistics.

http://professional.asha.org/resources/multcultural/reading_4.cfm

American Speech-Language Hearing Association Multicultural Issues Board: Intervention with multicultural populations. Includes references to guidelines for determining the most appropriate language of intervention, cultural factors that impact on intervention, and selecting culturally sensitive materials and activities.

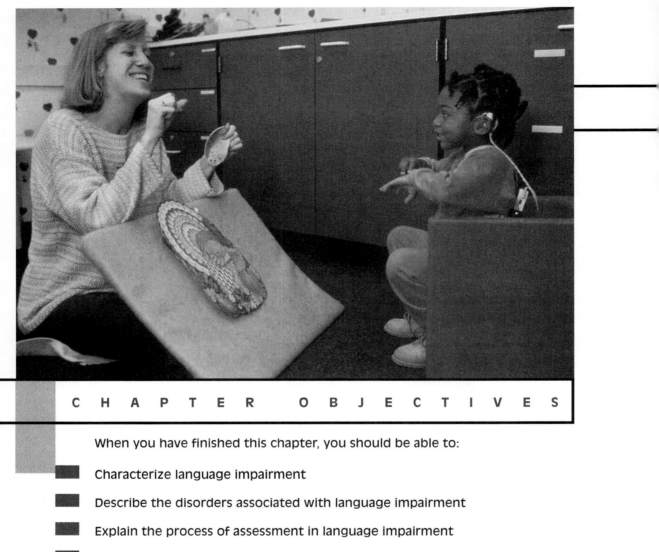

When you have finished this chapter, you should be able to:

- Characterize language impairment

- Describe the disorders associated with language impairment

- Explain the process of assessment in language impairment

- Describe the overall design of language intervention

Childhood Language Impairments

Language impairments are a complex group of diverse disorders and delays with a wide range of characteristics, levels of severity, and causes. Although some children may exhibit disorders in which language is inappropriate, inefficient, or ineffectual and others exhibit delays in which language is immature, in reality these differences are often difficult to isolate, and children may demonstrate both disorders and delays.

The term **language impairment** applies to a heterogeneous group of developmental and/or acquired disorders and/or delays that are principally characterized by deficits and/or immaturities in the use of spoken or written language for comprehension and/or production purposes that may involve the form, content, and/or function of language in any combination. Let's take this definition apart and examine it.

1. Children and adolescents with language impairment will be very different. The impairment may occur at any time within the life span of the individual and may vary in symptoms, manifestations, effects, and severity over time and as a consequence of context, content, and learning task.

2. The impairment may be the result of developmental abnormalities; may be acquired as the result of accident, injury, or other environmental factors; and/or may be delayed.

3. Deficits and/or immaturities may exist in one or more means of communication, such as listening/speech or reading/writing, and may affect receptive and/or expressive language. For example, preschoolers with language impairments are often less able to recognize and copy letters and less likely to write and draw every day, to pretend to read, and to ask questions during parental reading (Marvin & Wright, 1997).

4. One or more aspects of language—form, content, and use—may be affected. For example, as a group, children with language impairment have shorter, less elaborated sentences than typical children their age (Greenhalgh & Strong, 2001).

Box 6.1 presents an example of the somewhat scrambled language that we might find exhibited by children with language impairment. It is unclear whether most children with language impairment exhibit impairments in other areas of development as well (Casby, 1997). In the classroom, children with language impairments are reticent to speak. Boys are more likely to be withdrawn in both the classroom and on the playground (Fujiki, Brinton, Isaacson, & Summers, 2001; Fujiki, Brinton, Morgan, & Hart, 1999). In addition, they may lack social maturity.

BOX 6.1

Example of Conversation with a Language-Impaired Child

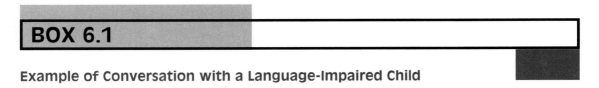

Teacher: Does your family have a pet?
Child: Yeah.
Teacher: Tell me about this pet.
Child: Got a pet.
Teacher: Um-hm, tell me about the pet.
Child: Got a pet.
Teacher: Yes, and I really want to hear about him.
Child: Go with my . . . ah, go with my . . . Dad go with . . .
Teacher: Your dad walks the pet.
Child: No, me.
Teacher: Oh, you and your dad walk the pet.

Child: No, me.
Teacher: Oh, just you walk the dog.
Child: No, me.
Teacher: I'm confused.
Child: Me dog.
Teacher: Oh, it's your dog. Who walks your dog?
Child: With one of them things, you know.
Teacher: What things? Who walks your dog?
Child: With them things like this.
Teacher: Yes, you use a leash.

Noticeably absent from our definition are language differences, such as those found in some dialectal speakers and in **limited English proficient** individuals learning English as a second language. Differences do not in themselves constitute language impairments and do not require clinical intervention by a speech-language pathologist, although elective intervention is possible at the client's request.

Theoretically, all speakers of a language should be able to communicate. Some differences are so great as to impair communication, but these differences still might not qualify as a disorder.

T H O U G H T   Q U E S T I O N

How's your Urdu or Farsi? Few Americans know these languages, which are spoken in parts of India and in Iran, respectively. If you don't speak either, do you have a language disorder? Of course not. But if you moved to Pakistan or Iran, you would need time to learn these languages or any of the others spoken there.

ASSOCIATED DISORDERS AND RELATED CAUSES

As you learned in Chapter 4, language and its use are extremely complex. It stands to reason, then, that language impairment would be even more so. So many things can go wrong at so many junctures that each child with a language impairment represents a unique set of circumstances. The speech-language pathologist is a detective trying to ascertain the type and extent of the problem and the appropriate method of intervention.

In this section, we discuss several disorders in which language impairment is a significant factor. Of necessity, we will be discussing groups of children under different categories of disorder. Categories are helpful for discussion of shared characteristics, but categories are not the same as individuals. Each individual is unique. We must be very careful when we label a child with a categorical name, because we might begin to expect less from that child.

T H O U G H T   Q U E S T I O N

Has anyone ever said to you "Oh, you're so intelligent"—or athletic, good-looking, or some similar trait? Did you then feel that you had to act a certain way around that person? Did you feel that this person treated you differently?

The effect that any disorder has on communication will vary with the severity of the disorder and the age of the client. As individuals mature, the communicative requirements change.

We will not be discussing all children with language impairment. The largest group to be excluded are individuals with hearing impairments. Many individuals who are deaf and not exposed to language early in life have language deficits. These individuals will be discussed in Chapter 14, "Audiology and Hearing Loss." Children may also exhibit impairments such as aphasia, which are generally considered to be adult disorders. Aphasia is a loss of language as the result of localized brain injury and will be discussed in Chapter 7, "Adult Language Impairments."

MENTAL RETARDATION/DEVELOPMENTAL DISABILITIES

According to the American Association on Mental Retardation, **mental retardation (MR)** is characterized by the following:

1. Substantial limitations in present functioning
2. Significantly subaverage intellectual functioning
3. Concurrent related limitations in two or more of the following applicable adaptive skill areas: communication, self-care, home living, social skills, community use, self-direction, health and safety, functional academics, leisure, and work
4. Manifestation before age 18 (American Association on Mental Retardation, 1992)

Mental retardation means more than just a low IQ. Values such as IQ usually measure past learning only.

Accounting for approximately 2.5 percent of the population, people with mental retardation/developmental disability are different from each other. The severity of the disorder will vary with causality and other factors such as the amount of home support, the living environment, education, mode of communication, and age.

T H O U G H T   Q U E S T I O N

Could you ever become mentally retarded? No, according to the definition, because you're over 18. You might acquire some other problem that would impair your performance, such as a head injury, but MR is a developmental disorder and, by age 18, most of development is complete.

Severity classifications are usually based on the level of IQ and range from mild to profound. Ranges of severity and characteristics are presenting in Table 6.1. However, a rating that is based only on IQ may reveal little about overall functioning. Each individual is different, and IQ is only one measure of overall functioning. For example, relatively high social skills may either mask or compensate for low intelligence. In addition, similar IQs in individuals with different ages will result in very different skill levels.

TABLE 6.1

Severities of mental retardation/developmental disability

Category	IQ Range	% of MR Population	Characteristics
Mild	52–68	89	Usually absorbed into the community where they work and live independently
Moderate	36–51	6	Capable of learning self-care skills and working within a sheltered environment; live semi-independently, with relatives, or in a community residence
Severe	20–35	3½	Capable of learning some self-care skills and are not totally dependent; often exhibit physical disabilities and deficits in speech and language
Profound	Below 20	1½	Capable of learning some basic living skills but require continual care and supervision; often exhibit severe physical and/or sensory problems

Source: Reprinted by permission from Owens, R. E. (1997). Mental retardation: Difference and delay. In D. K. Bernstein & E. Tiegerman (Eds.), *Language and Communication Disorders in Children* (4th ed.). Boston: Allyn and Bacon.

Causes of retardation are almost as varied as individuals with the disorder. Two large categories of possible causal factors are biological and socioenvironmental, although for many individuals, the cause is unknown. These factors are complicated by processing limitations that affect the cognitive handling of incoming and outgoing information. Biological factors include the following:

Genetic and chromosomal abnormalities, such as fragile X and Down syndromes
Maternal infections during pregnancy, such as rubella and sexually transmitted diseases
Toxins and chemical agents, such as fetal alcohol syndrome and lead poisoning

Nutritional and metabolic causes, such as inadequate diet and
phenylketonuria, an inability to synthesize an amino acid
present in many protein sources

Gestational disorders affecting development of the fetus, such as
malformation of the skull

Complications from pregnancy, such as extreme prematurity at
birth

Complications from delivery, such as anoxia, a loss of oxygen

Brain diseases, such as cancer and Huntington's disease.

Those with biological causes are likely to have more severe forms of MR.

Socioenvironmental factors include a stimulation-impoverished
environment, poor housing, inadequate diet, poor hygiene, and lack of
medical care. The exact effect of each of these factors is unknown and
varies with each child. It is clear that parental, especially maternal, behaviors are not a major cause of mental retardation. In general, parents
interact with their children at the child's language level, whether the
child has MR or is developing typically.

Information processing consists of four steps: attending, discriminating, organizing, and retrieving. In general, individuals with mild-
moderate MR can sustain attention as well as mental-age-matched
non-MR peers but have difficulty scanning and selecting stimuli to
which to attend.

The ability to discriminate likenesses and differences is related to
the severity of mental retardation. The more severe the mental retardation, the more difficulty the person will have in discriminating. In
general, individuals with MR are limited in their ability to identify relevant cues and attend to all dimensions of a task. For example, a child
may be able to match shapes but have difficulty matching both color
and shape.

Incoming linguistic information undergoes several types of decoding. Simultaneous synthesis occurs all at once and extracts overall meaning. Successive synthesis is more linear, occurring a piece at a time.
Although individuals with MR exhibit some difficulty with both types,
those with Down syndrome have much greater difficulty with successive processing, possibly reflecting poor short-term auditory memory.

Organization or the categorizing of information for storage is especially challenging for individuals with MR. In short, they do not rely
on strategies that link words and concepts to one another. Nor do they
spontaneously rehearse information for easy retrieval.

Memory or retrieval of previously stored information is poor and
operates more slowly within the MR population. Organizational
deficits contribute to this performance. Humans generally retain information by rehearsal, but those with MR do not seem to use this strategy spontaneously. To some extent, memory is affected by the type of

Individuals with mental retardation may process incoming sensory information differently from those without retardation.

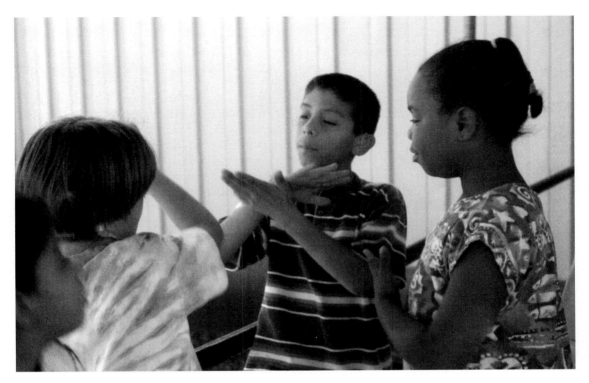

Some children with speech and language impairment
learn to communicate using alternative methods.

information (Kay-Raining Bird & Chapman, 1994). Individuals with MR
have more difficulty with auditory input, especially linguistic, than
with visual input.

LIFE SPAN ISSUES

Some neonates and infants with MR will be identified early because
of obvious physical factors, such as syndromes or anatomical anomalies, at-risk indicators such as low birthweight or poor physical responses, or delayed development. Intervention may begin at home or
in special early intervention centers. It is best for the child if intervention begins as soon as possible. Early intervention will focus on
sensorimotor skills, physical development, and social and communicative abilities. An Individualized Family Services Plan (IFSP) is written with specified services.

Some children with MR are not identified until age 2 or 3. These youngsters, along with those previously identified, will likely attend a special preschool. They may also receive some intervention services, such as physical therapy, special education, or speech-language therapy in the home.

Depending on the severity of a school-age child's mental retardation, she or he may attend a regular education class and receive special services within that environment. For some, this type of inclusion is not possible. These children will receive education in a self-contained classroom. Education and training will focus on academic skills, daily living and self-help activities, and vocational needs.

Only those children with the most profound MR accompanied by other disabilities are institutionalized. Usually, even these individuals are not placed in the huge warehouselike institutions of just a half-century ago. Generally, children who cannot reside at home live in community residences with eight to ten other children their age and houseparents.

Mike, a boy with profound MR and cerebral palsy, lived at home with his parents as an infant and preschooler. As he matured and his parents aged, Mike was placed in a community residence run by the Association for Retarded Citizens. He received daily care at this center and was able to continue his education at the same school. Most of his training involved daily living skills and use of a communication board to communicate.

In adulthood, living and working arrangements vary widely. People with milder retardation often live in the community and work competitively in minimally skilled jobs. More severely involved individuals may live with family or in community residences containing a small group of similar adults. They may work in a special workshop or be enrolled in a day treatment program in which education and training continue to be the focus.

LANGUAGE CHARACTERISTICS

For many individuals with MR, language is the single most important limitation. Low intellectual functioning alone, however, does not fully explain poor language. For 50 percent of the MR population, language comprehension and/or production is below the level of cognition (Miller, Chapman, & MacKenzie, 1981). This might be indicative of cognitive processing problems that accompany MR. For example, children with Down syndrome exhibit auditory short-term memory deficits (Seung & Chapman, 2000).

In general, both qualitative and quantitative differences exist between the language of children with MR and that of children who develop typically, although these differences vary across the life span (Weiss, Weisz, & Bromfield, 1986). In initial language development, in-

Very few individuals with mental retardation live in large institutions. Beginning in the 1970s, a philosophy called deinstitutionalization has been responsible for the movement of individuals with MR into small community residences.

dividuals with MR follow a similar but slower developmental path than that of typically developing children. Even so, children with MR produce shorter, less elaborated utterances—a quantitative difference. Individuals with MR use more immature forms (Boudreau & Chapman, 2000). In later development, the paths begin to differ more qualitatively. All areas of language exhibit some delay and disorder in children with MR.

LEARNING DISABILITIES

The National Joint Committee on Learning Disabilities (1991) defines learning disabilities (LD) as follows:

> a generic term that refers to a heterogeneous group of disorders manifested by significant difficulties in the acquisition and use of listening, speaking, reading, writing, reasoning, or mathematical abilities. These disorders are intrinsic to the individual and are presumed to be due to *central nervous system dysfunction.* Even though a learning disability may occur concomitantly with other handicapping conditions or environmental influences, it is **not** the direct result of those conditions or influences. (p. 19)

Approximately 15 percent of children with LD have their major difficulty with motor learning and coordination, while more than 75 percent primarily have difficulty learning and using symbols (Miniutti, 1991). This latter group is said to have a **language-learning disability.** Many children are atypical in both motor and language functioning.

Learning disabilities affect males four times as frequently as they do females. Approximately 3 percent of all individuals have LD, but the severity varies widely.

The characteristics of LD fall into six categories: motor, attention, perception, symbol, memory, and emotion. Few children will exhibit all of the characteristics described. Motor difficulties may include either hyperactivity or hypoactivity. Hyperactivity or overactivity is more prevalent, especially among boys. This results in difficulty attending and concentrating for more than very short periods. Children with hypoactivity may be deficient in their sense of body movement, definition of handedness, eye-hand coordination, and space and time conceptualization.

Attentional difficulties include a short attention span, inattentiveness, and distractibility. Irrelevant stimuli may capture the child's attention, and overstimulation easily occurs. Some children become fixed on a single task or behavior and repeat it, a process called *perseveration.*

Those who have hyperactivity and attentional difficulties but do not manifest other characteristics of LD may be labeled as having **attention deficity hyperactivity disorder (ADHD).** Children with ADHD

Children with language learning disabilities have difficulty learning and using symbols for speaking, listening, reading, and writing.

have an underlying impairment of the executive function in the brain that regulates behavior; as a result, they are impulsive. Although these children have difficulty using language socially and educationally, they may be missed on testing that ignores pragmatics (Oram, Fine, Okamoto, & Tannock, 1999).

Perceptual difficulties involve interpretation of incoming stimuli. This disorder is not a sensory one, such as deafness or blindness. Children with perceptual disabilities often confuse similar sounds, similar-sounding words, and similar-looking printed letters and words. In addition, children with LD may have difficulty both in determining where to focus their attention and in integrating sensory information from different sources, such as vision and hearing. Those children having particular difficulty in comprehending printed symbols may be labeled *dyslexic*. **Dyslexia** is characterized by word recognition and/or reading comprehension problems that may reflect underlying deficits. Slower letter- and word-naming speeds, reflecting insufficient phonological processing abilities, impede decoding and word-recognition processes (Kamhi, 1998). Children with dyslexia also exhibit delayed language development, listening comprehension problems, and poor phonological awareness (Catts, 1996).

Children who have difficulty producing written symbols are said to have **dysgraphia.** Often persisting into adolescence and adulthood, dysgraphia is characterized by spelling errors, word omission and substitution, punctuation errors, agrammatical sentences, and a lack of organization. A sample of the writing of a child with dysgraphia is presented in Figure 6.1.

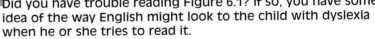

T H O U G H T   Q U E S T I O N

Did you have trouble reading Figure 6.1? If so, you have some idea of the way English might look to the child with dyslexia when he or she tries to read it.

Memory difficulties affect short-term retrieval, as in remembering directions, and long-term retrieval as in recalling names, sequences, and words. Some children also will exhibit word-finding problems. The resultant blocks and the use of fillers ("Ah, ah, you know . . . ") or circumlocutions ("Oh, it's that thing that does that stuff that goes round . . . ") may resemble similar behaviors in stutterers, discussed in Chapter 8 (German & Simon, 1991).

Emotional problems are usually an accompanying factor, not a causal factor. They are a reaction to the frustration that these children feel. Although most children with LD have normal intelligence, they perform poorly on language-based tasks and are told that they are not

Learning disabilities are not caused by emotional disorders; rather, the emotional problems result from misperception and from frustration.

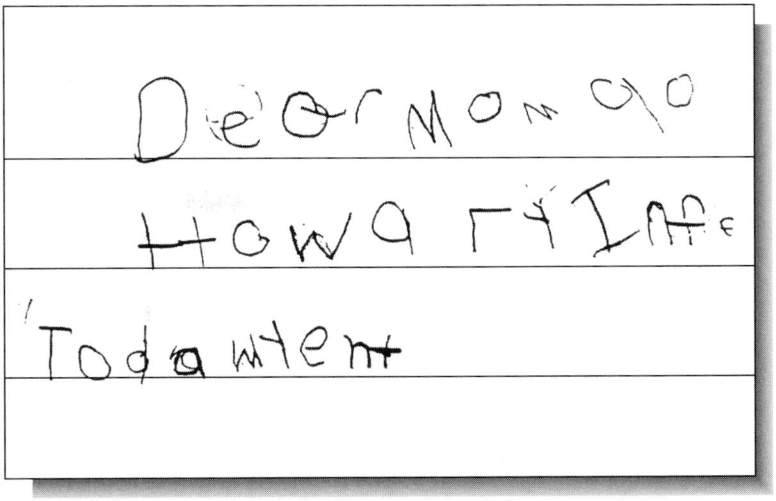

FIGURE 6.1 Sample writing of an 11-year-old child with dysgraphia

Dear mom and dad, How are you? I am fine. Today we went . . .

trying or that they're lazy or stupid. Emotional behavior may result in children being described as aggressive, impulsive, unpredictable, withdrawn, and/or impatient. These youngsters may exhibit poor judgment, unusual fears, and/or poor adjustment to change.

The fact that LD occurs more frequently in families with a history of the disorder and in children who had a premature or difficult birth suggests possible biological causal factors. The central nervous system or brain dysfunction mentioned in the definition is believed to involve a breakdown along the neural pathways that connect the midbrain with the frontal cortex, an area that is responsible for attention, regulation, and planning of cognitive activity (Bass, 1988).

Biological factors alone are insufficient to explain the characteristics seen in LD. Socioenvironmental factors may account for some of the behaviors. For example, misperceptions by the child affect interactions, which influence the child's development, especially language. Language difficulties, in turn, affect the child's interactions.

Processing difficulties are characterized by an inability to use certain strategies or to access certain stored information. In general, children with LD exhibit poor ability to selectively attend, concentrating on inappropriate or unimportant stimuli (Levine, 1987). They have difficulty deciding on the relevant information to which to attend. As we have seen, discrimination is extremely difficult because children with LD are not sure of the relevant aspects of a stimulus that make it similar or dissimilar to another.

Information that is poorly attended to and poorly discriminated will be poorly organized. The cognitive organization of children with LD reflects this confusion. In short, the organization is too inefficient for easy retrieval, so memory is less accurate and retrieval is slower.

LIFE SPAN ISSUES

Most learning disabilities are not discovered until children go to school, although some children may be enrolled in special preschool programs or may receive therapy services because of poor motor coordination, hyperactivity, or a failure to develop language typically. When they reach school and its accompanying demand for language skills, many children with LD require the services of special educators, speech-language pathologists, and reading specialists. Some children might not be identified in early grades and devise their own strategies for accomplishing academic tasks. Very bright children may "learn" to read by memorizing word shapes rather than using phonics-based word-attack skills.

Many children with LD receive special services while being included in regular classrooms. They can be successful if some adaptation, such as repeating instructions or allowing for a quiet work space, is made by the teacher to accommodate their needs. Box 6.2 tells the story of one child with language learning disability.

Some children with LD seem to outgrow their disability. Hyperactivity seems to fade in adolescence. Some adolescents succeed well enough to continue their education and graduate from college. We know adults with learning disabilities who are chemists, engineers, teachers, and speech-language pathologists. Even many successful adults have some lingering vestiges of their learning disability.

Other adults continue to have difficulty. Matt received special services throughout his school years and finished high school. His language difficulties were complicated by a volatile temper and frequent misinterpretations of the communicative intentions of others. After being fired from a series of jobs, he hit upon the idea of informing his new boss that he was "partially deaf" and needed all instructions and feedback repeated while he watched the speaker. He no longer flies off the handle when given a simple directive by his supervisor.

LANGUAGE CHARACTERISTICS

All aspects of language, spoken and written, usually are affected in children with language-learning disabilities (Wallach & Butler, 1995). These

BOX 6.2

Personal Story of a Child with Language Learning Disabilities

Darren's language learning disability went undetected until second grade. As a preschooler, he had some difficulty with speech sounds and displayed little interest in books, letters, or drawing. His mother considered his lack of interest and his overactivity to be a "boy thing." Darren received no preschool education. In first grade, he was slow to learn to read and write as were several of his classmates.

When Darren still seemed to be struggling in second grade, his teacher suggested an evaluation to determine whether he had a learning disability. He was evaluated by the school psychologist, a reading specialist, a special education teacher, and a speech-language pathologist. It was found that Darren's mother had received little, if any, prenatal care and that Darren was born preterm, weighing only 4 pounds, 10 ounces. After a stay in the hospital of several days, Darren went home with his mother. The rest of his preschool years were uneventful, and he remained at home with his older sister and younger brother, experiencing the occasional middle ear infection or childhood illness. Although his sister exhibits no signs of a learning disability, Darren's younger brother does exhibit hyperactivity.

At age 11, Darren is a very active child who enjoys sports, especially soccer, which he plays with his best friend Carlos. Darren has great difficulty reading and writing, and letter and word reversal and transposition are common in both. He has great difficulty sounding out new words. His speech is characterized by word retrieval problems and a limited vocabulary, peppered with "Ya know," "thing," and "one," as in "An' I got that one, ya know, that thing that goes like this."

Darren has had some difficulty behaving in school. His attention easily wanders and he fidgets in his seat often. If he is not kept busy, he bothers the other students and keeps them from working. He finds himself in frequent fights in school, usually because he has misunderstood some comment of another student. His temper flares easily, possibly because school can be very frustrating.

Although his schoolwork has improved somewhat, he is still well behind his classmates in his ability to read, write, and work independently. This deficit, in turn, has inhibited his ability to problem solve and to think critically in class. He continues to receive tutoring in reading and writing and to see the speech-language pathologist weekly to work on vocabulary, word retrieval, and language use skills.

children experience difficulty with the give-and-take of conversation and with the form and content of language. Synthesizing of language rules is particularly difficult, resulting in delays in morphological rule acquisition and in the development of syntactic complexity. As a result, overall oral language development may be slow, and frequent communicative breakdown is possible (MacLachlan & Chapman, 1988).

Attentional, discriminatory, and memory deficits along with both receptive and expressive symbol use problems can result in many communication breakdowns.

Word-finding problems are found in both conversations and narratives (German, 1987). As a result, greater time may be needed to respond verbally.

As preschoolers, children with LLD may exhibit little interest in language or even in books. When a child reaches school, the linguistic demands of the classroom are often well above her or his oral language abilities. The result is often academic underachievement. Language deficits are evident in written as well as spoken language. Poor working memory and attending may hinder recall of written material (Wright & Newhoff, 2001). Writing is characterized by grammatical errors, especially omission of morphological markers (Windsor, Scott, & Street, 2000).

Some children with LLD experience disfluent speech that on the surface might seem like stuttering. Called **cluttering,** the behaviors are characterized by overuse of fillers and circumlocutions associated with word-finding difficulties, rapid speech, and word and phrase repetitions. Unlike the situation with stuttering, the child seems barely to recognize his or her disfluency, and no fear of words or speech situations seems to exist.

SPECIFIC LANGUAGE IMPAIRMENT

Some children exhibit significant limitations in language functioning that cannot be attributed to deficits in hearing, oral structure and function, general intelligence, or perception. In other words, no obvious anatomical, physical, intellectual, or perceptual cause seems to exist. When this occurs, these children are said to possess a specific language impairment (SLI).

Similar to those with LLD, children with SLI exhibit language performance scores that are significantly lower than their intellectual performance scores on nonverbal tasks. The major distinction between those with LLD and SLI is that those with SLI do not exhibit perceptual difficulties, the misinterpretation of incoming information.

Although mostly preschoolers, children with SLI are a very heterogeneous group, especially in their language skills. Because the disorder is characterized primarily by the exclusion of other disorders, some professionals doubt the very existence of the disorder (Kamhi, 1998). Still, there are many children with language impairment for whom no readily identifiable causal factors exist.

If causal factors do exist, they may be very diverse. Biological factors point to a cortical or subcortical disorder, possibly brain asymmetry, in which language functions are located in different areas from those found in the majority of individuals (Aram & Eisele, 1994). A reported adeptness in analyzing visual spatial patterns may indicate greater reliance on the right hemisphere than found in most children.

Finally, language problems may also be the result of delayed myelination (Galaburda, 1989; Hynd, Marshall, & Gonzalez, 1991). Familial factors are also strong, especially for those with expressive difficulties (Lahey & Edwards, 1995).

Children with SLI do exhibit some information-processing problems with certain types of incoming sensory information, memory, and problem solving (Kamhi, 1998; Weismer & Hesketh, 1996). Short-term auditory sequential memory and problem solving in complex reasoning tasks are affected (Kamhi, Gentry, Mauer, & Gholson, 1990). Limits in verbal working memory suggest that children with SLI have a limited capacity for language processing (Weismer, Evans, & Hesketh, 1999).

> There is no single, obvious cause for specific language impairment.

LIFE SPAN ISSUES

Many children with SLI are later identified as having a language-learning disability. Lingering effects of SLI may result in reading difficulties that reflect difficulty with earlier language skills, such as rhyming, letter naming, and concepts related to print (Boudreau & Hedberg, 1999). In general, children with SLI exhibit slower and poorer processing of both linguistic and nonlinguistic material even in elementary school (Miller, Kail, Leonard, & Tomblin, 2001; Weismer, Tomblin, et al., 2000; Windsor & Hwang, 1999). Children with SLI are perceived negatively, even by other children, because their communication skills do not match expectations (Segebart DeThorne & Watkins, 2001). To date, long-term effects are unknown.

LANGUAGE CHARACTERISTICS

Children with SLI appear to be delayed in their language development but are unlike children developing typically at any stage of development. SLI is more than language delay. The language impairment may be primarily, but not exclusively, expressive or receptive or a combination of the two, and it may affect different aspects of language, although language form seems to be affected more than other aspects. The effect of the impairment changes with the age of and linguistic demands on the child.

In general, children with SLI have difficulty (1) extracting regularities from the language around them; (2) registering different contexts for language; and (3) constructing word-referent associations for lexical growth (Connell & Stone, 1992; Kiernan, Snow, Swisher, & Vance, 1997). As a result, these youngsters experience difficulty in morphological and phonological rule formation and application and in vocabulary development (Frome Loeb & Leonard, 1991; Oetting & Morohov, 1997). Pragmatic problems seem to result from an inability to use language forms effectively, resulting in more inappropriate utterances (Brinton, Fujiki, & Powell, 1997).

Language comprehension and processing are active processes, yet children with SLI do not appear to employ them actively. Auditory processing problems may result in difficulties with morphological inflections, such as past tense *-ed*, function words such as prepositions and articles (e.g., *a, the*), auxiliary verbs, and pronouns. Children with SLI exhibit persistent problems with morpheme use regardless of the language (Bedore & Leonard, 2001; Dromi, Leonard, Adam, & Zadunaisky-Ehrlich, 1999; Redmond & Rice, 2001), and they are less efficient in using syntax to aid in the acquisition of lexical items (Rice, Cleave, & Oetting, 2000).

AUTISM SPECTRUM AND PERVASIVE DEVELOPMENTAL DISORDERS

Autism spectrum disorder (ASD) is at the more severe end of an impairment known as **pervasive developmental disorder (PDD).** Depending on the severity of a child's disorder, the behavior might be labeled as ASD, or the child might be said to have varying levels of severity of PDD. Some children with PDD may have **hyperlexia,** an inordinate interest in letters and words, characterized by early ability to read but with little comprehension. Others have **semantic-pragmatic disorder,** characterized by limited vocabulary, concrete definitions, and poor conversational skills (Aram, 1997; Snowling & Frith, 1986).

Autism spectrum disorder is described as an impairment in reciprocal social interaction with a severely limited behavior, interest, and activity repertoire that has its onset before 30 months of age (American Psychiatric Association, 1987). It is characterized by disturbances in the following areas (Ritvo & Freeman, 1978):

- *Developmental rates and the sequence of motor, social-adaptive, and cognitive skills.* Development often proceeds in spurts and plateaus, rather than smoothly, and most areas of development are affected. Slightly more than half of the children with ASD have IQs below 50. The remainder are split evenly between IQs of 50–70 and IQs of 71 and above. These figures might not be accurate but rather represent our inability to test these individuals adequately.
- *Responses to sensory stimuli.* The same child may be both hypersensitive and hyposensitive in audition, vision, tactile stimulation, motor, olfactory, and taste. The child might have preferences for routines and become extremely upset with change. In addition, the child might engage in self-stimulatory behaviors, such as hand flapping, rocking, or spinning shiny objects.
- *Speech and language, cognition, and nonverbal communication.* Individuals with ASD may be nonspeaking, echolalic, or nearly typical in their communication.

- *Capacity to appropriately relate to people, events, and objects.* As infants, children with ASD are described as either lethargic, preferring solitude and making few demands, or highly irritable, with sleeping problems and screaming and crying. As they age, they may exhibit little affection and inappropriate play behaviors.

At this point, you may be suffering from *characteristics overload.* Stop briefly and try to recall the differences between MR, LLD, SLI, and ASD.

Early identification of children with ASD is often difficult because of the lack of obvious medical problems and the child's early development of motor abilities. Usually, between 18 and 36 months of age, the signs of ASD become pronounced, including frequent tantrums, repetitive movements and ritualistic play, extreme reactions to certain stimuli, lack of social play, and communicative difficulties. The toddler might avert her or his gaze or stare emptily and lack a social smile, responsiveness to sound, and anticipation of the approach of others. Often, parents are treated as things or, at best, no different from other people.

Few children are labeled as autistic. Usually, children are described as having "autistic-like" behavior or "autistic tendencies." More recently, children are described as having ASD or a severe form of PDD.

T H O U G H T   Q U E S T I O N

Might the world seem very different to you if you could perceive stimuli differently? Suppose that you had a dog's sense of smell. Could sensory differences alone explain the behavior of children with ASD?

The primary causal factors in autism are probably biological (Schreibman, 1988). Approximately 65 percent of all individuals with ASD have neurological differences and 20 to 30 percent experience seizures. In addition, some researchers have found unusually high levels of serotonin, a neurotransmitter and natural opiate, and abnormal development of the cerebellum, which regulates incoming sensations, and of sections of the temporal lobe responsible for memory and emotions. Finally, the incidence of ASD is higher among males—by a 4:1 ratio to females—and among those with a family history of autism. The family pattern suggests a genetic basis for the disorder, although no specific single gene has been directly linked to the disorder. The genetic basis is most likely complex and involves several genes in combination.

Some causal factors relate to processing incoming information. Individuals with ASD experience difficulty in analyzing and integrating information. Their responding is often very overselective, resulting in a tendency to fixate on one aspect of a complex stimulus, often some irrelevant, minor detail. As a result, discrimination is difficult.

Overall processing by children with ASD has been characterized as a gestalt in which unanalyzed wholes are stored and later reproduced in identical fashion, as in *echolalia*. The storage of unanalyzed wholes may account for the way in which individuals with ASD become quickly overloaded with sensory information. Storage of unanalyzed wholes also might hinder memory. It's difficult to organize information on the basis of relationships between stimuli if those stimuli remain unanalyzed. Lack of analysis would also hinder transferring or generalizing learned information from one context to another.

LIFE SPAN ISSUES

As was mentioned earlier, children with ASD are usually identified by the time they're 2 or 3 years of age. Parental concerns may involve lack of communication and/or lack of social skills. Toddlers may fail to begin gesturing or talking, seem uninterested in other people, lack vocal and verbal responding, or focus on an object intently. These young children are generally involved in early intervention and special preschooling.

Despite the lack of social and communicative behavior by their children, most parents of children with ASD are caring and concerned. When communicating, parents interact with their children with ASD at the appropriate language level.

School-aged children and adolescents with ASD or PDD may be included in regular education classes or be in special classes, depending on the severity of the disorder. For example, the child with mild hyperlexia might need the help of a reading specialist for interpreting the content of what he reads.

In some children, the severity of autism or ASD lessens with age. For example, as Jeffery became a teenager, his behavior seemed to be less disruptive, and there were fewer outbursts. Although he could engage in conversation easily, he continued to become annoyed and to begin flapping his hands if more than one person spoke at a time. People with milder forms of the disorder may be able to live on their own and hold competitive employment. For example, Dr. Temple Grandin, an individual with ASD, is employed as a college professor teaching agriculture. Unfortunately, the vast majority of people with ASD are not so successful and require supervision and care. Many have adult life patterns similar to those of adults with MR. Box 6.3 on page 180 presents the story of a young man with ASD.

LANGUAGE CHARACTERISTICS

Communication problems are often one of the first indicators of possible ASD. Between 25 percent and 60 percent of individuals with autism remain nonspeaking throughout their life. Those who speak often have a wooden or robotlike voice that lacks any musical quality. Many autistic children who use speech and language demonstrate some immediate or delayed echolalia, which is a whole or partial repetition of previous utterances, often with the same intonation. Mickey would say little during the day but store things said to him during the day and repeat them in sequence before he went to sleep at night. For some children, echolalia might either be a language processing strategy or signal agreement with the previous utterance. Even though echolalia may be outgrown, other problems, especially those related to pragmatics, persist in the child's language.

Pragmatics and semantics are affected more than language form (Lord, 1988). Conversations are particularly difficult. The range of intentions is often very limited and may consist solely of demands and seemingly self-entertaining gibberish. Some individuals incorporate entire verbal routines, called *formuli*, into their communication. For example, a child might repeat part or all of a television commercial to indicate a desire for the item that had been in the advertisement. A formula represents an attempt to overcome the difficulty of matching the content and form of language to the communicative context.

Individuals with ASD often have peculiarities and irregularities in their language, especially in the pragmatics of conversation. Adults with ASD who have good language skills might still misinterpret some of the subtleties of conversation. Syntactic errors seem to represent a lack of underlying semantic relationships. Phonological development appears not to be delayed, and the segmental aspects of phonology or sound characteristics are relatively unaffected. Prosodic phonology or suprasegmentals, such as stress, intonation, loudness, pitch, and rate, are often affected, giving the speech of children with ASD its sometimes mechanical quality.

Pragmatics is a continuing problem for individuals with autism, even those with seemingly typical language.

BRAIN INJURY

Brain injury can be confused with LLD, MR, or emotional disorders, although individuals with these disorders are very different. Injury and impaired brain functioning can result from **traumatic brain injury (TBI)**, cerebrovascular accident or stroke, congenital malformation, convulsive disorders, or encephalopathy, such as infection or tumors. Among children, the most common form of injury is TBI. Cerebrovascular accidents will be discussed in Chapter 7, "Adult Language Impairments." Individuals with brain injury differ greatly from one another as a result of the site and extent of lesion, the age at onset, and the age of the injury. In general, the smaller the damaged area, the better the chance of recovery.

Approximately one million children and adolescents in the United States have experienced TBI, which is diffuse brain damage as the result of external force, such as a blow to the head in an auto accident. Some individuals recover fully; others remain in a vegetative state.

Story of a Young Man with Autism Spectrum Disorder (ASD)

During high school and well into college, literal thinking and little imagination governed how I took a lot of information and interpreted much of the world. These factors also limited comprehension of what I read.

This was the central tenet of the larger picture: I suffered from autism. I was born with the disability. Compulsions and fixations changed with time, but varied little with intensity. My childhood was devoid of comfort, security, and pleasure; repetitious activities over which I exerted control filled a void . . . . For years I saw life's events in black and white, had a profound lack of imagination, and blocked out that which was not the compulsion of the moment.

My lack of imagination compounded my lack of self-esteem and other psychological problems that developed and fused as I got older . . . . I reacted angrily when someone inadvertently violated one of my arbitrary rules. I had a set no-tion of the order in which family members were to come to the breakfast table and where they should sit . . . My out-of-proportion anger when someone broke a rule that I could not articulate the need for caused . . . embarrassment . . . .

Numerous other life examples followed this pattern. I felt comfortable watching and being mesmerized by spinning objects such as a washing machine or a top. But a top's movement wasn't the only circular aspect of my autism. Later, the more severe my autistic behavior was, the more I alienated people; the more I alienated other kids, the more I withdrew. And the more I withdrew, the more my fragile self-esteem suffered, adding to the need to do repetitive activities for comfort.

All of this was my way of trying to relate to, and make sense of, a chaotic world. These behaviors provided short-term comfort and control . . . .

People with TBI exhibit a range of cognitive, physical, behavioral, academic, and linguistic deficits, any of which may be long-term in nature (Zitnay, 1995).

Cognitive deficits include difficulties in perception, memory, reasoning, and problem solving. Deficits vary and may be permanent or temporary and may partially or totally affect functioning ability.

Biological and physical factors affect functioning as well as informational processing. Children with TBI tend to be inattentive and easily distractible. All aspects of organization—categorizing, sequencing, abstracting, and generalization—may be affected. Children with TBI seem unable to see relationships, make inferences, and solve problems.

Unlike a fine wine, my life did not get better with age. Certain fixations disappeared over time, but were replaced with others. As a teenager, my speech, thinking, and relating to others was mechanical, rote, literal, and rigid . . . .[M]y most terrifying moments as a [h]igh [s]chool student occurred not in class, but between classes. My self-esteem was so low that when the halls exploded with 2,000 students, I felt on display. At times, I clung precariously to the wall's edge, holding on for dear life as I made my way to the next class . . . .

My slow recovery made me realize how much I missed and how much I didn't know. For years, I had little perspective about relationships; if people showed me positive attention, I would "absorb" them . . . . When I was flipping light switches off and on and doing numerous other compulsive activities, I wasn't bonding with other children. Years later, no sudden transformation took place that allowed me to naturally and spontaneously reach out to others . . . .

As my point of view expanded, I began to see how my behavior affected other people other than myself, and how socially inept I was. Soon, I began to turn years of unresolved anger and blame inward . . . . And I constantly feared I would one day regress. Such fears were "confirmed" whenever I reacted to stress in an autistic way . . . . Gradually, I reached a point where I could objectively discuss any aspect of my autism.

Unfortunately, not everyone will make a full recovery. Like most things in life, autism has varying degrees . . . . But I hope I've shown that there's nothing hopeless about it . . . . I'm free.

Source: From Barron, S. (2001, September 25). A personal story. *The ASHA Leader, 6*(17), 5, 7, 17. © American Speech-Language-Hearing Association. Reprinted by permission.

They have difficulty formulating goals, planning, and achieving their ends. Memory is also affected, although long-term memory before the trauma is usually intact.

Psychological maladjustment or "acting out" behaviors, called *social disinhibition,* may occur. Individuals with TBI may be incapable of inhibiting or controlling impulsive behavior. Other characteristics may include a lack of initiative, distractibility, inability to adapt quickly, perseveration, low frustration levels, passive-aggressiveness, anxiety, depression, fear of failure, and misperception.

Neural recovery over time is often unpredictable and irregular, and the variables that affect recovery of children with TBI are extremely independent. In general, a better recovery is signaled by a shorter, less severe period of unconsciousness following the injury, a shorter period of amnesia, and better posttraumatic abilities (Dennis, 1992; Russell, 1993). The age of the child at the time of injury is a less definitive factor because the child is developing when the injury occurs.

The age of the injury also can be an inaccurate predictor. In general, the older the injury, the less chance of change, although this can be complicated by the delayed onset of some deficits (Russell, 1993). For example, some neurological problems might not be manifested until later in recovery, making neural recovery unpredictable and irregular over time.

LIFE SPAN ISSUES

After the accident, an individual may be unconscious. The coma may last only a few minutes or much longer. Upon regaining consciousness, the individual usually experiences some disorientation and memory loss. Amnesia may involve only the time of the immediate accident or may be more extensive, including long-term memory. The disoriented individual might not recall what happened or understand the extent of his or her injuries or limitations. TBI may be accompanied by physical disability and personality changes.

When stabilized, the individual with TBI begins a long recovery process that can take years. Within the first few months, she or he might experience spontaneous recovery when large gains in ability are made.

Although the brains of younger children are more malleable or more adaptable, this does not mean that younger children will always recover more fully. In addition to recovering the language lost, younger children may still have much language to learn, a task that is possibly made more difficult by the brain injury.

Young children often recover quickly but experience difficulties learning new information later. Younger children may exhibit more severe and more long-lasting problems. Older children and adults have more to recover from their memory but less new information to learn. Even individuals who have made a seemingly full recovery may lack subtle cognitive and social skills. For example, Mary was a college student who had suffered TBI. She was able to succeed with minimal modifications in the classroom. Her main difficulties were in sustained attending and shifting tasks. In an evaluation, we found an inability to change *cognitive set* quickly. When you solve problems, you go about it systematically. If the problem changes, you change your way of thinking or your cognitive set. You can go easily from defining words to adding numbers. Mary could not.

THOUGHT QUESTIONS

Do you think intervention would be different for brain injury with a child who is learning language and an adult for whom development is complete? Why or why not? If so, how?

LANGUAGE CHARACTERISTICS

Language problems are evident even after mild injuries. Some deficits, especially in pragmatics, will remain long after the injury even when overall improvement is good. Overall, pragmatics seems to be the most disturbed aspect of language in both narratives and conversation. The child may lose the central focus or topic in both narratives and conversations (Chapman, Watkins, Gustafson, Moore, Levin, & Kufera, 1997). Utterances are often lengthy, inappropriate, and off topic, and fluency is disturbed.

Language comprehension and higher functions such as figurative language and dual meanings are also often impaired, although language form is relatively unaffected. Semantics, especially concrete vocabulary, is also relatively undisturbed, although word retrieval, naming, and object description difficulties may be present. Narration, especially maintaining story structure and providing enough information, may pose a problem (Chapman et al., 1997).

EARLY EXPRESSIVE LANGUAGE DELAY

Approximately 10 to 15 percent of middle-class U.S. children may be "late bloomers" whose early language development is delayed. Most outgrow it. Slightly fewer than half of these children, those with **early expressive language delay (EELD)** will continue to have problems. These children are at risk for academic failure when they begin school because they will not have the basic language skills for reading and writing in first grade.

Causal factors are difficult to identify. Nonverbal intelligence, birth and delivery, hearing, and self-help and motor skills all seem to be within normal limits (Paul, 1991). No obvious biological factors exist, although there is an increased prevalence in families with a history of speech and language problems. Otitis media, or middle ear infection, discussed in Chapter 14, may contribute, but it is not the sole cause. Nor are there any obvious socioenvironmental factors, although children with EELD are reportedly overactive and difficult to manage.

> Children with EELD will need some form of intervention in order to "catch up" with children developing typically. Children who are "late bloomers" catch up without professional help.

T H O U G H T   Q U E S T I O N S

Why might otitis media be a causal factor in EELD? Is hearing important for language learning? How?

LIFE SPAN ISSUES

Long-term data on children with EELD are sparse. Studies have indicated later academic difficulties, especially with language-based activities.

There is also some indication that even as adults, these individuals do not possess the language skills of their peers.

LANGUAGE CHARACTERISTICS

In general, children with EELD exhibit substantial delays in expressive language compared to their receptive understanding and nonverbal intelligence, although approximately 33 percent of these children also have poor comprehension. EELD manifests itself early, primarily as a lack of vocabulary development. As they mature, children with EELD begin to accelerate their vocabulary development, but language form greatly lags behind (Rescorla, Roberts, & Dahlsgaard, 1997). Although receptive language is not a good predictor of later expressive language, the gap between chronological age and expressive language at 30 months is (Ellis Weismer, Murray-Branch, & Miller, 1994; Rescorla & Schwartz, 1990). Problems persist in syntax and phonology (Paul, 1991). In turn, difficulties with language form affect pragmatics.

NEGLECT AND ABUSE

More than one million children are neglected or abused each year in the United States. Neglect and abuse are the outward signs of a dysfunctional family, the social environment in which these children learn language.

Although neglect and abuse are rarely the direct cause of the communication problem, the context in which they occur directly influences the child's development. Medical and health problems among poor Americans also can contribute, although neglect and abuse are not limited to poor families. Poor maternal health, substance abuse, poor or nonexistent pediatric services, and poor nutrition can all affect brain development and maturation.

Lack of maternal interaction rather than outright physical abuse accounts for much of the language impairment noted among children from abusive and neglectful environments.

The quality of the child-mother attachment is a more significant factor in language development than is maltreatment (Carlson, Cicchetti, Barnett, & Braunwald, 1989). Maternal attachment can be disturbed by childhood loss of a parent, death of a previous child, pregnancy complications, birth complications, current marital or financial problems, substance abuse, maternal age, and/or illness. The result is a lack of support for the development of meaningful communication skills with little active interaction, such as games, hugging, patting, nuzzling, and baby talk.

LIFE SPAN ISSUES

The affects of childhood abuse and neglect can remain with a child for life. There might be recurring physical, psychological, and emotional problems. Abuse or neglect, as was mentioned, is only a symptom of a dysfunctional family, and the situation might be complicated by drug and alcohol abuse, poverty, and poor health. Many children who have been abused abuse their own children later, thereby perpetuating this pattern with all its ill effects.

LANGUAGE CHARACTERISTICS

Although all aspects of language are affected, it is in pragmatics that children who have been neglected or abused exhibit the greatest difficulties. In general, they are less talkative and have fewer conversational skills than their peers. They are less likely to volunteer information or to discuss emotions or feelings. Utterances and conversations are shorter than those of their peers. In school, they have depressed oral and written language performance.

T H O U G H T   Q U E S T I O N

Why might an abused child have inappropriate pragmatics?

FETAL ALCOHOL SYNDROME AND DRUG-ADDICTED NEWBORNS

Within the last twenty years, there has been an increase in the prevalence of **fetal alcohol syndrome (FAS)** and drug-addicted newborns. FAS accounts for one in every 500 to 600 live births. Infants have a low birthweight and exhibit central nervous system problems. Later, they demonstrate hyperactivity, motor problems, attention deficits, and cognitive disabilities (Mallette, 1994). As a group, their mean IQ is in the borderline MR range.

The effects of drugs on the fetus vary with the drug, the manner of ingestion, and the age of the fetus (MacDonald, 1992). Crack is especially destructive and alters the fetus's neurochemical functioning. Like infants with FAS, those who are exposed to crack cocaine have low birthweight. They also have small head circumference and are jittery and irritable (Lesar, 1992).

LIFE SPAN ISSUES

Preterm babies, especially those with FAS or early drug exposure, are more likely to die during infancy and to experience developmental difficulties. The drug-exposed child's poorly coordinated behaviors and motor delays may disrupt caregiver-infant bonding (Crites, Fischer, McNeish-Stengel, & Siegel, 1992). In addition, caregivers who are addicted to alcohol or drugs might not attend or might reject the child. As a result, these children behave very much like children with learning disabilities. The limitations noted at birth remain with the child for life.

LANGUAGE CHARACTERISTICS

Children with FAS exhibit language problems characterized by delayed development of oral language, echolalia, and comprehension problems. Infants who were exposed to drugs have few infant vocalizations, inappropriate gestures, and delayed language. As preschoolers, they exhibit word-retrieval problems, short sentences, and inappropriate conversational turn taking and topic maintenance (Mentis & Lundgren, 1995). These difficulties persist and are compounded by problems with abstract meanings, multiple meanings, and temporal and spatial terms, such as *before* and *after*, *next* and *near*, *next to*, and *in front of*. Both children with FAS and those with fetal drug exposure are behind their peers in reading and other academic tasks.

CONCLUSION

There are so many disorders associated with language impairment that they probably all have begun to look similar to you. To help your memory, Table 6.2 presents the major characteristics of each disorder. In most cases, the child with a language impairment has other physical, cognitive, and psychological difficulties, too. In actual practice, speech-language pathologists treat each child as an individual, not as a member of a category. Of importance is each child's behavior and language features, not group characteristics.

ASPECTS OF LANGUAGE AFFECTED

In addition to the etiological categories we have just described, language impairments can also be characterized by the language features affected. For example, a child may have difficulty with word recall and with conversational initiation or possess a limited vocabulary and seemingly nonstop talking. Another child may have poor syntax and very short sentences or withdraw from conversational give-and-take. Table 6.3 presents the most common language features associated with language impairments. A sample of a school-aged child with a language impairment is presented on the accompanying CD-ROM. In an evaluation, speech-language pathologists assess many language features to determine where to begin intervention.

ASSESSMENT

Language assessment is a process of discovery and information gathering. As was noted in Chapter 5, good clinical practice requires that the

TABLE 6.2

Summary of disorders associated with language impairment

Disorder	Expected Deficit Area					Language Features Most Affected		
	Developmental	Cognitive	Perceptual	Affective	Unknown	Form	Content	Use
Mental retardation		X				X	X	X
Language learning disability			X			X	X	X
Specific language impairment					X	X		
Autism				X				X
Traumatic brain injury		X		X				X
Early expressive language delay	X					X		
Neglect and abuse	X							X

boundary between assessment and intervention be permeable. A portion of any good assessment is attempting to determine possible avenues for intervention. In turn, each intervention session should contain some assessment of the client's current skill level.

REFERRAL AND SCREENING

Referral may occur at any point in the life span. Some children, such as those with identifiable syndromes or those who are at risk for developing a language impairment, might be referred at birth or early infancy; others with LLD might go undetected until they begin

TABLE 6.3

Most common language characteristics of children with language disorders

Pragmatics

Difficulty answering questions or requesting clarification

Difficulty initiating, maintaining a conversation, or securing a conversational turn

Poor flexibility in their language when tailoring the message to the listener or repairing communication breakdowns

Short conversational episodes

Limited range of communication functions

Inappropriate topics and off-topic comments. Ineffectual, inappropriate comments

Asocial monologues

Difficulty with stylistic variations and speaker-listener roles

Narrative difficulties

Few interactions

Semantics

Limited expressive vocabulary and slow vocabulary growth

Few or decontextualized utterances, more here-and-now; more concrete meanings

Limited variety of semantic functions

Relational term difficulty (comparative, spatial, temporal)

Figurative language and dual definition problems

Conjunction (*and, but, so, because,* etc.) confusion

Naming difficulties may reflect less rich and less elaborate semantic storage or actual retrieval difficulties

Syntax/Morphology

Short, uncomplex utterances

Rule learning difficulties

Run-on, short, or fragmented sentences

Few morphemes, especially verb endings, auxiliary verbs, pronouns, and function words (articles, prepositions)

Overreliance on word order, which takes precedence over word relationships

Difficulty with negative and passive constructions, relative clauses, contractions, and adjectival forms

Article (*a, the*) confusion

Phonology

Limited syllable structure

Fewer consonants in repertoire

Inconsistent sound production, especially as complexity increases

Comprehension

Poor discrimination of units of short duration (bound morphemes)

Impaired comprehension, especially in connected discourse such as conversations

Reliance on context to extract meaning

Wh- question confusion

Overreliance on nonlinguistic for meaning

school; and those with either TBI or childhood aphasia may be of any age. Adults may also suffer either TBI or a cerebrovascular accident, resulting in the loss of language. Adults will be discussed in Chapter 7.

In a public school, the speech-language pathologist (SLP) may refer a child for further testing on the basis of results of screening testing for speech and language problems. Screening tests, used to determine only the presence or absence of a problem, are routinely administered to all kindergarten and first grade students.

Screening tests may be inappropriate for some children of color because they infrequently appear in the sample of children used in norming the test (Rhyner, Kelly, Brantley, & Krueger, 1999). Surveys and parental questionnaires, reporting toddlers' vocabulary and grammar in English, Spanish and other languages, are also effective diagnostic tools and compare favorably with other language measures (Patterson, 2000; Rescorla & Alley, 2001; Thal, Jackson-Maldonado, & Acosta, 2000).

Referral and subsequent evaluation may occur within an interdisciplinary team of child specialists. The nature of many of the disorders mentioned previously may necessitate input from a pediatrician, neurologist, occupational therapist, physical therapist, developmental psychologist, special education teacher, audiologist, and speech-language pathologist.

CASE HISTORY AND INTERVIEW

The case history questionnaire and interview are the first steps in a formal information-gathering process. In addition to asking the questions presented in Chapter 5, the SLP will want to ask more specific questions relevant to language impairment. Questions would relate to language development, the language environment of the home, and possible causes for language impairment. Table 6.4 presents predictors and risk factors for language change in toddlers (Olswang, Rodriguez, & Timler, 1998). Possible questions are presented in Table 6.5.

Information from referrals, questionnaires, and interviews provides needed background information from which to begin investigating for possible language impairment and determining what that impairment entails.

OBSERVATION

Language is heavily influenced by the context in which it occurs. It is helpful, therefore, to observe a child using language in as many contexts as possible. Although it is not always convenient to observe in multiple contexts, a school-based SLP might observe in the classroom, while a clinic-based SLP might observe in the waiting room or during a freeplay period between the mother and child. In all assessments, testing and sampling periods provide an additional observational period.

T H O U G H T   Q U E S T I O N S

What behaviors might we hope to observe? Might we be interested in the behaviors of others, too? Why or why not?

TABLE 6.4

Predictors and risk factors of language change in toddlers

Predictors

Language

Production:

Small vocabulary with few verbs

Verbs mostly general-purpose, such as *want, go, got,* and *look,* and transitive or verbs that take a direct object

Comprehension: Six-month delay with large gap between production and comprehension

Phonology:

Few prelinguistic vocalizations and limited variety in babbling

Vowel errors and limited number of consonants

Fewer than 50% of consonants correct

Restricted syllable structure

Speech Imitation

Limited spontaneous imitations and reliance on direct modeling and prompting

Nonspeech

Play: Manipulating and grouping toys with little combination of play schemes and/or little symbolic play

Gestures: Few gestures or gesture sequences

Social Skills:

Behavioral problems

Few conversational initiations

More interactions with adults than peers and difficulty gaining entrance to activities

Risk Factors

Otitis Media: Prolonged and untreated

Heritability: Family member with persistent language and learning problems

Parents

Low socioeconomic status

Directive style of interaction rather than responsive

Extreme concern

Source: Adapted from Olswang, Rodriguez, and Timler (1998).

TABLE 6.5

Possible questions for questionnaires/interviews when a language impairment is suspected

Language Use

Does the child . . .

Ask for information? How?

Describe things in the environment? How?

Discuss things in the past, future, or outside of the immediate contest?

Make noises when playing alone?

Engage in monologues when playing?

Prefer to play alone or with others?

Express emotions or discuss feelings? How?

Request desired items? How?

What emotions does the child express? How?

What does the child do when requesting that you do something?

When wants attention?

When wants to direct your attention?

Conversational Skills

Does the child . . .

Initiate conversations or interactions with others? What are the child's frequent topics?

Join in when others initiate conversational activities?

Get your attention before saying something? How does the child do this?

Maintain eye contact while talking?

Take turns easily while talking? Interrupt frequently? Are there long gaps between your utterances and the child's responses? Will the child take a turn without being instructed to do so or without being asked a question?

Demonstrate an expectation that you will respond when he or she speaks? What does the child do if you do not respond?

Respond meaningfully or are the responses mismatched, off-topic, or irrelevant?

Ask for clarification? How? How frequently?

Respond when asked to clarify? How?

Source: Adapted from Owens (1999).

Demonstrate frustration when not understood?

Relay sequential information or stories in an organized fashion so that they can be followed? Does the child relay enough information?

Have different ways of talking to different people, such as adults and smaller children? Does the child phrase things differently for different listeners? Is the child more polite in some situations?

Seem confused at times? What does the child do when confused?

React more readily to certain people and situations than to others? If so, please describe.

When does the child communicate best/most?

How does the child respond when you say something? How does the child respond to others?

Form and Content

Does the child . . .

Know the names of common events, objects, and people in the environment? What information does the child provide about these (actions, objects, people, descriptions, locations, causation, functions, etc.)?

Seem to rely on gestures, sounds, or immediate environment to be understood?

Speak in single words, phrases, or sentences? How long is a typical utterance? Does the child leave out words? Are the child's sentences simple or complex? How does the child ask questions?

Use pronouns and articles to distinguish old and new information?

Use words such as *tomorrow, yesterday,* or *last night*?

Use verb tenses?

Does the child put several sentences together to form complex descriptions and explanations?

Does the child follow simple directions?

Behaviors that are observed will vary with the age of the child and the reported disorder. In addition to observing the child's communicative behavior, the SLP is also interested in the child's interests and the caregiver's style of communicating and method of behavior control. Table 6.6 presents some behaviors that might be observed during an assessment.

Hypotheses about the child's language impairment are formed during observation. These are either confirmed or negated during the remainder of the assessment and during intervention.

It is important for the speech-language pathologist to remain focused during observation. This requires that she or he define very carefully the behaviors and/or language features that are observed and fully describe the events preceding and following them. For example, one adolescent we knew would scream "Don't hit me" repeatedly. It was observed that this occurred when she was asked a question. The behavior was inconsistent. It was hypothesized that the type of question influenced the response. The hypothesis was confirmed by careful data collection in which the type of question and the factual nature and personal or emotional quality of the potential response were modified systematically. The young woman was more apt to respond "Don't hit me" to questions that were more personal and emotional.

Few formal observational tools exist. Speech-language pathologists, recognizing the importance of observation as a vital portion of assessment, are developing reliable measures (Kaderavek & Sulzby, 1998).

TESTING

Testing does not begin immediately. Initially, the SLP and child spend some time getting to know each other and building *rapport*. Testing might begin with less threatening tasks such as pointing to pictures named or responding to pure tone auditory testing. Task variability can affect test results for some children (Fagundes, Haynes, Haak, & Moran, 1998).

Standardized tests are administered to compare the child's performance to others of the same age. Other test results are more descriptive and allow the SLP to explore a child's strengths and weaknesses. In addition, descriptive results can confirm or negate findings from standardized tests and provide useful information for treatment planning. Standardized, norm-referenced tests are appropriate for determining if a problem exists, but may be less useful in identifying specific language deficits (Merrell & Plante, 1997). It is important to go beyond scores and to supplement this information with a description of the child's performance.

The SLP bases test selection on many factors, including the hypothesized impairment, language features targeted by the test, norming population, method of testing, ease of administration and scoring, and test philosophy. It is best to use a series of tests to ensure that

TABLE 6.6

Possible behaviors to observe during an assessment of language impairment

With whom child communicates
Purposes for child's communication
Effectiveness of child's communication
    Obvious patterns of breakdown
Maturity of child's language
    Utterance length
    Verb usage
    Complexity
Relative amounts of initiative versus responsive communication
Relative amounts of nonsocial versus social communication
Responsiveness of caregiver
Turn allocation, relative size of child's and caregiver's turns

many features are tested (Gray, Plante, Vance, & Henrichsen, 1999). At the very least, receptive and expressive aspects of language form, content, and use should be tested or sampled in some way. Some widely used tests and their characteristics are presented in Table 6.7.

Approximately 25 percent of SLPs are dissatisfied with language tests and another 50 percent are neutral (Huang, Hopkins, & Nippold, 1997). Test scores do little to describe the child's language deficits.

Test methodology varies widely. Some tests employ nonsense words rather than real ones. Children may be asked to form syntactically similar sentences, to make judgments of correctness, to reconfigure scrambled sentences, or to imitate exactly what they hear. Children may have to supply definitions, form sentences, or point to words named. All these tasks require different language skills. Unfamiliar tasks may prejudice the results against the child (Peña & Quinn, 1997). Remember, testing is an extraordinary situation being used to measure typical language performance. Examples of language test tasks are presented in Table 6.8.

The knowledgeable SLP is familiar with many tests and chooses the ones that will yield the information required about the child being assessed. The SLP must remain flexible and open-minded in making a diagnosis until all possible information has been gathered.

During testing, the SLP will probe the child's performance to try to identify possible effective intervention procedures. Of interest are

Testing is an extraordinary situation for most children. Typical performance is more likely to be displayed in language sampling.

TABLE 6.7

Characteristics of common language tests

Test	Source	Target
Carrow Elicited Language Inventory (CELI) E. Carrow-Woodcock	DLM Teaching Resources	Identifies children with language problems and can be used to determine which specific linguistic structures may contributing to the child's problems
Clinical Evaluation of Language Fundamentals—Preschool (CELF-Preschool) (1992) E. Wiig, W. Secord, E. Semel	Psychological Corp.	Expressive and receptive language skills: basic concepts, sentence structure, word structure, naming, recalling sentence in context, linguistic concepts
Clinical Evaluation of Language Fundamentals III (CELF-3) (1995) E. Semel, E. Wiig, W. Secord	Psychological Corp.	Expressive and receptive language skills: semantics, syntax, morphology, and memory
Fullerton Language Test for Adolescents, second edition (FTLA-2) (1986) A. R. Thorum	Consulting Psychologists Press, Inc.	Assesses linguistic processing to identify language-impaired adolescents. Auditory synthesis, oral commands, convergent and divergent productions, syllabication, idioms, and morphological competency.
Peabody Picture Vocabulary Test, third edition (PPVT-III) L. & L. Dunn	American Guidance Service	Receptive vocabulary
Preschool Language Scale, fourth edition (PLS-4) (1992) I. L. Zimmerman, V. Steiner, R. Pond	Psychological Corp.	Auditory comprehension and verbal ability
Test of Adolescent and Adult Language, third edition (TOAL-3) D. Hammill, V. Brown, S. Larsen, J. Wiederholt	Pro-Ed	Expressive and receptive language, semantic and syntactic skills assessed in spoken and written form
Test of Auditory Comprehension of Language—third edition (TACL-3) (1999) E. Carrow-Woodcock	Pro-Ed	Auditory comprehension of word classes and relations, grammatical relations, and elaborated sentences
Test of Early Language Development, 3rd ed. (TELD-3) (1999) W. Hresko, D. Reid, D. Hammill	Pro-Ed	Receptive and expressive language
Test of Language Development—Primary, 3rd ed. (TOLD-P:3) (1997) P. Newcomer, D. Hammill	Pro-Ed	Receptive and expressive language, semantics, syntax, phonology
The Word Test—Adolescent L. Bowers, R. Huisingh, M. Barrett, J. Orman, C. LoGuidice	Lingui-Systems	Expressive vocabulary and semantics

Age	Notes
3–8 years	Administration of the test takes 10 minutes, and scoring takes 1 hour and 30 minutes. Child's responses must be transcribes phonetically.
3–6 years	Meets PL 99-457 and PL 94-142 guidelines.
6–21 years	Provides a guideline for areas of language that are in need of further observation and testing. Takes 45 minutes to score and administer. Provides supplementary oral and written expression sections for additional information.
11–18.5 years	Standardized: provides means and standard deviation for each subset and age group. Three score breakdowns: competence level, instruction level, and frustration level.
2.5–90 years	A standard. Child points to one of four black-and-white pictures named.
0–6 years	Widely used. Wide variety of receptive and expressive tasks using pictures and toys.
12–25 years	Test requires reading and writing for some of the subtests; 1–3 hours to administer; can be administered to a group for 6 of 8 of the subtests; requires several separate booklets to administer.
K to grade 4	Individually administered, no oral response required. Child points to one of three pictures named.
2 to 7–11 years	Individually administered in about 30 minutes; normed on children from 35 states, representing U.S. population.
4 years to 8–11 years	Administered in about one hour; computer scoring is available.
12–17 years	Administration time: 25 minutes. Results: standard scores, percentile ranks, age equivalencies, no basal or ceilings. Is designed to assess a subject's facility with language and word meaning using common as well as unique contexts, surveys 4 semantic and vocabulary tasks reflective of school assignment, as well as language usage in everyday life.

TABLE 6.8

Examples of language test tasks

Test Procedure	Example
Grammatical completion	I'm going to say a sentence with one word missing. Listen carefully, then fill in the missing word. *John has a dish and Fred has a dish. They have two _____.*
Receptive vocabulary	Look at the pictures on this page. I'm going to name one, and I want you to point to it. *Touch (Show me) the officer.*
Defining words	I'm going to say some words. I want you to tell me what each word means or use it in a sentence in a way that makes sense. For example, if I said "coin," you might respond "money made from metal" or "I put my coin in the vending machine."
Pragmatic functions	I'm going to tell you a story and ask you to imagine what the person in the story might say. *Mary lost her money and she must call home for a ride after band practice. She decides to borrow a quarter from her best friend Julie. Before practice begins, she sits down next to Julie and says _____.*
Sentence imitation	I'm going to say some sentences, and I want you to repeat exactly what I say. Let's try one. *We are going to play ball after school tomorrow.*
Parallel sentence production	Here are two pictures. I'll describe the first one, and then you describe the second one using the same type of sentence as I use. For example, for this picture I would say, "The girl is riding her bike," and for this one you would say, "The man is driving his car."
Grammatical correctness	I'm going to say a sentence, and I want you to tell if it is correct or incorrect. If it is incorrect, you must correct it. For example, if I say, "Thems is going to the dance," you would respond, "Incorrect. They are going to the dance."

strategies that either increase production or result in more correct production of a certain language feature (Peña, Iglesias, & Lidz, 2001). Sometimes called **dynamic assessment** (Olswang, Bain, & Johnson, 1990), this probe is invaluable in providing direction for subsequent intervention. Dynamic assessment and techniques that ask children to demonstrate skills that represent realistic learning demands are especially well suited for multicultural populations (Schraeder et al., 1999; Ukrainetz, Harpell, Walsh, & Coyle, 2000).

SAMPLING

If language is influenced by context, then the context of test taking should influence the language a child produces. For some, the extra structure will enhance performance; for others, it will detract. The latter is especially true for young children, children from minority populations, and those with disabilities. In either case, the child does not give her or his typical performance.

Although interested in a child's typical performance, the SLP should also engage a child in challenging conversation, so that he or she will attempt to "stretch" language abilities and in the process reveal difficulties (Hadley, 1998). A variety of discourse types, such as conversation, narration, explanation, and interview, should be included in the sample.

Typical performance may be enhanced if parents or teachers interact with the child in familiar settings. The experienced SLP can also be an excellent conversational or play partner for the child. Whenever possible, it is best to collect at least two samples of the child with different partners, locations, and activities or topics.

T H O U G H T   Q U E S T I O N

Does sampling ensure that we will get a child's typical performance? Can you think of some contexts in which a child's typical language performance would not occur?

Samples may be either very open ended, in which topics and interactions are not defined, or more closed, in which the SLP tries to elicit specific language features. Question-answer techniques are more restricted and elicit fewer complex utterances than more conversational strategies (Bradshaw, Hoffman, & Norris, 1998). Narratives are especially helpful for exhibiting deficits in older children or those with TBI because of the demands on a speaker who must create his or her own context linguistically while manipulating plot and characters (Chapman, 1997). Table 6.9 presents two very different types of language samples. In addition, narratives tend to elicit a large number and variety of syntactic structures (Gummersall & Strong, 1999).

Language samples are recorded on videotape and/or audiotape for later transcription as soon as possible. The SLP transcribes both the child's and caregiver's utterances and records important contextual information. The SLP is careful to transcribe the child's exact words.

The language transcript can be analyzed in several quantitative and qualitative ways to determine the extent and nature of the child's language difficulty. Values such as the average length of the child's utterances in morphemes, referred to as the *mean length of utterance (MLU)*,

TABLE 6.9

Examples of different types of language samples

Open-Ended

Clinician: I'll play with this farm set, and you can too or you can pick another toy.

Child: Want farm.

Clinician: Oh, you want the farm. We can share. I wonder what should we do first.

Child: Open door. Animals come out.

Clinician: Okay.

Child: You be horsie and I man.

Clinician: Oh, the farmer.

Child: Farmerman chase horsie in barn.

Clinician: Oh, he did. I better run fast.

Child: Man go fast in barn.

Structured

Clinician: Well, here's the puppy. What should we say to him?

Child: Hi puppy. [GREETING]

Clinician: Hi Timmy. I'm hungry. We need to get someone to help us get those cookies.

Child: You help. Want cookie. [REQUESTING]

Clinician: I wonder how I can reach it.

Child: Get chair. [HYPOTHESIZING]

Clinician: Oh, get on the chair. Should I (mumble).

Child: Yeah. [DOES NOT REQUEST CLARIFICATION]

Clinician: You want me to (mumble)?

Child: What's that? [REQUESTS CLARIFICATION]

Clinician: Which do you want, the cookie or the chair?

Child: Want cookie. No chair. [CHOICE MAKING]

the average number of clauses per sentence, and the number of different words used within a given period of time can be compared to the values for typical children of the same age or developmental level (Johnston, 2001). Samples might also provide information on the percent correct for a language feature, such as past tense -ed. More descriptive measures might be the variety of intentions expressed by the child, the number of conversational styles used, and the types of repair the child uses when the conversation breaks down (Yont, Hewitt, & Miccio, 2000). Being as thorough as possible, the SLP attempts to analyze the sample for all aspects of form, content, and use appropriate for the particular assessment. For example, with bilingual clients, the SLP might consider **code switching** or the movement between two languages, dialect, English proficiency, and contextual effects in addition to aspects of both languages (Gutierrez-Clellan, Restrepo, Bedore, Peña, & Anderson, 2000).

For some school-aged clients, especially those who might have dyslexia, the SLP also will want to collect samples of written language (Greene, 1996). Writing requirements vary greatly with the written task. For this reason, several first draft samples collected over time are more valuable than a single one. Samples of inventive spelling or early attempts to write prior to formal instruction may be collected for pre-reading children as a snapshot of reading readiness (Lombardino, Bedford, Fortier, Carter, & Brandt, 1997). In addition, multiple samples offer a more holistic view of the child's language. Within school, a variety of written assignments may be collected to evaluate the proficiency and flexibility of written language (Manning Kratcoski, 1998). Called a **portfolio evaluation,** it can provide a record of changes in writing ability over time (Kratcoski, 1998).

INTERVENTION

The complexity of language necessitates a multiplicity of intervention methods. Different intervention approaches target specific aspects of language and employ a variety of procedures. Within limits, we shall explore these diverse approaches to remediation of language impairments.

Increasingly, SLPs are including other individuals from the child's environment in the training. For example, without training, day care providers fail to finely tune their language for individual children's needs (Girolametto, Hoaken, Weitzman, & van Lieshout, 2000). With the aid of the SLP, parents may learn how to be better language partners for their young children. Many successful models of the classroom collaborative model mentioned in Chapter 5 have evolved (Prelock, 2000). Even peers can serve as effective tutors or models for children with language impairments (McGregor, 2000).

TARGET SELECTION AND SEQUENCE OF TRAINING

The goal of intervention is the maximally effective use of language to accomplish communication goals within everyday interactions. For most interactions, the context is conversation. Effective use requires an understanding of the rules of different contexts, a knowledge of the symbols and their meanings, and an ability to use grammar flexibly. Although most SLPs would agree on this overall goal, less unanimity exists on the route to achieving it. Decisions on target selection and training vary with each child and each SLP.

Using different criteria, several SLPs might not select the same targets for the same child. A strict developmental model might suggest that a child achieve all behaviors within a given stage of language development before progressing to the next stage. A less strict developmentalist would use language acquisition knowledge as a general guide. A functional model would suggest that training begin at the point of communication breakdown and frustration. Classroom approaches might

The criteria for target selection will vary with the child, the affected aspects of language, the child's disorder, and the needs of the environment.

suggest training for language used within the class. Another approach might be to begin with language features that are emerging. Emerging features are produced correctly between 10 percent and 50 percent of the time.

Decisions must be made as to where to begin once the target is selected. Once again, the SLP must determine the point at which communication breakdown occurs. Some SLPs prefer to begin with receptive language training and progress to expressive. Others will start with expressive training. Expressive training may be bottom-up, in which one begins at the symbol level and works toward conversational goals; top-down, in which training is placed within a conversational framework; or a combination of the two. Obviously, the child's abilities are an important determiner of the method selected. It would be inappropriate to begin at a conversational level with the child not yet using any recognizable symbols to communicate; however, even this child's training should be placed within meaningful communicative contexts.

T H O U G H T   Q U E S T I O N S

Can you think of reasons why you might begin with receptive training? Expressive? At the individual symbol level? With conversation?

Some communities have chosen to give a lower priority to services to children with low cognitive skills accompanied by language problems. This seems counterproductive given the benefit these children derive from intervention (Cole, Coggins, & Vanderstoep, 1999).

INTERVENTION PROCEDURES

It is important to remember that speech-language pathologists, wherever they may work, are teaching communicative skills. A few basic tenets of good teaching behavior include, but are not limited to, the following:

- *Model the desired behavior for the client.* Modeling may include multiple exposures, called *focused stimulation,* that occur before the child is required to produce the language feature (Cleave & Fey, 1997). The need for modeling decreases as the feature is learned. Older elementary school children and adolescents may also benefit from an explanation of the targeted behavior and a rationale for why its correct use is important.
- *Cue the client to respond.* Carefully selected cues, such as the use of the word *yesterday* to signal a past-tense response, will serve as aids for the client in conversation. Cues may range from very specific, such as *say, imitate,* or *point to,* to more general

conversational cues, such as *I wonder what I should say now* to elicit a specific linguistic structure in context or *Maybe Carol can help us if we ask* to elicit a question.

Cues may be verbal or nonverbal. Verbal cues attempt to elicit the language feature by providing a linguistic framework; nonverbal cues use the context of an event to evoke the feature.

- *Respond to the client in the form of reinforcement and/or corrective feedback.* Reinforcement varies from very direct and obvious forms, such as "Good, that was much better," to more conversational responses. Conversational responses come in many varieties, including imitating the child, imitating but expanding the child's utterance into a more mature version, replying conversationally, and asking for clarification. With some clients, especially those with vocabulary deficits, the relationship of the responsive to the content of the child's utterance has more effect on the child's language than the structural input of the clinician's feedback (Girolametto, Weitzman, Wiigs, & Steig Pearce, 1999).

  Natural reinforcers flow from the training target. The most obvious example is one in which a child obtains a desired object upon responding to the cue "What do you want?" Conversational responses can be very natural.

  Corrective feedback may range from a gentle reminder to instruction. In general, as a language feature is produced more correctly by the client, the SLP relies less on both direct forms. When a client is using a language feature correctly, conversational feedback, such as "What?" or "I don't understand," may be sufficient to cause the client to self-correct.

- *Plan for generalization of the learned feature to the everyday use environment of the client.* SLPs can help generalization by selecting training targets that are highly likely to occur in the client's everyday communication and by including in the training elements of the everyday use environment, such as familiar locations, people, and objects. Parents are often included in the training of young children, while teachers may be involved in the intervention of school-age children and adolescents.

SLPs are teachers of language. They must plan their behaviors well to teach without overly relying on less natural strategies such as drill and the use of edible reinforcers.

Specific examples of each teaching tenet are presented in Table 6.10.

INTERVENTION THROUGH THE LIFE SPAN

Targets of intervention will vary with the age and functioning level of the client. An infant in an early intervention program would have different training targets than an adolescent with LLD. However, an infant may be receiving some of the same training as an adolescent who has profound retardation and is functioning below age 1 year. Although reasonable professionals disagree, it seems best to use at least

TABLE 6.10

Examples of teaching methods

Method	Example
Modeling	
Focused stimulation	I'll pretend to make a cake first. Watch to see if I make a mistake. I'm *putting* the eggs in the bowl and *taking* them to the table. I'm *cracking* the eggs. Now I'm *beating* the eggs. Next, I'm *sifting* the flour. I'm *adding* the flour to the eggs and *mixing* them. Now I'm *measuring* the sugar and *pouring* it into the mix. . . .
Cuing	
Direct Verbal	
Imitation	Say "I want cookie."
Cloze	This is a _____.
	She should say _____.
Question	What should I say now?
	What's this?
	Which one's this?
Indirect Verbal	
Pass it on	I wonder if Joan knows the answer. How could we find the answer? [TARGET IS FORMATION OF QUESTIONS]
Nonverbal (Inherent in the activity)	Not giving child all the materials needed to complete a task. Not explaining how to accomplish an assigned task. Playing dumb.
Responding	
Direct Reinforcement	Good, I like the way you said that. Much better than the last time.
Indirect Reinforcement	
Imitation	*Child:* I go horsie.
	Clinician: I go horsie.
Expansion	*Child:* I go horsie.
	Clinician: I'm going to go on the horsie.
Extension	*Child:* I go horsie.
	Clinician: Yes, cowboys go on horses too.
Corrective Feedback	Remember, when we use a number like two, three or more, we say "/s/" on the word. Listen. One cat. Two cats.

some instruction in both languages with children experiencing difficulties in both (Gutierrez-Clellan, 1999).

Early intervention, especially for children with MR and autism, can have very positive benefit. Initial training may target presymbolic communicative skills and cognitive abilities, such as physical imitation, gestures, and receptive understanding of object names. The SLP may attempt to establish an initial communication system using an augmentative/alternative communication system, such as gesturing, a communication board, or an electronic device. Augmentative/alternative communication will be discussed in more detail in Chapter 15. Parents may be trained to treat their child's behaviors as having some communicative value or to interpret consistent behaviors as attempts to communicate.

Early symbolic training may focus on vocabulary acquisition, semantic categories, word combinations, and an array of early intentions. The beneficial effects of treatment for children with delayed language extend beyond the trained targets into other areas of linguistic and overall development (Brand Robertson & Ellis Weismer, 1999).

Children at the preschool language level usually work on language form in both conversations and narratives. Longer utterances, bound morphemes, and early phonological processes may be intervention goals. Vocabulary development will continue to be targeted, especially relational words, such as conjunctions (*and, if, so*), temporal terms (*tomorrow, next*), spatial terms (*in front of, next to*), and prepositions (*in, on, under*).

Intervention with higher functioning children may focus on pragmatic skills in conversations and semantic targets, such as figurative language, multiple meanings, abstract terms, and more advanced relational terms. Academic skills, including summarizing a reading and different types of writing and note taking, may also be targeted. SLPs may use computerized programs to supplement more face-to-face intervention. These must be used with caution and should mesh well with the SLP's overall clinical philosophy and the child's individual needs (Gillam, 1999). Language enhancement—metalinguistics, phonology, and language use—can be infused into the reading curriculum (Fleming & Forester, 1997). Speech-language pathologists may work with the child on both spoken and written language. It is also important for children with language impairment to learn to navigate the curriculum and to understand expectations (Westby, 1997).

Language intervention doesn't end with childhood. Adolescents may continue to exhibit language impairments and be in need of services (Nippold, 2000). Adults with severe autism or MR will most likely require continued intervention for language and communication deficits and a range of self-care, educational, and vocational needs. Individuals with LLD, dyslexia, or dyspgraphia may require additional support in postsecondary education (Downey & Snyder, 2000; Olivier, Hecker, Klucken, & Westby, 2000).

SUMMARY

In this chapter, we have discussed several disorders that are associated with language impairment. It is sometimes difficult for beginning students to remember the differences between children with mental retardation, learning disability, specific language impairment, autism and pervasive developmental disorder, brain injury, early expressive language delay, neglect and abuse, and fetal alcohol syndrome and drug addiction. Refer to Table 6.2 for the major differences between these disorders.

As the definition and the many associated disorders suggest, language impairments are very complex and many faceted. We have only touched the surface in this chapter. The number of associated disorders, the language features that are affected, and the individual differences among children result in each child's language being very individualistic. It is very important to remember that each child is a unique case. Given this fact, assessment becomes the search to find and describe each child's individual language abilities. This is accomplished through referral, collection of a case history, interviews, observation, testing, and language sampling.

As a result of the assessment process and through repeated assessment during intervention, the speech-language pathologist attempts to find the most efficient and effective method for teaching new skills. The SLP identifies targets for intervention and trains these through a combination of techniques in various settings with the aid of additional language facilitators. Some children may just be learning to communicate and may need to use augmentative and alternative communication methods, while others are working to become more efficient conversationalists, and still others are learning word retrieval strategies.

Obviously, every SLP needs thorough training and extensive experience with a variety of language impairments to serve children with these disabilities. With a firm foundation of speech and language development, speech-language pathologists take several courses in language impairment in both children and adults and complete practica with both populations.

REFLECTIONS

- What are the characteristics of language impairment?
- What disorders are associated with language impairment? Describe each one briefly.
- What are the steps in a typical assessment in language impairment?
- What is the overall design of language intervention?

SUGGESTED READINGS

Nelson, N. W. (1998). *Childhood language disorders in context: Infancy through adolescence* (2nd ed.). Boston: Allyn and Bacon.

Owens, R. E. (1999). *Language disorders: A functional approach to assessment and intervention* (3rd ed.). Boston: Allyn and Bacon.

Lloyd, L. L., Fuller, D. R., & Arvidson, H. H. (1997). *Augmentative and alternative communication: A handbook of principles and practices.* Boston: Allyn and Bacon.

Reed, V. A. *An introduction to children with language disorders* (2nd ed.). Boston: Allyn and Bacon.

Sanders, M. (2001). *Understanding dyslexia and the reading process.* Boston: Allyn and Bacon.

ON-LINE RESOURCES

gopher://gopher.sasquatch.com

Traumatic brain injury gopher with lots of information.

http://www.asha.org   American Speech-Language-Hearing Association.

Information for members, students, and others who are interested in careers in speech-language pathology or audiology, and anyone with a concern about communicative disorders.

http://www.chadd.org   Children and Adults with Attention Deficit/Hyperactivity Disorders

http://www.autism.org   Center for the Study of Autism

http://www.asel.udel.edu/at-online/   Augmentative/alternative communication. Links and pointers to a variety of AAC topics.

http://www/irsc.org/down.htm   Down syndrome.

Index with many web links.

http://www.ldresources.com/

Variety of writing on language learning disability and software to download.

http://www.ninds.nih.gov.healinfo/disorder/autism/autism.htm

Autism fact sheet from NIH.

http://www.autism-society.org   Autism Society of America.

Information on education and an on-line glossary. Good consumer and practitioner information.

http://cnet.shs.arizona.edu/childneuro_list.html   National Center for Neurogenic Communication Disorders

Children's language disorders.

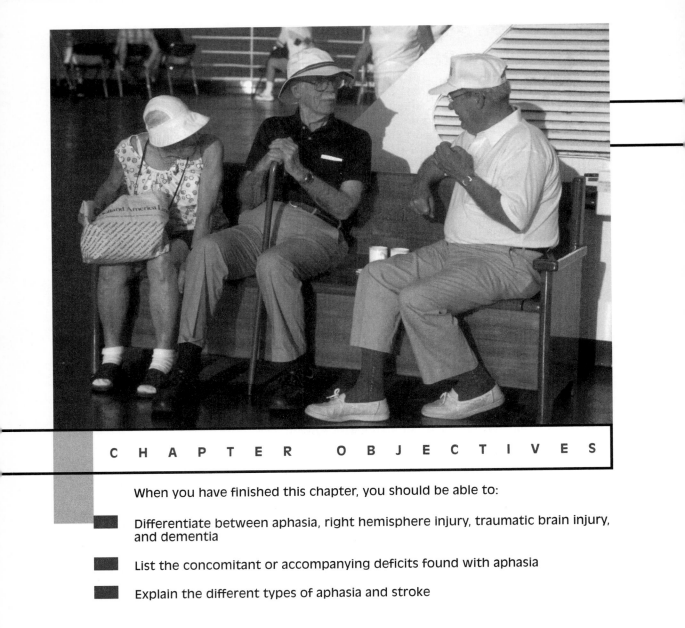

When you have finished this chapter, you should be able to:

- Differentiate between aphasia, right hemisphere injury, traumatic brain injury, and dementia

- List the concomitant or accompanying deficits found with aphasia

- Explain the different types of aphasia and stroke

Adult Language Impairments

Many language impairments found in childhood continue into the adult years. Mental retardation, autism, and learning disability do not disappear, although they may change or their effect on language may alter. Other language impairments may lessen or disappear, such as specific language impairment or early expressive language delay.

This chapter is not about those impairments. Rather, this chapter focuses on language disorders that occur or develop during adulthood. Specifically, we discuss aphasia, right hemisphere syndrome, traumatic brain injury, and degenerative neurological conditions. We will be describing language problems related to interruption of blood supply to the brain, direct destruction of neural tissue, or a pathological process. This will be your introduction, and, of necessity, it will only scratch the surface. Although the speech-language pathologist is concerned primarily with communication, the disorders described in this chapter necessitate an understanding of the medical conditions from which they originate.

In this chapter, we will explore four neurological impairments that affect adult language. Within each, we'll describe assessment and intervention considerations.

APHASIA

Aphasia means literally "without language," or "no language," a feature that describes the most severe varieties of the impairment. In some ways, it is the most difficult disorder for beginning students to comprehend. The aphasic population is extremely diverse. In addition, although aphasia results from localized brain damage, the exact locations and the resultant severity and type of aphasia are not a perfect match. Nor does all brain damage result in aphasia. Damage to the brain may result in loss of motor or sensory function, impaired memory, and poor judgment, while leaving language intact.

It is estimated that over one million Americans have aphasia (Klein, 1995). Over 200 individuals—primarily adults—become aphasic in the United States each day. For these people, language has suddenly become a jumble of strange and seemingly unfamiliar words that they are unable to comprehend and/or produce. In addition, they may be paralyzed or have severely weakened muscle use. Most of you, whether or not your chosen profession is speech-language pathology, are likely to have some experience with aphasia through a relative, friend, neighbor, if not firsthand.

Many severities and varieties of aphasia exist. Problems in two areas, auditory comprehension and word retrieval, seem to be common to varying degrees in all individuals with aphasia. Word retrieval difficulties suggest that memory may also be impaired in some way. Aphasia is not the result of a motor speech impairment, dementia, or the deterioration of intelligence.

Aphasia can cross all modalities and may affect listening, speaking, reading, and/or writing as well as specific language functions such as naming. Related language functions such as arithmetic, gesturing, telling time, counting money, or interpreting environmental noises such as a dog's bark may also be difficult. Given the great variation possible, it may be better to think of aphasia as a general term that represents several syndromes.

It is rare that brain injury is so precise as to affect only language. Other related areas of cognitive function and motor behaviors may also suffer damage.

Expressive deficits may include reduced vocabulary, either omission or addition of words, stereotypic utterances, either delayed and reduced output of speech or hyperfluent speech, and word substitutions. Each of these characteristics is an example of a deeper language-processing problem. **Hyperfluent speech,** very rapid speech with few pauses, may be incoherent, inefficient, and pragmatically inappropriate.

Language comprehension deficits, whether spoken or written, involve the impaired interpretation of incoming linguistic information. Aphasia is not a sensory disorder. Individuals with aphasia may have normal hearing and vision. Difficulty comes in the interpretation or the ability to make sense of the incoming signal.

Severity may range from individuals with a few intelligible words and little comprehension to those with very high-level subtle linguistic deficits that are barely discernible in normal conversation. Severity is related to several variables, including the cause of the disorder, the location and extent of the brain injury, the age of the injury, and the age and general health of the client. Differences in individual brains may account for different aphasic characteristics and for the lack of similar characteristics when similar areas of the brain are injured.

Although individuals with aphasia differ greatly, several patterns of behavior exist that enable us to categorize the disorder into numerous types or *syndromes.* Each aphasia syndrome is related to a corresponding site of cerebral damage, although, as was mentioned, a perfect match does not exist. It is important to remember that the classifications discussed in the following section are conveniences to aid our discussion. While categories of the disorder describe certain similarities among individuals with aphasia, they do not adequately characterize any one individual. Speech-language pathologists and other professionals, such as neurologists and psychiatrists, must thoroughly assess each individual and describe individual strengths and weaknesses.

It is rare to see an individual with pure aphasia of one type or another. In addition, other neurogenic disorders—those that affect the central nervous system—such as apraxia or dysarthria often exist along with aphasia, and these complicate classification. Apraxia and dysarthria will be discussed in Chapter 12.

Individuals with aphasia may also experience seizures and depression. Seizures may be of the *grand mal* type, which result in periods of unconsciousness, or the *petit mal* and psychomotor type, in which the client may lose motor control but remain conscious. Depression is a common condition in neurological disorders.

CONCOMITANT OR ACCOMPANYING DEFICITS

Physical and psychosocial problems may also accompany aphasia and be traced to the same cause. Physical impairments may include hemiparesis, hemiplegia, and hemisensory impairment. **Hemiparesis** is a weakness on one side of the body. Muscles still function, but strength and control are greatly reduced. In contrast, **hemiplegia** is paralysis on one side. Finally, **hemisensory impairment** may accompany either and is a loss of the ability to perceive sensory information. The client may complain of cold, numbness, or tingling on the affected side and may be unable to sense pain or touch.

Hemi means "half," as in "hemisphere."

Vision is one aspect of sensory impairment that may affect communication. Individuals with deep lesions in the left temporal or lower left parietal lobe may experience blindness in the right visual field of each eye. Called **hemianopsia**, this condition will affect the individual's ability to read.

When paresis, or paralysis, and/or sensory impairment involve the neck and face, the client may have difficulty chewing or swallowing. There may be accompanying drooling or gagging. This condition, known as **dysphagia**, is also the concern of speech-language pathologists and will be addressed in Chapter 13.

In addition, brain damage may result in seizure disorder or epilepsy. Approximately 20 percent of aphasic adults have some seizure activity.

The discussion of aphasia is complicated and uses terminology that might be unfamiliar to you. As we discuss each, try to think of it not as bizarre, but as an extreme form of some behaviors that you already manifest. For example, occasionally, we all have difficulty recalling a name or remembering a word. In its extreme form, we call this *anomia*. Some of the more common terms are listed below with a brief description. Examples of these expressive deficits of adults with aphasia are presented in Table 7.1 and Figure 7.1.

Agnosia: A sensory deficit accompanying some aphasias that makes it difficult for the client to understand incoming sensory information. The disorder may be specific to auditory or visual information.

Agrammatism: Omission of grammatical elements. Individuals with aphasia may omit short, unstressed words, such as articles or prepositions. They may also omit morphological endings, such as the plural -*s* or past-tense -*ed*.

TABLE 7.1

Examples of the expressive language deficits in the speech of adults with aphasia

Deficit	Characteristic	Example
Agrammatism	Omission of unstressed words; telegraphic speech	Take dog walk. Go home. Make instant coffee, watch T.V.
Anomia	Difficulty naming entities	It's a . . . a . . . thing . . . that thing that you do that with . . . you know, that thing for doing stuff with.
Jargon	Meaningless or irrelevant speech with typical intonational patterns	We went for the cookies to laugh in the elephants, didn't we?
Neologism	Novel word	Cow juice and cookies; that's what I like, especially mixed up chocolate (*chocolate milkshake*).
Paraphasia	Word and phoneme substitutions	I need the pen . . . pen . . . pencil and the sheet . . . peeper . . . peeper sheet to color on.
Verbal stereotype	An expression repeated over and over	I see, I see, I see, I see.

Agraphia: Difficulty writing. Writing may be full of mistakes and poorly formed. Clients may be unable to write what they are able to say. Agrammatism, jargon, and neologisms may be present in written language as well as in spoken.

Alexia: Reading problems. Clients may be unable to recognize even common words they use in their speech. Paraphasia and neologisms may be present.

Anomia: Difficulty naming entities. Clients may struggle greatly. Individuals who have recovered from aphasia report that they knew what they wanted to say but could not locate the appropriate word. An incorrect response may

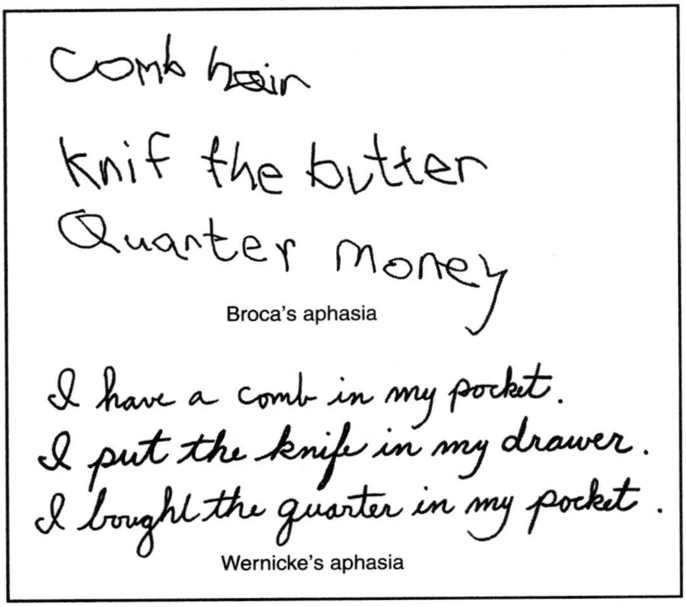

```
Comb hair

knif the butter

Quarter money
```
Broca's aphasia

```
I have a comb in my pocket.
I put the knife in my drawer.
I bought the quarter in my pocket.
```
Wernicke's aphasia

FIGURE 7.1 Examples of the expressive language deficits in the writing of adults with aphasia

continue to be produced even when the client recognizes that it is incorrect.

Jargon: Meaningless or irrelevant speech with typical intonational patterns. Responses are often long and syntactically correct although containing nonsense. Jargon may contain neologisms.

Neologism: A novel word. Some individuals with aphasia may create novel words that do not exist in their language, using these words quite confidently.

Paraphasia: Word substitutions found in clients who may talk fluently and grammatically. Associations to the intended word may be based on meaning, such as saying *truck* for *car*; on similar sound, such as *tar* for *car*; or on some other relationship.

Verbal stereotype: An expression repeated over and over. One young man responded to every question with "I know," occasionally stringing it together to form "I know I know I know." Sometimes the expression is an obscene word or expletive or a neologism. One Mother Superior, seen in the clinic, continually uttered the same obscene word with great gusto, to her total embarrassment but seeming inability to stop.

T H O U G H T   Q U E S T I O N

How does the term "jargon" as used here relate to the same term used to refer to the speech of a developing child of approximately 10 months? What are the similarities in meaning?

TYPES OF APHASIA

Aphasias can be classified into two large categories based on the ease of producing speech: **fluent aphasia** and **nonfluent aphasia.** In turn, these can be subdivided into *syndromes.* The most common syndromes and their characteristics are presented in Table 7.2.

TABLE 7.2

Characteristics of fluent and nonfluent aphasias

Aphasia Type	Speech Production	Speech Comprehension	Speech Characteristics	Reading Comprehension	Naming	Speech Repetition
Wernicke's	Fluent or hyperfluent	Impaired to poor	Verbal paraphasia, jargon	Impaired	Impaired to poor	Impaired to poor
Anomic	Fluent	Mild to moderately impaired	Word retrieval and misnaming, good syntax and articulation	Good	Severely impaired in both speech and writing	Good
Conduction	Fluent	Mildly impaired to good	Paraphasia and incorrect ordering with frequent self-correction attempts, good articulation and syntax	Good	Usually impaired	Poor
Transcortical Sensory	Fluent	Poor	Paraphasia, possible perseveration	Impaired to poor	Severely impaired	Unimpaired
Broca's	Nonfluent	Relatively good	Short sentences, agrammatism; slow, labored, with articulation and phonological errors	Unimpaired to poor	Poor	Poor
Transcortical	Nonfluent	Mildly impaired	Impaired, labored, difficulty initiating, syntactic errors	Unimpaired to poor	Impaired	Good
Global	Nonfluent	Poor, limited to single words or short phrases	Limited spontaneous ability of a few words or stereotypes	Poor	Poor	Poor, limited to single words or short phrases

FLUENT APHASIAS

Adults with fluent aphasia have typical rate, intonation, pauses, and stress patterns.

The fluent aphasias are characterized by word substitutions, neologisms, and often verbose verbal output. Lesions in fluent aphasia tend to be found in the posterior portions of the left hemisphere.

WERNICKE'S APHASIA   As a fluent aphasia, **Wernicke's aphasia** is characterized by rapid-fire strings of sentences with little pause for acknowledgment or turn taking. The nearly monologue nature of the delivery and the lack of concern for errors suggest little self-monitoring or error awareness. Content may seem a jumble and may be incoherent or incomprehensible although fluent and well articulated. Characteristics include the following:

1. Fluent or hyperfluent speech
2. Poor auditory and visual comprehension
3. Verbal paraphasia or unintended words and neologisms
4. Sentences formed by strings of unrelated words, called jargon
5. Mild to severe impairment in naming and imitative speech

To the casual listener, the individual with Wernicke's aphasia might not sound disordered because intonational patterns and sound-combination patterns of the language are maintained. Closer examination reveals the difficulties with content.

Poor comprehension extends to reading as well as listening. The underlying speech comprehension problems are evident in poor oral reading comprehension. In addition, poor auditory comprehension affects verbal repetition. The client might not be able to repeat back what was said to him or her. Further, clients may demonstrate reduced ability to comprehend their own speech as well as that of others.

Damage in Wernicke's aphasia is near Wernicke's area in the posterior portions of the left temporal lobe. The following is an example of the speech of a client with Wernicke's aphasia:

> I love to go for rides in the car. Cars are expensive these days. Everything's expensive. Even groceries. When I was a child you could spend five dollars and get a whole wagon full. I had a little red wagon. My brother and I would ride down the hill by our house. My brother served in World War II. He moved away after the war. There was so little housing available. My house is a split-level.

An audio sample of a person with Wernicke's aphasia is presented on the accompanying CD-ROM.

ANOMIC APHASIA   As the name suggests, the second type of fluent aphasia, called **anomic aphasia,** is characterized by naming difficulties. Most aspects of speech are normal with the exception of word retrieval. Because naming problems are common to most aphasias, you might not think that anomic aphasia is a separate syndrome. Other characteristics include the following:

1. Severe anomia in both speech and writing
2. Fluent spontaneous speech marred by word retrieval difficulties
3. Mild to moderate auditory comprehension problems

Names may be unavailable, or entities may be misnamed with both related and nonrelated words. As you might expect, imitated or repetitive language is less affected.

Brain damage seems to be at the convergence of the parietal-temporal-occipital cortex. Memory difficulties are evident and suggest damage near the angular gyrus. The following is an example of the speech of a client with anomic aphasia:

> It was very good. We had a bird . . . a big thing with feathers and . . . a bird . . . a turkey stuffed . . . turkey with stuffing and that stuff . . . you know . . . and that stuff, that berry stuff . . . that stuff . . . berries, berries . . . cranberry stuffing . . . stuffing and cranberries . . . and gravy on things . . . smashed things . . . Oh, darn, smashed potatoes.

CONDUCTION APHASIA Like the other fluent aphasias, **conduction aphasia** is characterized by conversation that is abundant and quick, though filled with paraphasia. Characteristics include the following:

1. Anomia
2. Only mild impairment of auditory comprehension, if any
3. Extremely poor repetitive or imitative speech
4. Paraphasia or the inappropriate use of words formed by the addition of sounds and incorrect ordering of sounds or by substituting related words

Paraphasia may be severe enough to make the individual's speech incomprehensible. Given the good comprehension skills of many individuals with conduction aphasia, self-correction attempts are frequent, although the client may be unable to benefit from the verbal cues of others.

Damage may be to the arcuate fasciculus. This is a subsurface band of neural fibers running between Wernicke's and Broca's areas. The following is an example of the speech of a client with conduction aphasia:

> We went to me girl, my girl . . . oh, a little girl's palace . . . no, daughter's palace, not a castle, but a pal . . . place . . . home for a sivit . . . and he . . . visit and she made a cook, cook a made . . . a cake.

TRANSCORTICAL SENSORY APHASIA **Transcortical sensory aphasia** is the rarest of the fluent aphasias. Although conversation and spontaneous speech are fluent, as in Wernicke's aphasia, they are filled with word errors. Characteristics include the following:

1. Unimpaired ability to repeat or imitate words
2. Verbal paraphasia or word substitutions
3. Lack of nouns and severe anomia
4. Poor auditory comprehension
5. Ability to repeat or imitate words, phrases, and sentences

The unimpaired imitative ability may be perseverative or may become so persistent as to seem echolalic. Echolalic speech is characterized by an immediate or delayed whole or partial repetition of the speech of another speaker.

Brain damage seems to isolate language areas from other areas of cortical control. The lesion is located in the posterior portions of the Sylvian fissure or lateral sulcus (see Figure 3.9).

SUBCORTICAL APHASIA Although its existence had been hypothesized, **subcortical aphasia** could not be confirmed until the advent or neuro-imaging techniques. Lesions occur in the thalamus and basal ganglia without involvement of the cerebral cortex. Characteristics include the following:

1. Fluent expressive speech
2. Paraphasia and neologisms
3. Repetition unaffected
3. Auditory and reading comprehension relatively unaffected

Additional language characteristics may include word-finding difficulties, perseveration, and spontaneous speech. Other characteristics, including dysarthria, have been related to specific sites in the basal ganglia (Alexander & Naeser, 1988; Kirshner, 1995).

NONFLUENT APHASIAS

Adults with nonfluent aphasia have slow rate, less intonation, inappropriately placed and abnormally long pauses, and less varied stress patterns than typical speakers.

Nonfluent aphasia is characterized by slow, labored speech and struggle to retrieve words and form sentences. In general, the site of lesion is in or near the frontal lobe.

BROCA'S APHASIA Broca's aphasia is associated with damage to the anterior or forward parts of the frontal lobe of the left cerebral hemisphere. Centered in Broca's area, the lesion must be somewhat larger for an individual to exhibit all the characteristics of this type of aphasia. The most common traits are the following:

1. Short sentences with agrammatism in which auxiliary or helping verbs, the verb *to be*, prepositions, articles, and morphological endings are omitted
2. Anomia

3. Problems with imitation of speech because of overall speech problems
4. Slow, labored speech and writing
5. Articulation and phonological errors

Auditory comprehension seems unimpaired, although careful testing may reveal subtle deficits in understanding.

The following is an example of the speech of a client with Broca's aphasia:

Foam, foam, phone, damn, phone . . . not ude . . . phone not ude . . . ude . . . ude . . . use . . . can't ude . . . no foam can ude.

TRANSCORTICAL MOTOR APHASIA   This is the nonfluent counterpart of transcortical sensory aphasia. Characteristics of this syndrome include the following:

1. Impaired speech, especially in conversation
2. Good verbal imitative abilities
3. Mildly impaired auditory comprehension

Individuals with **transcortical motor aphasia** may have difficulty initiating speech or writing.

Severely impaired speech is characteristic of damage to the motor cortex. Actually, the areas that are affected may go well below the surface of the brain.

GLOBAL OR MIXED APHASIA   As the name implies, **global or mixed aphasia** is characterized by profound language impairment in all modalities. It is considered the most severely debilitating form of aphasia. Mixed aphasia is a milder form. Other characteristics include the following:

1. Limited spontaneous expressive ability of a few words or stereotypes, such as overlearned utterances or emotional responses
2. Imitative speech and naming affected
3. Auditory and visual comprehension limited to single words or short phrases

Global aphasia has both the auditory comprehension problems found in some fluent aphasias and the labored speech of nonfluent aphasias. For this reason, some experts classify it as separate from both types.

These symptoms are associated with a large, deep lesion in the Sylvian region or in a deep subcortical area. Often, both the anterior speech and posterior language areas of the left hemisphere are involved.

T H O U G H T   Q U E S T I O N

Can you imagine how your life might change if you had global aphasia? What would happen to your social life? Family life? Career plans?

ADDITIONAL TYPES OF APHASIA

Not all aphasias can be neatly classified within the fluent-nonfluent system. Other aphasias may affect primarily one communication modality, such as writing. Examples of these specific aphasias include the following:

Alexia with agraphia: Reading and writing impairment
Alexia without agraphia: Reading impairment with no accompanying writing difficulty
Pure agraphia: Severe writing disorder
Pure word deafness: Lack of auditory comprehension with error-free spontaneous speech
Crossed aphasia: Aphasia accompanying right hemisphere damage

Aphasia classification and the loci of lesions are controversial issues and areas of continued study.

CAUSES OF APHASIA

The onset of aphasia is rapid. Usually, it occurs in people who have no former history of speech and language difficulties. The lesion or injury leaves an area of cortical tissue unable to function as it had just moments before.

Stroke is caused by an interruption of the blood supply to the brain.

The most common cause of aphasia is a **stroke** or **cerebrovascular accident,** the third leading cause of death in the United States. Strokes affect half a million Americans annually. Seventy percent of these are over 65 years of age (Bonita, 1992). Although some children suffer strokes, this is rare. In 1990, the National Institute on Neurological Disorders and Stroke estimated that as a result of strokes, approximately 80,000 people become aphasic each year.

T H O U G H T   Q U E S T I O N

Are you leading a healthy life that could reduce your chances of stroke?

Strokes are of two basic types: ischemic and hemorrhagic. **Ischemic strokes** result from a complete or partial blockage or occlusion of the arteries transporting blood to the brain as in cerebral arteriosclerosis, embolism, and thrombosis. **Cerebral arteriosclerosis** is a thickening of the walls of cerebral arteries in which elasticity is lost or reduced, the walls become weakened, and blood flow is restricted. The resulting ischemia, or reduction of oxygen, may be temporary—termed *transient ischemic* *attack* (TIA)—or may cause permanent damage through the death of brain tissue. An **embolism** is an obstruction to blood flow caused by a blood clot, fatty materials, or an air bubble. The obstruction may travel through the circulatory system until it blocks the flow of blood in a small artery. For example, a clot may form in the heart or the large arteries of the chest, break off, and become an embolus. As in cerebral arteriosclerosis, blockage results in a lack of oxygen-carrying blood, depriving brain cells of needed oxygen. Similarly, a **thrombosis** also blocks blood flow. In this case, plaque buildup or a blood clot is formed on site and does not travel. The result is the same.

A **hemorrhagic** stroke is one in which the weakened arterial walls burst under pressure, as occurs with an aneurysm or arteriovenous malformation. An **aneurysm** is a saclike bulging in a weakened artery wall. The thin wall may rupture, causing a cerebral hemorrhage. Most aneurysms occur in the meninges, the layered membranes surrounding the brain, and blood flowing into this space can damage the brain or cause death. Stroke is characterized by direct bleeding into the brain tissue.

Arteriovenous malformation is rare and consists of a poorly formed tangle of arteries and veins that may occur in a highly viscous organ such as the brain. Malformed arterial walls may be weak and give way under pressure.

Patterns of recovery differ with the type of stroke because of the differing nature of the resultant damage. Often, with ischemic stroke, there is a noticeable improvement within the first weeks after the injury. Recovery slows after three months. In contrast, the results of hemorrhagic strokes are usually more severe after injury. The period of most rapid recovery is at the end of the first month and into the second as swelling lessens and injured neurons regain functioning.

> The results of a stroke are further complicated by the prestroke storage patterns for language.

Damage from stroke may occur in any part of the brain. In all right-handed individuals and in some left-handed ones, injury to left hemisphere language areas produces aphasia. Injury to the right hemisphere results in aphasia in only 3 percent of the cases, usually left-handed individuals whose right hemisphere is dominant for language (Calvin & Ojemann, 1980).

Aphasia-like symptoms may be noted with head injury, neural infections, degenerative neurological disorders, and tumors. In most of these cases, however, other cortical areas are also affected, resulting in clinically different disorders.

The human brain is extremely complex. Categorizing the types of aphasias that we have discussed helps to bring some understanding to the subject of brain disorders but may have little practical clinical value. Most clients will present mixed aphasia. It is all the more important, therefore, that speech-language pathologists describe each client's abilities and disabilities carefully and clearly.

LIFE SPAN ISSUES

Most individuals with aphasia lived healthy productive lives until the incident that resulted in the impairment. The risk of stroke is increased if the individual has a history of smoking, alcohol use, poor diet, lack of exercise, high blood pressure, high cholesterol, diabetes, obesity, and previous strokes. Although children and adolescents can experience aphasia, especially accompanying brain tumors, most victims are adults in middle age and beyond. Usually, the onset of symptoms is rapid when the cause is vascular, but it can take months or years to become evident with tumor or degenerative disease. These patterns are presented in Figure 7.2.

In the most common situation, the individual suffers an ischemic stroke, depriving the brain of a needed supply of oxygenated blood. First indications may be loss of consciousness, headache, weak or immobile limbs, and/or slurred speech. This condition may be temporary in which function returns quickly or more permanent in nature. Some individuals may experience a series of "ministrokes" spaced over a period of years before they become alarmed. Some ministrokes go undetected by the individual.

Usually, the individual is rushed to the hospital. Approximately one-third of individuals will die from the stroke or shortly thereafter. For those

FIGURE 7.2 Severity of symptoms by neurological condition. Adapted from Brookshire, R. H. (1997). *Introduction to neurogenic communication disorders* (5th ed.). St. Louis, MO: Mosby-Year Book.

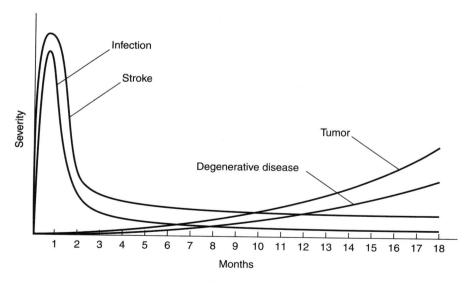

Individuals will differ in severity and path of the disorder.

who survive, there may be a period of unconsciousness, followed by confusion. Deep long-lasting periods of unconsciousness or coma are associated with poorer eventual recovery (Carlsson, Svardsudd, & Welin, 1987). Levels of consciousness can be measured in a consistent manner using the *Glasgow Coma Scale* (Teasdale & Jennett, 1974), which notes eye opening and motor and verbal responses. Categories are presented in Table 7.3.

Most individuals remain in acute care for only a few days until their condition stabilizes. Following this, an individual may receive a variety of care depending on the severity of the stroke. These include rehabilitative hospitalization, outpatient rehabilitation, or nursing home care. Most return home but with some impairment.

Intervention services may occur for years, but most individuals receive intervention services for several months. As mentioned previously, aphasia may be accompanied by neuromuscular deficits, seizures, and dementia. In addition, the individual with aphasia may

TABLE 7.3

The Glasgow Coma Scale

Category	Description (Least to most severe)
Eye Opening	Spontaneously
	To verbal command
	In response to pain
	No response
Motor Responses	Obeys verbal commands
	Attempts to pull examiner's hand away during painful stimulation
	Moves limb away from painful stimulus
	Flexes body in response to pain
	Extends limbs, becomes rigid in response to pain
	No response
Verbal Responses	Converses and is oriented
	Converses but is disoriented
	Utters intelligible words, but does not make sense
	Produces unintelligible sounds
	No response

Source: Adapted from Teasdale and Jennett (1974)

exhibit behavior changes. These may include perseveration, disinhibition, and emotional problems. *Perseveration* is the repetition of inappropriate responses. As was described in Chapter 6, the client may become fixed on a single task or behavior and repeat it. *Disinhibition*, also mentioned in Chapter 6, is a seeming inability to inhibit certain asocial or inappropriate behaviors, such as touching others. Finally, brain damage may contribute to exaggerated swings in emotion is appropriate but the magnitude of that emotion and the suddenness of the emotional shift are not. The appropriateness of emotional behavior must be considered in light of the extreme frustration experienced by some individuals with aphasia.

Given the variety of possible symptoms following a stroke, the individual will most likely receive services from a team of professionals. Team members may include a neurologist, physical therapist, occupational therapist, nutritionist, speech-language pathologist, and audiologist. Life changes and family concerns may necessitate the services of a counseling social worker, psychologist, psychiatrist, and/or pastoral counselor.

Immediately after the incident, neurological functioning is most severely affected. Within days, the body's natural recovery process begins. As swelling is reduced, injured cells may recover and begin to function normally. Adjacent areas of the brain that shared brain functions with the injured area may begin to play a larger role. The course and extent of this recovery process are difficult to predict, but the rate is fastest during the first few weeks and months after the stroke, then slows, and usually ceases after six months.

Recovery may be evident in cognitive, sensory, motor, and linguistic abilities. During this process, the entire syndrome that the client presents may change and most certainly will lessen in severity. Global aphasia often evolves into a less severe syndrome. The most frequent linguistic gains are in auditory comprehension (Kertesz & McCabe, 1997). In general, less severely affected individuals, those who are younger, in general good health, and left-handed recover from aphasia better and faster than those who are more severe, older, in poor health, and right-handed.

With or without spontaneous recovery, assessment and intervention should begin as soon as the client's individual condition permits. The clients who are most responsive to the environment are probably the best candidates for intervention services. A general rule is that the earlier the treatment, the better the rate of recovery, but clients do not all recover similarly (Robey, 1994, 1998). The SLP's first goal should be to determine the feasibility of clinical intervention. Although it is not possible to accurately predict how much gain will be the result of spontaneous recovery and how much the outcome of intervention, the

SLP must attempt to determine which clients will benefit most from clinical intervention (Marshall, 1997).

Loss of the ability to use language efficiently changes the social role of each individual with aphasia and can result in social isolation. This situation is complicated by the often incorrect assumption that cognitive abilities are also damaged. In addition, inability to communicate may cause the affected individual to become dependent on others for the simplest of daily tasks. Family roles and responsibilities may also change. Wives, husbands, and children may have to take on new responsibilities. If the individual supported the family prior to the incident, there may be economic problems in addition to medical ones. Box 7.1 presents the story of one individual with aphasia.

Communication is so entwined in our social interactions and in our very definition of who we are that the effects of aphasia reach well beyond speech and language.

ASSESSMENT FOR APHASIA

Assessment and intervention may begin in the hospital and continue as outpatient service. Successful intervention is a team effort. The relative importance of each specialist will change as the client recovers. In addition, a spouse, other family member, or close friend may be a critical participant in the recuperative process for a person with aphasia.

Before beginning any intervention, it is necessary to complete a thorough assessment of each client's abilities and deficits. This process may continue in several stages as the client stabalizes and experiences **spontaneous recovery,** a natural recovery process that proceeds without professional intervention.

The assessment procedures outlined in Chapter 5 provide a model. Especially important are the client's medical history, the interview with the client and family, the oral peripheral examination, the hearing testing, and direct speech and language testing. The medical history can reveal information about general health and previous cerebrovascular incidents. In addition, current neurological reports and progress notes provide valuable information on present and changing status.

During the interview, it will be necessary for the SLP to provide as much information as he or she receives from the client and family. The client may be confused and need reassurance. Family members will have many questions regarding recovery. Unspoken questions may center on family dynamics, income, medical expenses, and the like. It is important for families to know the extent of the injuries and to have a realistic appraisal of recovery with and without professional assistance. Although it is unethical to promise a "cure" (see Appendix 1.1, "Code of Ethics"), the SLP should give the family an honest estimate of expected progress.

BOX 7.1

Personal Story of an Adult with Aphasia

When Mr. W. was 55 years of age, he looked fitter than most men ten years his junior. Mr. W. had earned a master's degree in labor relations from Cornell University, and he had been employed for many years as a labor mediator by the small city in which he lived. Although he was very successful, his personal life had been disrupted by divorce after twenty years of marriage. Despite this, Mr. W. was viewed as cheerful by his circle of friends, primarily fellow hikers with whom he explored mountain trails almost every Saturday. Mr. W. has no children of his own, but he was beloved "Uncle John" to the teenaged children of his sister and brother-in-law, who lived less than a mile from his home.

Although Mr. W. had been rugged and capable of vigorous outdoor activity, he knew that he had high blood pressure, and he was taking medication under a doctor's care. Mr. W. was rarely ill, and he had been hospitalized only once, for acute appendicitis, before his stroke.

One Sunday afternoon, Mr. W. decided to lie down after a four-hour cross-country ski outing. He had a bad headache, and he hoped that a short rest would relieve it before a dinner date with skiing buddies. When he awoke from his nap, he got up to go to the bathroom but collapsed. His friends were concerned when he failed to meet them. They phoned and got no answer, so someone went to his home. The door was unlocked, and Mr. W. was found on the floor. He was breathing but unconscious. He had suffered a cerebrovascular accident (CVA), or stroke.

Mr. W. was taken to the emergency room of the local hospital. When he became conscious, he was confused, did not seem to understand what was said to him, and was unable to speak. The right side of his body was partially paralyzed. The medical report stated that he had "sustained a left CVA that resulted in right hemiplegia and aphasia." He remained hospitalized for six weeks. In addition to the attending neurologist and

THOUGHT QUESTION

Why is it unethical to promise to cure aphasia? Is there real danger, especially with this disorder, that the client and family may be vulnerable to such promises?

Such counseling with the family will be ongoing and should be a portion of all professional contacts with the client and family. In addition, the family and client will need separate, professional counseling to cope with the enormous changes that have occurred in their lives.

family physician, Mr. W. was seen by a speech-language pathologist and a physical therapist. The SLP performed an initial bedside assessment and counseled family members and friends. The SLP's initial report stated that "Mr. W. presented with severe expressive/receptive aphasia characterized by severe oral motor apraxia and a severe auditory comprehension deficit with moderate to severe reading comprehension deficits for single words."

When Mr. W. was discharged from the hospital, he moved in with his sister and her family. He was cared for largely by family and friends, and he was taken for medical appointments and twice-weekly physical and speech-language therapy. Early goals were simple auditory comprehension requiring yes/no head nods as responses, and the expression of needs such as "eat."

Two years after the stroke, Mr. W. was able to walk with a walker. Family members reported that they could under-stand 85 percent of his intentional speech. Strangers could understand only about 20 percent. He used gestures and largely unintelligible sounds to express himself. Mr. W.'s ability to comprehend language had improved dramatically, and he was now able to follow directions that contained three critical elements ("put the pencil on top of the card and then put it back"). Friends reported that he often seemed agitated, but he apparently liked their visits. Since Mr. W. had always enjoyed being outdoors, his friends frequently took him for short walks. Family members said that they tried to sing together on a regular basis and that Mr. W. joined in to the extent that he was able.

Recently, Mr. W. was evaluated for augmentative/alternative communication. He has received an electronic voice output system and is being taught how to use it. He will never be able to speak normally, but this device should greatly facilitate his ability to communicate.

The oral peripheral examination is important because of the potential for either neuromuscular paralysis or weakness. Speech disorders such as apraxia and dysarthria frequently are associated with aphasia and should be described or ruled out. See Chapter 12, "Neurogenic Speech Disorders," for a fuller discussion.

Possible hearing loss must be ascertained, especially given the older age of most individuals with aphasia. It is important to separate hearing loss from comprehension.

Finally, careful observation is essential, especially shortly after the incident, when more formal testing is not possible. It is important to observe the client's general speech and language behavior and to listen and observe what is communicated and how. Observing spontaneous language use in conversation can give the SLP important information on the nature and extent of the disorder (Davis, 1993; Helm-Estabrooks & Albert, 1991).

Initial testing, often at the bedside, may be very informal with probes of the client's knowledge of her or his name, date and year, personal history, and the ability to produce automatic language, such as counting or reciting the days of the week. Table 7.4 presents an outline of an informal bedside evaluation. More formal testing and sampling phases should assess overall communication skills as well as receptive and expressive language within all modalities—reading, writing, auditory comprehension, expressive language, and gestures and nonlinguistic communication—and across all five aspects of language: pragmatics, semantics, syntax, morphology, and phonology. With higher functioning clients, the SLP will want to assess higher language skills such as verbal reasoning and analogies, figurative language, categorization, and explanations of complex tasks. Table 7.5 is an overview of the areas that ASHA recommends be evaluated in a functional assessment of communication abilities.

Several standardized tests are available for assessing specific language skills. Table 7.6 presents some frequently used aphasia batteries. Formal tests must be selected carefully, given the varying range and scope of different instruments. Some attempt to assess performance in all modalities, while others are in-depth assessments of a single performance area, such as naming. Overall test construction varies from those

---

TABLE 7.4

Components of an informal bedside evaluation

What is your name?

How old are you?

Where do you live?

Count to 20 (or Tell me the days of the week or Tell me the months of the year).

Can you tell me the names of these objects? (Use common household objects.)

Point to the objects (or pictures) named.

Repeat the following sentences.

Read the following sentences.

TABLE 7.5

ASHA recommendations for a functional assessment of communicative abilities with adults with aphasia

Assessment Domains	Behaviors
Social communication	Use names of familar people
	Express agreement and disagreement
	Request information
	Exchange information on the telephone
	Answer yes/no questions
	Follow directions
	Understand facial expressions and tone of voice
	Understand nonliteral meaning and intent
	Understand conversations in noisy surroundings
	Understand TV and radio
	Participate in conversations
	Recognize and correct communication errors
Communication of basic needs	Recognize familiar faces and voices
	Make strong likes and dislikes known
	Express feelings
	Request help
	Make needs and wants known
	Respond in an emergency
Reading, writing, number concepts	Understand simple signs
	Use reference materials
	Follow written directions
	Understand printed material
	Print, write, and type name
	Complete forms
	Write messages
	Understand signs with numbers
	Make money transactions
	Understand units of measure
Daily planning	Tell time
	Dial telephone numbers
	Keep scheduled appointments
	Use a calendar
	Follow a map

Source: Adapted from American Speech-Language-Hearing Association. (1994). *Functional assessment of communicative skills for adults (FACS).* Washington, DC: Author.

TABLE 7.6

Frequently used aphasia batteries

Aphasia Assessment Battery
Boston Diagnostic Aphasia Exam (Goodglass & Kaplan, 1983a)
Boston Naming Test (Goodglass & Kaplan, 1983b)
Communication Abilities in Daily Living (Holland, 1980)
Minnesota Test of Differential Diagnosis of Aphasia (Schuell, 1972)
Porch Index of Communicative Abilities (Porch, 1981)
Western Aphasia Battery (Kertesz & McCabe, 1982)

that view aphasia as a multimodality disorder, such as the *Minnesota Test of Differential Diagnosis of Aphasia* (Schuell, 1972) and the *Porch Index of Communicative Abilities* (Porch, 1981), to those that consider performance in each modality to be somewhat distinct and help in describing different syndromes, such as the *Boston Diagnostic Aphasia Examination* (Goodglass & Kaplan, 1983a). Some measures, such as the *Functional Communication Profile* (Sarno, 1969) and *Communicative Ability in Daily Living* (Holland, 1980), follow neither model and attempt to describe the client's communicative abilities in daily living tasks. It is important for the SLP to remain flexible and to continue to probe the client's behavior for the duration of intervention.

Most tests include picture or object naming, pointing to pictures named, automatic language, repeating sentences, describing pictures and answering questions, reading and answering questions and/or drawing conclusions, and writing. Interpretation of client behavior during testing is extremely important. It is critical whether the client failed to respond because she or he could not retrieve the answer or because she or he did not comprehend the verbal cue. To some extent, the theoretical underpinnings of the test selected will influence the type of intervention attempted.

Most test tasks involve decision making or problem solving. In principle, these measures assess endpoints of several cognitive and linguistic processes. Subcomponents of the process are not assessed individually to determine the point of breakdown. It has been argued that *on-line* assessment, which measures effects at various points within the process, may be more sensitive to individual client strengths and weaknesses (Shapiro, Swinney, & Borsky, 1998). To date, most on-

Because most individuals with aphasia have some residual communication impairment, the goal of intervention is to maximize communication effectiveness in the face of this impairment.

line analysis is limited to research, but such procedures are slowly being adapted for clinical use.

INTERVENTION

The overall goal of intervention is to aid in the recovery of language and to provide strategies to compensate for persistent language deficits (Rosenbek, LaPointe, & Wertz, 1989). Individual intervention goals are determined by the results of the assessment and by the desires of both the client and family. Goals will be individualized according to the type and severity of the aphasia and upon the individual needs of each client. Ideally, the goals are mutually acceptable to the client, family, and SLP. All members of the team, including other professionals, coordinate their efforts to strengthen treatment received from others. Guidelines for working with individuals with aphasia are presented in Table 7.7.

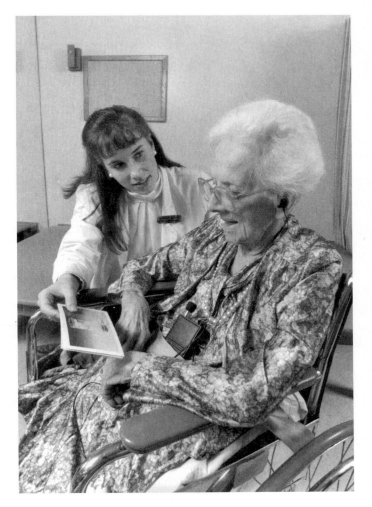

Speech and language sevices are part of a team approach to intervention.

Intervention approaches reflect the SLP's theoretical position on aphasia plus a strong dose of practical knowledge regarding the most effective techniques. Each clinician must decide whether to work on underlying skills, such as memory and auditory comprehension, or to begin with specific skill deficits, such as naming. The SLP must decide whether the brain needs help to reorganize, thus choosing cross-modality training, such as reading aloud while tracing the letters with one's finger.

TABLE 7.7

Guidelines for intervention with individuals with aphasia

Treat the client in an age-appropriate manner.

Keep your own language simple, clear, and unambiguous and control for length and complexity.

Adjust your language and the speed of production for the processing capabilities of the client.

Use everyday items and tasks and involve the family.

Use repetition and familiar routines, situations, and responses to facilitate learning.

Structure tasks to improve performance and adjust the amount of structure just enough to support the client's efforts but not foster dependency.

Provide a context to supportive the client's language processing.

Increase the demands made on the client gradually based on the client's abilities.

Teach the client to use his or her strengths to compensate for weaknesses.

The SLP can also take advantage of cross-modality generalization in which skills trained in one modality generalize to another. For example, individuals with agrammatism may benefit from cross-modality generalization following comprehension training more than following production training (Jacobs & Thompson, 2000). Comprehension training seems to generalize to comprehension and production.

Conversational techniques can provide language therapy and therapeutic support even in the first stages of intervention (Holland & Fridriksson, 2001). Within the conversation, the client carries as much of the "communication burden" as possible. Mindful of small improvements by the client, the SLP revises the demands made of the client and thus prevents chronic language problems. In short sessions using conversation, the SLP can reassure, explain what's happening to the client, and point out positive changes. As clients progress, the SLP provides less support and provides a variety of communication contexts and experiences.

Volunteers can also be trained to support the conversational attempts of individuals with aphasia (Kagan, Black, Duchan, Simmons-Mackie, & Square, 2001). These individuals need to acknowledge and respond the interactive aspects of a conversation, not just the content. Feedback to individuals with aphasia can affect motivation and performance and is an essential part of intervention (Simmons-Mackie, Damico, & Damico, 1999).

Intervention might also focus on cognitive abilities, such as memory and attention, in addition to more linguistic targets (Murray, Holland, & Beson, 1997, 1998). Clinician-assisted training may also be supplemented by more minimally assisted training, such as computer-provided reading tasks including visual matching and reading comprehension (Katz & Wertz, 1997).

Another method of intervention is to have the client attempt to access the language in the left hemisphere by bridging from the right. This might be attempted by teaching the client to gesture or sign and say the names of familiar objects. It is reasoned that gestures or signs, being visuospatial in nature, are stored in part in the right hemisphere. Another method, called *melodic intonational therapy* (Sparks, Helm, & Albert, 1974; Sparks & Holland, 1976), uses the client's usually intact right hemisphere ability to sing or produce intonational patterns. Words and phrases are taught by using different patterns of rhythm and melody. In either example, the signs or the intonational patterns are gradually faded as the client begins spontaneously to produce the targeted words and phrases without their aid.

As in many areas of language intervention, unanimity on cross-hemispheric treatment methods does not exist. Many SLPs prefer to remediate language deficits by multimodality stimulation of the affected cognitive processes (Heiss, Kessler, et al., 1999; Peach, 2001; Warburton, Price, et al., 1999). The goal is reactivation of speech areas in the dominant hemisphere.

Sign, gesture, or some other form of augmentative/alternative communication may become the primary communicative modality for clients who possess profoundly impaired language and/or speech disorders. Communication boards or electronic forms of communication may be appropriate for those who also have neuromuscular impairments. Amerind, or American Indian signs, may also be useful because many require only one hand and are easily guessable by others. See Chapter 15, "Augmentative and Alternative Communication."

Augmentative/alternative communication may become the primary mode of communication or may be used as a facilitative tool to access verbal language.

T H O U G H T   Q U E S T I O N

Might some forms of augmentative/alternative communication be utilizing the intact right hemisphere as in melodic intonational therapy?

Assuming that the family is amenable, it is best to involve them in an intense, around-the-clock communication training program. The familiar atmosphere of the home and the objects, actions, and people in it can provide a context that can facilitate a client's recovery and strengthen his or her relearned communicative behaviors. It is important for professionals to remember that the beneficial involvement of the family must not be at their emotional expense. Family members experience intense emotion when a loved one becomes ill. They must not be made to feel guilt if the client progresses little.

CONCLUSION

Aphasia is a complex impairment varying in scope and extent across individuals. In addition, clients may have other impairments, such as paralysis, as a result of their injury. Only a careful description of individual abilities and deficits in each specific modality of communication will enable the SLP to plan and carry out effective intervention. The individual variation in symptoms and severity, the team approach to intervention, and the possibility of spontaneous recovery complicate our efforts to measure intervention effectiveness and offer opportunities for those of you interested in research.

RIGHT HEMISPHERE INJURY

The term **right hemisphere injury or syndrome (RHI)** refers to a group of deficits that result from damage to the right hemisphere of the brain, the nondominant hemisphere for nearly all language functions. Deficits may be neuromuscular, perceptual, and linguistic. Neuromuscular impairments may include epilepsy, hemisensory impairment, and hemiparesis or hemiplegia, which were discussed previously. In addition, individuals may exhibit unusual behaviors. One client would regularly take a shower with his clothes on and try to go outside nude. Families report personality and mood changes including indifference and apathy. Even less-involved clients can have unrealistic estimates of their own condition and prognosis. An apparent lack of concern may actually mask a client's confusion.

Less information exists on RHI than on damage to the left hemisphere, although approximately half the individuals who have suffered stroke have right hemisphere involvement. The communication disorders that clients with RHI experience are not language based. Rather, a combination of cognitive deficits results in the communication problem. As a result, the efficiency, effectiveness, and accuracy of communication are affected.

Approximately 4 percent of the population are right hemisphere dominant for language or have bilateral language processing. If these individuals become aphasic as a result of left hemisphere damage, they usually experience milder impairment and quicker recovery than those who are left hemisphere dominant. The role of the right hemisphere is unclear in the recovery of left dominant individuals with aphasia.

CHARACTERISTICS

Deficits in RHI are not as obvious as those that result from left hemisphere damage. The most common include the following (Meyers, 1999):

1. Neglect of all information from the left side
2. Unrealistic denial of illness or limb involvement
3. Impaired judgment and self-monitoring
4. Lack of motivation
5. Inattention

FIGURE 7.3 Drawings of an individual with mild RHI that demonstrate left side neglect

Deficits may be very subtle but can have a great effect on everyday life.

Although these deficits may seem nonlinguistic in nature, they can have a great effect on communication (Meyers, 1999; Tompkins, 1995).

Disturbances can be grouped into attentional, visuospatial, and communicative. Attentional disturbances are characterized by client's lack of response to information coming from the left side of the body. Much less frequent in individuals with left hemisphere damage, this phenomenon is exhibited in the drawings of individuals with mild RHI who may omit all or provide few left side details. Figure 7.3 shows an example of left side neglect in a drawing. More severely impaired individuals may even refuse to look to the left side.

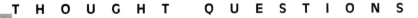

T H O U G H T   Q U E S T I O N S

Does it seem odd that the damaged right hemisphere would ignore information from the left side? What can you recall about contralateral neural pathways and sensory information?

Visuospatial deficits may include poor visual discrimination and poor scanning and tracking. The client may have difficulty recognizing

About half of individuals with RHI have communication impairments.

familiar faces, remembering familiar routes, and reading maps. Some clients not only fail to recognize family members, but may be convinced that they are actually impostors (Bienemann, 1989).

Attentional deficits have a great impact on communication. Communication impairments can be further divided into linguistic and paralinguistic deficits. Linguistic difficulties occur in both reception and expression. Of the various aspects of language, pragmatics seems to be the most impaired. For example, topic maintenance, appreciation of the communication situation, and determination of listener needs are impaired. Clients with RHI may exhibit poor auditory and visual comprehension of complex information and limited word discrimination and visual word recognition. They may also incorrectly interpret complex information, possibly because of a tendency to respond to superficial qualities of stimuli and not to observe relationships among them. In general, individuals with RHI fail to suppress irrelevant or inappropriate information, which in turn affects comprehension (Tompkins, Baumgaertner, et al., 2000). In addition, clients may fail to make use of other contextual, paralinguistic, and nonlinguistic cues (Meyers, 1999). Contextual information may be misinterpreted and the client may fail to integrate sensory information.

Understanding may be very concrete with literal interpretation of humor, indirect requests, and common figurative expressions, such as *hit the roof*. In indirect requests, the speaker does not state his or her request or demand directly. For example, a speaker might say, *I think I'll get my sweater* when meaning *Please turn up the heat*. Clients with RHI also exhibit poor judgment in determining which incoming information is important and which is not.

A similar pattern of difficulty with selectivity is noted in expressive use of language. Clients may include unnecessary, irrelevant, repetitious, and unrelated information, seemingly unable to organize their language in meaningful ways or to present it efficiently. Other problem areas include naming, repetition, and writing, especially letter substitutions and omissions.

Paralinguistic deficits include difficulty comprehending and producing emotional language. The speech of individuals with RHI lacks normal rhythm or prosody and the emphasis used to express joy or sadness, anger or delight.

ASSESSMENT

As with aphasia, the assessment of individuals with RHI is a team effort involving many of the same professionals and diagnostic tasks. The SLP is interested in visual scanning and tracking, auditory and visual comprehension of words and sentences, direction following, response to emotion, naming and describing pictures, and writing. For example, the client may be asked to re-create patterns with blocks or to find two objects or pictures that are the same; to recall words or sentences heard, seen in print, or both; and to describe a picture accurately enough for the SLP to recreate it. Sampling and observational data are essential in assessing the client's pragmatic abilities in conversational contexts.

Portions of aphasia batteries, standardized tests for RHI, and nonstandardized procedures may be used in the assessment. Standardized batteries include the *Right Hemisphere Language Battery* (Bryan, 1989) and the *Mini Inventory of Right Brain Injury* (Pimental & Kingsbury, 1989). Tasks include reading and writing, affective language, and figurative language. The *Rehabilitation Institute of Chicago Evaluation* (RICE) *of Communicative Problems in Right-Hemisphere Dysfunction* (Burns, Halper, & Mogil, 1985) is a nonstandard testing procedure that includes interviewing, observation, and ratings of the client's behavior along with testing of communication.

INTERVENTION

Intervention often begins with visual and auditory recognition. These skills are essential before progressing to more complex tasks, such as naming, describing, reading, and writing. Self-monitoring and paralinguistics are introduced, and the complexity of the content is gradually increased.

Because of the diffuse effects on behavior seen in RHI, we know less about the treatment of these patients.

Clients are helped to respond appropriately to common communicative initiations and to track increasingly complex information in conversations. Beginning with questions from the SLP that require precise information, the client learns to make responses that come to the point. These questions become more open-ended as the client learns to make less frequent off-topic responses. Similarly, time restraints may limit conversational turns to keep the client from rambling.

Sequencing tasks and explanations of common multistep actions, such as making coffee, will be introduced to help the client organize linguistic content and make relevant contributions. Cues such as objects or pictures may be used initially to aid organization.

Finally, within conversations, the SLP will help the client to synthesize these many skills. Visual and verbal cues may aid in turn taking. Important nonlinguistic markers such as eye contact, body language, and gestures may be targeted. Topic maintenance and relevant conversational contributions are stressed.

TRAUMATIC BRAIN INJURY (TBI)

Although the news media and auto safety agencies stress the importance of child restraints in motor vehicles, it is adolescents and young adults (15–24 years of age) who are most at risk for head injury. The increase in motor vehicles, motorcycles, and off-road vehicles is directly related to the increase in TBI. Another disturbing increase is the rise in attempted homicides and gun-related injuries, especially in urban areas. We have seen adult clients with TBI as the result of automobile, motorcycle, and bicycle collisions; falls; violent crime; and failed suicide attempts involving firearms.

Every minute, nearly four people in the United States suffer head injury. Approximately 500,000 individuals sustain TBI annually (Kraus, 1993). Of these, approximately 200,000 die. Most others are treated for concussion and recover. Approximately 50,000–100,000 have significant impairment requiring further care and have altered their lives for the foreseeable future (Kraus, 1993). Approximately 70 percent of these are males. The statistics tell a chilling story but do not begin to explain the pain and suffering or the long struggle to recover. Box 7.2 presents the personal story of one young man with TBI.

You will recall from our discussion of children that, unlike stroke, which injures a specific area of the brain, TBI is a diffuse injury to the entire brain; it is nonfocused. Damage may result from bruising and laceration of the brain caused by forceful contact with the relatively rough inner surfaces of the skull and from secondary **edema** or swelling due to increased fluid, which can lead to increased pressure; infection; hypoxia (oxygen deprivation); intracranial pressure from tissue swelling; **infarction,** or death of tissue deprived of blood supply; and **hematoma,** or focal bleeding (Sohlberg & Mateer, 1989). Aphasia-like symptoms are rare, but linguistic impairments related to cognitive damage are not. In addition, the individual with TBI may have sensory, motor, behavioral, and affective disabilities. Neuromuscular impairments may include epilepsy, hemisensory impairment, and hemiparesis or hemiplegia. The symptoms and the life changes that result can be profound.

CHARACTERISTICS

The behavioral characteristics of adults with TBI are similar to those of children who are similarly injured. Attention and memory are affected, and the client exhibits *disinhibition*. Individuals with TBI are a heterogeneous group with a diverse collection of physical, cognitive, communicative, and psychosocial deficits. Usually, the most devastating aspect

BOX 7.2

Personal Story of a Young Man with TBI

His family called him Felipe, but he preferred to use the more Americanized nickname "Chip" that his friends had given him. He was excited to be leaving home for college. Thoughts of being on his own thrilled him with endless possibilities. Even though he was only a freshman, he planned to live with some older friends in their off-campus apartment.

A few weeks after school began, Felipe decided to hitchhike home to surprise his mother, who missed him a great deal. He stuck out his thumb early on Friday afternoon but never made it home. After his first ride, he bought a soda and began to thumb anew. Shortly afterward, he was struck in the head by the mirror on a pickup truck. Luckily, Felipe was carrying identification in his backpack, and his family was alerted shortly after he was admitted to the hospital.

When he regained consciousness, a few hours after the accident, Felipe was extremely disoriented. He made no attempt to speak and was very lethargic. Although he seemed to recognize his family, he made no attempt to communicate with them. Over the next few weeks, his condition slowly stabilized. Physicians were initially concerned about swelling in the area of the injury. There was evidence of some internal bleeding, but it was not a major problem.

Once the swelling began to recede, Felipe's abilities slowly returned. He began to recall the names of family members and common objects. Walking was extremely difficult because of paralysis on the right side of his body. He dropped out of college and remained at home, where he received intervention services. As an outpatient, he was seen by the speech-language pathologist, physical therapist, and occupational therapist.

After a year's absence from school, Felipe returned and was able to be successful with some adaptations, such as the use of a tape recorder and extra time for completing written tests. He retains a slight limp in his right leg and some minimal weakness in his right arm. His language and speech skills have returned, although he has some mild word-finding difficulties. His cognitive abilities are more concrete than those he had before the accident, and problem-solving tasks require a greater effort. All indications are that he will be successful in his academic pursuits, although his physical and cognitive limitations will continue to affect him.

is an inability to resume interests and daily living tasks to the level that existed before the injury. Some clients exhibit near total dependence on others. Cognitive difficulties may be evident in orientation, memory, attention, reasoning and problem solving, and executive function, or the planning, execution, and self-monitoring of goal-directed behavior (Sohlberg & Mateer, 1989).

Language may be affected in three out of four individuals with TBI (McKinlay, Brooks, Bond, Martinage, & Marshall, 1981). The estimated percentage of these with aphasia-like characteristics may be close to one-third (Sarno, Buonaguro, & Levita, 1986). The two most commonly reported symptoms for TBI are anomia and impaired comprehension (Coelho, 1997).

As with children, the most disturbed language area and that with the most pervasive problems is pragmatics (Sohlberg & Mateer, 1989). Most published tests target language form and content and may miss pragmatic deficits that are evident in conversation. Pragmatic impairments result from the inability to inhibit behavior and from errors of judgment. The result may be rambling speech and incoherence, as manifested by off-topic and irrelevant comments and inability to maintain a topic, and poor turn-taking skills, such as frequent interruption of others. In addition, communication may be marked by poor affective or emotional language abilities and inappropriate laughter and swearing.

Deficits are not limited to language and may include speech, voice, and swallowing difficulties. Approximately one-third of all individuals with TBI exhibit dysarthria, a disorder resulting from weakness or incoordination of the muscles that control speech production (Sarno et al., 1986). The exact type of dysarthria (see Chapter 12) varies with the areas of the brain that are most affected. Language deficits reflect underlying disruptions in information-processing, problem-solving, and reasoning abilities. In addition, psychosocial and personality changes may include disinhibition or impulsivity, poor organization and social judgment, and withdrawal or aggressiveness. Physical signs may include difficulty walking, poor coordination, and vision problems. A more complete list of the possible outcomes of TBI is presented in Table 7.8.

Severity seems to be related to altered levels of consciousness and posttraumatic amnesia. Consciousness levels can be classified along a continuum from extended states of unconsciousness or coma, in which the body responds only minimally to external stimuli, to consciousness with disorientation, stupor, and lethargy. Amnesia, or memory loss, is a frequent result of TBI. The duration of both coma and amnesia has been used successfully, but not infallibly, as a predictor of severity and prognosis. In general, the shorter both are, the less severe the resultant deficits of TBI and the better the potential outcome.

TABLE 7.8

Possible outcomes of TBI

Cognition
Inattentive
Disoriented
Poor memory
Poor problem-solving abilities

Language, Speech, and Oral Mechanism
Dysphagia
Dysarthria
Possible mutism
Pragmatic difficulties (talks better than can communicate)
Confused language—irrelevant, confabulatory, circumlocutionary, tangential to the topic, lacks logical sequencing, misnaming

Emotion/Personality
Aggression/withdrawal
Apathy and indifference
Denial
Depression
Disinhibition and impulsivity
Impatience
Phobias
Socially inappropriate behavior and comments
Suspiciousness and anxiety

LIFE SPAN ISSUES

Most adults with TBI are young and have experienced an auto or motorcycle accident. Imagine that you, a college student, are riding in a friend's car. The next thing that you remember is waking in the hospital, dazed, confused, and unaware of your surroundings. You may have language or other impairments that will change your life forever or at least for the immediate future.

Several stages of recovery have been described and clinical intervention varies with each (Hagen & Malkamus, 1979). Most individuals will not reach full recovery and some residual deficits will most likely remain. Initially, the individual may be nonresponsive to stimuli and need total assistance in a hospital setting.

When the individual does begin to respond, his or her responses may be undifferentiated, whole body responses that do not reflect the varying nature of the stimuli. Responses may be delayed. Vocalizations will seem purposeless.

Gradually, the individual will begin to respond differently to different stimuli and to recognize some familiar individuals. Response to commands will be inconsistent.

As the individual becomes more alert, he or she may be confused or agitated. Short-term memory and goal-directed behaviors will be poor. Although able to sit and walk, these behaviors are performed without purpose. Subject to violent mood swings, the individual may have incoherent, inappropriate, or emotional language. The individual will still need rehabilitative hospital care but will have recovered enough to move from intensive care.

As agitation fades and language continues to return, the individual can remain alert for short periods of time and hold brief conversations with strong external cues. There are still periods of nonpurposeful behavior. Short-term memory is still severely impaired. With structure, the individual can perform learned tasks but is unable to learn new behaviors.

As the individual continues to improve, he or she needs less assistance. Able to attend for up to 30 minutes with redirection, the individual is aware of the appropriate responses to self, family, and basic needs, which become more goal-directed. Relearned tasks exhibit some carryover, although new learning exhibits none. Language is used appropriately in highly familiar contexts.

Gradually, the individual becomes oriented to persons and place. Time is still confusing and the individual demonstrates only superficial understanding of his or her condition. Usually in outpatient status, the individual is able to learn and carry over this learning to other tasks and to monitor his or her own behavior with minimal assistance. Still unable to recognize inappropriate social behavior, the individual is often uncooperative, unrealistic in his or her expectations, and unaware of the needs and feelings of others.

As the individual gains more of an understanding of his or her condition and is able to plan and initiate routine tasks, frustration builds, and the individual becomes depressed, argumentative, irritable, or overly dependent or independent. Living at home and possibly having returned to work, the individual is able to concentrate for an hour even with distractions, to recall past and present events, and to learn new tasks with only minimal assistance.

Increasing abilities may not reduce the individual's low tolerance for frustration, although behavioral responses may be less. In the later stages of recovery, the individual can shift between tasks for up to two hours and initiate and carry out familiar tasks. Able to acknowledge his or her impairment, the individual is able to consider the consequences of his or her actions and to recognize the needs and feeling of others.

Finally, the individual may be able to consistently act in a socially appropriate manner, to respond appropriately to others, and to plan, initiate, and complete both familiar and unfamiliar tasks. Periodic depression may occur and irritability may reappear with illness, inability to perform a task, and in emotional situations.

The individual with TBI may face a long period of rehabilitation. Even those who have made a near-full recovery will have some lingering deficits. The authors have worked with college students who were able to gain their degrees with only minimal adaptations.

ASSESSMENT

The SLP is a member of an interdisciplinary team of rehabilitation specialists who collaborate in assessment of and intervention with persons with TBI (Ylvisaker, 1994). As such, the SLP is responsible for assessing all aspects of communication, cognitive-communicative functioning, and swallowing.

Unlike individuals with aphasia, those with TBI progress through recognizable stages of recovery. Assessment must be ongoing and varies with each stage. Background information is extremely important in determining the extent of loss. Neurological, psychiatric, and psychological reports will aid in the planning of both assessment and intervention. Observation can aid the SLP in deciding which areas to probe, especially in determining pragmatic deficits that may be missed in formal testing.

To date, few comprehensive tools exist for assessment of language skills in individuals with TBI. Many SLPs working with this population have compiled a series of individual tests for aspects of both language and cognition. These tests are often portions of larger test batteries. Language testing must be comprehensive. Tests that emphasize language form and content may fail to adequately assess pragmatics, thus underestimating the extent of the language impairment.

Sampling is essential because pragmatic behavior that varies across communicative contexts cannot be adequately assessed in a testing context alone (Starch & Falltrick, 1990). Sampling contexts should include functional activities, such as talking on the phone or grocery shopping, in natural environments, such as the home. Sampling should occur within a discourse unit, a series of related linguistic units that convey a message (Coelho, Liles, & Duffy, 1995).

INTERVENTION

With or without intervention, the pattern of recovery for individuals with TBI is predictable. Unlike those with focal damage such as a stroke, who progress smoothly, those with TBI recover in a stepwise or plateau fashion characterized by periods of little or no change interspersed with periods of rapid improvement. After a period of unconsciousness, the person often responds indiscriminately and seemingly without purpose. Attention may be fleeting, and overall level of arousal may fluctuate. The client is often hyperresponsive to stimuli and easily irritated and agitated. Clients may become very emotional and exhibit shouting, biting, and repetitive, stereotypic movements such as rocking. With recovery, clients become more clear thinking, and their behavior becomes more purposeful, although restlessness and irritability may persist.

Cognitive rehabilitation promotes independent functioning in daily life by focusing on specific cognitive processes such as memory and language processing.

As the client becomes more oriented in place and time, he or she is better able to respond to simple requests, although attention span is short and distractibility high. Memory and abstract reasoning may continue to be a problem even as the client becomes better able to manage daily living and to begin to function independently.

Intervention for cognitive-communicative deficits with individuals with TBI is called **cognitive rehabilitation,** a treatment regimen designed to increase functional abilities for everyday life by improving the capacity to process incoming information. The two primary approaches are restorative and compensatory (Ben-Yishay & Diller, 1993). The restorative approach attempts to rebuild neural circuitry and function through repetitive activities, while the compensatory approach concedes that some functions will not be recovered and develops alternatives. Restorative techniques might include classification tasks and word associations. In contrast, compensatory strategies to improve memory might include focused attending and rehearsal of new information. Traditionally, restorative strategies are attempted first and may include rehearsal and encoding strategies and the use of memory aids (Hutchinson & Marquardt, 1997). Compensatory methods are used when the restorative attempts have failed. Slowly, professionals are recognizing that compensatory strategies aid in restorative development, and both methods are being used simultaneously (Coelho, 1997).

The SLP is responsible for designing and implementing treatment programs to decrease the effects of impairment. In addition to providing direct intervention, the SLP helps to identify functional supports, such as memory logs, and work adjustments that aid in successful independent living.

Intervention programs vary depending on the stage of recovery. During the early stages, intervention focuses on orientation, sensorimotor stimulation, and recognition of familiar people and common objects and events. Early intervention results in shorter rehabilitation and higher levels of cognitive functioning (Mackay, Bernstein, Chapman, Morgan, & Milazzo, 1992).

In the middle stages, training becomes more structured and formal. The goals are to reduce confusion and improve memory and goal-directed behavior. Much of the training involves increasing the client's orientation to the everyday world. Consistency and routines are important in orientation training. The SLP may target active listening and auditory comprehension and following directions with increasingly more complex information. Word definitions, descriptions of entities and events, and classification of objects and words are also targeted. Conversational speech training is also attempted. One SLP, recognizing that the act of taking a turn is too difficult for some clients, begins by using a beanbag or other object, which is passed back and forth to signal turn changes.

During the late stages of recovery, the goal is client independence. Targets include comprehension of complex information and directions and conversational and social skills. The SLP helps the client to explore alternative strategies for word recall, memory, and problem solving. Conversational problem-solving tasks are also targeted, along with self-inhibition and self-monitoring. Real-world contexts are emphasized, especially those that are potentially confusing or emotional.

DEMENTIA

We live in a youth-oriented culture. Commercial images lead to the stereotype of older people with deteriorated bodies and minds. While physical decline with age is inevitable, intellectual capacity is frequently unimpaired. Fewer than 15 percent of the elderly experience dementia, and as many as 20 percent of these positively respond to treatment (Shekim, 1990). The incidence of dementia is increasing rapidly as the percentage of the U.S. population over age 65 increases.

T H O U G H T   Q U E S T I O N S

Do you ever assume that seniors have lost some of their cognitive abilities? Is occasional confusion always a sign of deteriorating cognitive abilities? Do you equate physical frailty with mental frailty?

Dementia is an umbrella term for a group of both pathological conditions and syndromes. It is acquired and is characterized by intellectual decline due to neurogenic causes. Memory is the most obvious function affected (American Psychiatric Association, 1994). Additional

Dementia is an impairment of intellect and cognition.

deficits include poor reasoning or judgment, impaired abstract thinking, inability to attend to relevant information, impaired communication, and personality changes.

Dementia can be divided into cortical and subcortical types based on patterns of neurophysiological impairment (Cummings & Benson, 1992). The characteristics of cortical dementias, such as Alzheimer's and Pick's diseases, resemble those of focal impairments such as aphasia and RHI. These include visuospatial deficits, memory problems, judgment and abstract thinking disturbances, and language deficits in naming, reading and writing, and auditory comprehension. Alzheimer's disease accounts for over 50 percent of the dementia cases and may affect 20 million people worldwide.

Subcortical dementias may accompany multiple sclerosis, AIDS-related encephalopathy, and Parkinson's and Huntington's diseases. A slow, progressive deterioration of cognitive functioning occurs with deficits in memory, problem solving, and language. Those disorders that involve neuromuscular functioning will be discussed in Chapter 9, "The Voice and Voice Disorders," and Chapter 12, "Neurogenic Speech Disorders."

The language functions that are most dependent on memory seem to be primarily affected. A significant decline is noted in naming and word retrieval. Language form—phonology, morphology, and syntax—is generally less disordered, although syntax may be less coherent than before as the client struggles with anomia. As a consequence, conversations may lack coherence and may be filled with repetitions, stereotypic utterances, false starts, verbal repairs, jargon, neologisms, and the use of phrases such as *that one* and *you know* (Shekim & LaPointe, 1984).

ALZHEIMER'S DISEASE

Alzheimer's is characterized by microscopic changes in the neurons of the cerebral cortex.

Alzheimer's disease is a cortical pathology that affects approximately 6 percent of individuals over age 65 and 15 percent of those over age 80 (Clarke & Witte, 1991). A heterogeneous population, individuals with Alzheimer's may be primarily impaired in memory, language, or visuospatial skills (DeSanti, 1997). Alzheimer's is two or three times as common in women as in men.

The cause of Alzheimer's disease is unknown but may be a combination of genetic and environmental factors. The neuropathology is characterized by the presence of twisted neurofilaments in the cytoplasm of neurons that deteriorate cell functioning. These tangles are most pronounced in the temporal lobe and in associational areas of the brain. Nerve fibers degenerate, resulting in brain atrophy that may decrease brain weight as much as 20 percent, especially in the temporal, frontal, and parietal lobes (Kemper, 1984; Koo & Price, 1993). Other physical changes include extensive damage to the hippocampus, located on the interior portion of the temporal lobes and formation of senile plaques within the cortex that affect dendrite and axon function.

Memory problems are the most obvious changes that accompany Alzheimer's disease. Retention of newly learned information is most impaired (Convit, deLeon, Tarshish, DeSanti, Tsui, Rusinek, & George, 1995). Long-term memory is unimpaired initially but deteriorates as the disease progresses.

Mild dementia may be characterized by name recall difficulties, occasional disorientation, and memory loss. For those with Alzheimer's, there is a slow decline with severe cognitive consequences.

Language is not affected in all individuals initially. Early problems involve word finding, off-topic comments, and comprehension. Later characteristics include paraphasia and delayed responding. In more severe stages, expressive and receptive vocabulary and complex sentence production becomes reduced, pronoun confusion is evident, topic digression and inability to return to and to shift topic are more pronounced, and writing and reading errors occur (Mentis, Briggs-Whittaker, & Gramigna, 1995). In its most severe form, the language of individuals with Alzheimer's is characterized by naming errors and the use of generic words (this, that), syntactic errors, minimal comprehension, jargon, echolalia, or mutism (DeSanti, 1997). As might be expected, increased severity results in more conversational breakdowns (Orange, Lubinsky, & Higginbotham, 1996).

LIFE SPAN ISSUES

Alzheimer's disease is a genetic disorder that lies in hiding, although early screening is possible in some cases. Environmental factors also seem to be important. Often the person who will be afflicted with the disease is unaware and/or ignores early signs. At present there are no cures, but some early drug therapies seem to lessen the effects.

In the early stages, the individual experiences memory loss, especially of new information. The individual experiences word retrieval problems and some difficulty with higher language functions, such as humor and analogies. The individual may seem indifferent and initiate little communication. Able to live at home, the individual can become an increasing burden on an elderly spouse or on adult children with families of their own.

As the disease progresses, memory loss increases with the effect that vocabulary decreases. Comprehension is reduced. Language production may be reduced to ritualistic or high usage phrases accompanied by poor topic maintenance and repair of errors, frequent repetition and word retrieval problems, and insensitivity to conversational partners. Irritability and restlessness may increase. The individual may be able to live at home with visiting nurse care to help with daily living routines.

In the most advanced stages of the disease, all intellectual functions including memory are severely impaired and almost all individuals reside in nursing homes. Language may be meaningless or the individual may be mute or echolalic. Most clients cannot recall the names of loved ones and may undergo radical personality changes. Motor function is also severely impaired and the individual will need total care.

ASSESSMENT

Definitive diagnosis of Alzheimer's is difficult in the early stages of the disease. Use of magnetic resonance imaging (MRI) may help in early identification once the course of the disease has been studied more closely. Pupil dilation tests may also indicate the presence of the disease in the early stages.

SLPs usually help identify changes in language performance that may signal intellectual deterioration. The results of this assessment may help differentiate Alzheimer's disease from other neuropathologies.

Genetic history and general and neurological health data are important elements in the assessment process. In the early stages, dementia may be confused with other disorders, such as depression. The progressive nature of the disorder makes it imperative that the SLP remain current on the changing condition of a client.

Although few language tests for this population exist, the *Arizona Battery for Communicative Disorders of Dementia* (Bayles & Kazniak, 1987) has been specifically designed to assess the retrieval, perceptual, and linguistic deficits common to dementia. Several scales exist for rating the severity of a client's loss. Of particular importance are the memory deficits that are common to many forms of dementia (Azuma & Bayles, 1997). In addition, many of the assessment batteries that are used with individuals with aphasia can be helpful in evaluating the communication skills of persons with dementia. Detailed understanding of a client's strengths and weaknesses is essential for helping family members choose the most effective communicative strategies (Causino Lamar, Obler, Knoeful, & Albert, 1994).

INTERVENTION

Intervention with those with progressive disorders can sometimes feel like trying to hold back the tide. Decline is inevitable, given the present state of our knowledge. That does not mean that we throw up our hands in dismay and give up. Quite the contrary, clinical intervention by an SLP can help to maintain the client at her or his highest level of performance and help others to maximize the client's participation in conversational interactions.

Intervention is not undertaken in isolation. As in the other disorders discussed in this chapter, the SLP is a member of a team. Professionals consult with one another and with the client and family on the best course of action.

The SLP may target memory or word retrieval by working on word associations and categories, auditory attending and comprehension in conversational contexts, coherent verbal responses, and formation of longer, more complex utterances with the help of memory aids. Family members can be helped to keep conversations focused on the present, to reduce distractions and limit the number of participants, and to foster comprehension and participation by slowing the rate and decreasing the complexity of their utterances, and using nonlinguistic cues (Shekim, 1990).

New drug therapies and bioengineering techniques hold the promise that many of the diseases that cause dementia may one day be controllable. At present, most of these new medical interventions are experimental or extremely expensive.

> Appropriate and effective intervention requires that the SLP understand what the family of the client is experiencing.

▌ SUMMARY

Aphasia, right hemisphere injury, traumatic brain injury, and dementia result in very different types of language impairment. Aphasia, the result of a focal brain injury, most likely a stroke, may result in a wide variety of impairments that may affect one or more modalities of communication, although comprehension, speech, and naming are usually impaired. Stroke is also the primary cause of right hemisphere injury. Comprehension and production of paralinguistics and complex linguistic structures are affected. Pragmatics is the most affected aspect of language. This is also true for traumatic brain injury, which, in contrast to the previous two, is a nonfocused rather than a focal injury. Finally, dementia, particularly that caused by Alzheimer's disease, is a degenerative disease. Word-finding difficulties, off-topic comments, and comprehension deficits are the most common characteristics.

In the adult language impairments discussed, the SLP functions as a member of a multidisciplinary collaborative team. The role of the SLP includes assessment of communicative abilities and their implication of other cognitive deficits, swallowing, and associated neurological disorders. Other responsibilities include treatment planning and programming, direct intervention services, interdisciplinary consultation, and family training and counseling. Intervention usually focuses on retrieval of language skills and on compensatory strategies.

REFLECTIONS

- What are the major differences between aphasia, right hemisphere injury, traumatic brain injury, and dementia?
- What are the concomitant or accompanying deficits found with aphasia?
- What are the two main types of aphasia and the characteristics of each?
- Describe the different types of stroke or CVA.

SUGGESTED READINGS

Brookshire, R. H. (1997). *Introduction to neurogenic communication disorders* (5th ed.). St. Louis, MO: Mosby.

ON-LINE RESOURCES

alzheimer@wubios.wustl.edu   Alzhemer's discussion group.

cnet_strode_dem_head_injury@listserv.arizona.edu   Stroke discussion group. TBI gopher points to other sites.

http://www.asha.org/fact_14.htm   #14 Neurological/Fluency/Voice Disorders in Multicultural Populations

http://www.nyneurosurgery.org/

Head injury tutorial with information on classification and treatment for head injury.

http://www.ninds.nih.gov/healinfo/disorder/alzheimr/alzheimers.htm

NIDCD publication on Alzheimer's disease including information and a current bibliography.

http://www.stroke.org/

Information on causes and treatment of stroke with available low-cost materials.

tbi-sprt@maelstrom.stjohns.edu   TBI discussion group.

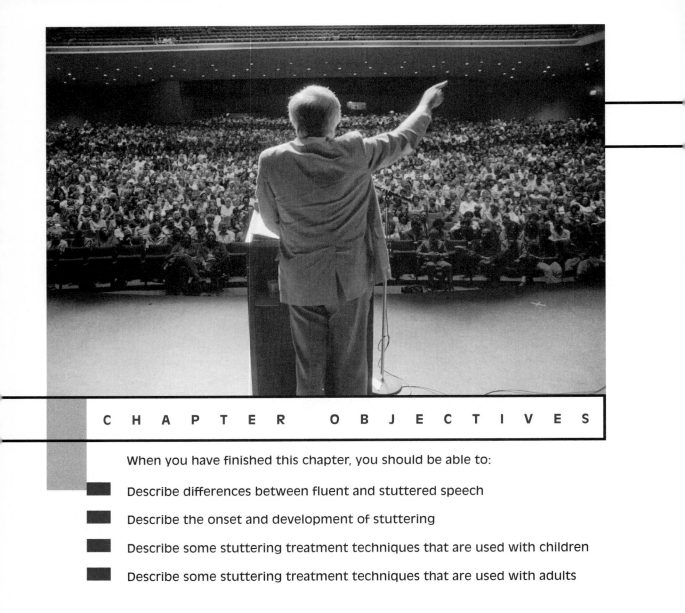

C H A P T E R   O B J E C T I V E S

When you have finished this chapter, you should be able to:

Describe differences between fluent and stuttered speech

Describe the onset and development of stuttering

Describe some stuttering treatment techniques that are used with children

Describe some stuttering treatment techniques that are used with adults

Fluency Disorders

Fluent speech is the consistent ability to move the speech production apparatus in an effortless, smooth, and rapid manner resulting in a continuous, uninterrupted forward flow of speech. Several conditions that adversely influence speech and language production can have a disruptive effect on the fluency of speech. Dysarthria, apraxia, cerebral palsy, and some forms of aphasia affect the fluency of speech. These disorders and their effects on speech and language production are discussed in Chapters 6, 7, and 12 of this book. Another condition called *cluttering* also adversely affects speech fluency. Cluttering is characterized by rapid bursts of unintelligible speech. The pri-

mary focus of this chapter is on a disorder of speech called "developmental stuttering." Developmental stuttering, or simply "stuttering," primarily influences the speaker's ability to produce fluent speech. Stuttered speech is characterized by involuntary repetitions of sounds and syllables (i.e., b-b-b-ball), sound prolongations (i.e., mmmmm-mommy), and broken words (i.e., b——oy). All three of these interruptions are considered to be stuttering behaviors, and they have a negative impact on the speaker's ability to produce fluent speech.

In this chapter, we define stuttering and discuss how stuttering begins and develops as a disorder, paying particular attention to how stuttered speech differs from fluent speech. Consideration will be given to some of the major theories regarding stuttering, the clinical diagnosis of stuttering, stuttering treatment, and, finally, treatment efficacy. As you begin reading this chapter, consider carefully the thoughts of the late Charles Van Riper, a pioneer in the treatment of stuttering. His words set the tone for this chapter. In the dedication to his 1992 book entitled *The Nature of Stuttering*, Van Riper wrote:

Dr. Charles Van Riper was a distinguished professor of speech-language pathology for many years at Western Michigan University. Dr. Van Riper learned to control his stuttering and spent most of his life searching for the cause and cure of stuttering. Therapy techniques that he developed are still in use today.

> To the ancient birch tree to whom, when I was a youth and it was a sapling, I swore an oath to find the cause and cure of the stuttering that afflicted me and so many others. Though I have failed and we have both grown old I did my utmost and am content. Others will take up my quest. (dedication page)

Many people have indeed taken up Van Riper's quest to find the cause of stuttering and a cure for it, but neither has been discovered. The cause of stuttering is elusive, and our understanding of stuttering is incomplete, despite its long and diverse history. Stuttering has been part of the human condition for all recorded time. Clay tablets found in Mesopotamia dating from centuries before the birth of Christ record the disorder, hieroglyphics from the twentieth century B.C. depict stuttering, and poems written in China more than 2,500 years ago allude to stuttering (cf. Van Riper, 1992). Stuttering affects people worldwide. Physicist Sir Isaac Newton, author W. Somerset Maugham (*Of Human Bondage*), and statesman Winston Churchill stuttered. Performers James Earl Jones, Carly Simon, Marilyn Monroe, and Bruce Willis stuttered. Stuttering is insensitive to race, creed, color, intellect, and virtually any other attribute that could be used to distinguish one human being from another.

How many people stutter? There are two ways to answer this question. The first way of determining how many people stutter is to consider the *incidence* of stuttering; the second way is to consider the *prevalence* of stuttering. The incidence of stuttering is typically determined by the number of adults who report that they stuttered at some time in their life, and the prevalence of stuttering is determined by ascertaining the number of cases in a given population (usually school-age children) during a given period of time.

The number of adults who report that they had stuttered at some time in their life is 5 percent (Andrews et al., 1983; Conture & Guitar, 1993). However, this 5 percent incidence rate includes the high percentage of children who spontaneously recover from the disorder before the age of 6 (Conture, 1996). Relatively new information indicates that 65 to 75 percent of children will recover from stuttering within the first two years after its onset and 85 percent will recover within the next few years. Given a recovery rate of about 85 percent (i.e., more than four out of five children), the 5 percent lifetime incidence percentage reduces down to about a 1 percent incidence (Conture, 1996; Yairi & Ambrose, 1992a; Yairi, Ambrose, & Nierman, 1993). It is not well understood why some children spontaneously recover from stuttering and others do not. For example, females appear to recover from stuttering more frequently than males.

Prevalence estimates of stuttering are obtained through demographic research studies. Research findings of many studies conducted in various regions around the United States suggest an average prevalence rate of 0.97 percent for school-age children (Bloodstein, 1995). This figure is consistent with the 1 percent incidence estimate and with prevalence estimates from European and Near East countries. The prevalence of stuttering is stable from the first to the ninth grade with a precipitous decline in stuttering during grades 10, 11, and 12.

T H O U G H T   Q U E S T I O N

What might be some of the reasons for the decline in stuttering during grades 10, 11, and 12?

Stuttering affects more males than females, the reported sex ratio differences ranging from 2.3 to 1 to 3.0 to 1. This difference has been attributed to differences in the physical maturation rates of boys and girls and to differences in speech and language development, but genetic factors may also be involved.

Stuttering has a high degree of familial incidence. Fifty percent of people who stutter report that they have a relative who stuttered at some time in his or her life. Fifteen percent of first-degree relatives (parents, sisters, and brothers) of people who stutter are current or recovered stutterers. This threefold increase over the reported 5 percent lifetime incidence for the general population is genetically significant (Felsenfeld, 1997; Kidd, 1984). Additionally, if one twin stutters, there is a high probability that the other twin will stutter, and the rate of concordance (both twins exhibiting the disorder) is higher for monozygotic twins (genetically identical) than for dizygotic (fraternal) twins.

Recent genetic research has indicated that stuttering may be linked to a specific single gene, although the location and nature of such a gene is unknown (Ambrose, Yairi, & Cox, 1993). Continued genetic research will ultimately play a role in our understanding of stuttering, but the actual contributions of such research "remain over the horizon" (Felsenfeld, 1997, p. 20).

EFFECTS OF STUTTERING ACROSS THE LIFE SPAN

Using a model developed by the World Health Organization, we can conceptualize the effects of the disorder of stuttering on daily life activities

(Conture, 1996; Curlee, 1993). From within the context of this model, stuttering is considered to be a *handicap* or a *handicapping condition*. Specifically, a handicap comprises "the disadvantages that result from reactions to the audible and visible events of a person's stuttering, including those of the person who stutters" (Conture, 1996, p. S20). Both informal and formal observations suggest that stuttering has a negative effect on a wide variety of daily life activities, especially in three main venues of life, school, work, and social interactions. Children may withdraw and refuse to communicate orally in school, adults may select professions that require little or no oral communication, and both children and adults may avoid social contact because of a fear of speaking.

EFFECTS OF STUTTERING ON SCHOOL PERFORMANCE

Let us first consider the negative impact stuttering can have on a child's school performance. Stutterers, on the whole, are poorer in educational adjustment than normal speakers. This conclusion is based on the amount of retention in grade at school. On average, children who stutter are delayed about half a year or half a grade level. Schoolchildren who stutter are older than their classmates who do not stutter, a finding suggesting that children who stutter are more likely to be held back in school. If so, timely and appropriate treatment should be expected to improve the academic performance of children who stutter (Bloodstein, 1995; Conture, 1996).

EFFECTS OF STUTTERING ON WORK

Stuttering can also have a negative impact in the workplace. Stuttering is a vocationally handicapping condition because employers view it as a disorder that decreases employability and opportunities for promotion (Hurst & Cooper, 1983). Despite this view, when an employee who stutters seeks treatment, there is an attendant improvement in the employer's perception of the employee (Craig & Calvert, 1991). This enhanced perception is reflected by increased numbers of job promotions among employees who sought treatment and were successful in maintaining fluency following treatment.

EFFECTS OF STUTTERING ON SOCIAL INTERACTIONS

Stuttering's potential effects on an individual's social interactions and quality of life are not well understood. Clinical observations suggest that successfully treated individuals, particularly adults, experience an improvement in their social interactions, but the nature and significance of these changes in social behavior are not well documented (Conture, 1996). However, considerable research has indicated that people who stutter do not as a group exhibit consistent, recognized patterns of psychoneurotic disturbance, but mild forms of social maladjustment are frequently reported (Bloodstein, 1995). Further research is needed to determine whether and to what extent stuttering treatment influences psychosocial adjustment (Conture, 1996).

T H O U G H T   Q U E S T I O N

What kinds of jobs require a great deal of speaking? What kinds of jobs do not require a great deal of speaking? Do you think it likely that people who stutter might choose to avoid jobs that require a great deal of speaking? Explain.

FLUENT SPEECH VERSUS STUTTERING

Anyone who has listened carefully to a young child speak can attest to the fact that the flow of most children's speech is not continuously forward and uninterrupted. Children exhibit many hesitations, revisions, and interruptions in their utterances. Children are not born as fluent speakers. Fluency requires some degree of physical maturation and language experience, but it does not develop linearly as the child matures. Longitudinal research indicates that children around 25 months of age are more fluent than they will be at 29 months and at 37 months of age (Yairi, 1981, 1982). There is a gradual increasing in disfluent behaviors beginning around 2 years of age that peaks around the third birthday. Fluency then improves after the third birthday, and the types of disfluency change.

NORMAL DISFLUENCIES

The type of disfluency exhibited by the normally developing child changes between the ages of 25 and 37 months. At approximately 2 years of age, typical disfluencies are whole-word repetitions (I-I-I want a cookie), interjections (Can we-uhm-go now?), and syllable repetitions (I like ba-baseball). Revisions such as "He can't—he won't play baseball" are the dominant disfluency type when the child is approximately 3 years old (Yairi, 1982). Normal disfluencies persist throughout the course of one's life, but they do not tend to adversely affect the continuous forward flow of speech. Normally fluent speakers frequently interrupt the forward flow of speech by repeating whole multisyllablic

Some parenthetical interjections or asides that are common interruptions in adult speech are devices that help to maintain listener interest. An example of a parenthetical interjection is "When John slipped on the stairs—like Mary slipped in the same spot last week—he broke his ankle."

words (I really-really like hockey), interjecting a word or phrase (He will, uhhhhh, you know, not like that idea), repeating a phrase (Will you, will you please stop that), or revising a sentence (She can't—She didn't do that).

THOUGHT QUESTION

What are some normal speech disfluencies that you might exhibit under conditions such as speaking in front of a large audience or to a professor whom you find intimidating?

STUTTERED DISFLUENCIES

What is stuttering and how is it different from normally fluent and normally disfluent speech? These are not simple questions, and there are no simple answers. Consider the words of English literary genius Samuel Johnson (1709–1784) when he mused about poetry: "Sir, what is poetry? Why, sir, it is much easier to say what it is not" (Gregory, 1981, p. 416). We might say the same about stuttering.

The chances are that you know what stuttering is, but could you explain what it is? For example, if you viewed a cartoon featuring Porky Pig and were then asked to classify Porky's speech, it is highly likely that you would classify it as stuttering. But what exactly are you reacting to? What aspects of Porky's speech led you to such a conclusion? Your best friend might also classify Porky's speech as stuttering, but is your friend reacting to the same aspects of speech as you are? Clinical and research evidence suggests that even though both of you classify Porky as a stutterer, you might be using different aspects of his speech to lead you to that classification.

The issue of what stuttering is and how to define it lies at the center of some unresolved issues (Ingham & Cordes, 1997). Can clinicians determine reliably if and when stuttering has occurred? Do normal disfluencies and stuttered disfluencies lie along the same continuum or are they categorically different behavioral events? There are no absolute answers to these questions. At present, no universally accepted definition of stuttering exists. However, a reasonable framework from which one can begin to distinguish between normal disfluencies and those that are likely to be regarded as stuttered disfluencies has been proposed:[1]

> Speech, like many other human behaviors, is occasionally produced by speakers with hesitations, interruptions, prolongations and repetitions. These disruptions in . . . ongoing speech behavior are termed

[1]See also Guitar's (1998) definition of stuttering.

disfluency and the frequency, duration, type, severity and so forth of these speech disfluencies vary greatly from person to person and from speaking situation to speaking situation. Some speech disfluencies, particularly those which involve within-word disruptions (such as sound or syllable repetitions), are most apt to be classified or judged by listeners as *stuttering*. (Conture, 1990a, p. 2)

Specifically, stuttering or stuttered speech involves part-word repetitions, sound prolongations, monosyllabic whole-word repetitions, and/or within-word pauses (Conture, 1990b). Tense pauses and hesitations between words may also be regarded as stuttering. In other words, stuttering is "any cessation in the forward flow of speech marked by audible or inaudible repetitions or prolongations of word/syllable fragments, including periods of silence between words/syllables" (Prins, Hubbard & Krause, 1991, p. 1012). Examples of stuttered speech can be heard and seen on the book's CD-ROM.

Disfluencies that occur within a word unit that are likely to be regarded as stuttering include monosyllabic whole-word repetitions (he-he-he-he-hit me), sound repetitions (p-p-p-p-pail), syllable repetitions (ba-ba-ba-ba-baseball), audible prolongations (sssssss-snow), and inaudible prolongations, (g——irl). Table 8.1 lists some between-word and within-word disfluency types. More than one type of within-word disfluency may be present in a given disruption that interferes with the forward flow of speech. Consider the following disfluent production of the word "mommy" that contains elements of both a sound repetition and an audible prolongation: "m-m-m-mmmommy" (Yaruss, 1997). Such productions, called "clustered disfluencies," are quite common in the speech of children who stutter. Some researchers have suggested that the presence of clustered disfluencies may indicate incipient (just beginning, in an early stage) stuttering and that they may help to differentiate children who stutter from children who do not stutter.

Within-word disfluencies and some between-word disfluencies are considered to be the cardinal, universal features of stuttering, but there are other behaviors that may accompany instances of disfluency. Behaviors that occur concomitantly with stuttered disfluencies are called secondary symptoms, or accessory behaviors, and are widely varied and idiosyncratic. Some common secondary symptoms include blinking of the eyes; facial grimacing; facial tension; and exaggerated movements of the head, shoulders, and arms. Interjected speech fragments that are superfluous to the utterance are also considered to be secondary symptoms, particularly when they are in connection with a disfluency. An example of an interjected speech fragment is the superfluous phrase "that is to say" in the utterance "I met her in T-T-T-T, that is to say, I met her in Toronto." An example of secondary symptoms can be seen on the book's CD-ROM.

TABLE 8.1

Types of within-word (stuttered) and between-word (normal) speech disfluencies

Disfluency Type	Within-Word	Between-Word	Examples
Sound/syllable repetitions	X		He's a b-b-b-boy. G-g-g-g-go away. Yes, puh-puh-please.
Sound prolongation	X		Ssssssee me swing! T——oronto is cool.
Broken word	X		Base-(pause)-ball.
Monosyllabic whole-word repetitions	X	X	I-I-I-hit the ball. It's my-my-my-turn.
Multisyllabic whole-word repetitions		X	I'm going-going home.
Phrase repetition/ interjection		X	She hit—she hit me. I like, uh, ya know, big boats.
Revisions		X	He went, he came back.

Source: Adapted from Conture (1990b).

The speaker may have adopted these behaviors in an effort to minimize stuttering (Bloodstein, 1995). The person who stutters discovers through trial and error that some action (e.g., bodily movements) momentarily distracts from the act of speaking and that action appears to help terminate or avoid an instance of stuttering. Behaviors such as eye blinking, however, soon lose their apparent power to reduce stuttering, and the individual is forced to replace the ineffective behavior with a new behavior, such as shrugging the shoulders, to reduce stuttering. Unfortunately, the eye blinking behavior may have become so strongly habituated that it will remain permanently associated with a person's stuttering. How do these cardinal stuttering behaviors and secondary symptoms develop and how do they change over the course of an individual's life?

THE ONSET AND DEVELOPMENT OF STUTTERING THROUGH THE LIFE SPAN

Although stuttering can develop at any age, the most common form of stuttering begins in the preschool years and is called **developmental stuttering.** Developmental stuttering is contrasted with the second form of stuttering, called **neurogenic stuttering,** which is typically associated with neurological disease or trauma. Neurogenic stuttering differs from the more common developmental stuttering in several ways.

Disfluencies associated with developmental stuttering usually occur on content words (e.g., nouns, verbs), whereas disfluencies associated with neurogenic stuttering tend to occur on function words (e.g., conjunctions, prepositions) and content words. People who have developmental stuttering frequently exhibit secondary symptoms and anxiety about speaking, whereas neurogenic stutterers do not. Finally, developmental stuttering tends to occur on the initial syllables of words, whereas neurogenic stuttering is more widely dispersed throughout the utterance (Ringo & Dietrich, 1995). We will focus primarily on developmental stuttering in this chapter.

It is generally accepted that the onset of developmental stuttering occurs between the ages of 2 and 5 and that the risk of developing stuttering is mostly over by the time the child is 3½ years old (Yairi, 1983; Yairi & Ambrose, 1992a, b). The onset of stuttering is gradual for the majority of children who develop the condition, with stuttering severity increasing as the child grows older. When stuttering develops in a gradual manner, some general trends regarding stuttering behaviors, reactions to stuttering, and conditions that seem to promote stuttering can be observed. We will outline some of these developmental trends (Bloodstein, 1995). Not all children will exactly follow this developmental framework of stuttering, but it generally does capture the onset and progression of the disorder. This developmental framework is divided into four phases that have a sequential relationship to each other.

Phase One corresponds to the preschool years, roughly between the ages of 2 and 6. During Phase One, periods of stuttering are followed by periods of relative fluency. The episodic nature of stuttering is an indication that stuttering is in its most rudimentary form. The child may stutter for weeks at a time between long interludes of normally fluent speech. The child will tend to stutter most when he or she is upset or excited, and in conditions of communicative pressure, such as when a parent forces a child to recite in front of friends or relatives. Sound and syllable repetitions are the dominant feature of stuttering during Phase One, but there is also a tendency to repeat whole words. Stuttering tends to occur at the beginnings of sentences, clauses, and phrases on both content words (e.g., nouns, verbs) and function words (e.g., articles, prepositions, etc.) unlike more advanced forms of stuttering, in which disfluencies are generally confined to content words. Finally, during Phase One, most children are unaware of the interruptions in their speech.

Phase Two represents a progression of the disorder and is associated with children of elementary school age. In Phase Two, stuttering is essentially chronic, or habitual, with few intervals of fluent speech. The child has developed a self-concept as a person who stutters and will refer to himself or herself in that way. Stuttering in Phase Two occurs primarily on content words with much less tendency to stutter only on the initial words of sentences and phrases. Stuttering is more widely dispersed throughout the child's utterances. Although the child has a self-concept as a person who stutters, he or she exhibits little or no concern about the stuttering. Stuttering in Phase Two also increases under conditions of excitement.

Phase Three is associated with individuals who can range in age from about 8 years to young adulthood. Stuttering in Phase Three seems to be in response to specific situations such as speaking to strangers, speaking in front of groups, or talking on the telephone. Certain words are regarded as more difficult than others, and the person who stutters will attempt to avoid such words by using word substitutions and circumlocutions. An example of a word substitution is "I want a ni-ni-ni—five cents"; the child substitutes "five cents" for the originally intended word "nickel." Circumlocutions are roundabout or indirect ways of speaking. A circumlocution used to avoid the term "fire truck" in a child's request for a toy might take on the following form "I want a——ya know——red thing——sirens and ladders——truck for my birthday." Despite the individual's awareness of stuttering, he or she will present little evidence of fear or embarrassment and will not avoid specific speaking situations.

In Phase Four, the apex of development, stuttering is in its most advanced form. A primary characteristic of Phase Four is vivid and fearful anticipation of stuttering. Certain sounds, words, and speaking situations are feared and avoided, word substitutions and circumlocutions are frequent, and there is evidence of embarrassment. Stuttered words may have associated audible vocal tension and rising pitch, which can be seen on the book's CD-ROM. Bloodstein's phases are summarized in Table 8.2. See Box 8.1 for the personal story of a young man whose fear of speaking prevented him from eating his favorite food.

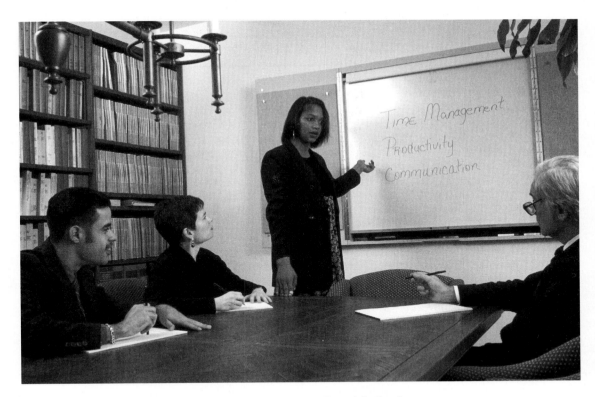

Speaking in public often causes an increase in disfluent behaviors.

T H O U G H T   Q U E S T I O N S

What factors might contribute to the changes in a person's reactions to his or her stuttering? What speaking situations do
you have that are fearful or very difficult?

Stuttering does not always develop gradually. For some individuals, stuttering first appears in a severe form with characteristics of advanced stuttering. A number of investigators have reported that when
stuttering is first diagnosed in some young children, the symptoms
appear to be very advanced and secondary symptoms may be present
(Van Riper, 1982; Yairi & Ambrose, 1992a, b; Yairi, Ambrose, & Nierman, 1993). In one longitudinal study of stuttering, the onset was a distinct and sudden event for 36 percent of the children, and the stuttering

Personal Story of a Young Man Who Stuttered

Geoff was a teenage boy who was first seen at the speech and hearing clinic on his thirteenth birthday. His parents explained, during an initial interview, that Geoff had begun stuttering when he was around 4 years old. They further explained that the stuttering would come and go, and he would sometimes have fluent periods that lasted two months. Although the parents were concerned about Geoff's stuttering behaviors, they thought that he would outgrow the stuttering. This belief was reinforced by his long periods of fluency.

Geoff was evaluated by an SLP. Formal tests of stuttering placed him as a severe stutterer, most of his stuttering behaviors taking the form of long sound prolongations. Geoff told the SLP that his grades in school were falling because he would not speak in class and that he didn't like to interact with his classmates because they "always make fun of the way I talk." He also reported that there were certain words that he could not say without stuttering severely.

The SLP recommended that Geoff enroll in therapy twice a week for a trial period of six months. The parents and Geoff agreed. He made good progress during this trial period and stayed in therapy for an additional four months. At the end of ten months of therapy, he was dismissed, exhibiting good control over his stuttering.

Two months later, he and his mother came back to the clinic for a reevaluation of his fluency skills. During the reevaluation, Geoff told the SLP that he was happy with his new speech because he could say any word he wanted without stuttering. He told the SLP that he loved to go to McDonald's or Burger King to eat cheeseburgers and French fries. But before therapy, if he had to place his own order, he wouldn't order the French fries because he knew he would stutter on the word "French." He went without the fries more times than he cared to recall. Nowadays, Geoff is enjoying his cheeseburgers *with* the French fries that he orders himself. According to Geoff, that makes him the "happiest kid on the planet."

behaviors were considered to be moderate to severe (Yairi & Ambrose, 1992a).

More research is needed on the onset and development of stuttering. Such research could provide clues that could distinguish children who exhibit incipient, or beginning, stuttering from those who will spontaneously recover from the disorder. Additionally, such research could shed light on the cause or causes of stuttering in children.

TABLE 8.2

Summary of Bloodstein's four phases of the onset and development of stuttering

Phase	Age	Highlights
One	2–6 years	Stuttering is episodic.
		Most stuttering occurs when the child is upset or excited.
		Sound/syllable repetitions are the dominant speech feature.
		Child seems unaware of the stuttering.
Two	Elementary school age	Stuttering is chronic.
		Stuttering occurs on content words (nouns, verbs).
		Child regards himself or herself as a stutterer.
Three	8 years to adulthood	Stuttering is situational (speaking on the telephone, speaking to large groups).
		Certain words are regarded as more difficult than others.
		Circumlocutions and word substitutions are frequent.
Four	8 years to adulthood	Stuttering is at its apex of development.
		There is fearful anticipation of stuttering.
		Certain sounds, words, and speaking situations are avoided.
		Increased circumlocutions and word substitutions are present.

THEORIES AND CONCEPTUALIZATIONS OF STUTTERING

An examination of some of the more prominent etiological theories of stuttering will provide you with an appreciation of the various models that have influenced stuttering research and treatment for over seventy years in this country. Additionally, various aspects of some of the theories we will consider are implicitly present in contemporary stuttering research and treatment. Etiological theories of stuttering can be classified into three categories: organic, behavioral, and psychological.

ORGANIC THEORY

Organic theories propose an actual physical cause for stuttering. Speculations about a physical cause for stuttering date back to the writings of Aristotle, who suggested that stuttering was a disconnection between the mind and the body. Aristotle theorized that the muscles of the tongue were weak and could not follow the commands of the brain (Rieber & Wollock, 1977). Many organic theories have been proposed since Aristotle's writings, but they have all failed in one manner or another to explain stuttering satisfactorily. Perhaps one of the best-known organic theories of stuttering is the *theory of cerebral dominance* or the "handedness theory" proposed by Samuel Orton and Lee Travis in the 1930s (Bloodstein, 1995). The theory assumed that one of the cerebral hemispheres was dominant over the other for issuing the neural impulses that controlled the temporal sequencing of speech. If one hemisphere was not dominant, both would send competing neural impulses to their respective muscles of speech. As a result, a discoordination between the right and left halves of the speech musculature would exist. This discoordination was believed to result in stuttering. Subsequent research and clinical observation ultimately led to the demise of this theory.

Speculations about potential organic origins of stuttering reemerged in the 1970s, based largely on the observations of Marcel Wingate. Wingate (1969, 1970) developed the modified vocalization hypothesis, which asserted that stuttering was reduced greatly in conditions in which voicing was absent (whispering) or modified in some way (singing or speaking with delayed auditory feedback). (Delayed auditory feedback is discussed later this chapter.) A great deal of research conducted in the 1970s indicated that the amount of stuttering was reduced proportionally as the rapid shift between voiced and unvoiced sounds associated with spontaneous speech was reduced. Such research findings led Wingate and other investigators to suggest that stuttering was a discoordination between the muscles used for phonation and other muscles that are used during speech production.

The continued search for a specific organic cause of stuttering has been enhanced recently by developments in medical technology. Researchers are currently studying the central nervous system of people who stutter using techniques such as computerized tomography, magnetic resonance imaging, and the measurement of regional cerebral blood flow. The findings of this research, although preliminary, indicate that stuttering may be linked to the failure of a neurophysiological system that integrates motoric, linguistic, and cognitive processes (Watson & Freeman, 1997). Future brain imaging research may facilitate the development of a comprehensive neurophysiological model for both fluent and stuttered speech that could lead to new stuttering prevention and treatment methods.

BEHAVIORAL THEORY

Behavioral theories assert that stuttering is a learned response to conditions external to the individual. A prominent behavioral theory, the *diagnosogenic* theory, was developed by Wendell Johnson of the University of Iowa during the 1940s and 1950s. Johnson contended that the speech hesitations of children whose parents believed their children to be stuttering did not differ from the speech hesitations of children whose parents did not consider them to be stuttering. The differences between these two groups of children lay in the parental reactions to these hesitations. Three of Johnson's conclusions stand as a formal statement of his theory:

1. Practically every case of stuttering was originally diagnosed, not by a speech expert, but by a layperson—usually one, or both, of the child's parents.
2. What these laypersons had diagnosed as stuttering was, by and large, indistinguishable from the hesitations and repetitions known to be characteristic of the normal speech of young children.
3. Stuttering . . . as a definite disorder was found to occur, not before being diagnosed, but after being diagnosed (Bloodstein, 1995, p. 77).

For Johnson, stuttering began in the parent's ear, not in the child's mouth, through a series of events similar to the following scenario: Overly concerned parents would react to the child's normal speech hesitations and repetitions with negative statements admonishing the child to speak more slowly and not to stutter. Such parental behaviors made the child anxious about speaking, and the child's anxiety fostered further hesitations and repetitions. The parents would react with increased criticism and punishment, which in turn raised the child's anxiety level about speaking and increased disfluent speech behaviors. The child's disfluent behaviors soon became a habitual manner of speaking.

Johnson's diagnosogenic theory has not been verified, and some of the basic premises of the theory have been called seriously into question (McDearmon, 1968). Nonetheless, parent-child communicative interactions play a pivotal role in certain contemporary therapeutic regimes; this will be discussed later in this chapter.

THOUGHT QUESTION

In what ways could a parent's speech pattern influence the speech pattern of his or her child? For example, could the rate of a parent's speech affect the child's speech?

PSYCHOLOGICAL THEORY

Psychological theory contends that stuttering is a neurotic symptom with ties to unconscious needs and internal conflicts, treated most appropriately by psychotherapy. Some psychological theories regard people who stutter as individuals with neuroses; other theories regard stuttering as a phobic manifestation. However, research indicates that psychotherapy is not an effective method for the treatment of stuttering. Some people who stutter may indeed have neuroses, but psychological theory has yet to provide a cogent explanation for the underlying cause of stuttering or its onset and development.

CURRENT CONCEPTUAL MODELS OF STUTTERING

Postma and Kolk (1993) introduced a conceptualization of stuttering called the *covert repair hypothesis,* which is based on a language production model. The basic assumption of the covert repair hypothesis is that stuttering is a reaction to some flaw in the phonetic plan of speech. Speakers have the capability of monitoring their speech as it is being formulated and detecting errors in the speech plan. People who stutter have poorly developed phonological encoding skills that cause them to introduce errors into their speech plan. If there are more errors in the speech plan, there will be more occasions for error correction. Postma and Kolk (1993) suggest that stuttering is not the error. Rather, stuttering is a "normal" repair reaction to an abnormal phonetic plan.

Another relatively new conceptualization of stuttering is the *demands and capacities model* (DCM) (Starkweather, 1987, 1997). This model asserts that stuttering develops when the environmental demands placed on a child to produce fluent speech exceed the child's physical and learned capacities. The child's capacity for fluent speech depends on a balance of motor skills, language production skills, emotional maturity, and cognitive development. Children who stutter presumably lack one or more of these capacities for fluent speech. Some children who stutter may lack the required motor skills, other children who stutter may lack the required language skills, and so on. Parents of a child who lacks the required motor skills for fluency might talk rapidly; rapid rates of speech may put a time pressure on the child that exceeds his or her motoric ability to respond. Other parents might insist on the use of advanced language structures that are in excess of the child's language development. In every case of stuttering within the DCM, there is an imbalance between the environmental demands that are placed on the child and the child's capacity for fluent speech.

The DCM is not a theory of stuttering, and it does not suggest a cause for stuttering. Rather, the DCM is a useful tool that helps clinicians to understand the dynamics of forces that contribute to the development of stuttering. Therapeutically, the DCM provides useful guidelines for understanding what capacities a child may lack for fluent speech production and the elements of the child's environment that may be challenging those capacities.

T H O U G H T   Q U E S T I O N

Your professor has called on you in class to explain a problem that was part of the homework assignment that you didn't complete. What happens to your speech patterns?

THERAPEUTIC TECHNIQUES USED WITH YOUNG CHILDREN

When parents present a child to the speech-language pathologist (SLP) with the concern that the child is stuttering, it is the SLP's responsibility to determine whether there should be concern about the child's speech behaviors and, if so, to plan an appropriate course of action. Two important components of the evaluation of a child suspected of stuttering are observations of the child and parents interacting with one another and a detailed parental interview (see Table 8.3 for some common questions for parents with a disfluent child).

THE EVALUATION OF STUTTERING

A number of aspects of parent-child interactions have been identified as contributing to stuttering in children, including excessive parental speech rates exceeding 200 words per minute, the use of complex linguistic structures that are too sophisticated for the child, and frequent parental interruptions. Although these parental behaviors do not cause stuttering, they are quite likely to exacerbate or perpetuate the stuttering (Conture, 1990b). Careful observation of parent-child interactions will provide vital information that will be used later in parent counseling.

A second important component of the stuttering evaluation is a detailed analysis of the child's speech behaviors. The SLP determines the average number of each type of disfluency the child produces (e.g., within-word repetitions, sound prolongations). Three or more within-

TABLE 8.3

Common questions for parents of a disfluent child

Introduction

Why are you here today?

Tell us (me) about your child's problem.

General Development

Tell us (me) about your child's development from birth to present.

How does this compare with his or her siblings?

Family History

Do any other family members have speech, hearing, or language problems?

Did they receive speech therapy?

Speech/Language Development

When did your child say his or her first words?

When did your child say his or her first phrases and sentences?

History/Description of the Problem

Describe your child's speaking problems.

When did the problem start?

What was your reaction? Did you bring the problem to your child's attention?

Can you describe your child's stuttering when it first began?

Has it changed over time?

Does your child lose eye contact when talking to you?

Does your child have excessive body movements when talking?

Does he or she avoid speaking situations?

Have you done anything to help your child stop stuttering?

Family Interactions

What do you and your child do when you spend time together?

What kind of things do you do as a family?

How do you handle sibling hostilities?

Wrap Up

If you could wish for three things for your child, what would you wish for?

Source: Adapted from Conture (1990b).

word disfluencies per 100 words spoken may indicate that the child has a fluency problem (Conture, 1990b). The percentage of the total disfluency that each type of disfluency contributes is another important evaluative measure. For example, if the child produces 10 disfluencies per 100 words spoken and 6 of them are sound prolongations, then 60 percent of all the disfluencies are sound prolongations. A high percentage of sound prolongations may indicate a chronic fluency problem. The SLP will also measure the duration of several disfluencies. Longer durations and/or multiple sound or syllable repetitions may represent an increase in the severity of the stuttering problem. Standardized tests such as the *Stuttering Prediction Instrument* (SPI; Riley & Riley, 1981) may also be used in the fluency evaluation. The SPI yields a numerical score that ranges from 0 to 37 based on a number of stuttering-related behaviors such as the duration of disfluencies and stuttering frequency. The numerical score is converted to a verbal stuttering severity rating. Numerical scores of 10–11 indicate very mild stuttering, whereas scores of 36–37 indicate very severe stuttering. Finally, the SLP will record the types of secondary symptoms that the child presents. A wide assortment of secondary symptoms may indicate a progression of the disorder.

The SLP's decision to recommend therapy is not based on any single behavior or test result. Therapy may be recommended if two or more of the following behaviors are observed:

1. Sound prolongations constitute more than 25 percent of the total disfluencies produced by the child.
2. Instances of sound or syllable repetitions or sound prolongations on the first syllables of words during iterative speech tasks (e.g., iterative productions of pa-ta-ka, pa-ta-ka, pa-ta-ka).
3. Loss of eye contact on more than 50 percent of the child's utterances.
4. A score of 18 or more on the SPI (Conture, 1990b).

INDIRECT AND DIRECT STUTTERING INTERVENTION

If the SLP determines that the child has a stuttering problem or a high probability of developing stuttering, therapeutic intervention is indicated. In general, two broad intervention strategies can be used with young children who stutter: indirect therapy and direct therapy. Indirect approaches are considered viable for children who are just beginning to stutter and whose stuttering is fairly mild. Direct approaches are typically reserved for children who have been stuttering for at least a year and whose stuttering is moderate to severe.

An indirect approach does not explicitly try to modify or change the child's speech fluency, focusing instead on the child, the child's parents, and the child's environment. Important aspects of indirect therapy are information sharing and counseling in which the parent is encouraged to reduce communicative pressure on the child and provide a slow, relaxed speech model for the child. Play-oriented activities that encourage slow and relaxed speech are the central component of such intervention. There is no explicit discussion about the child's fluent or stuttering speaking behaviors. The goal of indirect therapy is to facilitate fluency through environmental manipulation.

T H O U G H T   Q U E S T I O N

What kinds of activities might be used to encourage slow, relaxed speech?

Direct approaches involve explicit and direct attempts to modify the child's speech and speech-related behaviors. In direct therapy, concepts such as "hard" and "easy" speech are introduced. Hard speech is rapid and relatively tense (such as a tense sound prolongation of /s/ in sssssssssss-snake), whereas easy speech is slow and relaxed. The terms "hard" and "easy" are simple and carry little negative connotation for the child. Children are taught to identify both types of speech by first monitoring their tape-recorded utterances and later by identifying these types of speech in their ongoing productions. Once the child is able to accurately and reliably identify hard and easy speech segments, the SLP teaches the child strategies that will help him or her increase easy speech and change from hard speech to easy speech when required. The therapeutic sequence of identification followed by identification/modification forms the core elements of many strategies for children and adults.

PARENTAL COUNSELING

Whether or not the child is recommended for therapy, parental counseling is almost always indicated. In addition to providing the parents with information about normal speech and language development, the SLP needs to suggest ways that will help their child to speak in an easy, effortless manner. Perkins (1992) has summarized some important issues that need to be stressed in a parental counseling session. First, parents and other family members should provide relaxed and slow speech models for the child. Relaxed and slow speech can be accomplished by prolonging vowels, delaying response times, and pausing frequently during conversational speech. Simply telling the child to "slow down" or "relax" might cause the child to feel self-conscious or anxious about speaking, which in turn might increase stuttering behaviors. Slow and relaxed communicative situations facilitate fluency by reducing pressure on the child to compete for time on the floor. Another way to reduce communicative pressure is to have one parent spend time with the child in a one-to-one context. One-to-one speaking situations provide an opportunity for the child to communicate without interruptions from other children or adults. Parents should also be counseled to reduce the general level of excitement in the home and to avoid negative verbal interactions between the child and other family members. Finally, parents should not pressure the child to talk or perform verbally.

T H O U G H T   Q U E S T I O N

What are some other ways a parent could reduce communicative pressure on his or her child?

THERAPEUTIC TECHNIQUES USED WITH OLDER CHILDREN AND ADULTS WHO STUTTER

Individuals who continue to stutter into their teenage years and beyond are considered to be adults who stutter. The adult who stutters will likely have many negative reactions to speaking situations that may affect his or her social life and vocational goals. Many of these individuals will have had previous unsuccessful speech therapy and perhaps other forms of remediation to combat the fluency problem. The adult who stutters "brings a complexity of attitudes, experiences, and coping attempts to the therapeutic process, and these must be dealt with directly or indirectly" (Gelfer, 1996, p. 160).

The primary focus of this section of the chapter is on several of the therapeutic techniques that are used to manage adulthood stuttering. In particular, we will explore direct techniques that are used to establish fluency in the adult stutterer. Changing certain aspects of one's speaking behavior is of fundamental importance in stuttering intervention and is often a source of confusion among clinicians who treat the adults who stutter (Sommers & Caruso, 1995).

Therapeutic techniques designed to modify stuttering behaviors are classified generally into two broad categories: *fluency-shaping techniques* and *stuttering modification techniques.* When used properly, both techniques have a powerful effect in reducing stuttering. Fluency-shaping techniques involve changing the overall speech timing patterns of the individual. This is typically accomplished by lengthening the duration of sounds and words and greatly slowing down the overall rate of speech. Stuttering modification techniques involve changing only the stuttering behaviors. This is typically accomplished by lengthening the duration of or in some way modifying only the speech segment on which the stuttering is occurring.

A different and perhaps more useful way of classifying therapeutic techniques considers those that modify the "timing of speech movements" and those that modify the "physical tension of speech movements" (Max & Caruso, 1997). Although we will be discussing various techniques that modify speech timing and physical tension as individual entities, combinations of these various individual techniques can be used therapeutically. That is, many of these techniques are not mutually exclusive, and elements of several techniques can be used simultaneously in the treatment of stuttering. It is not well understood exactly how these various techniques reduce stuttering, and their genesis has come largely from the clinical trenches of trial and error. Techniques that modify the timing of speech movements will be discussed first.

Delayed Auditory Feedback systems use a microphone and earphones. A person wearing the earphones speaks into the microphone, which transmits the speech to a device that electronically delays sending the speech to the earphones. If the delay were set at 0 milliseconds, there would be no delay, much like hearing yourself talk. However, if the delay were set at 250 milliseconds (or ¼ second) the speaker would hear his or her utterance ¼ of a second after it was uttered. Delaying the auditory feedback causes the speaker to reduce the rate of speaking.

MODIFYING THE TIMING OF SPEECH MOVEMENTS

Reducing the rate of speech, known as *prolonged speech,* is one of the most frequently used techniques to reduce stuttering. Prolonged speech may be a specific therapeutic goal, or it may be used as strategy to control the occurrence of stuttering (Max & Caruso, 1997). The term "prolonged speech" arose from research conducted in the 1960s regarding the effects of delayed auditory feedback (DAF) on speech production. DAF is a condition in which a speaker hears his or her own speech after an instrumental delay of some finite period of time, such as 250 or 500 milliseconds. When a person speaks under DAF, his or her speech is slowed down involuntarily because the duration of syllables is prolonged. For example, when people who stutter speak under conditions of DAF, speaking rates decrease dramatically, and the longer the delay, the slower the speech. The slowed speaking rate associated with DAF is accompanied by a substantial decrease in stuttering.

When DAF is used clinically to prolong speech, the feedback delay is set to promote speaking rates of approximately 30–60 syllables per minute. During this initial phase, the person who stutters is taught to prolong the duration of each syllable but not to increase the duration of pauses between syllables (Boburg & Kully, 1995; Max & Caruso, 1997). This prolonged speech pattern is systematically altered over the course of intervention by adjusting the DAF times to reduce the magnitude of syllable prolongation while maintaining fluent speech. Speech rates ranging from 120 to 200 syllables per minute are typical targets for the termination of therapy. An example of DAF-facilitated prolonged speech can be seen on the book's CD-Rom.

Another clinical rate reduction technique, called *pausing/phrasing,* is designed to lengthen naturally occurring pauses (clause and sentence boundaries) and to add pauses between other words or phrases. Additionally, pausing/phrasing techniques may attempt to limit utterance length to 2–5 syllables. Both this strategy and DAF have an ameliorative or lessening effect on the frequency of stuttering. A formal stuttering treatment known as the *Gradual Increase in Length and Complexity of Utterance* (Ryan, 1974) capitalizes on the underlying principles of pausing/phrasing techniques.

Three techniques developed by Charles Van Riper can be placed under the general rubric of modifying the timing of speech movements. These techniques are well established and widely used for stuttering modification. Van Riper conceptualized stuttering as a disorder of speech timing, and he later proposed that his techniques were designed to improve the sequential ordering and timing of speech motor acts (Van Riper, 1982). As such, his three techniques known as *cancellations, pull-outs,* and *preparatory sets* are considered under modifying speech timing movements. Examples of these techniques can be seen on the website.

These three techniques are introduced therapeutically in sequential order, beginning with stuttering cancellation. During the cancellation phase of therapy, an individual is required to complete the word that was stuttered and pause deliberately following the production of that stuttered word. The individual pauses for a minimum of three seconds and then reproduces the stuttered word in slow motion. This ostensibly provides practice with the motoric integration and speech timing movements that are required for a fluent production of that word. When the individual reaches a criterion level of cancellation proficiency, he or she will move to the second technique, known as pull-outs.

During the pull-out phase of therapy, the individual does not wait until after the stuttered word is completed to correct the inappropriate behavior. Rather, the individual modifies the stuttered word during the actual occurrence of the stuttering. This modification involves slowing down the sequential movements of the syllable or word when stuttering occurs in a fashion similar to the slowed and exaggerated movements that were learned in the cancellation phase of therapy. In essence, the individual is modifying the stuttering on-line, "pulling out" of the stuttering behavior and completing it with a more fluent production of the intended word. Once again, when the individual reaches a criterion level of proficiency, he or she will move to the last stage, known as preparatory sets.

Preparatory sets involve using the slow motion speech strategies that were learned during the first two phases of therapy, not as a response to an occurrence of stuttering, but in anticipation of stuttering. A person who stutters typically knows when and on what word a stuttering will occur. When an individual anticipates a stuttering, he or she will start preparing to use the newly learned fluency producing strategies before the word is attempted. The goal of this phase of therapy is to initiate the word in a more fluent manner even though the individual is producing consecutive speech movements and transitions in a slowed manner.

MODIFYING THE PHYSICAL TENSION OF SPEECH MOVEMENTS

Techniques designed to modify the physical tension of speech movements reduce the amount of physical tension in the speech musculature before and during occurrences of stuttering. Some of the common forms of these techniques are discussed below.

Light articulatory contacts are particularly germane to the production of stop consonants (/b/, /p/, /t/, /d/, /k/, and /g/) because production of this class of speech sounds requires a complete constriction somewhere in the vocal tract (Max & Caruso, 1997). The therapeutic use of light articulatory contacts involves instructing an individual to use less tension in the articulators used for the constriction. It is believed that reducing articulatory tension will prevent the occurrence of prolonged articulatory

People who stutter frequently use excessive articulator pressure when producing sounds. They may, for example, press the tongue very hard on the roof of the mouth during the production of /t/ and /d/ sounds. Teaching the individual to reduce such pressure, or make light articulatory contacts, promotes fluency.

postures that interfere with smooth articulatory transitions from sound to sound. In summary, "Light touches promote continuity and ease of articulation. They are intended to prevent the development of excessive pressure and tension in the articulators" (Boburg & Kully, 1995, p. 305).

There are two related intervention techniques that are used to modify the manner in which a person who stutters initiates his or her voice; both are powerful fluency enhancers. These two techniques are called *gentle voicing onsets* (GVOs) and *speaking after exhalation has begun* (Max & Caruso, 1997). Gentle voicing onsets are a cardinal feature of many therapy programs, and they are known by many different names, such as Fluency Initiation Gestures (FIGS) (Cooper, 1984). The basic characteristic of GVOs is a tension-free onset of voicing that gradually builds in intensity. One can appreciate the dynamics of this technique by initiating production of the vowel /a/ in a whisper, gradually engaging the vocal folds such that the vowel is produced with a breathy voice quality, and finally increasing the vowel's intensity. The apparent fluency enhancing effects of GVOs are presumably related to reduced vocal fold tension, which reduces tense adduction of the vocal folds. In most therapeutic programs, GVOs are learned in a hierarchical fashion beginning with vowel production, followed by syllable productions, and then word productions.

T H O U G H T   Q U E S T I O N

Can you initiate a vocalization using GVO? Try producing the /a/ or any vowel as described above.

A technique related to GVOs is speaking after exhalation has begun. This technique modifies voicing onset by delaying the initiation of speech until after exhalation has begun rather than initiating voicing at the onset of exhalation (Max & Caruso, 1997; Neilson & Andrews, 1993). In clinical application, an individual is taught to inhale, begin to exhale, and then initiate speech shortly after the exhalation has begun. This technique is first taught in single syllables with gradual increases in utterance length up to the conversational level (Culatta & Goldberg, 1995; Max & Caruso, 1997).

SELECTING INTERVENTION TECHNIQUES

The SLP's selection of a specific fluency-establishing technique will depend on many factors, including the severity of the stuttering problem, the motivation and specific needs of the person who stutters, and the SLP's knowledge of the specific techniques available. Careful and detailed observation of an individual's stuttering behaviors before initiating treatment and during the treatment process is an essential component of successful clinical management. Such observation will assist the SLP in "selecting, combining, and modifying available techniques in order to teach the client how to alter timing and tension aspects of his or her speech movements" (Max & Caruso, 1997, p. 50). In short, a one-size-fits-all clinical program does not and should not exist. Inherent differences among individuals within the stuttering population prohibit the use of inflexible clinical protocols that cannot be modified to meet the individual's needs.

THE EFFECTIVENESS OF STUTTERING INTERVENTION THROUGH THE LIFE SPAN

Determining how effective stuttering treatment is depends largely on how "effectiveness" is defined. This is a complex issue. However, a "treatment for stuttering might be considered *effective* if it resulted in the individual's being able to speak with disfluencies within normal limits whenever and to whomever he or she chose, without undue concern or worry about speaking" (Conture, 1996, p. S20). The treatment of stuttering differs across an individual's life span in terms of frequency and nature of therapy, and rates of recovery. Therefore, the review of treatment efficacy is probably best considered relative to four age groups: preschoolers, school-age children, teenagers, and adults.

EFFICACY OF INTERVENTION WITH PRESCHOOL-AGE CHILDREN

In general, the findings of most recent studies are quite encouraging and indicate the potential benefits of early diagnosis and treatment of stuttering. As many as 91 percent of preschool children who had been in a stuttering treatment program maintained their fluent speech five years subsequent to their initial evaluation (Fosnot, 1993). Among preschool-age children enrolled in a parent-conducted therapy program, all maintained their fluent speech four years after dismissal from treatment (Lincoln & Onslow, 1997). In another study, 100 percent of 45 preschool-age children who stuttered had maintained fluent speech two years following dismissal from treatment (Gottwald & Starkweather, 1995).

EFFICACY OF INTERVENTION WITH SCHOOL-AGE CHILDREN

One noteworthy study of stuttering treatment effectiveness utilized four different treatment approaches with school-age children and reported an average 60 percent posttreatment improvement (Ryan & Van Kirk Ryan, 1983). Even better results were found in another study in which 96 percent of the school-age children enrolled in two treatment programs maintained fluent speech fourteen months after treatment (Ryan & Van Kirk Ryan, 1995).

The findings of nine investigations of the effectiveness of stuttering treatment involving 160 school-age children are mildly encouraging. The findings of these studies indicated a 61 percent average (range of 33% to over 90%) decrease in stuttering frequency and/or stuttering severity across the nine studies. As with the stuttering treatment efficacy findings among preschool-age children, these studies suggest cautious optimism (Conture, 1996).

EFFICACY OF INTERVENTION WITH ADOLESCENTS AND ADULTS

Teenagers who stutter can be difficult to manage clinically, and very little information is available regarding specific therapy programs for this age group (Daly, Simon, & Burnett-Stolnack, 1995; Schwartz, 1993). In sharp contrast, many reports of treatment outcomes for the adult who stutters are available. A wide variety of adult stuttering treatment techniques have been investigated, ranging from operant conditioning techniques to drug therapies. Collectively, these studies suggest a 60 to 80 percent improvement rate regardless of the therapeutic technique that was used. However, two specific treatment techniques seem to yield superior benefits for the adult stutterer. These two treatments use the techniques of prolonged speech and/or gentle voicing onsets (Andrews, Guitar, & Howie, 1980; Conture, 1996; Ingham, 1990). Both of these techniques seem to result in both short- and long-term reductions in stuttering frequency and severity.

In summary, stuttering intervention across all age groups results in an average improvement for about 70 percent of all cases, with preschool-age children improving more quickly and easily than people who have a longer history with stuttering. The clinical research that we have considered indicates that effective treatment of stuttering is increasingly able to improve the daily life of people who stutter by increasing their ability to communicate whenever and with whomever they choose without undue concern about speaking.

SUMMARY

Stuttering is a handicapping condition primarily characterized by sound and syllable repetitions and sound prolongations that interrupt the smooth forward flow of speech. Stuttering is a universal problem that affects males more than females. In most cases, stuttering appears between the ages of 2 to 4 years, and as the disorder progresses, it increases in severity. Stuttering can adversely affect an individual's school performance, employment, and social interactions. The treatment of stuttering is most effective when it is initiated in early childhood, although treatment at any age can reduce stuttering.

A number of theories—organic, behavioral, and psychological—attempt to account for the onset and development of stuttering, but its cause is unknown. Solving the riddle of stuttering will undoubtedly require expertise from many specialists including SLPs, neurolinguists, geneticists, and medical specialists. Perhaps one of you reading this text will find your own birch tree and take up Van Riper's quest to find the cause and a cure for stuttering.

REFLECTIONS

- What is the difference between the incidence and the prevalence of stuttering? What are the incidence and prevalence of stuttering?
- How can stuttering affect one's life in school, at work, and in one's social interactions?
- What are normal disfluencies and how do they differ from stuttering?
- Briefly describe the onset and development of stuttering using Bloodstein's phases.
- What are the general stuttering treatment procedures that are used with children who stutter?
- What are rate reduction techniques and what are cancellations, pull-outs, and preparatory sets?
- How effective is stuttering treatment for preschool-age children, school-age children, and adults?

SUGGESTED READINGS

Bloodstein, O. (1995). *A handbook on stuttering.* San Diego: Singular Publishing Group.

Conture, E. G. (1990). *Stuttering* (2nd ed.). Englewood Cliffs, NJ: Prentice-Hall.

Curlee, R. F., & Siegel, G. M. (1997). *Nature and treatment of stuttering: New directions.* Boston: Allyn and Bacon.

Guitar, B. (1998). *Stuttering: An integrated approach to its nature and treatment* (2nd ed.). Baltimore, MD: Williams and Wilkins.

Yaruss, J. S. (1997). Clinical measurement of stuttering behaviors. *Contemporary Issues in Communication Science and Disorders, 24,* 33–44.

ON-LINE RESOURCES

http://www.stuttersfa.org   Website of the Stuttering Foundation of America. Available catalogs, referral lists, videotapes, and excellent information about stuttering.

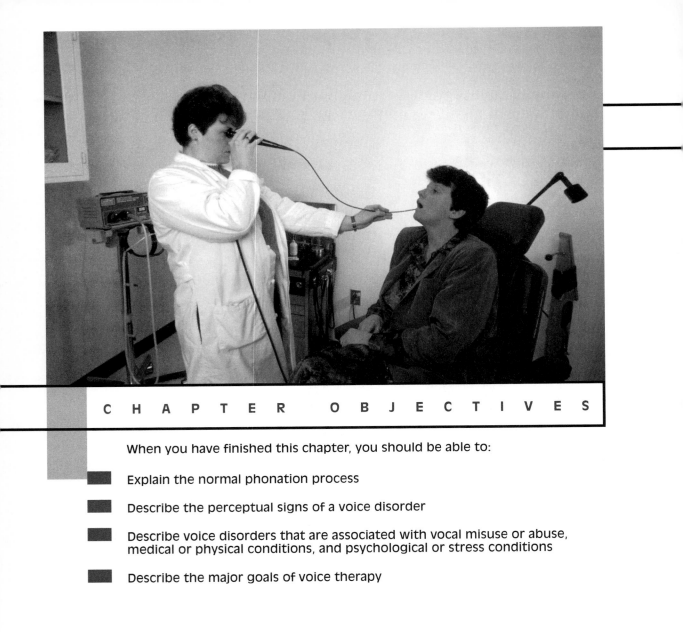

When you have finished this chapter, you should be able to:

- Explain the normal phonation process

- Describe the perceptual signs of a voice disorder

- Describe voice disorders that are associated with vocal misuse or abuse, medical or physical conditions, and psychological or stress conditions

- Describe the major goals of voice therapy

The Voice and Voice Disorders

Voice is our primary means of expression and is an essential feature of the uniquely human attribute known as speech (Boone & McFarlane, 2000; Colton & Casper, 1996; Titze, 1994). One's voice reflects gender, personality, personal habits, age, and the general condition of health. Research has shown that certain characteristics of the voice reflect various personality dimensions, and these vocal characteristics correlate well with standardized tests of personality (Colton & Casper, 1990; Markel, Meisels, & Houck, 1964). The voice is an emotional outlet that mirrors one's moods, attitudes, and general feelings. Expressions of anger can be achieved by shouting, and expressions of affection can be achieved by speaking softly; these types of vocal expression have great potential to evoke emotional responses from a listener. Evoking emotional responses from listeners through controlled vocal expression is key to a successful operatic performance. Dramatic actors achieve pathos through deliberate and controlled vocal expression. The evocative nature of vocal expressions, however, is hardly limited to stage performances. We constantly vary the tone of our voices to achieve some specific meaning or intention. The voice is a powerful tool that delivers a message and simultaneously adds to the meaning of that message (Colton & Casper, 1990).

T H O U G H T Q U E S T I O N

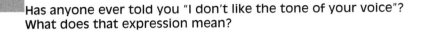

Has anyone ever told you "I don't like the tone of your voice"?
What does that expression mean?

From this brief introduction, it should be clear that the human voice is a dynamic multidimensional tool that is central to verbal communication.[1] In Chapter 3, we discussed the basic concepts related to normal voice production. We will extend some of these basic concepts in this chapter with a discussion of how one changes the pitch and loudness of the voice. Next, we will discuss voice disorders in children and adults associated with vocal misuse and hyperfunction, abnormal medical and physical conditions, and psychological and stress conditions. Finally, assessment, treatment, and treatment efficacy issues will be discussed.

PITCH AND THE PITCH-CHANGING MECHANISM

During one complete vibratory cycle of vocal fold vibration, the vocal folds move from a closed or adducted position to an open or abducted position and back to the closed position.

You are probably aware that the relative pitch of one's voice is somewhat dependent on the person's sex and age. *Pitch* of the voice is the perceptual counterpart to fundamental frequency associated with the speed of vocal fold vibration. As the speed of vocal fold vibration increases, the perceived pitch of the voice increases. As we discussed in Chapter 3, the speed at which the vocal folds vibrate is called the fundamental frequency of the voice. Frequency is measured in **hertz (Hz),** or the number of complete vibrations per second. The fundamental frequency of the voice varies considerably during speaking, but each individual speaker has an average fundamental frequency, or *habitual pitch.* Each individual also has a particularly suitable pitch level known as the **optimal pitch level,** which is largely determined by vocal fold structure. For example, on average, adult men have fundamental frequencies of around 130 Hz (the vocal folds open and close 130 times per second), whereas adult women have fundamental frequencies around 250 Hz. Therefore, the perceived pitch of male voices is, on average, lower than the perceived pitch of female voices. The fundamental frequency of young children's voices can be as high as 500 Hz,

---

[1] It should be noted that the primary biological functions of laryngeal structures, including the vocal folds, are to prevent foreign objects from entering the trachea and to impound air for forceful expulsion (coughing) of such objects.

resulting in a very high-pitched voice. The difference in vocal fundamental frequency (and resulting vocal pitch) among men, women, and children is due largely to the structure of the vocal folds themselves.

At birth, the infant larynx is positioned relatively high in the neck, at about the level of the third cervical vertebra. The epiglottis is in contact with the soft palate. The elevated laryngeal position allows the infant to breath while nursing and reduces the risk of choking (Kent, 1997; Zemlin, 1998). The infant larynx begins to descend in the neck shortly after birth, reaching the level of the sixth cervical vertebra by about 5 years of age. Laryngeal descent continues until the larynx reaches the level of the seventh cervical vertebra between 15 and 20 years of age.

At birth, the vocal folds are approximately 3 mm long for both sexes. The growth rate of the vocal folds is approximately 0.4 mm/year in females and 0.7 mm/year in males, but this difference in growth rate does not result in appreciable average pitch differences between boys and girls (Titze, 1994). Males and females have similar fundamental frequencies until about 12 years of age. During puberty, however, male vocal folds rapidly increase in length by about 10 mm and, importantly, they also thicken. The increase in vocal fold length and thickness during the pubertal period results in a large drop in the male's vocal fundamental frequency. In comparison, female vocal folds lengthen by approximately 4 mm during puberty with no significant thickening of the folds. Female fundamental frequency drops only about three musical tones during puberty. Postpubertal vocal fold length ranges from 17 mm to 20 mm in males and from 12.5 mm to 17 mm in females (Zemlin, 1998). In general, because of their larger structure, male vocal folds vibrate with a lower fundamental frequency than female vocal folds, resulting in a lower-pitched male voice. The structural changes of the vocal folds and the relationship to vocal fundamental frequency are summarized in Table 9.1.

T H O U G H T   Q U E S T I O N

Think about the strings on a piano or a guitar. What is the relationship between the thickness of the string and the sound it produces when it vibrates?

Although individuals have a habitual speaking frequency (average pitch), the frequency of the voice constantly varies during speech production. A monotonous or **monotone** voice is the result of not varying the habitual speaking frequency during speech production. People who use a monotone voice are not terribly interesting to listen to, and listeners

TABLE 9.1

Summary of laryngeal development and fundamental frequency characteristics across the life span

Time	Structural Development	Fundamental Frequency
Birth	Larynx positioned high in the neck; vocal fold length is 3 mm	Average is about 400 Hz; unstable
4 years	Little sex difference in vocal fold length until about 10 years	Stable from 4 to 10 years with little sex influence
Puberty	10 mm increase in vocal fold length for males; 4 mm increase for females	One octave decrease for males; decreases 3 musical tones for females
Adulthood	Vocal fold length is 20 mm in men; vocal fold length is 17 mm in women	Males' average is 130 Hz; females' average is 250 Hz

Source: Adapted from Kent (1997).

will quickly lose interest in what is being said. Varying the pitch of the voice also has linguistic significance. Consider these two sentences:

Tom has a dog.

Tom has a dog?

The words in these two sentences are identical, but the sentences' meanings are quite different. "Tom has a dog" is a statement of fact (a declarative), whereas "Tom has a dog?" is a question (an interrogative). Say those two sentences out loud, paying particular attention to what happens to your pitch at the end of each sentence. For the declarative, the pitch of your voice will decrease or fall off as you are saying the word "dog." In contrast, for the interrogative, the pitch of your voice will increase when you are saying the word "dog."

How does one change the pitch of the voice? Modifications in the length and tension of the vocal folds are necessary to produce pitch change. Lengthening and tensing the vocal folds via intrinsic muscle contraction will increase the pitch of the voice, whereas relaxing these muscles will decrease pitch.

VOCAL INTENSITY AND THE INTENSITY-CHANGING MECHANISM

Like changing the pitch of the voice, changing vocal intensity is also necessary for adequate communication. Vocal intensity is measured in **decibels (dB),** and in general, as vocal intensity increases, the perceived loudness of the voice increases. The loudness of normal conversational speech, such as conversations at the dinner table, averages around 60 dB. Changes in vocal intensity require the vocal folds to stay together longer during the closed phase of vibration, but subglottic pressure is the major determinant of vocal intensity (Kent, 1997; Zemlin, 1998). As discussed in Chapter 3, subglottic pressure is the pressure placed on the inferior aspects of the vocal folds by the lungs. Every time subglottic pressure doubles, there is an 8 to 12 dB increase in vocal intensity. The *Guinness Book of World Records* reports that the loudest scream ever recorded was produced at 123.2 dB, and a man named Anthony Fieldhouse won the World Shouting contest with a yell that was registered at 112.4 dB (Kent, 1997). Unless you are a record seeker, this kind of behavior is not recommended, as we will see later in the chapter.

CHANGES IN VOICE PRODUCTION THROUGH THE LIFE SPAN

The manner in which one uses the voice changes with each major stage of life: infancy and childhood, adulthood, and advanced age. Changes in the voice are related to biological, cognitive, social, and emotional maturation.

INFANCY AND CHILDHOOD

Crying is how an infant uses the voice to express pain, hunger, or displeasure. Crying is purposeful, and it is the major avenue for infant communication. Cooing is how the infant uses the voice to express pleasure, happiness, and contentment. Both crying and cooing reflect the beginning of the infant's ability to control his or her voice and, in turn, his or her environment.

As children mature, they begin to use voice for the production of speech sounds and to express ideas and moods. Mature intentional patterns are mimicked before children learn words to fit these patterns. Later, pitch and intensity changes are used to denote differences of meaning and intention.

ADULTHOOD

The adult voice is achieved by about the age of 18 years (Kahane, 1982; Titze, 1994). At this age, the individual has full control over the voice and is capable of using many variations of pitch, loudness, and vocal expression. Under normal circumstances, the average speaking pitch or frequency of the voice will remain constant for the next several decades, and the way the voice is used will be determined by specific situational demands.

Adults frequently abuse their voice through excessive misuse. Some jobs, for example, require speaking in the presence of loud machinery or background noise. Such conditions might require the use of very loud vocal production, which can affect the voice negatively. Smoke and alcohol adversely affect the voice. Even if one recognizes that he or she is engaging in abusive vocal habits, making the necessary changes to eliminate the aggravating condition is frequently difficult. In addition to vocal abuse, certain disease processes such as cancer or neurological dysfunctions can adversely affect the adult voice (Colton & Casper, 1990).

T H O U G H T   Q U E S T I O N

Do you like the music of Elton John? He had trouble with his voice during a tour of the United States in 1986 and was forced to cancel engagements. Fortunately, his voice problem was associated with a nonmalignant lesion that was corrected surgically. Do you think that vocal performing might injure vocal fold tissue?

ADVANCED AGE

The voice begins to decline in much the same way that other body functions begin to decline after the age of 60 or so. Typical voice changes include increases or decreases in vocal pitch, a decreased capacity to control the vocal loudness, and diminished vocal quality (Colton & Casper, 1990; Kahane, 1982; Titze, 1994). For example, with advanced age, the pitch of the voice tends to decrease in females and to increase in males. Such unidirectional gender-linked voice pitch changes have been associated with decreased estrogen levels in females and decreased testosterone levels in males (Hollien, 1987; Kent, 1997; Titze, 1994).

By simply listening to someone's voice, even untrained listeners can make reasonable estimates of that person's chronological age. Additionally, physiological age, which is determined by standard measures of blood pressure, heart rate, vital capacity, and the like, more closely determines the quality of one's voice than chronological age (Ramig & Ringel, 1983; Shipp, Qi, Huntley, & Hollien, 1992; Titze, 1994). Staying in shape pays many dividends.

Demands on the voice are different for the adult of advanced age than for younger adults. For example, the retired college professor no longer needs to deliver lengthy lectures that can strain the voice in large classrooms. The decline of body function is generally accompanied by reduced demands on the system. Despite the general physiological decline in aged individuals, the voice retains its central importance for communication. Verbal communication may be the only manner in which a person of advanced age can "maintain human contact and control the environment" (Colton & Casper, 1990, p. 5).

DISORDERS OF VOICE

Normal voice production requires that voice quality, pitch, loudness, and flexibility be relatively pleasing and audible to a listener. Disordered voice production involves deviations of voice quality, pitch, loudness, and flexibility that may signify illness and interfere with communication (Aronson, 1990). Voice disorders can affect people of any age. It is estimated that approximately 3 to 6 percent of school-age children have voice disorders (Ramig & Verdolini, 1998), although estimates as high as 23.4 percent have been reported (Silverman & Zimmer, 1975). Children's voice disorders are characterized by abnormal pitch, loudness, quality, or combinations thereof (Aronson, 1990). Such voice disorders are related generally to vocal misuse or abuse and in most cases are temporary. The primary focus of the remainder of this chapter will be concerned with voice disorders that develop in adulthood.

It is estimated that 3 to 9 percent of the adult population of the United States have a voice disorder and that males are more commonly affected than females. Data from the National Center for Voice and Speech (Ramig & Verdolini, 1998) suggest that approximately 3 percent of the working population in the United States have occupations (e.g., police, air traffic controllers, pilots) in which use of their voice is necessary for public safety. Given this statistic, it is clear that the occurrence of voice disorders in adults is "potentially one of great magnitude from a health, as well as an economic standpoint" (Laguaite, 1972, p. 151). In contrast to children, adult voice disorders are quite varied; we will discuss some of the specific disorders later in the chapter.

Perceptual signs of a voice disorder are related to specific characteristics of a person's voice, which can be evaluated by a clinician. Clinically, perceptual signs in conjunction with a person's case history serve as the initial benchmarks in the differential diagnosis of a voice disorder. Perceptual signs of the voice can be divided into five broad categories: pitch, loudness, quality, nonphonatory behaviors, and aphonia, or the absence of phonation (Colton & Casper, 1996).

DISORDERS OF VOCAL PITCH

As we stated earlier in this chapter, pitch is the perceptual correlate of fundamental frequency. Three aspects of pitch may suggest a voice disorder. The first is **monopitch.** A monopitch voice lacks normal inflectional variation and, in some instances, the ability to change pitch voluntarily. Monopitch may be a sign of a neurological impairment or a psychiatric disability, or it may simply reflect the person's personality. **Inappropriate pitch** refers to the voice that is judged to be outside the normal range of pitch for age and/or sex. A vocal pitch that is too high may indicate underdevelopment of the larynx, whereas a vocal pitch that is excessively low may be related to endocrinological problems such as hypothyroidism. It is also possible that a vocal pitch that is excessively high or low may be related to personal preference or habit.

Pitch breaks are sudden uncontrolled upward or downward changes in pitch. Pitch breaks are common among males who are going through puberty, but this condition usually resolves itself over time. Certain types of laryngeal pathologies and/or abnormal neurological conditions can be related to pitch breaks.

DISORDERS OF VOCAL LOUDNESS

Loudness is the perceptual correlate of vocal intensity. Two aspects related to vocal loudness may indicate a voice disorder. The first is **monoloudness.** A monoloud voice lacks normal variations of intensity that occur during speech, and there may be an inability to change vocal loudness voluntarily. Monoloudness may be a reflection of neurological impairment or psychiatric disability or merely a habit associated with the person's personality. **Loudness variations** are extreme variations in vocal intensity in which the voice is either too soft or too loud for the particular speaking situation. The inability to control vocal loudness may reflect a loss of neural control of the respiratory or laryngeal mechanism. Psychological problems may also contribute to abnormal variations in vocal loudness.

DISORDERS OF VOCAL QUALITY

Several perceptual characteristics of the voice are related to vocal quality. *Hoarseness/roughness* is the first. A hoarse/rough voice lacks clarity, and the voice is noisy. Pathologies that affect vocal fold vibration can result in a hoarse/rough vocal quality. Some of these pathologies are discussed later in this chapter. A hoarse/rough voice can also be a temporary condition that results from minor forms of vocal misuse or abuse that produce vocal fold swelling called edema.

T H O U G H T   Q U E S T I O N S

Have you ever attended a sporting event or rock concert at which you shouted or yelled excessively to root for your team or to overcome the loud background noise and music? How did your voice sound the following day? What do you think happened to make your voice sound that way?

Breathiness is the perception of audible air escaping through the glottis during phonation. Excessive airflow through the glottis usually indicates inadequate glottal closure during vocal fold vibration. The inability to close the glottis during vocal fold vibration may be related to the presence of a lesion on the vocal folds that prevents closure or some form of neurological impairment.

Tremor involves variations in the pitch and loudness of the voice that are not under voluntary control. **Vocal tremor** is usually an indication of a loss of central nervous system control over the laryngeal mechanism. **Strain and struggle** behaviors are related to difficulties initiating and maintaining voice. During speech production, the voice fades in and out, and actual voice stoppages may occur. Strain and struggle behaviors are usually related to neurological impairment, but psychological problems may also cause them.

Some research suggests that normal female voices are perceived to be more breathy than normal male voices. Research also suggests that young women use more air than young males to produce a syllable.

NONPHONATORY VOCAL DISORDERS

Stridor is noisy breathing or involuntary sound that accompanies inspiration and expiration. Stridor is indicative of a narrowing somewhere in the airway. Stridor is always abnormal and serious because its presence represents a blockage of the airway.

Excessive throat clearing, a frequent accompaniment to many voice disorders, is an attempt to clear mucus from the vocal folds. Although throat clearing is a normal behavior, it is considered abnormal when it occurs with excessive frequency.

Consistent aphonia is the persistent absence of voice and is perceived as whispering. Aphonia may be related to vocal fold paralysis, disorders of the central nervous system, or psychological problems. **Episodic aphonia** is uncontrolled, unpredictable aphonic breaks in voice that can last for a fraction of a second or longer. Central nervous system disorders and psychological problems can contribute to episodic aphonia. The perceptual signs of voice disorders are summarized in Table 9.2.

Before we turn our attention to specific voice disorders, it should be noted that many of the perceptual signs of voice disorders can be objectively quantified with clinical instruments that are readily available to the SLP (Behrman & Orlikoff, 1997). Briefly, quantitative assessments of the voice are easily made by using specially designed computer hardware and software. Kay Elemetrics, for example, manufactures a computer-based instrument called the VisiPitch®. It is a user-friendly instrument that permits numerous objective assessments of

---

TABLE 9.2

Perceptual signs of voice disorders

I. Pitch
   A. Monopitch
   B. Inappropriate pitch
   C. Pitch breaks
II. Loudness
   A. Monoloudness
   B. Inappropriate loudness (soft, loud, uncontrolled)
III. Quality
   A. Hoarseness/ roughness
   B. Breathiness
   C. Tremor
   D. Strain/struggle
IV. Nonphonatory Behaviors
   A. Stridor
   B. Excessive throat clearing
V. Aphonia
   A. Consistent
   B. Episodic

Source: Adapted from Colton and Casper (1990).

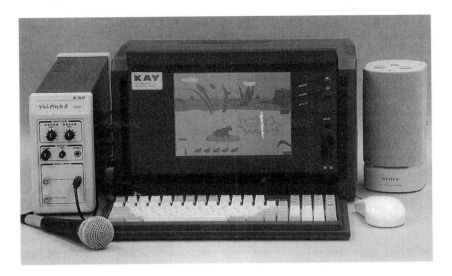

Kay Elemetrics VisiPitch®.

the physical correlates of pitch, loudness, and hoarseness/roughness. Objective assessments are valuable for diagnostic purposes as well as monitoring improvements during voice therapy. VisiPitch operations can be seen on the book's CD-ROM.

Instruments are also available that measure airflow and air volume exchanges during phonation that can be used to objectively assess vocal breathiness. These instruments can be interfaced with specially designed computer hardware and software for vocal assessment. Normative data exist for many objective correlates that are related to the perceptual signs of voice disorders (see, for example, Baken & Orlikoff, 2000).

Three general etiologies of voice disorders are vocal misuse or abuse (functional) conditions, medical or physical (organic) conditions, and psychological or stress conditions (Ramig, 1994). The exact etiology of a specific voice disorder is not always easy to determine, and some voice disorders may have multiple causes. With this caution in mind, we use these three general etiologies to examine some of the more common disorders of voice

VOICE DISORDERS ASSOCIATED WITH VOCAL MISUSE OR ABUSE

Vocal misuse and abuse are frequently claimed to contribute to structural damage of vocal fold tissue, which in turn affects vocal fold vibratory behavior. Although there is a fine distinction between vocal misuse and abuse, vocal abuse is considered to be the harsher of the two with a greater risk of injuring vocal fold tissue (Colton & Casper, 1996). Conditions and behaviors that are considered to be vocal misuse and abuse are listed in Table 9.3 and discussed below.

Vocal nodules are a common vocal fold pathology that is secondary to vocal misuse/abuse. Nodules are localized growths on the vocal folds resulting from frequent, hard vocal fold collisions that occur, for example, during yelling or shouting (Colton & Casper, 1996; Gray, Titze, & Lusk, 1987). They are generally bilateral (appearing on both vocal folds), although they can appear on only one vocal fold. Nodules are soft and pliable early in their formation. Over time, however, they become hard and fibrous, interfering greatly with vocal fold vibration. Nodules usually appear at the juncture of the anterior one-third and posterior two-thirds of the vocal folds where contact is greatest. Nodules occur more frequently in adult women, particularly those between 20 and 50 years of age. However, children who are prone to excessive loud talking or screaming may also develop vocal nodules; in this age group, they are more likely to develop in boys (Colton & Casper, 1996).

The primary perceptual voice symptoms of vocal nodules are hoarseness and breathiness. People who have vocal nodules may complain of soreness in the throat and an inability to use the upper third of their pitch range. Newly formed nodules are treated effectively with vocal rest (no talking). To prevent their return, however, people with vocal nodules need to alter the vocal behaviors that produced the nodules. Consulting a SLP for voice therapy and education is usually recom-

---

TABLE 9.3

Common conditions and behaviors that are considered to be misuse or abuse of the voice

Misuse	Abuse
Abrupt voicing onsets	Screaming or yelling
High laryngeal position	Excessive use of alcohol
Lack of pitch variability	Excessive throat clearing and coughing

Source: Adapted from Colton and Casper (1990).

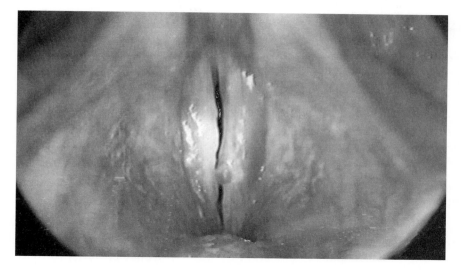

Unilateral vocal fold nodule. (Photograph courtesy of Robert Orlikoff, Ph.D., Memorial Sloan-Kettering Cancer Center, New York, NY)

mended. Longstanding nodules may require surgical removal followed by voice therapy designed to eliminate vocally abusive behaviors. See Box 9.1 for the personal story of a college music student with nodules that were effectively treated with therapy and vocal rest. A voice sample of a woman with bilateral vocal nodules can be heard on the book's CD-ROM.

Contact ulcers are reddened ulcerations that develop on the posterior surface of the vocal folds in the region of the arytenoid cartilages. Contact ulcers, like vocal nodules, are usually bilateral, but unlike nodules, they can be painful. Pain is usually unilateral, and it may radiate into the ear. It was once believed that contact ulcers, which occur predominantly in males over the age of 40, resulted from forceful and aggressive speaking behaviors (Colton & Casper, 1996; Titze, 1994). Contemporary thought, however, suggests that the regurgitation of stomach acids into the esophagus and throat (gastric reflux) during sleep may be an important predisposing condition for the development of contact ulcers. Stomach acids irritate vocal fold tissue, promoting excessive throat clearing, which is abusive to the tissue and causes the ulcerations (Colton & Casper, 1996).

The primary voice symptoms of contact ulcers are vocal hoarseness and breathiness. Throat clearing and vocal fatigue accompany the

BOX 9.1

Personal Story of a College Woman with Vocal Nodules

Jessica, a music major, decided to pledge a sorority in the fall semester of her sophomore year. A talented vocal performer, Jessica had aspirations to teach singing and to perform professionally. During the fall semester, her course work was demanding, requiring several vocal performances and long hours of rehearsal. Pledging turned out to be demanding vocally also. Jessica was talking excessively all day long and well into the night, in addition to shouting loudly at sorority events.

During the fifth week of the semester, Jessica noted that her voice fatigued easily, she sounded hoarse, and she could not reach some of the high notes required in her singing. Her vocal teacher suggested that she be evaluated at the university's speech and hearing clinic in an effort to determine the cause of her diminished vocal capacity. A perceptual and instrumental evaluation of Jessica's voice was performed by two graduate students enrolled in the university's communication disorders program. The findings of this evaluation suggested the possibility of vocal nodules. During the consultation after the evaluation, the supervising professor and the two graduate students explained their findings to Jes-

sica and told her that she needed to be examined by an otolaryngologist before they could proceed further. Otolaryngologic examination is required to confirm or disconfirm the presence of nodules, and speech-language pathologists are required ethically to ensure that such an examination has been performed before they initiate therapy.

The otolaryngologic examination confirmed the presence of newly formed bilateral vocal nodules. Her physician prescribed complete vocal rest for a week followed by voice therapy. Jessica enrolled in voice therapy at the university for six weeks. Vocal hygiene was stressed during therapy sessions. Jessica was examined by her otolaryngologist at the end of the sixth week of therapy. Her vocal nodules were significantly reduced in size and were no longer adversely affecting her voice.

Jessica completed her academic semester and sorority pledging successfully, graduated two years later, and went on to graduate school at the Julliard School of Music in New York City. She maintains contact with the university's speech clinic and reports that she continues to practice good vocal hygiene. Jessica and her voice are doing very well.

disorder. Although some individuals claim that contact ulcers can be treated effectively with voice therapy (e.g., Boone & McFarlane, 2000), others suggest that successful treatment is questionable and not well documented. Quite frequently, contact ulcers reappear after surgical removal. A voice sample of a man with contact ulcers can be heard on the book's CD-ROM.

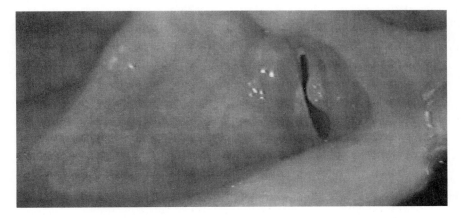

Sessile polyp. (Photograph courtesy of Robert Orlikoff, Ph.D., Memorial Sloan-Kettering Cancer Center, New York, NY)

Vocal polyps, like vocal nodules, are caused by trauma to the vocal folds associated with vocal misuse or abuse. Polyps develop when blood vessels in the vocal folds rupture and swell, developing fluid-filled lesions. Polyps tend to be unilateral, larger than nodules, vascular, and prone to hemorrhage (Colton & Casper, 1996). Unlike vocal nodules, polyps can result from a single traumatic incident such as yelling at a sporting event.

Two general types of polyps have been identified: sessile and pedunculated (Colton & Casper, 1996; Titze, 1994). A **sessile** (closely adhering or attached to vocal fold tissue) **polyp** can cover up to two-thirds of the vocal fold. A **pedunculated polyp** appears to be attached to the vocal fold by means of a stalk and can be found on the free margins of the vocal folds as well as on the upper and lower surfaces of the folds.

Hoarseness, breathiness, and roughness are the typical vocal symptoms, and individuals who have a vocal polyp may report the sensation of something in the throat. The combination of surgical removal of the polyp and voice therapy to eliminate vocal misuse or abuse is effective in treating this condition (Ramig, 1994).

T H O U G H T   Q U E S T I O N

Have you or anyone you know had a voice disorder? What were the symptoms and how was it treated?

Acute and **chronic laryngitis** are the last disorders that we will consider that are associated with vocal misuse or abuse. Laryngitis is an inflammation of the vocal folds that can result from exposure to noxious agents (tobacco smoke, alcohol, etc.), allergies, or vocal abuse (Colton & Casper, 1996). Acute laryngitis is a temporary swelling of the vocal folds that can result in vocal hoarseness.

Chronic laryngitis is the result of vocal abuse during periods of acute laryngitis, and it can lead to serious deterioration of vocal fold tissue. The vocal folds appear thickened, swollen, and reddened because of excessive fluid retention and dilated blood vessels in the vocal folds. If chronic laryngitis persists, a marked atrophy (wasting away of tissue) of the vocal folds will occur. The vocal folds become dry and sticky, resulting in a persistent cough, and the individual reports frequent throat aches (Boone & McFarlane, 2000). The voice symptoms of chronic laryngitis range from mild hoarseness to near aphonia. Surgery and subsequent voice therapy are usually both necessary to treat chronic laryngitis effectively.

VOICE DISORDERS ASSOCIATED WITH MEDICAL OR PHYSICAL CONDITIONS

The second major group of voice disorders is those caused by central nervous system (CNS) disorders, organic disease, or laryngeal trauma. A number of the conditions discussed in this section of the chapter have a general deleterious impact on bodily functions. We will focus primarily on how these conditions affect voice production.

Disorders of the CNS can result in speech and voice disorders that are characterized by muscle weakness, discoordination, tremor, or paralysis. Generally, such disorders are called *dysarthrias*, and most forms of dysarthria involve generalized neurological damage resulting in complex patterns of speech and voice symptoms. It is useful to broadly separate CNS disorders that affect the voice into two categories: those that result in **hypoadduction,** or reduced vocal adduction, and those that result in **hyperadduction,** or increased adduction (Ramig, 1994).[2] These categories are related generally to the anatomical location of CNS lesions or disease. CNS disorders will be discussed in more detail in Chapter 12, "Neurogenic Speech Disorders."

VOICE DISORDERS ASSOCIATED WITH HYPOADDUCTION

Parkinson's disease is a CNS disease that results in vocal fold hypoadduction. Muscle rigidity, tremor, and an overall slowness of movement,

---

[2]Ramig (1994) also proposes a third category, called phonatory instability, which is characterized by involuntary variations of pitch and loudness.

or hypokinesia, are characteristics of Parkinson's disease (Aronson, 1990; Colton & Casper, 1996). Facial appearance is unemotional and sometimes referred to as masklike. Head trauma, viruses, and carbon monoxide poisoning have been implicated as potential causes of this disease. The voice symptoms associated with Parkinson's diesease include monopitch, monoloudness, harshness, and breathiness (Aronson, 1990).

Parkinson's disease is a serious medical condition that is treated aggressively with a variety of drugs (neuropharmacological). Neuropharmacological treatments have a positive effect on limb movement, but speech and voice symptoms are not consistently improved. Intensive voice therapy aimed at improving vocal fold adduction has been successful in improving vocal loudness and speech intelligibility (Ramig, 1994). A voice sample of a man with Parkinson's disease can be heard on the book's CD-ROM.

Unilateral and bilateral **vocal fold paralysis** is another common hypoadductory disorder that can result from CNS damage. The **recurrent branch** of the tenth cranial nerve (vagus) is the nerve supply for most of the laryngeal muscles associated with voice production. This nerve leaves the brain stem and travels down into the chest cavity, loops around the heart's aorta, and then courses upward, inserting into the larynx from below. Damage to this nerve can occur through injuries to the head, neck, or chest; from viral infections; and sometimes during neck or chest surgery. If the recurrent laryngeal nerve is damaged on one side, unilateral vocal fold paralysis results. If it is damaged on both sides, bilateral vocal fold paralysis results.

The recurrent branch of the vagus nerve was severed frequently in the early days of open heart surgery, resulting in postoperative aphonia. Improved surgical procedures have minimized this problem, although the risk still exists.

The voice symptoms of unilateral vocal fold paralysis include a hoarse, weak, and breathy voice quality. The paralyzed vocal fold is flaccid (limp or weak) in comparison to the nonparalyzed vocal fold. Therefore, the two vocal folds vibrate at different speeds, resulting in **diplophonia,** the perception of two vocal frequencies. The voice is very weak or totally absent in cases of bilateral vocal fold paralysis. If nerve regeneration and improved function are not observed within six months after the injury, surgical treatment may be required to facilitate vocal fold closure. Collagen or Teflon can sometimes be injected surgically into a paralyzed vocal fold to build up its mass. Vocal fold implantation helps to promote vocal fold contact. Voice therapy after surgery will be aimed at increasing vocal fold closure and vocal loudness. Three examples of vocal fold paralysis can be heard on the book's CD-ROM.

VOICE DISORDERS ASSOCIATED WITH HYPERADDUCTION

Pseudobulbar palsy is a neurological condition that results in vocal fold hyperadduction. This condition can be caused by strokes, brain injuries, and multiple sclerosis (Colton & Casper, 1996). People who suffer from pseudobulbar palsy have great difficulty swallowing and producing speech. These individuals also exhibit emotional lability, breaking into fits of crying or laughing for no apparent reason. Such behaviors appear to be uncontrolled (Colton & Casper, 1996). The prominent voice symptoms include hoarseness, pitch breaks, and a strained or strangled vocal quality; these are characteristic of vocal fold hyperadduction.

Huntington's chorea (a hyperkinetic disorder characterized by abrupt, jerky movements of the head, neck, and limbs), a genetically transmitted disease of the basal ganglia, is also a disorder that results in vocal fold hyperadduction during phonation. The voice symptoms associated with this vocal fold hyperadduction are harshness, mono-pitch, and a strained or strangled voice quality. People who suffer from this disease also exhibit sudden phonatory arrests that are probably associated with uncontrolled adductory or abductory vocal fold gestures (Ramig, 1986).

The last disorder that we will consider in the hyperadductory category is **spastic dysphonia.** Spastic dysphonia occurs with equal incidence in men and women. This disorder is typically associated with middle age, but it has been observed in people as young as 20 years of age. There is some controversy about the etiology of spastic dysphonia. Some authors claim that the etiology of the disorder is psychological; others believe that the etiology is neurological (Colton & Casper, 1996).

Spastic dysphonia is typically characterized by hyperadduction of the vocal folds resulting in a strained or strangled voice production with intermittent stoppages of the voice that resemble stuttering (Titze, 1994). Associated symptoms include hoarseness, harshness, and vocal tremor. Surgical resecting (cutting) of the recurrent laryngeal nerve and drug therapy have been used to treat spastic dysphonia. Voice therapy has also been a treatment option for spastic dysphonia to provide relief from the hyperadductory behaviors. A voice sample of a woman with spastic dysphonia can be heard on the book's CD-ROM.

OTHER CONDITIONS THAT AFFECT VOICE PRODUCTION

A number of other conditions unrelated to CNS disorders can affect the larynx and, in turn, voice production. **Laryngeal papillomas** are small wartlike growths that cover the vocal folds and the interior aspects of the larynx. These lesions are caused by a papovavirus and are common in children under the age of 6 years (Boone & McFarlane, 2000; Colton & Casper, 1996). Papillomas are noncancerous, but they can obstruct the airway, hindering breathing. Children with the disorder exhibit stridor during inhalation and may be aphonic (Wilson, 1987). Papillomas must be surgically removed, but they have a strong tendency to reappear, requiring multiple operations that may damage vocal fold tissue.

Congenital laryngeal webbing is present at birth. Congenital webs typically form on the anterior aspects of the vocal folds and can interfere with breathing. Laryngeal webbing must be removed surgically. Webs may produce a high-pitched, hoarse voice quality.

Laryngeal cancer is the most serious organic disorder of the voice; it has been linked to cigarette smoking and the excessive use of alcohol. One of the early signs of laryngeal cancer is persistent hoarseness in the absence of colds or allergies (Ramig, 1994). Once cancer is diagnosed, it is frequently necessary to remove the entire larynx to prevent the spread of the cancer to other parts of the body. When the larynx is removed surgically, the trachea is repositioned to form a stoma (mouthlike opening) on the anterior aspect of the throat for breathing purposes. Two voice samples of a man and a woman with laryngeal cancer can be heard on the book's CD-ROM.

Removal of the larynx requires alternate methods of producing voice. Some alaryngeal (without larynx) speakers use a technique called **esophageal speech,** which uses the esophagus as a vibratory source. Essentially, these individuals learn to speak using "burps" as a substitute for actual voice production. Some individuals are incapable of producing esophageal speech. Several prosthetic devices are available to produce an alternative form of voicing for these alaryngeal speakers. One such device is a battery-powered **electrolarynx.** The electrolarynx has a vibrating diaphragm that is placed on the lateral aspects of the neck. This vibration excites the air in the vocal tract and thus serves as an alternate form of voicing. Some alaryngeal speakers may be candidates for devices that are inserted through a surgical opening in the throat. A device called a **tracheo-esophageal shunt (TEP)** directs air from the trachea into the esophagus, allowing the speaker to use respiratory air and a muscle of the esophagus, the cricopharyngeous muscle, for voice production (Ramig, 1994). This device enhances esophageal speech. Voice samples of a man and a woman using a TEP can be heard on the book's CD-ROM.

Trauma can damage the nerve supply to the larynx or cause structural damage to laryngeal cartilages and vocal folds. For example, a condition associated with surgical intubation of the larynx (respiratory tube placed between the vocal folds) is called **granuloma** (see photo on page 298).

The severity of this condition is directly related to the size of the tube and the length of time it is in place between the vocal folds (Titze, 1994). Granulomas are ruptured capillaries covered with epithelial tissue (Colton & Casper, 1996). The preferred treatment for granuloma is surgical removal followed by voice therapy.

Over 75 percent of people who are diagnosed with cancer of the larynx are or were heavy cigarette smokers. Particles in tobacco smoke are a major irritant to vocal fold tissue.

VOICE DISORDERS ASSOCIATED WITH PSYCHOLOGICAL OR STRESS CONDITIONS

The voice involuntarily responds to emotional changes. Strong emotional reactions such as extreme sadness, fear, anger, or happiness are reflected by the voice. The individual experiencing strong emotions might not be able to control his or her voice.

T H O U G H T   Q U E S T I O N S

Have you ever given a presentation to a large group of people? When you first started speaking, did your voice tremble and quaver? What might cause such vocal behaviors?

Strong emotions, when they are suppressed, can cause *psychogenic* voice disorders. Psychogenic voice disorders that are the result of psychological suppression of emotion are called **conversion disorders** because the person is converting emotional conflicts into physical symptoms (Aronson, 1990). In these cases, the vocal folds are structurally normal, and they function normally for nonspeech behaviors. One type of vocal conversion disorder is called **conversion aphonia.** People who suffer from conversion aphonia whisper to produce voice. Although these individuals are capable of coughing and clearing the throat, indicating the capability of glottal closure, they do not approximate the vocal folds for speech production. In many cases, people with conversion aphonia believe that they have a physical condition that prevents them from using their voice.

It is believed that conversion aphonias develop out of a desire to avoid some type of personal conflict or unpleasant situation in the person's life (Aronson, 1990). Conversion aphonia is not a common con-

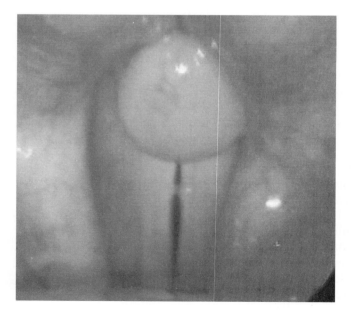

Granuloma. (Photograph courtesy of Robert Orlikoff, Ph.D., Memorial Sloan-Kettering Cancer Center, New York, NY)

dition, and it will likely persist until the person is willing to resolve the emotional conflict. People with deep-rooted psychological problems may require psychotherapy or psychiatric treatment.

THE VOICE EVALUATION AND INTERVENTION

Evaluation and treatment of voice disorders requires a multidisciplinary team approach. The specific nature of the presenting voice disorder will determine the precise composition of the team. At the very least, however, the team needs to comprise an otolaryngologist and a SLP.

THE VOICE EVALUATION

The first step in the evaluation of any suspected voice disorder is an examination performed by an otolaryngologist. The otolaryngologic examination will provide information about vocal fold tissue damage, presence of nodules, polyps, or other abnormal growths. A direct examination of the vocal folds and other laryngeal structures is essential to determine whether the voice disorder has an organic basis. The otolaryngologist makes direct observation of the laryngeal structures using laryngeal mirrors (similar to the mirror used by a dentist) or with an **endoscope.** An endoscope (see photo on page 300) is basically a lens coupled with a light source. The light source[3] illuminates the larynx, and laryngeal structures are viewed through the lens. The use of an endoscope is illustrated in the photograph at the beginning of this chapter. Biopsies of vocal fold tissue may be taken if laryngeal cancer is suspected.

Fiber optics are specially constructed flexible, tubular-shaped rods of glass that conduct light in only one direction. In an endoscope, small fiber optics transmit light from a source to illuminate an object, and a larger fiber optic transmits light from the illuminated object to a camera lens or viewing instrument.

The SLP's role in the voice evaluation typically begins by obtaining a case history. Information regarding the nature of the voice disorder, how it affects daily life activities, the developmental history and duration of the disorder, the person's social and vocational use of the voice, and his or her overall physical and psychological condition are important areas of interest in taking a case history (Colton & Casper, 1996).

A perceptual evaluation will also be conducted to describe the pitch, loudness, and vocal quality characteristics of the voice. In some clinical situations, detailed acoustic and physiological data regarding vocal function will be collected and compared to normative data. The

[3]The light source can be a stroboscopic light that flashes light rapidly in synchrony with vocal fold vibration.

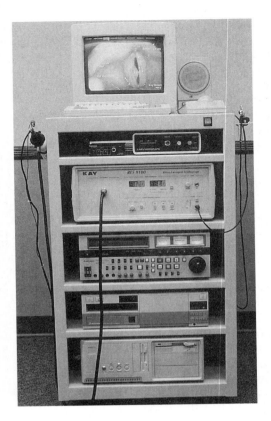

An endoscope system.

data obtained by the otolaryngologist and the SLP will be considered collectively, and a therapeutic plan will be recommended.

INTERVENTION FOR VOICE DISORDERS ASSOCIATED WITH VOCAL MISUSE OR ABUSE

Treatment of any voice disorder may involve behavioral voice therapy, surgical intervention, psychological or psychiatric counseling, drug treatments, or various combinations of these. Treatment protocol decisions are based on the specific needs of the individual and the established clinical efficacy of the treatment (Ramig, 1994). Voice therapy is frequently the clinical method of choice for voice disorders that have resulted from vocal misuse or abuse.

When voice therapy is the primary treatment method, the SLP will work toward several goals: (1) restore the vocal fold tissue to a healthy condition, (2) regain clear and full vocal function, (3) identify and eliminate behaviors that are abusive to the voice, and (4) establish improved vocal habits (Colton & Casper, 1996). Table 9.4 lists some suggestions for good **vocal hygiene** that the SLP might recommend during a counseling session. When voice therapy is a secondary treatment method, as after the surgical removal of vocal nodules or polyps, the SLP will work toward these goals: restore healthy vocal function, help the individual discover the "best" voice of which he or she is capable, and make environmental changes as necessary (Colton & Casper, 1996).

The SLP will use a number of therapeutic techniques in an effort to reach the goals outlined above: breathing and relaxation exercises, soft glottal attacks (initiation of voice with a whisper), reducing vocal loudness, and a variety of other techniques that facilitate healthy use of the voice. The therapeutic process may also involve discussions regarding personal concerns and it is important that the SLP listen in nonjudgmental fashion. It is also essential that the SLP provide support and encouragement that will help an individual accept a changed or restored voice (Colton & Casper, 1996).

TABLE 9.4

Behaviors that promote good vocal hygiene

Drink plenty of fluids, especially water.

Limit the intake of caffeine.

Limit the intake of alcoholic beverages.

Avoid tobacco products.

Avoid yelling and screaming.

Speak at a comfortable loudness level; don't "push" your voice.

Avoid loud, dry, or smoky environments.

Do not use "unnatural" voices, such as imitating cartoon characters.

Practice vocal rest.

Avoid excessive throat clearing and coughing.

T H O U G H T   Q U E S T I O N

Complete vocal rest for a given period of time is often a therapeutic goal. Consider your own life and think how hard it would be not to talk for a week or two.

INTERVENTION FOR VOICE DISORDERS ASSOCIATED WITH MEDICAL OR PHYSICAL CONDITIONS

Treatment of voice disorders associated with disease processes does not focus on elimination of the disorder (such as reducing the size of a nodule) or on precipitating conditions (frequent yelling at sporting events), but rather on assisting the individual to achieve the best voice possible or on establishing alternative manners to produce voice. For example, voice disorders associated with neurological problems are usually not the primary disability. Therefore, direct treatment of voice disorders associated with certain types of neurological disease may be a secondary concern to the SLP's treatment of related disabilities such as apraxia, aphasia, or dysphagia (Colton & Casper, 1996).

If voice therapy is indicated, the overriding therapeutic goal is to assist the individual to produce the best voice possible to remain communicatively functional in vocational and social settings. Additionally, the SLP can be helpful in assessing the effects of medications or surgery on voice production. Some of the specific techniques that the SLP uses to establish the best voice possible include increasing breath support, changing the rate of speaking, and changing the overall prosody of speech. It is essential that the SLP recognize the limitations of voice therapy for certain medical or physical conditions and help the individual to achieve the best possible means of communication (Colton & Casper, 1996).

INTERVENTION FOR VOICE DISORDERS ASSOCIATED WITH PSYCHOLOGICAL OR STRESS CONDITIONS

Treatment of voice disorders associated with psychological or stress conditions can be effective if the SLP succeeds in convincing the individual that there is nothing wrong physically with his or her voice. Individuals who have recognized conditions of stress or emotional conflict in their life and the relationship of this stress to their voice problem are the best candidates for voice therapy (Boone & McFarlane, 2000). These individuals want the ability to use their voice again.

A recommended therapeutic technique for voice disorders associated with psychological or stress conditions (conversion aphonia) begins by having the individual initiate voice from a prolonged throat clearing. This strategy is followed by having the individual initiate voice from the production of an "uh-huh." Such techniques provide solid evidence to the individual that he or she is capable physically of normal voice production (Boone & McFarlane, 2000).

Unfortunately, many individuals with conversion aphonia are highly resistant to changing their vocal patterns and habits. For these individuals, psychological counseling is imperative, and the SLP and psychologist should work as a team in an effort to restore the voice.

EFFICACY OF VOICE THERAPY

Assessing the efficacy of the treatment of voice disorders is complex because of the variety of conditions that produce voice disorders; varying severity levels of specific types of voice disorders; the variety and combinations of behavioral, pharmacological, and surgical treatments available; and the manner in which treatment efficacy is defined. Despite these complexities and the fact that not all voice disorders respond well to voice therapy, an impressive amount of clinical and experimental data compiled recently by Ramig and Verdolini (1998) suggest a general clinical effectiveness. In particular, voice disorders associated with vocal misuse or abuse, including those with structural tissue damage, some voice disorders associated with medical or physical conditions like Parkinson's disease, and voice disorders associated with psycho-logical or stress conditions, respond reasonably well to treatment. Ramig and Verdolini stress the need for continued research regarding voice therapy efficacy.

SUMMARY

The human larynx is a versatile instrument that, in addition to its primary biological function of protecting the lower airways from invasion of foreign substances, serves as the primary sound generator for spoken communication. The human voice reflects one's personality, general state of health and age, and emotional condition. Vocal function changes in predictable ways as one matures. The infant's crying to satisfy some particular need soon gives way to more purposeful communication designed to control his or her environment. Most adults have full control over their voices and are capable of a wide assortment of differentiated vocalizations that convey meaning, attitude, and emotion.

Disorders of the voice affect a substantial number of people in the United States. These disorders can range from relatively uncomplicated abnormalities such as vocal hoarseness resulting from yelling excessively at a sporting event to life-threatening cancer of the larynx. Voice disorders vary in both etiology and severity, and the specific method of treatment will in large measure be dictated the etiology and severity of the disorder.

SLPs play a pivotal role in the treatment of voice disorders, but effective and ethical intervention demands a team approach. In many instances, surgical intervention followed by voice therapy is the treatment protocol of choice; in other instances, voice therapy may precede surgery, perhaps rendering surgery unnecessary. Dealing effectively with individuals with voice disorders requires detailed and specific knowledge about normal and abnormal laryngeal functioning. Because many voice disorders respond well to techniques used by SLPs, it can be a rewarding and exciting clinical endeavor.

REFLECTIONS

- Explain the normal phonation process.
- Describe how the pitch of one's voice changes with age.
- Explain how one changes the pitch of the voice.
- Explain how one changes the loudness of the voice.
- Describe the perceptual signs of a voice disorder.
- Describe voice disorders that are associated with vocal misuse or abuse.
- Describe voice disorders associated with certain medical or physical conditions.
- Describe voice disorders associated with certain psychological conditions.
- Describe the major goals of therapy for voice disorders associated with misuse or abuse.
- Discuss the efficacy of voice therapy.

SUGGESTED READINGS

Colton, R. H., & Casper, J. K. (1996). *Understanding voice problems: A physiological perspective for diagnosis and treatment* (2nd ed.). Baltimore: Williams & Wilkins.

Hollien, H. (1987). Old voices: What do we really know about them? *Journal of Voice, 1,* 2–17.

Titze, I. R. (1994). *Principles of voice production.* Englewood Cliffs, NJ: Prentice-Hall.

ON-LINE RESOURCES

http://www.bgsm.edu/voice/index.html   Center for Voice Disorders of Wake Forest University.

One of the first multidisciplinary voice centers in the United States, the Center is housed in the Department of Otolaryngology of the Bowman Gray School of Medicine. The site features extensive links to information about a variety of voice disorders.

http://www.nyee.edu/otolaryn/voicefaq.htm New York Eye and Ear Infirmary, Department of Otolaryngology: FAQs about Voice Disorders.

Voice disorders are discussed in terms of conditions that influence vocal quality, loudness, pitch, or serviceablility of the voice.

http://www.asha.org/ Voice disorders.

Click on the "search site" button and type "voice." Many different voice disorders and therapeutic techniques are discussed.

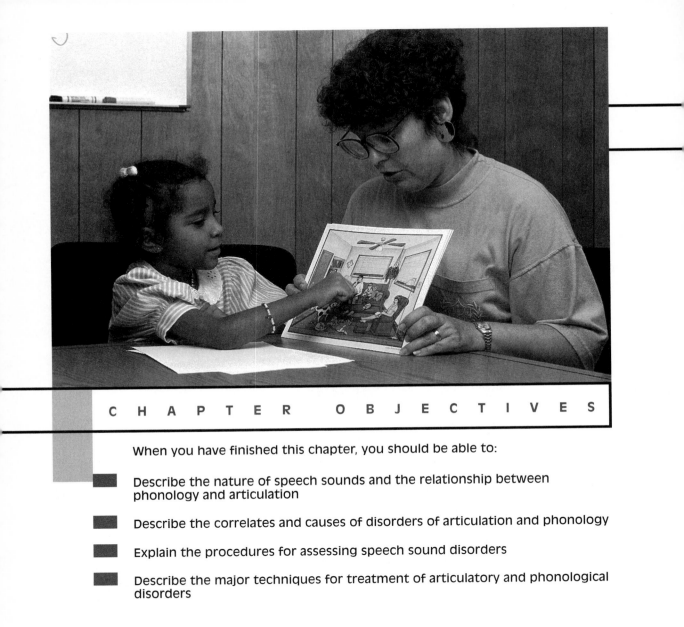

When you have finished this chapter, you should be able to:

Describe the nature of speech sounds and the relationship between phonology and articulation

Describe the correlates and causes of disorders of articulation and phonology

Explain the procedures for assessing speech sound disorders

Describe the major techniques for treatment of articulatory and phonological disorders

10

Disorders of Articulation and Phonology

While the written alphabet that we use contains twenty-six letters, spoken English has about forty-one different speech sounds. In this chapter, we are concerned primarily with speech sounds, called phonemes, which are combined to form spoken words, phrases, and sentences. For example, the word "cat" contains three phonemes [kæt]. Be careful; phonemes and letters are not the same. The word "that" also has three phonemes [ðæt]. Phonemes are generally written between two slashes, as in /p/, while transcribed phonemic combinations such as words are often transcribed between brackets as in [ðæt]. Some phonemes are universal and are found in all languages;

other phonemes are used in only a few languages. For example, the tongue clicks that are used in some African languages are not used as phonemes in English. In general, the more phonemes two languages have in common, the more similar the languages sound. The phonemic symbols for standard American English speech sounds are shown in Table 10.1.

In addition to phonemes, which are the building blocks of speech, *phonotactic* rules exist that specify acceptable sequences and locations. For example, the "ks" combination is never used at the beginning of an English word, but it is fine at the end in words such as "books" [bʊks]. Many Polish and Russian names

TABLE 10.1

Phonemic symbols for standard American English speech sounds

Consonants				Vowels			
Phoneme	Example	Phoneme	Example	Phoneme	Example	Phoneme	Example
/p/	put	/ʃ/	shoe	/i/	eat	/ɔ/	all
/b/	book	/ʒ/	treasure	/ɪ/	it	/ɑ/	hot
/t/	talk	/h/	hello	/e/	ate		
/d/	door	/tʃ/	chair	/ɛ/	elbow	**Diphthongs**	
/k/	kiss	/dʒ/	gym	/æ/	apple		
/g/	get	/m/	me	/ʌ/	up	Phoneme	Example
/f/	fun	/n/	no	/ə/	ahead	/aɪ/	eye
/v/	very	/ŋ/	sing	/ɝ/	her	/aʊ/	out
/θ/	thumb	/l/	lime	/ɚ/	mother	/ɔɪ/	boy
/ð/	the	/w/	wick	/u/	who		
/s/	see	/j/	yes	/ʊ/	could		
/z/	zoo	/r/	red	/o/	go		

Source: Adapted from Edwards (1997).

Allophonic variations contribute to regional and foreign dialects. The examples given in the text do not apply to all English speakers.

are difficult for English speakers to pronounce because these Slavic languages permit consonant combinations that are not found in English.

Each phoneme is really a family of related sounds and may be said with some variation but still be considered to be that particular phoneme. These variations are called **allophones.** Say the words "letter" and "better" out loud. When "tt" is found between two vowels, it is usually pronounced similar to a "d," which is quite different from the way you would say the "t" in "talk." Now compare the "p" in the words "pot" and "spot." When "p" is at the beginning of a word and followed by a vowel it is pronounced with a little puff of air (**aspiration**), but in most regions of the United States, when "p" is immediately preceded by "s," it is not aspirated. If the wrong allophone is used, the spoken words do not sound right.

We begin our discussion of articulation and phonology with information about how sounds are produced and classified. We examine the distinction between articulation and phonology, then we go on to describe impairments that may be related to articulatory and phonological disorders. The second half of the chapter is devoted to assessment and treatment.

UNDERSTANDING SPEECH SOUNDS

Although speech is largely an automatic process (we do not intellectually plan which sounds we'll produce or where we'll place our tongue and teeth), the command center is in the human brain, which stimulates neural impulses to the muscles involved in breathing, phonating, and articulating speech. Figure 10.1 is a simplified model of speech production. You'll notice that the processes of respiration, phonation, and articulation/resonation, which were described in Chapter 3, work together in response to neural impulses and are monitored by auditory and kinesthetic feedback At this point we'll focus on *articulation*, which is the shaping of speech sounds by the lips, tongue, and other

FIGURE 10.1   A simplified view of speech production. *Source:* Adapted from Zemlin (1998).

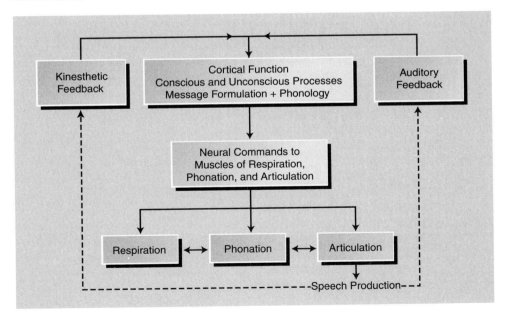

articulators. Phonemes are often categorized as either **vowel** or **consonant.** Very generally, we can say that vowels are produced with a relatively open or unobstructed vocal tract, and consonants are made with some degree of constriction.

All spoken languages have vowels and consonants. The intelligibility of the utterance is determined largely by the consonants, while the sound energy comes primarily from the vowels.

Consonant phonemes may be classified according to which articulators are used (place of articulation), how the sound is made (manner of production), and whether they occur with laryngeal vibration (voicing). Vowels are normally described according to tongue and lip position and relative degree of tension in these articulators. In addition, the concept of **distinctive features** is sometimes used to describe both vowels and consonants. These methods of characterizing phonemes are described in the next few pages.

CLASSIFICATION OF CONSONANTS BY PLACE AND MANNER

As was mentioned, consonants are characterized by constriction somewhere along the vocal tract. This point of contact or constriction, usually identified by its anatomical name, is used to classify consonants. Consonants in which constriction is made with both lips are called **bilabial,** meaning "two lips." **Labiodental** consonants are made with the bottom lip and upper teeth in contact. **Interdental** consonants are produced with the tongue between the teeth and are sometimes called **linguadental. Alveolar** sounds are made when the tongue tip is touching the alveolar or upper gum ridge. In **palatal** consonants, the center of the tongue is near the hard palate. The rear of the tongue approaches the velum or soft palate in the production of **velar** consonants. When the constriction occurs at the level of the vocal folds, the phonemes that are produced are called **glottal.**

Consonants may be *voiced* or *voiceless,* that is, produced with or without laryngeal vibration. Most English consonants are **nonresonant,** since resonance occurs only in a small portion of the vocal tract. Nonresonants are also known as **obstruents,** because the airflow is blocked or obstructed, Nonresonants include stops, fricatives, and affricates. In the production of **stops,** air pressure is built up behind the point of constriction, momentarily stopped, and then released, as in the /p/ sound. **Fricatives** are nonresonants that are made with a narrow passageway for the air to pass through, creating a frictionlike sound. **Affricates** are obstruents that begin as stops, and then are released as fricatives. **Resonants** are the **nasals** and **approximants.** The special characteristic of nasals is that they are produced with resonance in the nose. Approximants include **glides** and **liquids.** Glides occur when the articulatory posture changes gradually from consonant to vowel. Liquids include the **lateral** phoneme /l/ and the **rhotic** phoneme /r/. A lateral is a sound in which air is released on both sides of the tongue. Rhotic phonemes are made with the tongue in either a bunched or a turned-back posture.

Before looking at Table 10.2, say the phonemes /p/ and /m/. Which one is a stop? How do you know? Which one is nasal? How did you tell? Now place two fingers on the side of your throat and say the following speech sounds: /s/, /z/, /t/, /d/, /f/, /v/. Can you tell which are voiced and which are not voiced?

Table 10.2 depicts the classification of consonants by manner and place of production.

CLASSIFICATION OF VOWELS BY TONGUE AND LIP POSITION AND TENSION

Vowels are produced by resonating the exhaled air within the oral cavity. The exact sound that is made is dependent upon which part of the

TABLE 10.2

Classification of American English consonants by manner and place of production

Manner	Place						
	Bilabial VL V*	Labio- dental VL V*	Inter- dental VL V*	Alveolar VL V*	Palatal VL V*	Velar VL V*	Glottal VL V*
Nonresonants							
Stops	p b			t d		k g	
Fricatives		f v	θ ð	s z	ʃ ʒ		h
Affricates					ʧ ʤ		
Resonants							
Nasal	m			n		ŋ	
Approximants							
Glides	w				j	w	
Liquids				l	r		

*VL = voiceless; V = voiced.
Note: Affricates are not listed in the 1996 update of the International Phonetic Alphabet; however, the term is still widely used.
Adapted from Small (1999). Used with permission.

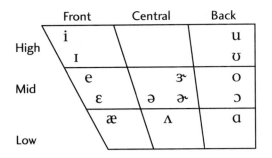

FIGURE 10.2 Classification of American English vowels by height and frontness/backness of tongue. *Source:* Adapted from Shriberg & Kent (1995) and Yavas (1998).

tongue is elevated (front, center, or back), its relative height (high, mid, or low), and the amount of tension (tense or lax) in the articulators. Whether the lips are rounded (pursed) or retracted (pulled back into a sort of smile) also influences the sound that is produced. All English vowels are normally voiced and not nasal. Exceptions occur when you whisper and when nasal resonance occurs for any number of reasons including proximity to a nasal phoneme, such as /m/ or /n/. Figure 10.2 is a diagram of vowel production. In the figure, the higher vowel of the front and back paired vowels and /ɝ/ are relatively tense; all other vowels are lax. High and mid back vowels and the back central vowels are produced with the lips somewhat rounded. All other English vowels are unrounded.

When two vowels are said in close proximity, they produce a special type of phoneme called a **diphthong.** In English, the vowels in the words "sigh," "now," and "boy" are diphthongs. "Sigh" contains /aɪ/, "now" has /aʊ/, and "boy" contains /ɔɪ/.

T H O U G H T   Q U E S T I O N

Can you think of additional words containing the phonemic diphthongs /aɪ/, /aʊ/, and /ɔɪ/?

DISTINCTIVE FEATURE ANALYSIS

In an attempt to provide a system for describing phonemes found in all languages, linguists identified the components of individual sounds and called these distinctive features. Each phoneme can then be theoretically identified by the presence or absence of each of these features (Chomsky & Halle, 1968). For example, three English phonemes (/m/, /n/, and /ŋ/) are produced with nasal resonance. They are considered + nasal. All other English phonemes are – nasal. To further distinguish among the nasal phonemes, we might note that /m/ and /n/ are produced with obstruction in the front portion of the mouth; they are + anterior, while /ŋ/ is – anterior. The phonemes /m/ and /n/ can be differentiated on the basis of the distinctive feature "distributed." If the constriction extends for some distance along the direction of the airflow, it is + distributed. In the example we are using, /m/ is considered + distributed, while /n/ is – distributed.

The concept of distinctive feature analysis has been helpful in finding patterns of speech sound errors and thereby facilitating their correction. Table 10.3 on page 314 contains brief definitions and examples of some of the more commonly used distinctive features.

THOUGHT QUESTIONS

Contrast the use of distinctive features with classification by place and manner of production. How are the systems similar? How are they different?

PHONOLOGY AND ARTICULATION

The correct use of speech sounds within a language requires knowledge of the sounds of the language and the rules that govern their production and combination. This somewhat theoretical concept is called *phonology*. Speech also requires neuromotor coordination to actually say sounds, words, and sentences; this is considered *articulation*. To help you understand this distinction, visualize learning a new language such as French. You will be exposed to new words and sound combinations and begin to grasp the nature of that language's sound system or phonology. But you must also be able to form the words with your lips, tongue, and so on. You might find this very difficult because your neuromotor pathways have been trained to make English words; the inability to coordinate your muscles to correctly produce the words is a problem of articulation.

The distinction between phonology and articulation is often difficult to understand. Articulation refers to the actual production of speech sounds; phonology is knowledge of speech sounds within a language and the ways in which they are combined.

Phonological impairments are disorders of conceptualization or language rules. Remember that phonology is concerned with classes of sounds and sound patterns within words. For example, English has both open and closed syllables at the ends of words. An **open syllable** is one that ends in a vowel—for example, "ba-na-n<u>a</u>"; a **closed syllable** ends in a consonant ("kum-qua<u>t</u>"). A child who uses only open syllables and deletes all final consonants would be exhibiting a disorder of phonology. In this example, the child would say "banana" correctly but produce "kumquat" as "kuqua."

Articulation impairments are disorders of production. A child whose only speech error is incorrect production of the /s/ phoneme has a disorder of articulation. Disorders of articulation are typically characterized as

- Substitutions
- Omissions
- Distortions
- Additions

TABLE 10.3

Definitions and examples of some common distinctive features

Anterior: Sounds that are produced with an obstruction in the front portion of the mouth—specifically, labials, dentals, and alveolars

Examples of + anterior: /m, p, b, f, v, θ, ð, n, t, d/

Consonantal: Sounds that are produced with obstruction in the oral cavity—specifically, obstruents and nasals

Examples of + consonantal: /s, z, t, d, m, n, r, l/

Examples of – consonantal: /æ, i, e, o, u/

Continuant: Sounds in which the air may flow without interruption—specifically, fricatives, glides, liquids, vowels.

Examples of + continuant: /f, v, s, z, h, j, r, l, i, e, o, u/

Examples of – continuant: /p, t, k, b, d, g/

Distributed: Consonants that are produced with a constriction that extends a relatively long distance along the direction of airflow

Examples of + distributed: /m, p, b, ʃ, ʒ, ʧ, dʒ/

Nasal: Phonemes that are produced with a lowered soft palate

Examples of + nasal: /m, n, ŋ/

Sonorant: Sounds that are produced with a relatively open vocal tract, such that spontaneous voicing is possible—specifically, vowels, nasals, liquids, glides

Examples of + sonorant: /æ, o, m, n, l, r, w, j/

Examples of – sonorant: /p, b, t, d, k, g, ʃ, ʧ/

Strident: Sounds in which the airstream is constricted in such a way as to produce a high-intensity noise

Examples of + strident: /s, z, f, v/

Examples of – strident /p, b, i, e, o/

Syllabic: Sounds that serve as the nucleus of a syllable—specifically vowels, syllabic liquids, syllabic nasals

Examples of + syllabic: [bʌ tn̩] as in "button"

Examples of – syllabic: the /b/ and /t/ in "button."

Voiced: Sounds that are produced with vocal fold vibration—specifically all vowels, nasals, glides, voiced consonants

Examples of + voice: /i, e, o, m, n, j, w, b, d, g, z, v/

Examples of – voice: /p, t, k, s, f/

Source: Based on Chomsky and Halle (1968).

Substitutions occur when one phoneme is replaced with another. For example, a person who says "shair" for "chair" would be substituting "sh" for "ch." An omission is the deletion of a phoneme, as in "chai" for "chair." Distortions occur when a nonstandard form of the phoneme is used. An example of an addition would be "ch<u>uh</u> air" for "chair." Some individuals have disorders of both phonology and articulation. We will talk more about specific patterns and types of errors later in this chapter.

ASSOCIATED DISORDERS AND RELATED CAUSES

The causes of phonological and articulatory disorders in most children are not readily identifiable. In these cases, when no cause is known, it may be termed a *functional disorder*. Recognizing the limited usefulness of this concept, researchers have directed their attention to **correlates,** or factors that tend to be present in individuals with phonological disorders. Correlation means that two or more things occur together but one does not necessarily cause the other(s). Nevertheless, correlates may offer some clues to causality that should prompt further research. Table 10.4 on page 316 lists some correlates of phonological impairment. In the next few sections, we describe the characteristics associated with a few well-established correlates of phonological and articulatory impairment.

The term "functional articulation disorder" is commonly used. The majority of children with disordered articulation and phonology do not exhibit an identifiable physical reason for the problem.

T H O U G H T   Q U E S T I O N S

Can you think of any two things that are correlated but not causally related? What may account for the correlation? Why is it important to distinguish between causality and correlation?

DEVELOPMENTAL IMPAIRMENT IN CHILDREN

As you discovered in Chapters 4 and 6, language and speech learning is not easy. In addition to understanding what is said to them, children must figure out how to use meaningful words and how to put these words into grammatically correct fluent utterances. Words are composed of phonemes that are typically acquired gradually between 1 and 8 years of age. Many children with articulation and phonological difficulties are not easily classifiable. These children may exhibit

TABLE 10.4

Possible correlates of phonological and articulatory impairments

Hearing loss

History of otitis media during the first few years of life

Diminished speech sound perception and discrimination ability

Atypical tooth alignment and missing teeth

Impaired oral-motor skills

Eating problems

Tongue thrust swallow after 6 years of age

Neuromotor disabilities

Mental retardation

Language problems

Reading disorders

Family history

---

a developmental impairment in speech sound production with no readily identifiable corollary factors.

CHARACTERISTICS OF ARTICULATION

Table 4.4 in Chapter 4, "Communication Development," lists the consonants that are typically mastered at various ages. When the cause of poor articulation is a delay in speech development, you would expect that children are not yet producing the phonemes expected for their age. For example, a 7-year-old who misarticulates the "sh" sound (/ʃ/), for no apparent reason, might be considered delayed in speech sound development. This child's speech might sound as follows:

TARGET: "She made a wish."
CHILD'S PRODUCTION: "Si made a wis."

Children with developmental impairments may be idiosyncratic in their phoneme use. Some researchers identify these children as "deviant" in their development, while those whose speech is like that of much younger children are considered "delayed." This dichotomy is a difficult one, however, because of the wide range of behaviors in young children (Howell & Dean, 1994; Stoel-Gammon & Dunn, 1985).

PHONOLOGICAL PROCESSES

As we discussed in Chapter 4, children simplify adult speech in many ways. They use shorter sentences, simpler grammar, more everyday words, and an immature but generally systematic way of producing speech sounds in words and sentences. Children's phonological and phonotactic simplifications are called **phonological processes.** Table 4.3 in Chapter 4 provides explanations and examples of phonological processes of young children. When these processes persist, they constitute phonological impairments. A child who regularly produces stop phonemes instead of fricatives would be exhibiting the phonological process called **stopping of fricatives.** An example would be as follows:

TARGET: "They saw five violets."
CHILD'S PRODUCTION: "Dey taw fibe biolet."

Fronting, producing front phonemes for back ones, is another common process. Following is an example:

TARGET: "What color is the car?"
CHILD'S PRODUCTION: "What tolor is the tar?"

The reverse process, known as **backing,** using back phonemes for front ones, is less typical but also occurs in children who have functional phonological disorders. An example would be as follows:

TARGET: "Tom told Tim."
CHILD'S PRODUCTION: "Kom kolk Kim."

Box 10.1 describes a young girl who exhibited the phonological process of backing.

Phonological processes involve more than individual phonemes. Final consonant deletion can involve any consonant, as when the target "Give him the book" is produced as "Gi- hi- the boo." Similarly, reduplication is the repetition of any syllable, as when "water" is said as "wawa." Many children exhibit multiple processes.

LIFE SPAN ISSUES

The average age of diagnosis of a developmental phonological disorder is 4 years, 2 months (Shriberg & Kwiatkowski, 1994), although the roots of these problems may be seen in infancy and toddlerhood. With maturation and therapy, immature patterns of articulation tend to diminish (Gierut, 1998). If they do not, they may have a negative impact on the individual's academic and professional accomplishments as well as on personal relationships. What was considered "cute" in childhood may be viewed negatively in adulthood.

Children who were unsuccessful in correcting immature speech patterns through therapy may become rebellious and feel punished by continued intervention efforts. These youngsters sometimes benefit from a break from treatment. When they return for therapy, SLPs must be careful to use age-appropriate materials and activities. Although speech sound production can be modified at any stage in life, as we age, old habits become more firmly entrenched, and so change is more difficult.

Personal Story of a Child with a Phonological Disorder

Brandi was just over 3 years of age when she was first brought to the University Speech and Hearing Center by her mother, Mrs. A. Brandi had been identified in a preschool screening program as needing further evaluation. Mrs. A. noted that Brandi mispronounced many words and could not be understood by people outside of the family, and "people say her mouth looks stiff." Brandi's 5-year-old brother frequently interpreted Brandi's speech so that others could understand her. Examination at the center revealed that Brandi had normal hearing and physical structure for speech. Her receptive and expressive language skills were above average in all areas but phonology. Brandi was diagnosed with a moderate-to-severe phonological disorder of unknown cause.

A cycles approach was used in therapy that first targeted the phonological processes cluster simplification, stopping of fricatives, and backing to velars. An example of Brandi's speech at the beginning of therapy is as follows:

Target: Stop playing with my toy.
Brandi: Kop payin' wid my koy.

Because of her young age and her high spirits, therapy was presented through structured play activities. Brandi enjoyed beanbag tosses and musical chairs. She also demonstrated that she understood the purpose of the speech sessions and attempted to do as the SLP requested of her. By the end of three months, Brandi frequently self-corrected in the clinical setting. At the end of a year of therapy, Brandi's mother reported that Brandi was self-correcting at home. Although Brandi had made good progress, she would receive speech therapy for two more years. She entered first grade with easily intelligible speech and only a few articulation errors.

LANGUAGE IMPAIRMENTS

Children who have language impairments, as described in Chapter 6, may also be disordered and/or delayed in their production of the sounds of the language. It has been estimated that a general impairment in expressive language is present in about 60 percent of children who are hard to understand and who have multiple speech sound errors (Shriberg & Kwiatkowsi, 1994; Tyler & Watterson, 1991). These children have more complicated problems than those of youngsters with isolated phonological or articulatory deficiencies. Some children with language learning disabilities have difficulties not only with listening and speaking, but also with reading, writing, reasoning, and mathematics (National Joint Committee on Learning Disabilities, 1991). They may be classified with a **learning disability** and exhibit many of the behaviors including distractibility and impulsivity described in Chapter 6.

ARTICULATION AND PHONOLOGICAL PROCESS CHARACTERISTICS

The speech sound productions of children with language learning disabilities are similar to those with developmental impairments, although complex syllable structures may be especially challenging for those with language learning difficulties (Orsolini, Sechi, et al., 2001). Those with language learning disabilities may also have difficulty understanding language and will use simpler and less grammatically correct speech. They are also more likely to exhibit phonological errors that also affect morpheme production (Owen, Dromi, & Leonard, 2001).

T H O U G H T   Q U E S T I O N

What bound morphemes are affected by omission of the final /s/ in words in the sentence "Tom like<u>s</u> to read Pete'<u>s</u> book<u>s</u>"?

LIFE SPAN ISSUES

Individuals with learning disabilities of any type are of normal intelligence. Despite this, phonological impairments may have a deleterious effect on the acquisition of reading and writing skills. Children with specific language impairments are more likely than their peers to struggle with academic subjects through the grades and even into college and beyond. They may require support and the use of various strategies to achieve to their full potential (Owens, 1999).

HEARING IMPAIRMENTS

Because hearing is the primary way in which we acquire the speech sounds of a language, it is no surprise that individuals with hearing impairments may have disordered articulation and phonology. Not only are those with hearing loss limited in their ability to hear others, but their ability to monitor their own speech production may be inadequate. It must be recognized that phonology will not be impaired alone, but all parameters of speech, including voice quality, pitch, rate, and rhythm, will similarly be affected. (This is discussed in further detail in Chapter 14, "Audiology and Hearing Loss." As we noted in Chapter 2, auditory disorders may range in severity from mild to profound, and they may be classified as conductive, sensorineural, mixed, or central.

ARTICULATION AND PHONOLOGICAL PROCESS CHARACTERISTICS

Although the specifics vary, in general, the more severe a person's hearing loss, the less intelligible his or her speech is likely to be (Wolk & Schildroth, 1986). Although researchers point out that an exact relationship between type and degree of hearing impairment and speech cannot be made, certain patterns are frequently observed (Bankson & Bernthal, 1998a).

Articulation errors that tend to occur in the speech of children who are deaf include voicing confusion, as when "toy" is said as "doy," and vowel substitutions, as when "ill" is pronounced as "eel" (Calvert, 1982). More examples are provided in Table 10.5.

Although it is not always the case, children who have a history of frequent bouts of **otitis media** (middle ear infections), resulting in transient conductive hearing loss, are more likely than youngsters who have not had these infections to exhibit the phonological and articulatory errors shown in Table 10.6 (Bankson & Bernthal, 1998a).

LIFE SPAN ISSUES

The age at onset and the degree and type of hearing impairment influence the nature of the articulation and phonological disability. Individuals who are born deaf or with severe hearing impairment typically have poorer speech than those who lose hearing later in life. Speech deteriorates over time, however, for those who are initially hearing and become hard-of-hearing or deaf after they have learned to talk. Accuracy of

---

TABLE 10.5

Typical speech sound errors in children who are deaf

Sound Substitution Pattern	Examples
Voiced for voiceless sounds	"see" → "zee" [zi]
	"can" → "gan" [gæn]
Nasal for oral consonants	"dog" → "nong" [nɔŋ]
Sounds with easy tactile perception for those difficult to perceive	"run" → "wun" [wʌn]
Tense vowels for lax vowels	"sick" → "seek" [sik]
Diphthongs for vowels	"miss" → "mice" [maɪs]
Vowels for diphthongs	"child" → "chilled" [tʃɪld]

Sources: Adapted from Bankson & Bernthal (1998a) and Calvert (1982).

TABLE 10.6

Phonological processes often observed in children with history of otitis media

Phonological Process	Phonemes Involved	Examples
Stopping of fricatives	/s/, /z/, /ʃ/, /ʒ/, /tʃ/, /dʒ/ /f/, /v/, /θ/, /ð/	"see" → [ti] "John" → [dɑn] "thumb" → [tʌm]
Initial consonant deletion	Any consonant	"see" → [i] "John" → [ɑn]
Glottal fricative replacement	/h/ used for initial consonant	"see" → [hi] "John" → [hɑn]
Glottal stop replacement	Any consonant	"see" → [ʔi] "John" → [ʔɑn]
Nasal replacement	/m/, /n/, /ŋ/	"my" → [naɪ] or [baɪ]

Source: Bankson, J. E., & Bernthal, N. W. (1998). Factors related to phonologic disorders. In Bernthal, J. E., & Bankson, N. W., *Articulation and phonological disorders.* Fourth Edition. Boston: Allyn and Bacon. Copyright © 1998 by Allyn and Bacon. Reprinted by permission.

speech sound production can be enhanced by the use of hearing aids (for individuals with some hearing) and appropriate training. (See Chapter 14, "Audiology and Hearing Loss.")

T H O U G H T   Q U E S T I O N S

Why do people who lose hearing later in life have less impaired speech than those who were born deaf? Which phonemes do you think a deaf or severely hard-of-hearing person would find most difficult to learn? Why?

NEUROMUSCULAR DISORDERS

Dysarthrias are speech problems that are due to neuromuscular impairment that results in poor coordination, weakness, or paralysis of the speech mechanism. Cerebral palsy (CP) is the term for numerous congenital neuromotor disorders that are described in more detail in Chapter 12, "Neurogenic Speech Disorders." About two-thirds of people with cerebral palsy have impaired speech or language. Because it is not a unitary problem, no single pattern of articulation or phonology can be identified; however, disorders in articulation are often related to some form of CP or *dysarthria* (Air, Wood, & Neils, 1989). The precise symptoms depend largely on the type and extent of the brain lesion. Dysarthrias commonly also affect respiration, phonation, resonance, and the rate and rhythm of speech. Clients with dysarthria may also have chewing, sucking, and swallowing problems. (See Chapter 13, "Disorders of Swallowing.")

CHARACTERISTICS OF ARTICULATION

Most people with dysarthric or cerebral palsied speech are imprecise in their articulation of consonants. The errors that an individual exhibits tend to be similar whether she or he is reading aloud, speaking to a group, or in an intimate conversation. In general, the location of the motor neuron impairment in a particular speaker determines which phonemes are involved. For example, a person with loss of lip strength and coordination would likely misarticulate such phonemes as /p/, /b/, and /m/. Someone with primarily tongue tip **paresis,** that is, muscle weakness or partial paralysis, might incorrectly produce /t/, /d/, /l/, and /n/ (Crary, 1993).

LIFE SPAN ISSUES

In cerebral palsy, the symptoms are present from earliest childhood onward. Muscular dystrophy also has an early beginning, typically between the ages of 2 and 5 years. Dysarthrias that are the result of a stroke, tumor, or disorders such as Parkinson's disease most often occur in adulthood. At any age, dysarthrias are but one aspect of an individual's diminished physical condition.

APRAXIA OF SPEECH

People with dysarthric speech have a neuromuscular impairment resulting in muscle weakness and poor coordination that interferes with accurate production of speech sounds. Individuals with speech apraxia may have adequate muscle strength and often have satisfactory articulation when engaging in automatic speech such as counting, but they exhibit errors in volitional speech that requires motor planning.

As we noted earlier, production of speech sounds requires both a mental image of phonology and the ability to move the articulators to achieve the correct phoneme. Some individuals have no difficulty in conceptualizing speech sounds and have adequate muscle strength and coordination, but their speech is characterized by multiple speech sound errors. These errors may be attributable to an impairment in programming the speech musculature to select, plan, organize, and initiate a motor pattern. This deficiency is termed *apraxia of speech.* The causes of apraxia are probably neurological. Apraxia is not due to hearing loss, muscle weakness, low intelligence, impaired receptive language, or an apparent organic condition, although it may coexist with other disorders (Hall, Jordan, & Robin, 1993).

CHARACTERISTICS OF ARTICULATION

A person with apraxia of speech does not have a typical pattern of mis-articulated phonemes; in fact, an individual's errors tend to be inconsistent. However, a commonality of speech production activity can be described. These behaviors include the following:

- Poor speech sound imitation
- Difficulty initiating speech movements characterized by initial consonant deletion
- Vowel misarticulations
- Groping and struggle behavior in producing speech sounds on command
- Rate and rhythm abnormalities
- Poor diadochokinetic performance (ability to rapidly repeat syllables)
- Inconsistent vowel and consonant errors (Bankson & Bernthal, 1998a; Strand & McCauley, 1997)

In addition, clients with apraxia often do not respond readily to speech therapy; their rate of improvement may seem frustratingly slow (Hall et al., 1993).

LIFE SPAN ISSUES

Brain damage at any age can result in apraxia of speech. When the behaviors described above are observed in a child, it may be called **developmental apraxia of speech (DAS)** or **developmental verbal dyspraxia (DVD),** although the injury to the brain may never be documented. Apraxia in adults is caused by damage to the left side of the brain, which may be due to a degenerative neurological disease, tumor, stroke, or other trauma. An adult with apraxia of speech may also have aphasia, dysarthria, and/or limb apraxia (difficulty moving fingers, arms, or legs in a purposeful manner). **Aphemia,** which is the result of a stroke, is characterized by marked speech abnormality. When aphemia occurs without language involvement, it may be considered a severe form of apraxia of speech (Fox, Kasner, Chatterjee, et al., 2001). The articulatory patterns noted above may be seen in adults or children with apraxia. However, older individuals are more likely to exhibit automatic speech—such as counting or naming the days of the week—that is free of error, while words and sentences that are linguistically and intellectually complex show more deterioration. Younger children may not have had the opportunity to develop this automaticity.

Many writers suggest that developmental apraxia of speech and adult onset apraxia are clearly distinct disorders because of the differences in etiology (Bankson & Bernthal, 1998a; Bloom & Ferrand, 1997).

CLEFT PALATE

Children who are born with a cleft palate frequently exhibit articulatory errors in their speech. These errors may be due not only to the nature of the cleft, an inadequate or too short palate, and inability to sufficiently close the oral/pharyngeal passageway to the nose, but also to frequently related factors such as misaligned teeth, hearing loss, and delayed development. The type of cleft, the age of the client, and the age at the time of surgical repair(s) also influence the precise nature of the articulatory impairment. For this reason, the SLP must not assume a particular pattern of errors but must take care to assess the child's articulation and phonology fully (Air et al., 1989; Grunwell, 1993). In addition, as we'll see in Chapter 11, "Cleft Lip and Cleft Palate," aspects of voice and resonance are typically also impaired.

CHARACTERISTICS OF ARTICULATION

Despite the variability noted above, certain speech sound errors are particularly common among those with a history of cleft palate. Phonemes that require the buildup of intra-oral pressure are typically affected. These include stops, fricatives, and affricates. Vowels may sound especially nasal. Minor variations of the dimensions of the hard palate and velum do not appear to affect speech articulation; however, surgical removal of any portion of the roof of the mouth and congenital clefts seriously compromise speech intelligibility. Surgery and/or the use of prosthetic devices, called **obturators,** have been found to be effective intervention and, along with speech therapy, permit significant gains in speech articulation.

LIFE SPAN ISSUES

Although a person may be born with a cleft palate, simple clefts are usually surgically repaired between the ages of 12 and 18 months. More involved clefts may require a number of surgical, orthodontic, and other procedures. In these cases, and if surgery is delayed past the age of 2 years, the child's articulation becomes more disordered and harder to correct. This is because the individual is likely to develop *compensatory* movements to produce sounds that are intended to resemble target phonemes. These maladaptive errors are sometimes labeled "cleft palate speech." Beyond 10 years of age, surgery without speech therapy is insufficient to alter disordered articulation. Although therapy is never guaranteed, it results in positive changes for many speakers. Some individuals with early surgery develop unimpaired speech without formal training; however, therapy tends to enhance progress. (Grunwell, 1993). Some compensatory articulations are included in Table 10.7.

Cleft palate is a congenital condition; it is something you are born with. Occasionally, however, similar impairments to the roof of the

TABLE 10.7

Compensatory articulations often present among individuals born with a cleft palate

Target	Phonemes Involved	Compensatatory Articulation
Stop	/p/, /b/, /t/, /d/, /k/, /g/	Glottal stop /ʔ/, stop produced at the glottis
		Pharyngeal stop, stop produced near pharynx
		Middorsum stop, stop produced in middle of tongue
Fricative	/s/, /z/, /ʃ/, /ʒ/	Pharyngeal fricative, closure occurs near pharynx
		Velar fricative, posterior nasal fricative
Affricate	/ʧ/, /dʒ/	Pharyngeal fricative, velar fricative, posterior nasal fricative

The overall effect is speech that is hypernasal and contains nasal emission and weak and distorted consonants.

Source: Adapted from text material in Air, Wood, and Neils (1989).

mouth or ability to achieve velopharyngeal closure occur later in life. These disruptions may be due to removal of tumors, adenoidectomy, or neurological disorders such as muscular dystrophy. In these cases, speakers probably will not develop compensatory movements, but their speech will contain some misarticulations. This subject is addressed in greater detail in Chapter 11, "Cleft Lip and Cleft Palate."

OTHER ORGANIC ABNORMALITIES

Speech sounds are produced by making subtle adjustments that involve the lips, teeth, tongue, hard and soft palate, larynx, and respiratory system. In this section, we review the impact of structural and functional variations on articulation.

LIPS

If you were to systematically examine the lip structure of every student in your class, you would observe considerable variation in appearance.

Although speech articulation requires rapid and accurate movements involving the tongue, teeth, and lips, some individuals with organic problems can compensate and produce acceptable speech in atypical ways.

These structural differences do not affect speech sound production (Fairbanks & Green, 1950). On the other hand, neuromotor problems that impair the ability to purse and retract the lips might slightly affect the way vowels are said. Remember, in English, front vowels usually are said with the lips pulled back, and back vowels typically require lip rounding. (Refer to Figure 10.1 and related discussion.)

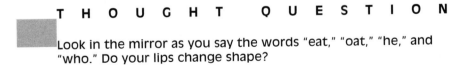

T H O U G H T   Q U E S T I O N

Look in the mirror as you say the words "eat," "oat," "he," and "who." Do your lips change shape?

TEETH

Both occlusion (tooth alignment) and missing teeth may affect articulation, but this is not always the case. Most individuals with malocclusions or rotated or absent teeth are able to compensate for these deficiencies. Although an open bite, in which the front teeth do not meet, occurs more often in speakers with articulatory errors, many people with open bite speak normally. Similarly, more children with missing front incisors misarticulate /s/ and other phonemes than children with a full set of teeth. On the other hand, most children whose front incisors are missing do not make articulatory errors (Bankson & Bernthal, 1998a).

Adults with dentures may exhibit misarticulations, particularly of the /s/ phoneme. Readjustment of these prostheses, with particular attention to the upper incisors so that they mimic the original position of the person's natural teeth, is generally effective (Runte, Lawerino, Dirksen, et al., 2001). If this is insufficient, the SLP may work with the client to compensate for any misalignment.

TONGUE

Technically, a person who is "tongue-tied" has **ankyloglossia,** or a relatively short lingual frenum (the tissue that connects the underportion of the tongue to the floor of the mouth), which restricts tongue movement. Several decades ago, frenums were frequently clipped soon after birth if there was apparent ankyloglossia. Physicians have become more conservative with this procedure. In fact, although the tip of the tongue must be free to move to produce tongue tip sounds such as /l/, /t/, /d/, it is quite rare for misarticulation to be caused by ankyloglossia (Bankson & Bernthal, 1998a).

Complete or partial **glossectomy** (surgical removal of the tongue) is likely to impair speech sound production, but again, humans are remarkably adaptable and can often compensate. As might be expected, the greater the amount of tongue that is removed, the more impaired speech intelligibility will be. Fricatives such as /s/, /z/, /f/, /v/, /ʃ/, /ʒ/,

/θ/, and /ð/ and stops such as /p/, /b/, /t/, /d/, /k/, and /g/ are more affected than nasals (/m/, /n/, /ŋ/), liquids (/r/ and /l/), and glides (/w/ and /j/) (Leonard, 1994). Speech therapy typically is helpful in assisting clients improve their speech intelligibility (Furia, Kowalski, Latorre, et al., 2001).

During the first few years of life, because of the size of the tongue relative to the oral cavity, all youngsters have tongue placement somewhat forward in the mouth with the tongue tip resting against the back of the front teeth. Swallowing during this time also involves a forward movement of the tongue. This pattern has been termed **tongue thrust, myofunctional disorder,** or **reverse swallow.** By age 5, tongue thrust should no longer be apparent; its perpetuation has been associated with dental malocclusion and speech misarticulation. The phonemes that are most likely to be affected by tongue thrust are /s/, /z/, /ʃ/, /ʒ/, /tʃ/, /dʒ/, /t/, /d/, /l/, and /n/ (Hanson, 1994).

LANGUAGE AND DIALECTAL VARIATIONS

Although the United States was once considered a "melting pot," with people from different countries and cultural backgrounds blending into one homogenous group, during the final decades of the twentieth century, the concepts of "salad bowl" and "multiculturalism" have emerged. Today, many Americans take pride in their regional and linguistic backgrounds and cherish the cultural diversity that characterizes this country.

If you are a native speaker of American English and went to another country, such as Greece, to live, you would learn Greek to communicate with those around you. When you spoke in Greek, your speech would reveal your American background. You would speak Greek with an "American accent." This is not a speech disorder.

Similarly, if you are from Georgia and moved to Massachusetts, you would bring your Georgia regionalism with you. Again, this is not a disorder but a dialectal difference to those in your new environment.

T H O U G H T   Q U E S T I O N S

What do you think the role of speech-language pathologists should be for individuals from diverse linguistic, regional, and cultural backgrounds? Have you ever wanted your speech to sound more "mainstream"? Why or why not?

"In assessing phonological skills in bilingual speakers, speech-language pathologists must guard against both over- and underdiagnosis"

A person whose speech reflects a regional or foreign language influence may also have a speech disorder. However, the regionalism or foreign dialect in itself is not a disorder.

(Yavas & Goldstein, 1998, p. 51). The SLP must differentiate between disordered phonology and that which is simply different due to foreign language influences. The SLP must do the following:

1. Recognize cultural differences
2. Evaluate phonological competence in all relevant languages whenever possible
3. Select appropriate assessment tools
4. Use nonstandard assessments often with the help of bilingual assistants
5. Describe phonological patterns
6. Diagnose any phonological disorders that exist (Yavas & Goldstein, 1998)

When these have been accomplished, the SLP must plan and engage in intervention as appropriate. If dialect differences are targeted, the SLP must assess the client's attitude toward his or her dialect and the individual's motivation (or lack of motivation) for accent reduction. Some generalizations can be made regarding the speech of individuals from various linguistic and regional backgrounds; see Table 10.8.

CHARACTERISTICS OF ARTICULATION AND PHONOLOGY

It is impossible to describe all the variations in articulation and phonology that reflect non-English or dialectal influences. Table 10.8 highlights just a few of these. A general principle is that the first language learned will interfere with languages that are learned later. For example, in Spanish, /d/, and /ð/ are allophones or variations of the same phoneme, whereas in English, these are two separate phonemes, as can be seen in the words "dough" [do] and "though" [ðo]. Native Spanish speakers, however, may confuse the /d/ and /ð/ and pronounce both words the same way (Yavas, 1998).

T H O U G H T   Q U E S T I O N

How does your articulation differ from that of someone from another part of the country or a different linguistic or dialectal background?

LIFE SPAN ISSUES

Some adults for whom English is a second (or third or fourth) language choose to modify their foreign accent. Often this desire is based on professional considerations. Teachers of English as a second language and speech-language pathologists may contribute to the improvement of Eng-

TABLE 10.8

Sample phonological characteristics of American English dialects and non-English language influences on spoken English

Rule	Example
African American Vernacular	
Final cluster reduction	"presents" → "presen"
Stopping of interdental initial and medial fricatives	"they" → "dey"
	"nothing" → "noting"
Deletion of "r"	"professor" → "puhfessuh"
Appalachian English	
Addition of "t"	"once" → "oncet"
Addition of initial "h"	"it" → "hit"
Addition of vowel within clusters	"black" → "buhlack"
Portugese, Italian, Spanish	
Final consonant deletion	"but" → "buh"; "house" → "hou"
Cantonese	
Confusion of /i/ and /ɪ/	"heat" → "hit"; "leave" → "live"; "hit" → "heat"; "live" → "leave"
Spanish	
Confusion of /d/ and /ð/	"they" → "day"
Devoicing of "z"	"lies" → "lice"
Affrication of /ʃ/	"shoe" → "chew"

Sources: Adapted from Iglesias and Goldstein (1998) and Yavas and Goldstein (1998).

lish expression and comprehension. However, once a person is teenaged and beyond, the articulatory patterns of a first language are often firmly established and are difficult to entirely eliminate. The goal, then, is not to make a nonnative speaker sound like a native, but rather to improve intelligibility and thereby the person's communicative effectiveness. Many individuals are not inclined to rid their American speech of its foreign language influence.

What regional or foreign dialect patterns have you heard in the media? Do you think certain variations occur more often than others? If so, why might this be?

ASSESSMENT

Disorders of articulation and phonology sometimes, but not always, co-occur with other communication impairments.

No matter what the cause of the speech sound disorder, assessment should be comprehensive. The standard procedures described in Chapter 5, "Assessment and Intervention," including written case history report, interview, hearing screening, and oral peripheral examination, are important when articulation and phonology appear to be disordered. Specific formal and informal measures are essential in obtaining a complete picture of the speech of an individual with articulatory and phonological deficits.

The goals of phonological assessment parallel those for any communication disorder and have been described as follows:

- To describe an individual's phonological status
- To identify the differences between the client's articulatory patterns and nondisordered speech
- To determine the communicative implications of the client's phonology
- To assess the client's pronunciation patterns from a developmental viewpoint
- To identify factors that may relate to the etiology and maintenance of the phonological disability
- To plan treatment when appropriate
- To make a prognosis without and with treatment
- To monitor change over time (Bankson & Bernthal, 1998b; Grunwell, 1985)

These objectives may be achieved by assessment that results in a description of phonological status including the following:

- A speech sound inventory
- Characterization of syllable and word structure
- Listing of phonemic errors
- Phonological process analysis when warranted
- An evaluation of intelligibility

From the data reported in the description, the SLP will identify differences in the client's speech that warrant attention based on interference with communication, developmental information, and other factors. The SLP also will have baseline data from which to measure change over time with or without intervention. The case history, interview, hearing screening, and oral peripheral examination may provide insight into the etiology of the disorder. Predictions for improvement are based on the foregoing and on measures of consistency, stimulability, and error sound discrimination. Typical assessment procedures are briefly described and explained in the following sections.

DESCRIPTION OF PHONOLOGICAL STATUS

The speech-language pathologist should obtain data on several aspects of speech that relate to articulatory performance. Samples of three children with phonological impairments are presented on the accompanying CD-ROM.

SPEECH SOUND INVENTORY

A speech sound inventory and description of word and syllable shapes are highly appropriate for children who are at a very early stage of development and for others whose speech is markedly unintelligible. A recommended system for listing phonemes is by manner of production and syllable and word position (Grunwell, 1987; Klein, 1997). Table 10.9 on page 332 shows a speech sound inventory for Pablo, a 4-year-old boy who is receiving speech and language therapy.

SYLLABLE AND WORD STRUCTURE

A listing of the consonant-vowel (CV) patterns that have been produced in words suggests their complexity. The SLP might list the word and syllable shapes that are most characteristic of the client's speech as well as the reductions or simplifications that have occurred. Table 10.10 on page 333 provides a list of the words in Pablo's language sample in both standard orthography and phonetic transcription.

PHONEMIC ERROR INVENTORY

In all cases, the SLP needs to make a list of the phonemes that the client misarticulates. This list is typically compiled on the basis of formal testing of sounds in words. The *Goldman-Fristoe Test of Articulation-2* (GFTA-2) (Goldman & Fristoe, 2000) and the *Photo Articulation Test–3* (Lippke, Dickey, Selmar, & Soder, 1997) are two commonly used published tests. Phoneme errors are reported as **substitutions, omissions, distortions,** and **additions** in the syllable/word initial or final position. For example, if 8-year-old Amanda pronounced "lemon" as "wemon," the SLP might record

> w/l (I) [meaning "w" was substituted for "l" in the initial position; i.e., at the beginning of a word]

If a client has only one or two speech sound errors and all other phonemes are correctly produced, a statement to that effect is sufficient. A listing of all the correct phonemes is not needed.

TABLE 10.9

Phonemes produced in various word positions by Pablo, age 4 years

Manner of Production	Syllable Initial Word Initial	Syllable Initial Word Within	Syllable Final Word Within	Syllable Final Word Final
Nasals	/m/ /n/ "more," "no"	/n/ "nana"	/m/ "Sam-uel"	/m/ "drum"
Stops	/p/ /b/ /t/ /d/ "put," "ball," "top," "drum"	/p/ /b/ /d/ "happy," "Toby," "lady"		
Fricatives	/h/ /f/ /s/ "house," "face," "see"	/f/ "coffee"		
Glides	/w/ /j/ "wet," "you"	/j/ "yo-yo"		

Note: Words were taken from spontaneous language sample. Words in quotes are exemplars of produced phoneme in given word position. Accuracy of articulation of the entire word is not suggested.

Errors are compared with norms for the individual's age. A sample of an administration of the GFTA-2 is presented on the accompanying CD-ROM.

T H O U G H T   Q U E S T I O N

Go back to Chapter 4 to determine whether Amanda's substitution is typical for her age. At what age do most children correctly produce the /l/ phoneme in all positions of words?

PHONOLOGICAL PROCESS ANALYSIS

Many research studies have shown that targeting a process rather than an individual phoneme has the advantage of encouraging generalization of learning to similar phonemes and phonological contexts (Gierut, 1998). Therefore, if an individual has numerous errors, it is helpful to identify which phonological processes are apparent. The ten most common processes are shown in Chapter 4, Table 4.3. They are assimilation, fronting, final consonant deletion, weak syllable deletion, stopping, glid-

TABLE 10.10

Words in Pablo's language sample in standard orthography and phonetic transcription

"more" → [mɔə]	"happy" → [hæpi]	"baseball" → [bebɔ]
"no" → [no]	"Toby" → [tobi]	"ice cream" → [aɪtim]
"banana" → [nænə]	"lady" → [ledi]	"face" → [fe]
"Samuel" → [sæmu]	"house" → [hau]	"wet" → [wɛ]
"put" → [pʊ]	"face" → [fe]	"you" → [ju]
"ball" → [bɔ]	"see" → [si]	"yoyo" → [jojo]
"top" → [tɑl]	"shoe" → [su]	"light" → [jaɪ]
"drum" → [dʌm]	"coffee" → [tɔfi]	"balloon" → [bʌju]

The word shapes produced include CV ([no]), CVCV ([jojo]), CVC ([dʌm]), and VCVC ([aɪtim])

The word shapes that were reduced are

CVC → CV	("put" → [pʊ])
CVCVCV → CVCV	("banana" → [nænə])
CVCCVC → CVCV	"baseball" → [bebɔ])
VCCCVC → VCVC	("ice cream" → [aɪtim])

ing, cluster simplification, deaffrication, and vocalization. Phonological process information may be analyzed by the SLP on the basis of transcriptions of the child's conversational or single word utterances. Often SLPs will use a published test such as the *Khan-Lewis Phonological Analysis-2* (Khan & Lewis, 2002), which analyzes phonological processes on the basis of the findings of the *Goldman-Fristoe Test of Articulation-2* (Goldman & Fristoe, 2000). Other published tests for determining phonological processes include the *Assessment of Phonological Processes—Revised* (Hodson, 1986) and the *Bankson-Bernthal Test of Phonology* (Bankson & Bernthal, 1990). One version of the *Comprehensive Test of Phonological Processing* addresses the needs of older individuals ages 7 through 24 years (Wagner, Torgesen, & Rashotte, 1999).

Phonological processes may be analyzed by using a computerized program. These systems often save the SLP time and provide more detailed information than hand-scored procedures. Examples of computerized phonological analysis programs include *Diagnostic Report Writer 2000* (Weiner, 2000) and *Macintosh Interactive System for Phonological Analysis* (Mac-ISPA; Masterson & Pagan, 1993). The

While computer analysis of phonological processes might save time, once the program is learned, the SLP must still understand the nature of the processes to effectively work with the client.

Assessment of Phonological Processes noted in the previous paragraph is also available in a computerized version called *Computerized Analysis of Phonological Processes* (Hodson, 1985).

In the case of Amanda above, if her only phoneme error was /l/ → /w/ (I), this would not be indicative of a phonological process; it is a *single* phonemic substitution. However, if Amanda produced /l/ → /w/ (I,M) and /r/ → /w/ (I,M), this *pattern* could be described as the phonological process gliding of liquids, since /l/ and /r/ are liquids and they were said as the glide /w/.

T H O U G H T   Q U E S T I O N

Why was final position not included in the examples of Amanda's use of /w/ for /l/ and /r/?

INTELLIGIBILITY

Speech **intelligibility** refers to how easy it is to understand the individual. Poor intelligibility has a negative impact on communicative effectiveness. Intelligibility depends on such articulatory factors as the number, type, and consistency of speech sound errors. The person's voice, fluency, rate, rhythm, language, and use of gesture also contribute to ease of comprehension, and these should be noted. Other factors, such as the listener's hearing acuity, familiarity with the speaker, and experience listening to disordered speech, also influence ease of deciphering what was said. In addition, environmental noise, the complexity of the message, and environmental cues play a role in overall intelligibility. Often, a listener does not need to understand each word, as intelligibility and the message may be inferred from a few words and situational comprehension. Table 10.11 illustrates a commonly used subjective way of reporting intelligibility.

TABLE 10.11

Subjective descriptors of intelligibility

1. Readily intelligible even when the context is not known
2. Intelligible with careful listening when the context is not known
3. Intelligible with careful listening when the context is known
4. Unintelligible with careful listening even when the context is known

A more objective measure of intelligibility is percentage of intelligible words. If speech is exceedingly poor, intelligibility may be measured in terms of syllables or consonants (Strand & McCauley, 1997). A tape-recorded sample of continuous speech is transcribed, and the symbol # may replace each word that is not understood. The percentage of intelligible words is then computed:

$$\text{Percentage of Intelligible Words} = \frac{\text{Number of Intelligible Words}}{\text{Total Number of Words}} \times 100$$

The percentage of intelligible syllables or consonants is computed in the same way, using those units rather than words. These measures are becoming increasingly common in research and clinical use (Shriberg, Austin, Lewis, McSweeney, & Wilson, 1997). On the *Children's Speech Intelligibility Measure* (CSIM), a published test designed for children between the ages of 3 and 10, intelligibility is determined from a taped sample of a child repeating 50 stimulus words that are modeled by an examiner (Wilcox & Morris, 1999).

In general, highly unintelligible speech signals a severe disorder, while readily intelligible speech suggests that the disorder may be mild. Severity is also based on expectations for a child's age and the presence of additional communication impairments.

PROGNOSTIC INDICATORS

The detailed description of the client's speech will provide some insights into the likelihood of improvement without and with therapy. For example, if the speech sound errors and phonological processes that the client exhibits are expected for a person of that age, it is probable that they will self-correct with maturation. In addition, background information on family models and support, illnesses, ear infections, and the like may help the SLP to predict the client's improvement. Prognosis may also be determined by the consistency of the phoneme errors, the stimulability of the client, and possibly the individual's ability to discriminate error sounds from target phonemes.

CONSISTENCY

Think about your own speech. If you are reading aloud in front of a class, you are likely to be very careful in how you produce all the sounds of the words. On the other hand, when you are speaking casually to a friend, your articulation is probably far less precise. Inconsistency is normal, and it may be a clue to the exact nature of an articulation or phonological error. Let's go back to Amanda. If her misarticulation of /l/ occurs only when she is in conversational speech and then only at the beginning of words, her speech sound error may be more amenable

Intuition suggests that the easier it is for a person to produce a target phoneme, the more likely it is that the individual will make rapid progress. However, researchers have found that improvement in nontargeted phonemes, in addition to those that are taught, is often made when the targets are relatively difficult.

to change than it would be if it were present both initially and medially and when she was just saying a list of words containing /l/. Lack of consistency is considered a positive prognostic indicator. However, an individual with consistent errors may be easier to understand than someone whose error pattern is inconsistent. Consistency of phoneme errors is achieved by evaluating the client's speech during more than one task and in more than one word position and phonemic context (Bernhardt & Holdgrafer, 2001).

STIMULABILITY

Assessment should always include trial therapy. **Stimulability** is the ability of an individual to produce the target phoneme when given focused auditory and visual cues. Typically, the SLP will say, "Look at me. Listen to me. Now say exactly what I say: _____ ." The SLP will first prompt correct production of the error phoneme or pattern within the word in which it had been misarticulated. If the client does not correctly imitate the SLP, the prompt is moved to the syllable or phoneme level. For example, the SLP would have Amanda watch the SLP's face and listen carefully as he or she said "lemon." If Amanda correctly produced the word, she would be stimulable for /l/ in words. If she did not correctly imitate the SLP but correctly followed the model for /l/ in the nonsense syllables /la/, /lo/, /li/, Amanda would be stimulable at the syllable level. Stimulability is often a positive prognostic indicator; however, research studies suggest a more complex relationship. Children who are stimulable may respond more quickly to correction of the target phoneme and may also be more likely to self-correct without therapy than those who are not stimulable. Those sounds for which a child is not stimulable are highly unlikely to change without treatment. On the other hand, among children in therapy, those with low stimulability scores often make more progress, especially with untreated sounds, than do those who are more stimulable. Stimulability training may be provided as part of therapy (Powell & Miccio, 1996).

ERROR SOUND DISCRIMINATION

It is possible that a child does not perceive the difference in his or her speech. This would be a weakness in **external error sound discrimination.** A fairly common exchange between a parent and five-year-old child goes something like this:

Child: Oh, I see a wabbit

Parent (exaggerating the /r/): You see a rabbit!

Child: Yeah, I see a wabbit!

Parent: Say "er."

Child: "er."

Parent: say "er abbit."
Child: "er wabbit."

While the above dialogue is an example of a parent trying to stimulate the child to correctly produce a word, it may also probe whether a child hears the difference between the parent's and the child's utterances.

T H O U G H T   Q U E S T I O N S

Do you think the child can discriminate between his or her production of the word "rabbit" and the parental model? Why? What other explanations could account for the differences?

Error sound discrimination is often assessed both externally and internally. External discrimination, or **interpersonal error sound discrimination,** refers to the ability to perceive differences in another person's speech. For example, in external discrimination, the SLP might ask the client, "Are these the same or different: 'wemon'—'lemon'?" Sometimes two real words are contrasted, and the client is asked to point to pictures that can be labeled using either the targeted phoneme or the one that was substituted; for example, shown two pictures, the client is told "Point to awake. Now point to a lake." **Internal error sound discrimination,** sometimes termed **intrapersonal error sound discrimination,** is the ability to judge one's own ongoing speech. The client may be asked to judge the accuracy of her or his phoneme productions while self-monitoring with the use of headphones.

Much has been written about the relationship of speech sound discrimination to articulation and phonology, but its nature remains unclear.

A multimodality approach is often helpful in teaching speech sounds.

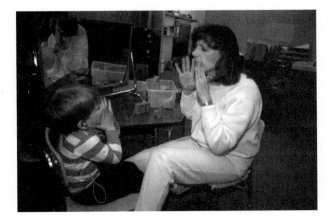

Do individuals have to be able to "hear" the difference between correct and incorrect productions of a phoneme to correctly say a given sound? While not universally true, perception of a contrast such as /r/ or /l/ and /w/ usually precedes production in children who are developing typically (Strange & Broen, 1980). In addition, children who are better at internal discrimination have been reported to have more correct articulations (Lapko & Bankson, 1975). From this, we might conclude that error sound discrimination ability signals a more favorable prognosis than the absence of this ability. Two warnings about phoneme discrimination testing are warranted: (1) Only the error phonemes appear to relate to therapeutic prognosis, so only these should be routinely assessed. (2) Many young children do not understand the concept of same versus different; therefore, their error sound discrimination is difficult to judge.

INTERVENTION

Parents may be enlisted to reinforce therapy under the guidance of a speech-language pathologist. Carefully structured homework assignments can provide a client with additional beneficial practice.

If the results of the assessment suggest that treatment is appropriate, the SLP must determine how to proceed. Initial questions to be answered include the following:

- Where will therapy occur? (Clinic, center, school, or home setting?)
- How frequently will the client be seen? (Once or twice a week or three, four, or five times weekly?)
- How long will the sessions be? (Twenty to sixty minutes is the typical range.)
- Will therapy be individual, group, or within a classroom?

Answers to these questions will be related to the facilities that are available as well as to the needs of the child. In addition to such administrative type decisions, the SLP must determine the following:

- What should be the therapy targets?
- What treatment approach appears most suitable?

As described in Chapter 5, "Assessment and Intervention," therapy and evaluation are cyclical; adjustments in intervention will be made on the basis of ongoing assessment.

T H O U G H T   Q U E S T I O N

What might be some relative advantages and disadvantages of different therapy settings and schedules?

TARGET SELECTION

The major goal of therapy should be to make the client easier to understand, that is, to improve his or her intelligibility in a way that will have a positive impact on the person's life. For example, if a client named Larry consistently says /wæwi/ when asked what his name is, correction of /l/ and /r/ (phonological process gliding of liquids) is likely of major importance and should be targeted early. Important to intelligibility is also the frequency of a particular misarticulated phoneme within the language: For example, /ʒ/, as in "treasure" ([trɛʒɚ]), does not occur in many American English words, so it would not normally warrant early attention. On the other hand, targets that may generalize to correction of phonological processes would be extremely helpful in improving intelligibility. If a child exhibits the process stopping of fricatives, as in saying "see" as [ti] and "five" as [paɪb], intervention for correct production of /s/ may generalize to other fricatives, including /f/ and /v/.

A second factor in target selection is likelihood of success. The SLP might initially choose targets that the client will probably master relatively quickly. The best predictors of ease of mastery are stimulability and inconsistency. If the client can produce the target phonemes when prompted to imitate with increased visual and auditory stimulation, this is a favorable sign. In addition, if the client does not misarticulate a particular target in all words or situations, this demonstrates that successful intervention is likely (Edwards, 1983).

Some current research studies have demonstrated that greater generalization to nontarget phonemes occurs when the targets are more difficult for the child—that is, not stimulable, consistent, later developing, and more phonetically complex (Gierut, 1998). It is up to the SLP to determine whether early success on a few targets or more long-term progress on multiple phonemes is best for the individual client.

INTERVENTION APPROACHES

A variety of therapy approaches and techniques exist. The SLP might target one phoneme at a time, work with phonological processes, emphasize motor movements, or focus on the nonsegmental aspects of speech such as rate, rhythm, and melody. Most SLPs will adjust their approach to suit each client and combine procedures to provide individually tailored therapy. In the next few sections, we provide highlights of just a few of the well-known therapy approaches.

SINGLE PHONEME TARGETS

A single phoneme target approach may be valuable for individuals who have a limited number of phoneme errors and who do not have significant neuromotor impairment. This approach consists of four stages, each one following the previous or overlapping (Van Riper & Erickson, 1996).

Perceptual or **ear training** is normally the first stage. It in turn contains four steps:

1. Identification of a target sound
2. Location of target sound
3. Stimulation
4. Discrimination

First, the client is made aware of the target phoneme. If the target is /s/, it might be called the "snake sound," and a picture might be used to highlight this association. Second, the client might first signal every time she or he hears the target. Soon the client might specify whether the target phoneme occurred at the beginning, middle, or end of a presented word. Third, the SLP stimulates the client by reading sentences that contain multiple examples of the target. For example, if the target is /f/, the SLP might say "Find the funny fox." Naturally, for children, these utterances would be accompanied by appropriate activities. Fourth, ear training culminates with the client learning to discriminate correct from incorrect productions.

Production training refers to teaching the client to say the target phoneme first in isolation, then in syllables, words, phrases, and sentences. Exercises, drills, and games are used to provide opportunities for learning and practice in progressively more difficult utterances. At the phrase level, carrier phrases are often used. For example, if the target is /f/, the client may be instructed to say "I found X," X being a variety of items beginning with /f/, such as "five," "fork," "foot," and "finger." Phonemic contexts are also varied so that the client practices the target in all positions of words and in all combinations.

Stabilization involves activities that will reinforce and review the learned target. Many different activities will be used to ensure stabilization. Structured conversations will give way to more spontaneous situations always with the goal of correct production of the previously misproduced phonemes. The client will be expected to engage in self-monitoring and self-correction of errors.

Finally, the client needs to transfer or **carry over** correct production into everyday conversation. Most SLPs encourage their clients to use what they have learned in conversation outside of the clinical setting as early as feasible. Homework assignments and activities that are naturalistic are used to ensure that what was accomplished clinically becomes automatic and habitual. In doing this, it is important that adequate guidance is provided to parents, teachers, or others who are to assist in carryover.

What should parents, caregivers, teachers, and others know to effectively assist in carryover? Can you think of a situation in which an untrained person might do more harm than good?

STIMULABILITY TRAINING

Since the ability to imitate sounds is an important predictor of success in producing these sounds spontaneously, some SLPs work to enhance the stimulability of their clients. This is particularly useful for children who have few phonemes in their repertoire and are not stimulable for many sounds. In working with preschoolers, one method uses stimulus characters and associated gestures in playlike activities. For example, to teach the child to imitate /s/, the clinician would present a picture of a "silly snake" and slinkily move a finger up his or her arm, while modeling the sound and encouraging the child to repeat it. Since the clinician wants to avoid frustrating the child by only presenting sounds that the child is unable to produce, stimulable sounds are also included in the sessions (Miccio & Elbert, 1996).

PHONOLOGICAL PROCESS TARGETS

Children who have multiple phonemic errors and are highly unintelligible may benefit from phonologically based treatment that focuses on phonological processes, rather than individual phonemes as the primary targets. In the **cycles approach,** the basis for choosing targets is the ease with which the client is likely to master them (Hodson & Paden, 1991). The first target would be the pattern for which the child is most *stimulable.*

When a youngster has multiple phonemic errors, these generally can be described as phonological processes. It is more efficient to target a process than to attempt to correct one phoneme at a time.

Each session in the cycles approach follows a particular structure. First, the previous session's target words are reviewed. Then the child listens to about twelve words containing the target pattern, which are presented with slight amplification (**auditory bombardment**). The child is asked to say three to five production practice words that contain the target in a carefully selected phonemic context. These words are then used in carefully planned play activities. Some conversation is introduced each session so that the SLP can observe whether targets are being generalized to spontaneous speech. Possible targets for the next session are probed, and the most stimulable target is selected for the next session. Auditory bombardment is repeated, and the list of words is given to the parent or caregiver to read aloud to the child for about two minutes each day.

The **metaphon** approach is also based on phonological processes. The special contribution of this approach is incorporation of the child's active cognitive participation in remediation of the disorder. For therapy to be effective, metaphon theorists state that the client must be aware that his or her articulatory production is inappropriate, want to modify it, know the relevant articulatory targets, and have the neuromotor capability of accurately producing the targets with adequate speed in a variety of phonetic contexts (Hewlett, 1990).

Metaphon therapy is divided into two basic phases. In Phase One, the client develops phonological awareness. The goal is to make the client interested in the sound system of the language and prepared to learn about how sounds are produced and how they differ from one another. During Phase Two, the client transfers the knowledge acquired in Phase One to communicative situations and learns to self-monitor and modify output to improve message transmission. The concept of minimal pairs (described later in this chapter) is a useful tool in metaphon and other therapy (Howell & Dean, 1994).

ARTICULATORY TRAINING

Both single-phoneme and phonological process approaches depend heavily on auditory stimulation and the ability to hear and then reproduce target speech sounds. Some individuals for various reasons are unable to imitate what they've heard even when they understand the objective. Consider, for example, that you are learning to speak Mandarin Chinese, a language that uses melodic patterns or tones to communicate word meaning. In Mandarin Chinese, the English words "cat" and "hair" are both pronounced "mao"; however, to say "cat," you must use the melodic pattern known as the first tone, and to say "hair," you must use the second tone. Although you "hear" what is said to you and you understand what is required, you may have difficulty correctly imitating and differentiating between these two words. You simply cannot get your vocal mechanism to act the way it must to say the Chinese words.

Articulatory techniques focus on the neuromotor processes needed in phoneme production. We will briefly describe two approaches that are sometimes used particularly with children who do not respond easily to auditory stimulation. These approaches are sensory-motor and oral-motor.

In **sensory-motor training** the client is made aware of the tactile and proprioceptive sensations associated with the production of sounds in syllables and words. The client is asked to imitate targets and then describe, for example, where the tongue is placed, where air can be felt, and so on. The focus is not on the individual phoneme but on overlapping movements that occur in connected speech (McDonald, 1964).

Oral-motor training goes beyond the mouth and provides suggestions for appropriate body posture and breathing for speech. Six principles of oral-motor dynamics have been suggested (Boshart, 1998):

1. Motor development is continuous, sequential, and cumulative. We move from generalized movements and reflexes to more precise voluntary oral gestures. If this process is interrupted for any reason, later speech sound production may be impaired.

2. Correct speech sound production depends on the correct oral-facial resting posture. The lips are closed, the tongue is up, and the jaw is gently relaxed. This is essential for stabilization from which movement is possible.

3. Speech requires adequate muscle strength, tone, and endurance. Although it likely seems easy to you, consider the muscular strength required to bring your tongue tip from a resting position up to the alveolar ridge to say /t/. Tone refers to the muscle's state of readiness to act, and endurance means that the movement can be held and/or repeated many times.

4. Tactile and proprioceptive feedback permit the speaker to self-monitor. Remember the last time you were at the dentist and received novocaine? Your sense of touch (tactile) and position (proprioception) within your mouth were impaired. You probably had difficulty speaking normally. Speakers constantly make tiny adjustments based on how things feel as well as how they sound (auditory feedback).

5. Stability is critical to movement. Try to say the word "temperature" while moving your jaw from side to side. You will find it difficult. Speakers learn to isolate one part of the oral mechanism while holding everything else stable. For example, if the tongue is not resting at the bottom of the mouth in a stable position when you say the /l/ phoneme in "listen," the /l/ might sound more like [gl], a distortion of the target.

6. Speech requires well-coordinated, subtle movements. The lips must be able to move independently of the jaw. Movement of the tongue tip must be isolated from that of the back of the tongue.

Specific exercises are recommended for accomplishing each of these principles. In essence, the SLP prepares the client motorically before actually teaching speech sounds. The oral-motor principles identified above relate broadly to speech production. Diminishment of oral apraxia without relating this to speech motor control may do nothing to improve speech movements (Hall et al., 1993).

MINIMAL PAIRS

Minimal pair contrasts are used in many types of articulation and phonological therapy. Two words are presented that are the same with the exception of a single phoneme, for example, boy/toy, chip/ship, or fine/pine. At least three types of contrasts are possible: error phoneme/target phoneme, **minimal contrast,** and **maximal contrast** or **maximal opposition.**

In error phoneme/target phoneme minimal pairs, the SLP attempts to reproduce the target as normally said by the client and contrast this with a correct production. For example, if the client typically pronounced "chair" as "share," the SLP might begin by presenting both utterances and asking the client whether they are the same or different. From there, the SLP may have the client point to pictures representing each member of the pair. Additional exercises include using both words in sentences and asking the client whether the sentences make sense or not—for example, "He sat on the share." Production exercises follow, in which the client is expected to produce the minimal pair in designated contexts.

In minimal contrasts, the phonemes that are contrasted differ in a single distinctive feature. Actually, the example above of error phoneme contrast is also a minimal contrast. An additional example of a minimal contrast would be "Sue" and "zoo." The "s" and "z" differ only in that the "s" is voiceless and the "z" is voiced.

Maximal contrasts, sometimes called maximal opposition, pair two phonemes that differ in more than one distinctive feature. For example, in the words "man" and "fan," "m" and "f" differ in manner of production, voicing, and nasality. Maximal contrasts are sometimes used earlier in therapy, since they might be easier for a client to differentiate. In addition, maximal contrast training may lead to modification of error phonemes beyond that which is immediately targeted (Gierut, 1989).

When minimal pair contrasts are used in the metaphon approach, the client is asked how he or she knows whether the utterance and picture match (or whether the sentence makes sense). Focus of discussion is always on the communicative success of the transaction rather than on the "correctness" of the articulation. When the client is asked to name pictures, the clinician responds on the basis of what is said, whether or not it is what the client intended (Howell & Dean, 1994).

However minimal pairs are used, they are a valuable tool in the remediation of articulation and phonology (Bauman-Waengler, 2000).

COMPUTER APPLICATIONS

Computer programs are available that can be used as an adjunct to intervention by the SLP. These programs provide exercises in both perception of phonemic targets and production. They are helpful in providing immediate feedback on the client's performance. School-age children with few phonemic errors often respond especially well to drills that are presented in computer game format. Computer exercises provide an opportunity for independent practice as well as for variety within a therapy session. It is up to the SLP to ensure that mastery goes beyond simple exercises and that improvement is reflected in conversational speech (Gierut, 1998).

COMBINATION

Most speech-language pathologists use a combination of approaches and select features of each that are appropriate to the needs of the particular client. Table 10.12 outlines the basic steps of intervention.

GENERALIZATION AND MAINTENANCE

Once the client has achieved an acceptable level of correct phoneme production, the SLP must ensure that slippage does not occur and that the new speech pattern becomes habitual. Many SLPs introduce self-monitoring exercises from the very beginning of therapy. In this way, clients understand that they are ultimately responsible for their own success. Once the SLP believes that the client is ready for dismissal from therapy, follow-up sessions may be scheduled at progressively longer intervals. If the progress has been maintained over time, the remediation has been effective.

Success of therapy is determined by the application of what has been learned in a clinical setting to everyday life.

TABLE 10.12

A basic progression in phonemic therapy

1. Prepare the client for correct phoneme production.
   a. Auditory, visual, and oral-motor training are applied as necessary.
   b. Listening exercises and oral-motor drills may be used.
2. Facilitate target production in a minimally complex context.
   a. Auditory, visual, and oral-motor training provide techniques for correct productions.
   b. Isolated phonemes and processes may be targeted.
3. Increase the level of complexity as the client is ready.
   a. Target words become longer and more phonologically challenging.
   b. Target words are embedded in phrases and sentences.
4. Encourage self-monitoring, self-correction, and generalization.
   a. The client is challenged to take responsibility for correct productions.
   b. Situations for using targeted phonemes are extended to conversations and different communicative partners and settings.

SUMMARY

Producing the sounds of a language during speech is a complex process. It involves an inner conceptualization of phonemes and phonotactic rules so that in our "mind's ear" we know how the language we are speaking should sound. Speech production also requires the neuromotor ability to move our articulators to form the desired sounds in a smooth, rapid, and automatic fashion. As children develop spoken language, they typically employ phonological processes that simplify adult forms. If these persist beyond the expected ages, they may present difficulties. Hearing disorders, neurological impairments, and organic abnormalities may contribute to phonological and articulatory disorders. Foreign language background and regional dialects contribute to variations in speech. Assessment of articulation and phonology includes a detailed description of the individual's phonological output, as well as investigation of etiology and determination of prognosis. Intervention strategies may include ear training, oral-motor facilitation, and production enhancement techniques. The general goal is improved intelligibility in spontaneous speech.

REFLECTIONS

- What systems are used for classifying speech sounds? Why is it important to do this?
- What disorders are associated with articulatory and phonological impairments?
- Identify the steps in the assessment of articulation and phonology.
- What factors are considered in selecting targets for articulatory and phonological improvement?
- How do speech-language pathologists modify articulatory and phonological production?
- What is the major goal of articulatory and phonological intervention?

SUGGESTED READINGS

Ball, M. J., & Kent, R. D. (1997). *The new phonologies: Developments in clinical linguistics.* San Diego, CA: Singular.

Baumann-Waengler, J. (2000). *Articulatory and phonological impairments: A clinical focus.* Boston: Allyn and Bacon.

Bernthal, J. E., & Bankson, N. W. (1998). *Articulation and phonological disorders* (4th ed.). Boston: Allyn and Bacon.

Crary, M. A. (1993). *Developmental motor speech disorders.* San Diego, CA: Singular.

Grunwell, P. (1985). *PACS: Phonological assessment of child speech.* San Diego, CA: College-Hill.

Hodson, B., & Paden, E. (1991) *Targeting intelligible speech: A phonological approach to remediation* (2nd ed.). Austin, TX: Pro-Ed.

ON-LINE RESOURCES

http://www.americandialect.org/   Home page of the American Dialect Society.

Dedicated to the study of the English language in North America and its relationship to other languages. Highlights related news such as recent books and conferences on language.

http://www.tandf.co.uk/journals/ft/02699206.html   *Clinical Linguistics & Phonetics.*

The tables of contents of recent issues are available on-line. Articles are featured on such topics as phonetic disorders of speech, clinical dialectology, phonetics of hearing impairment, and disordered communication in multicultural settings. If you sign up, you also can view a free sample issue.

http://www.arts.gla.ac.uk/IPA/   The International Phonetic Association.

Web site contains the latest version of IPA, phonetic fonts for word-processing, and information about the International Congress of Phonetic Sciences and the *Journal of the International Phonetic Association.*

http://www.ling.upenn.edu/phono_atlas/NationalMap/NationalMap.html   A national map of the regional dialects of American English.

A phonological atlas showing the major dialect regions of the United States and linguistic features that characterize the areas.

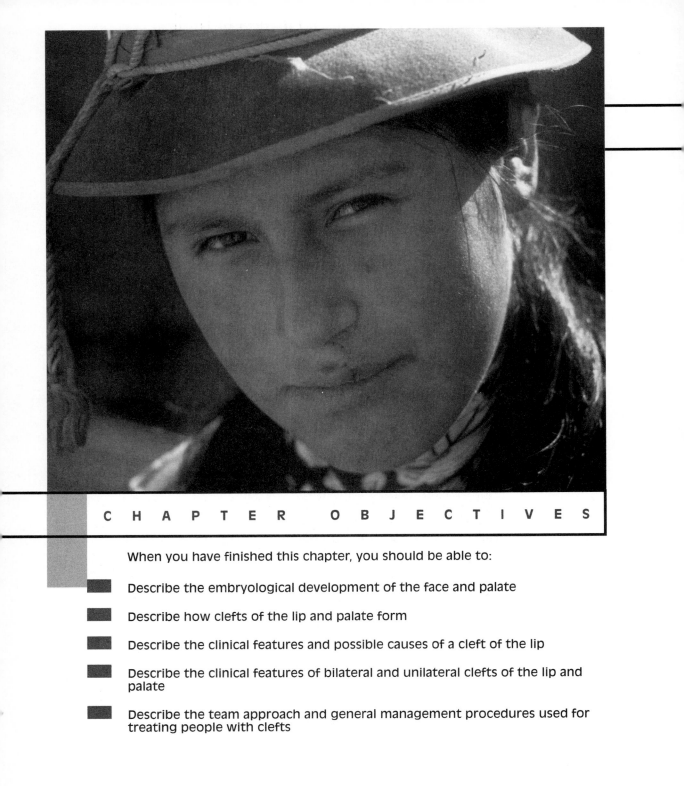

C H A P T E R   O B J E C T I V E S

When you have finished this chapter, you should be able to:

Describe the embryological development of the face and palate

Describe how clefts of the lip and palate form

Describe the clinical features and possible causes of a cleft of the lip

Describe the clinical features of bilateral and unilateral clefts of the lip and palate

Describe the team approach and general management procedures used for treating people with clefts

11

Cleft Lip and Cleft Palate

In Chapter 3, you learned that the roof of your mouth is called the palate. The anterior two thirds of the palate is the hard palate, which is composed of bony plates that are fused along their midline. If you run the tip of your tongue along the roof of your mouth in a front-to-back direction, you will trace roughly the fusion line of your hard palate. The hard palate is stationary and serves to separate the anterior aspects of the oral and nasal cavities. **Mucosal tissue,** pinkish-colored tissue lining the inside of the mouth, covers the hard palate.

The soft palate, called the *velum*, constitutes the posterior one-third of the palate and is composed of muscle and mucosal tissue. The velum and muscles in the back of the throat, or **pharynx**, constitute the **velopharyngeal mechanism.** This mechanism acts like a valve; it can be open, allowing a coupling between the oral and nasal cavities, or it can be closed, partitioning the oral and nasal cavities. For example, when you breathe through your nose, the soft palate hangs like a curtain coupling the nasal and oral cavities. Air passes through the nose into the pharynx, trachea, and lungs.

Put your index finger under your nose and say the /p/ sound several times. You will observe that no air escapes from your nose. During production of the /p/ sound, your velopharyngeal mechanism closed, separating the oral and nasal cavities. Separation of the oral and nasal cavities is required during swallowing and for the production of most speech sounds. This separation is accomplished through muscle contraction that moves the velum in a superior (upper) and posterior direction. The **velopharyngeal portal,** or conduit connecting the oral and nasal cavities, is closed, and separation of the oral and nasal cavities is complete when the velum makes contact with the posterior and lateral aspects of the pharynx. In addition to elevation of the velum, closure of the velopharyngeal portal is assisted by active movement of the lateral walls of the pharynx.

The term **velopharyngeal competence** means that the velopharyngeal mechanism adequately closes the portal during swallowing and speech production. **Velopharyngeal incompetence (VPI)** is a term that we will be using frequently in this chapter. It means that the mechanism is incapable of separating the oral and nasal cavities during swallowing and speech production. VPI is a frequent result of palatal clefts and is associated with velar soft tissue and muscle tissue deficiencies. We will have more to say about VPI later in the chapter.

You can see a portion of your soft palate by looking into a well-illuminated bathroom mirror. You will also see a structure projecting inferiorly (downward) called the **uvula;** the uvula is the termination of your soft palate.

THOUGHT QUESTION

When you swallow, your velum elevates, separating the oral and nasal cavities. What would happen if your velum didn't close the velopharyngeal portal during swallowing?

In this chapter, we will explore **craniofacial anomalies** that are congenital malformations involving the head (*cranio:* above the upper eyelid) and face (*facial:* below the upper eyelid). There are hundreds of different craniofacial anomalies, many of which are accompanied by malformations of the upper lip, hard palate, and soft palate. Malformations of the upper lip and hard and soft palate are called **clefts.** A cleft is an abnormal opening in an anatomical structure (Shprintzen, 1995), representing a failure of structures to fuse early in embryonic development. This fusion (merging) process will be discussed later in this chapter.

Clefts may involve an entire anatomical structure, such as the entire hard palate, or only a part of it. Clefts of the lip that may involve the dental arch (**alveolus**) and the anterior aspect of the hard palate (**premaxilla**) develop between the fifth and eighth weeks of gestation. Isolated clefts of the hard and/or soft palate develop between the eight and twelfth weeks of gestation.

Clefts of the lip and palate create a condition that interferes with basic biological functions such as breathing and swallowing, and they can inhibit severely a child's development of speech and language. We will discuss some of the unique communicative problems associated with palatal clefts and the wide range of medical, dental, and behavioral treatments that children with clefts require. We will also discuss the necessity of an interdisciplinary treatment approach for people with clefts.

DEVELOPMENT OF THE FACE AND PALATE

To begin our discussion of cleft lip and palate, we will focus on the normal development of the face and the palate. A brief examination of how the face and palate are formed will shed light on the underlying nature of clefts and how they form. The **embryological period** (the third week through the eighth week of gestation) and early fetal period (the ninth week through the twelfth week)[1] are when the face and the palate are formed. The formation of cleft lip with or without cleft palate and of isolated cleft palate are well understood.

During the embryonic and fetal periods of life, humans are at a higher risk of death than at any other period of life except extreme old age. Half of all conceptions are not recognized clinically, and approximately 15 percent of clincally recognized pregnancies result in miscarriage (Peterson-Falzone & Imagire, 1997).

FACIAL DEVELOPMENT

The face and anterior aspects of the mouth are formed between the fifth and eighth weeks after conception. Normal development of the face and mouth is a result of a complex fusion among five embryonic processes: the right and left **mandibular processes,** the **frontonasal process,** and two **maxillary processes.** These processes are illustrated in Figure 11.1a.

Fusion of the right and left mandibular processes that forms the mandible and the lower lip occurs early in the development of the face, during the fourth and fifth weeks of gestation. The right and left mandibular processes grow toward one another and fuse in the midline of the face. This fusion process has been completed in the 6-week-old embryo shown in Figure 11.1a. Mandibular fusion is relatively simple when considered in light of fusion processes that occur above the mandible.

During the fifth week of gestation, the frontonasal processes grow in a downward direction, separating into two distinct tissue masses on both sides of the face called the **nasomedian processes** and the **lateral nasal**

[1]The complete fetal period extends from the ninth week of gestation to delivery of the child.

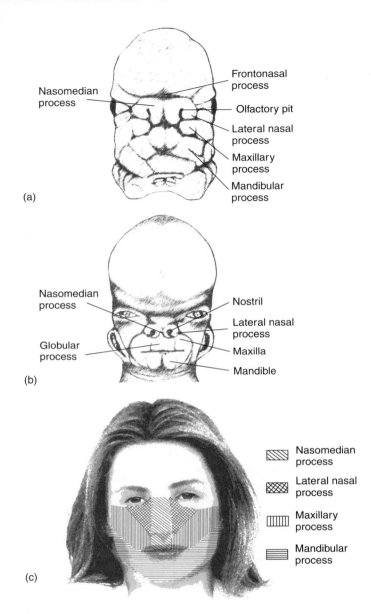

processes. Depressions between the nasomedian and lateral nasal processes called the **olfactory pits** will ultimately become the right and left nasal cavities. The lateral nasal processes fuse with the maxillary processes to form the **nasal alae** (the flared portion of the nostrils) and the anterior aspects of the face just beneath the eyes as shown in Figure 11.1b.

The nasomedian processes also fuse with the paired maxillary processes. Primitive tissue contained in the nasomedian processes will become the anterior portion of the upper lip, the anterior aspect of the alveolus (the portion of the maxilla or upper jaw that holds teeth) containing the upper frontal incisor teeth, and the anterior aspect of the hard palate, called the premaxilla. Facial development is completed during the eighth week of gestation, as shown in Figure 11.1b. Clefts of the lip that may include a cleft alveolus and premaxilla occur when the fusion process between the nasomedian and maxillary processes has been interrupted by some abnormal genetic condition or by environmental agents (e.g., certain drugs, chemicals, nicotine, irradiation) called **teratogens** that adversely affect the developing child.

FIGURE 11.1 Embryonic face at six weeks of development (a), embryonic face at eight weeks of development (b), adult face illustrating fusion of embryonic processes (c)

Given that development of the face begins around the fourth week of pregnancy, why is it important for couples planning on having a child to be as drug-free as possible?

DEVELOPMENT OF THE SECONDARY PALATE

The secondary palate includes the bony hard palate and the soft palate. Although development of the anterior aspects of the face is complete by the end of the eighth week of gestation, complete separation of the oral and nasal cavities has not yet been achieved. Between the eighth and twelfth weeks of gestation, embryonic processes that give rise to the hard and soft palate will fuse, separating the oral and nasal cavities.

Two **palatal shelves,** which are wedge-shaped tissue masses, grow downward from the inner aspects of the maxillary processes. Up to the ninth week of gestation, the tongue projects into the nasal cavity. A rapid growth spurt during the eighth and ninth weeks of gestation increases the length and width of the mandible, pulling the tongue downward and away from its position between the palatal shelves, which then begin fusing with one another in an anterior to posterior fashion. Figure 11.2 shows the general aspects of this anterior to posterior fusion process. As the palatal shelves are fusing, the nasal septum grows downward to meet the palatal shelves in the midline, separating the left and right nasal cavities.

Muscles of the soft palate also evolve from the palatal shelves. The soft palate begins forming during the tenth week of gestation, and fusion of the secondary palate is completed by the end of the twelfth week. Aberrations that prevent fusion of the palatal shelves will result in an isolated cleft of the hard and/or soft palate. As with cleft lip, genetic and nongenetic factors have been identified as causing an isolated cleft of the secondary palate. These factors will be discussed later in this chapter.

CLEFT LIP AND PALATE CLASSIFICATION SYSTEMS

Clefts vary in size and severity, and it is important clinically and for clinical research to accurately classify clefts. At present, there is no universally accepted classification system, but there are some classification systems that are widely used and are useful for clinical reference (Bzoch, 1997).

Contemporary cleft palate classification systems are based on the embryological development of the face and palatal structures.

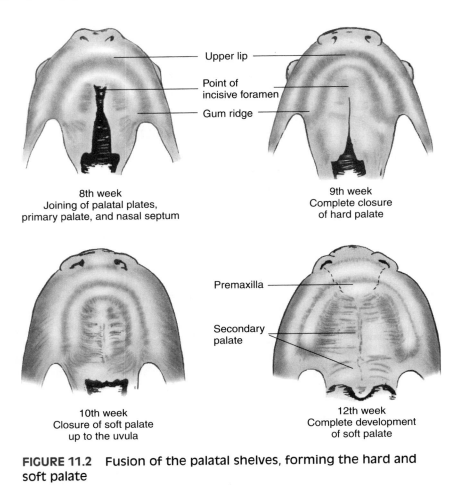

8th week
Joining of palatal plates,
primary palate, and nasal septum

9th week
Complete closure
of hard palate

10th week
Closure of soft palate
up to the uvula

12th week
Complete development
of soft palate

Upper lip

Point of
incisive foramen

Gum ridge

Premaxilla

Secondary
palate

FIGURE 11.2 Fusion of the palatal shelves, forming the hard and soft palate

A cleft lip and palate classification scheme that was developed originally in the 1930s is still in use today. The **Veau system** is useful for a quick general reference regarding the nature and extent of clefts (Bzoch, 1997). Four classes of clefts, identified by Roman numerals, comprise the Veau system. The Roman numerals and their associated descriptors are listed in Table 11.1.

More modern clinical classification systems include **Kernahan's Striped Y** and one developed by the American Cleft Palate Association (ACPA), now called the American Cleft Palate-Craniofacial Association. The ACPA recommends generally that different classification systems at least follow the principles of their system.

TABLE 11.1

The Veau cleft lip and palate classification system

Class	Descriptor
I	Cleft of the soft palate only
II	Cleft of the hard and soft palate to the incisive foramen
III	Complete unilateral cleft of the soft and hard palate and of the lip and alveolar ridge on one side
IV	Complete bilateral cleft of the soft and hard palate and/or the lip and alveolar ridge on both sides

CLINICAL FEATURES OF CLEFTS

Clefts vary greatly in type and severity, ranging from a small V-shaped notch of the lip to a complete separation of the upper lip, dental arch, and the right and left sides of the hard and soft palate. Clefts are classified commonly as: (1) unilateral or bilateral cleft of the lip, (2) unilateral cleft of the lip and palate, (3) bilateral cleft of the lip and palate, (4) submucous cleft, or (5) bifid uvula. Some of the clinical features of these clefts are discussed below.

CLEFT OF THE LIP

A cleft of the lip involves the reddish (**vermilion**) portion of the upper lip and may extend through the lip toward the nostril. For example, an **incomplete cleft** of the lip may be a minor V-shaped notch in the vermilion portion of the lip, whereas **complete cleft** of the lip continues through the upper lip into the floor of the nostril. A cleft of the lip has an adverse affect on the shape of the nose characterized by a flattening of the nose and a flaring of the nostril on the side of the cleft. Additionally, the **columella,** the strip of tissue connecting the base and tip of the nose, is short and misaligned. Clefts of the lip may be unilateral or bilateral. When the cleft lip is unilateral, it most commonly occurs on the left side. If the cleft lip is bilateral, it is generally accompanied by a cleft of the palate as well.

An isolated cleft of the lip is rare, accounting for less than 5 percent of all cleft cases (Shprintzen, 1995). Usually, clefts of the lip extend posteriorly through the alveolus. Such clefts may be minor notches

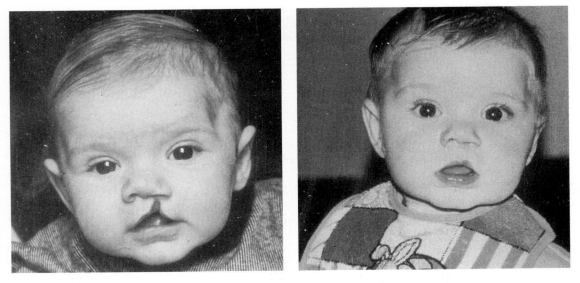

Unilateral cleft of the lip presurgery (a) and postsurgery (b). Note the "V" shaped notch in the vermilion border of the lip extending toward the left nostril and the flattening of nose and flaring of the nostril on the side of the cleft. (Photographs courtesy of Donald Warren, D.D.S., Ph.D., University of North Carolina, Chapel Hill.)

in the alveolus, or they may extend completely through the alveolus and involve the premaxilla.

UNILATERAL CLEFT OF THE LIP AND PALATE

A unilateral complete cleft of the lip and palate extends from the external portion of the upper lip, through the alveolus, and through the hard and soft palate. The nasal septum attaches to the larger of the two palatal segments.

As was discussed above, a cleft of the secondary palate alone without a cleft lip is sometimes observed. Clefts of the secondary palate alone vary in severity, involving all of the hard and soft palate or only a small portion of the hard or soft palate.

BILATERAL CLEFT OF THE LIP AND PALATE

A bilateral complete cleft of the lip and palate is the most severe type of cleft due primarily to a severe tissue deficiency. The lip and the alveolus are cleft under both nostrils and the central portion of the lip (**pro-**

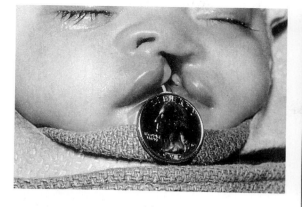

(a)

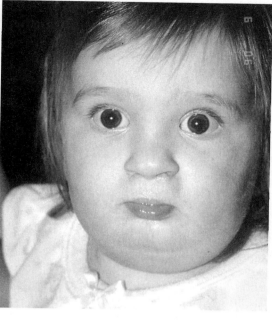

Unilateral cleft of the lip and palate presurgery (a) and postsurgery (b). Observe that this cleft extends completely through the lip into the left nostril and the alveolus is also cleft. The cleft of the hard and soft palates cannot be seen in this photograph. (Photographs courtesy of Donald Warren, D.D.S., Ph.D., University of North Carolina, Chapel Hill.)

(b)

labium), alveolus, and the premaxilla is positioned abnormally at the tip of the nasal septum as a protruding mass of tissue that is sometimes called the free-floating premaxilla (Seagle, 1997; Shprintzen, 1995). In bilateral complete clefts, the columella is usually absent, resulting in the tip of the nose attaching directly to the lip. The nasal septum is not attached to either of the palatal shelves in bilateral clefts.

THOUGHT QUESTIONS

What are your impressions of the postsurgical results of the clefts you have seen? How do you think these repaired clefts will function during speaking or eating?

SUBMUCOUS CLEFT

A submucous cleft is a muscular cleft in the region of the soft palate. The cleft is covered by a thin layer of mucosal tissue that can conceal

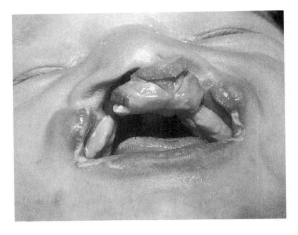

(a)

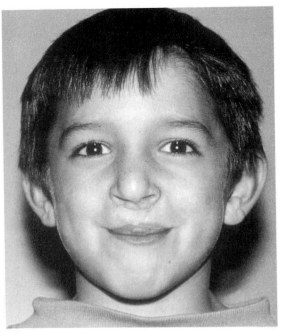

(b)

Bilateral cleft of the lip and palate presurgery (a) and postsurgery (b). Note the clefts on both sides of the face and the protruding tissue mass in the central position of the upper lip. (Photographs courtesy of Donald Warren, D.D.S., Ph.D., University of North Carolina, Chapel Hill.)

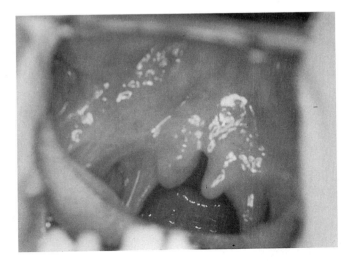

Submucous cleft. (Photograph courtesy of Donald Warren, D.D.S., Ph.D., University of North Carolina, Chapel Hill.)

the underlying lack of muscular fusion. Unlike the clefts discussed above, the submucous cleft may not be discovered until late in childhood. Physical characteristics such as a **bifid uvula** (the uvula appears to be split in half) may indicate the presence of a submucous cleft. However, a bifid uvula may be present in the absence of a submucous cleft. In fact, about one in eighty people has a bifid uvula (Bradley, 1997).

Another symptom of a submucous cleft is a bluish coloration in the middle of the soft palate where the muscles failed to fuse; this may be accompanied by a notch on the posterior border of the hard palate that can be felt. Submucous clefts may lead to velopharyngeal incompetence.

ETIOLOGIES OF CLEFTS

We have already seen that a cleft of the lip, palate, or both results from a fusion failure among primitive embryonic structures. But what causes such a fusion failure? It is generally accepted that there are four different categories of etiologies that can produce cleft lip, cleft palate or both cleft lip and cleft palate (Shprintzen & Goldberg, 1995): genetic disorders, chromosomal aberrations, teratogenically induced disorders, and mechanically induced abnormalities.

GENETIC DISORDERS

Genetic disorders account for a substantial percentage of clefting. Clefting is associated with over 400 multiple anomaly **syndromes,** or combinations of symptoms, that occur together in predictable and consistent combinations of traits.[2] Some of the major syndromes that SLPs are likely to encounter include Pierre Robin syndrome (Robin sequence), Treacher Collins syndrome, velocardiofacial syndrome, and Apert syndrome.

The primary symptoms of Pierre Robin syndrome, or, more properly, Robin sequence, include **micrognathia** (an underdeveloped mandible), a retrusion of the tongue into the pharyngeal airway, an isolated cleft of the hard and soft palate, congenital heart problems, digital anomalies, conductive hearing loss, and developmental deficits. Communication deficits are related to minimal brain dysfunction, and severely delayed language development is common (McWilliams, Morris, & Shelton, 1990). The small mandible is believed to interfere with the descent of the tongue around the eighth or ninth week of gestation. Position of the tongue between the palatal shelves prevents palatal fusion. The isolated palatal cleft is a result of the tongue's failure to descend.

Treacher Collins syndrome is characterized by **malar hypoplasia,** or an underdevelopment of the cheekbones, underdevelopment of the mandible, malformation of the external ear and the ear canal, conductive hearing loss, cleft palate, and a projection of scalp hair onto

[2]Another definition for syndromes is "A syndrome may be defined as the presence of multiple anomalies in a single individual with all those anomalies having one primary cause" (Shprintzen, 1995).

the cheek. Brain dysfunction is rare with these individuals, and the major communication problems result from conductive hearing loss and VPI.

Of special interest to the SLP is velocardiofacial syndrome because of the universality of language deficits and learning disabilities in conjunction with a palatal cleft. People with this syndrome are usually of small stature with a broad, flattened nose and have underdeveloped cheekbones and heart problems. A delayed onset of expressive language and persistent language difficulties are primary communication problems among these individuals. The cognitive behavior of individuals with velocardiofacial syndrome is concrete, and they sometimes demonstrate perseverative behaviors (Peterson-Falzone, Hardin-Jones, & Karnell, 2001).

Apert syndrome has an invariable feature called **craniosynostosis** (a premature closing of the sutures of the skull) that greatly disfigures the forehead and **syndactyly** (webbing of the fingers and toes with bone fusion). The palate is very high and narrow, giving the appearance of a cleft, but actual clefts occur in only 30 percent of people with Apert syndrome. Conductive hearing loss is frequent, and language development is commensurate with mental ability. Expressive language development is typically delayed.

Before turning our attention to chromosomal aberrations, some mention of general familial inheritance patterns associated with clefting should be made. The risk factors for having a child with a cleft are summarized in Table 11.2.

T H O U G H T   Q U E S T I O N S

Put yourself in the position of a parent under each of the conditions listed in Table 11.2. What would you decide about having another child? Would your decision be the same as that of the person sitting next to you in class?

CHROMOSOMAL ABERRATIONS

Within the nucleus of human cells are forty-six chromosomes arranged in twenty-three pairs. Abnormalities of these chromosomes are associated with a wide variety of disorders. A chromosomal aberration known as trisomy 13 results in a cleft lip with or without cleft palate in 60 to 70 percent of cases. Trisomy 13 is a rare condition resulting from the appearance of a third #13 chromosome. This condition occurs about once in 6,000 births. Like syndromes, disorders associated with chromosomal aberrations are characterized by multiple congenital abnormalities (Peterson-Falzone et al., 2001).

TABLE 11.2

Risks for cleft lip with or without cleft palate (CL [+/−] CP) and cleft palate (CP)

Situation	(CL [+/−] CP)	(CP)
Frequency of defect in the general population	0.1%	0.04%
My spouse and I are unaffected. We have an affected child. What is the probability that our next baby will have the same condition if:		
We have no affected relatives?	4%	2%
We have an affected relative?	4%	7%
We have two affected children.		
What is the probability that our next child will have the same condition?	9%	1%
I am affected or my spouse is. We have no affected children.		
What is the probability that our next child will be affected?	4%	6%
We have an affected child.		
What is the probability that our next child will be affected?	17%	15%

Source: Adapted from Grabb, Rosenstein, & Bzoch (1971).

TERATOGENICALLY INDUCED DISORDERS

Environmental teratogens are agents that interfere with or interrupt normal development of a fetus and create congenital malformations. Recognized teratogens associated with clefting include drugs such as dilantin (an anticonvulsant), thalidomide (a drug that was formerly used as a sedative), excessive use of aspirin, and retinoids (nontopical acne medication). In excessive amounts, ingestion of alcohol, nicotine, and caffeine are also considered to be teratogens responsible for clefting. In addition, X-rays, certain viruses, and some naturally occurring environmental substances have teratogenic properties. The effects of teratogens vary with an individual's unique genetic makeup, the time during pregnancy when the agent was encountered, the amount, and the mother's metabolism (Kummer, 2001; Shprintzen & Goldberg, 1995).

Thalidomide caused thousands of birth defects, including clefting, in the 1960s when the drug was administered to pregnant women. As a result, the drug was outlawed for over thirty years. In 1998, the Food and Drug Administration approved its use for the treatment of certain serious conditions such as leprosy and some cancers associated with AIDS.

MECHANICALLY INDUCED ABNORMALITIES

Mechanical factors that cause clefts are those that impinge directly on the embryo. With such clefts, the embryo is developing in a normal fashion, and the cleft is induced by something external to the embryo (Shprintzen & Goldberg, 1995). The most frequent cause of mechanically induced clefts is amniotic rupture (loss of amniotic fluid). Intrauterine crowding as when there is a twin, a uterine tumor, or an irregularly shaped uterus can also result in clefts.

INCIDENCE OF CLEFTS

Clefts occur in approximately one in every 750 live births. Clefts of the lip with or without cleft palate occur more frequently than clefts of the palate alone. Submucous clefts occur in approximately one in every 1,200 births (Peterson-Falzone et al., 2001). There are some indications that the incidence rate for clefts may be increasing because improved prenatal treatment is resulting in the birth of more high-risk fetuses. Additionally, improved postnatal treatment results in adults with clefts who look, speak, and function in a typical manner, making it more likely than it once was that they will have children of their own. Both these factors could serve to increase the size of the genetic pool that carries the cleft trait, resulting in more children being born with clefts (McWilliams et al., 1990; Peterson-Falzone et al., 2001).

GENDER AND RACIAL DIFFERENCES

Clefts of the lip with or without clefts of the palate occur about twice as frequently in males and tend to be more severe. Clefts of the palate alone, however, occur more frequently in females than males. Submucous clefts occur at approximately the same frequency in males and females. In the United States, Native Americans have the highest incidence rates, followed by people of Asian descent, Caucasians, and people of African descent. These incidence differences have been attributed to genetic and environmental factors (McWilliams et al., 1990).

Regardless of gender and race, individuals with clefts present many different interrelated problems that require the cooperation of a wide variety of specialists for effective treatment and management (McWilliams et al., 1990; Shprintzen, 1995). The group of specialists working together providing care for persons with cleft palate is referred to as a **cleft palate team.**

THE CLEFT PALATE TEAM AND GENERAL MANAGEMENT ISSUES ACROSS THE LIFE SPAN

The concept of a cleft palate team, sometimes called the craniofacial team, was developed originally at the Lancaster Cleft Palate Clinic in Lancaster, Pennsylvania, in the 1930s. Today the Membership-Team Directory of the American Cleft Palate-Craniofacial Association lists 250 cleft palate teams in the United States. Table 11.3 lists the professions that constitute a typical cleft palate team.

Clinical management of people with clefts requires the efficient integration of information among professionals. For example, a surgeon might require information about speech production ability from the SLP when deciding whether to perform a particular operation.

Practical advantages of a team approach include the following: (1) The family can see several specialists during one appointment, (2) the family associates all aspects of care with one setting, (3) only one contact is required if an emergency arises, and (4) follow-up is managed in a controlled manner (McWilliams et al., 1990).

The needs of a person with a cleft and his or her family change during the life span, requiring team member compositions and roles to change accordingly. These changing needs are managed effectively with the team approach. Table 11.4 summarizes briefly the function of a few

---

TABLE 11.3

Composition of a cleft palate team

Anesthesiologist	Nurse practitioner	Plastic surgeon
Audiologist	Oral surgeon	Prosthodontist
Coordinator	Orthodontist	Psychiatrist
Educator	Otolaryngologist	Psychologist
Endodontist	Parents	Radiologist
Geneticist	Pediatrician	Social worker
Genetic counselor	Periodontist	Speech-language pathologist

TABLE 11.4

Functions of the cleft palate team as the needs of the person with a cleft change during the life span

Age in Years	Team Function
Birth	Pediatrician discusses cleft with parents with cooperation of geneticist and social worker. Surgeon discusses cleft type and operative procedures.
Birth to 1	Surgeon closes lip. Pediatrician discusses general health issues. Audiologist begins hearing testing. Otolaryngologist watches for middle ear pathology. Surgeon and SLP discuss possible velopharyngeal incompetence.
1 to 2	Surgeon closes hard palate. SLP evaluates velopharyngeal function. Otolaryngologist watches for possible middle ear problems. Audiologist tests hearing. Dental specialists are consulted.
2 to 6	Surgeon works with SLP on the effect of surgery for velopharyngeal function. Geneticist role minimal. Dental specialist begins corrections. SLP, surgeon, and dental specialist work closely together during this important period of speech and language development.
6 to 12	Pediatrician watches general health and development. Surgical follow-up for secondary repairs of the lip and palate. Dental specialist, SLP, and audiologist work closely together noting speech and language development.
12 to 18	Focus on orthodontic care. Geneticist may give premarital counseling. Otolaryngologist and audiologist continue monitoring middle ear and hearing status. Speech therapy and counseling as indicated.
18 to Adult	A general practitioner deals with health concerns. Surgical role is moot. A general dentist deals with dental care. Geneticist and social worker counsel regarding risk of having a cleft palate child. Hearing and speech services as required.

Source: Adapted from McWilliams, Morris, & Shelton (1990).

select members of a cleft palate team as an individual's needs change from birth to adulthood.

SLPs, surgeons, dental specialists, and audiologists work closely together on the team. Therefore, the SLP needs to have some familiarity with the specific roles and concerns of the other team members. In the next four sections of this chapter, we will discuss surgical, dental, audiological, and psychosocial concerns regarding clefts. This discussion will be followed by a detailed account of the communicative problems faced by persons with clefts and the SLP's role as a member of a cleft palate team.

SURGICAL MANAGEMENT OF CLEFTS

Although the recorded history of clefts dates back to the Ching dynasty (390 B.C.), surgical repair of clefts did not occur until the nineteenth century. Surgical repair of clefts, or **palatoplasty,** is divided into two stages: primary surgical correction followed by secondary procedures to correct velopharyngeal incompetence.

PRIMARY SURGICAL CORRECTION

The first stage of primary surgical correction is lip surgery if the child has a cleft of the lip and palate. Lip surgery is performed generally before 3 months of age (Seagle, 1997). Some surgeons prefer to defer surgical correction of the lip until the parents have lived with the baby long enough to understand and accept the cleft. These surgeons hope that during this waiting period, the parents will adjust and develop a realistic attitude about the benefits of surgery and the inevitable scar (Peterson-Falzone et al., 2001).

Surgical correction of a cleft palate is designed to create a velopharyngeal valving mechanism that is capable of separating the oral cavity from the nasal cavity during speech production. Early surgical closure of the palate also improves swallowing function and reduces the number of middle ear and upper respiratory infections. Recent surgical trends advocate closure of the palatal cleft between 6 and 18 months of age. Early closure has a positive influence on velopharyngeal function, midfacial symmetry, and overall appearance (Seagle, 1997).

SECONDARY SURGICAL CORRECTION

The efficacy of primary palatal surgery is assessed by the adequacy of the velopharyngeal mechanism for speech production. Approximately one in four individuals who have primary palatal surgery fails to achieve velopharyngeal competence for speech production, requiring additional surgical management to correct the velopharyngeal incompetence (Riski, 1995).

A commonly used secondary surgical procedure designed to correct VPI is called a **pharyngeal flap** operation. A pharyngeal flap is created by cutting a flap of soft tissue from the posterior pharyngeal wall, as shown in Figure 11.3. One end of the flap remains attached to the posterior pharyngeal wall, and the other is sutured to the velum. To permit nasal breathing and the production of nasal speech sounds, small

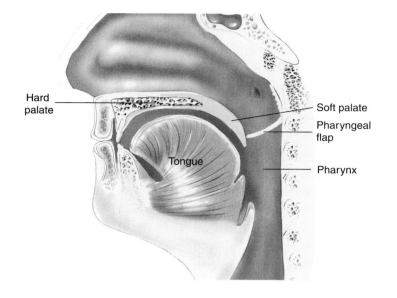

Hard palate

Soft palate

Pharyngeal flap

Tongue

Pharynx

FIGURE 11.3   Stylized drawing of a pharyngeal flap

openings are maintained between the flap and the lateral walls of the pharynx. Closure of these openings during swallowing and the production of nonnasal speech sounds is accomplished by active **medial** (toward the midline) movement of the lateral walls of the pharynx (Riski, 1995). Pharyngeal flap procedures are performed generally between the ages of 6 and 12, and it has been reported that "normal" speech is realized following the majority of these operations (Peterson-Falzone et al., 2001).

DENTAL MANAGEMENT OF CLEFTS

People with cleft lip and palate have significant dental problems that can interfere with chewing, swallowing, and speech production. During the life span, various dental specialists will be involved in a "time-ordered agenda" of dental care ranging from developing devices to assist the infant's swallowing to treatment focusing on improving the positions of teeth and maxillary bone segments (Peterson-Falzone et al., 2001, p. 123). **Orthodontists** are crucial members of cleft palate teams who are concerned primarily with the alignment of teeth and dental **malocclusions.** A malocclusion is the improper alignment of the maxillary and mandibular dental arches. Orthodontic techniques for the correction of a malocclusion are based on the premise that steady amounts of pressure over time will result in tooth movement and/or dental arch expansion. Pressure is applied to the teeth and/or the dental arches with metal bands and various dental appliances.

T H O U G H T   Q U E S T I O N S

Did you have dental braces as a child? Do you still have braces? Do you remember how your mouth felt after visiting the orthodontist? The discomfort you probably experienced was the pressure being applied to your misaligned teeth.

Abnormal **dentition** based on the kind, number, and arrangement of teeth and malocclusions can have very adverse effects on speech production. Nearly 90 percent of all English consonants are made in the anterior portion of the mouth, the area of the mouth that is most affected by clefts. Missing or misaligned teeth and malocclusions can affect adversely the production of sounds that require accurate tongue placement on the teeth or dental arch, such as /t/, /d/, and /l/. Sounds that require a constriction between the tongue and teeth, such as /s/, /th/, and /sh/, will be adversely affected by the absence or misalignment of teeth (Le Blanc & Cisneros, 1995).

A **prosthodontist,** a dental specialist, is frequently involved in the care of individuals with clefts. Prosthodontics is a dental specialty concerned with the replacement of missing teeth and other oral structures with various appliances. For some individuals with clefts, palatoplasty is not recommended because of other complicating medical conditions, religious beliefs, or simply personal choice. In such circumstances, closure of the cleft can be achieved by a prosthodontic *obturator.* An obturator is a special kind of dental prosthesis designed to occlude or fill the cleft and partition the oral cavity from the nasal cavity. Obturators may be used as primary management of a cleft or as a secondary procedure after unsuccessful palatoplasty (Peterson-Falzone et al., 2001).

Obturators are made of acrylic material and custom built to conform to the general configuration of an individual's oral cavity. The obturator is held in place by clasps that anchor it to the teeth. The palatal portion of the obturator covers the cleft, and the posterior portion extends into the pharynx and terminates in a bulblike structure, called a **speech bulb,** that fills the velopharyngeal space. Velopharyngeal closure is achieved by medial movement of the lateral pharyngeal walls making contact with the bulb.

AUDIOLOGICAL MANAGEMENT OF CLEFTS

People with clefts exhibit a higher incidence of hearing disorders and middle ear disease than the general population. Middle ear disease is universal during a cleft palate child's infancy, resulting in a conductive hearing loss that may persist into adulthood (Peterson-Falzone et al., 2001). It has been estimated that 58 percent of the cleft palate population has some degree of hearing loss (Kemker, 1995). Later in this section, we will discuss the potential impact of hearing loss on speech and language development, but first we will consider how middle ear disease leads to conductive hearing loss in the cleft palate population.

The middle ear is an air-filled cavity in the temporal bone of the skull bounded on the outside by the tympanic membrane (eardrum) and on the inside by the cochlea, a spiral-shaped structure that contains the nerve endings for hearing. A tube runs from the middle ear down into the nasopharynx (the portion of the pharynx above the velum). This tube, called the **auditory tube,** permits drainage from the middle ear into the pharynx and serves to equalize air pressure in the middle ear with atmospheric pressure.

T H O U G H T   Q U E S T I O N S

You are a passenger in an aircraft. When the aircraft is taking off or landing, do you feel pressure in your ears? What happens to the sense of pressure when you swallow, yawn, or chew gum vigorously?

The auditory tube is normally closed, opening only when one swallows or yawns widely. The tube is opened by a reflexive contraction of the **tensor veli palatine** muscle. The tensor veli palatine muscle is a muscle of the soft palate. When a cleft of the soft palate occurs, it does not function properly and will not open the tube. Dysfunction of the auditory tube results in poor middle ear ventilation, which, in turn, leads to inflammation and abnormal fluid accumulation. This fluid accumulation is a disease called *otitis media,* which causes mild to moderate hearing loss. Otitis media frequently needs to be treated with a **myringotomy,** which is a surgical puncture of the tympanic membrane and insertion of a ventilating tube for pressure equalization.

You can develop some appreciation of how a mild conductive loss affects your hearing sensitivity by occluding (plugging) your ears gently with your fingers. Note that you still hear some sounds but not others. In general, loud sounds can be heard, but soft sounds cannot. Try this little experiment with a friend: Have your friend stand behind you and produce a vowel sound such as /a/ for three seconds and then produce an /s/ for three seconds. If you have normal hearing, you will hear both these sounds clearly. With your friend still standing behind you, plug your ears gently and have him or her produce those sounds again in the same manner. With your ears plugged, you probably heard the /a/ but not the /s/. If you did hear the /s/, it was very muffled and distorted.

Your little experiment demonstrates that even a mild conductive loss can prevent a listener from hearing many of the sounds of spoken English. Longstanding conductive hearing loss associated with otitis media can have a devastating effect on speech and language development, compounding the already adverse conditions created by the cleft.

The audiologist is a vital member of the cleft palate team who provides critical information to the SLP about an individual's hearing status. For people with clefts, hearing testing should be done routinely every three to six months. During episodes of active otitis media, hearing should be checked more frequently.

PSYCHOSOCIAL MANAGEMENT OF CLEFTS

There is no strong evidence that children with repaired clefts are more maladapted psychosocially than their noncleft peers, and they have no documented personality deviations. Frequently, however, these children suffer from social isolation owing to discrimination by peers and teachers who overemphasize the residual evidence of the cleft condition and underestimate the child's real capabilities. Such social isolation may lead to low self-esteem, decreased participation in group activities, inhibited behavior, and lowered expectations on the part of parents, teachers, and peers (McWilliams et al., 1990).

Children with clefts encounter unusual social pressures, and there is a continuing need to ensure their psychological well-being. The SLP needs to be keenly aware of the child's psychological and social needs and "provide treatment or referral as required in individual cases" (McWilliams et al., 1990, p. 144).

Table 11.5 highlights some of the psychosocial concerns as they change during the life span of individuals with cleft palate.

COMMUNICATION PROBLEMS ASSOCIATED WITH CLEFTS

Approximately 80 percent of people born with clefts that are not associated with a syndrome and receiving palatal repair by 18 months can be expected to develop reasonably good speech without therapeutic intervention. For the other 20 percent born with clefts and for children with associated syndromes, "the road to normal speech often seems long and arduous" (Golding-Kushner, 1995, p. 327). The child with a cleft palate may have voice disorders, resonance disorders associated with VPI, articulation disorders associated with VPI, dental malocclusions, and possible hearing loss. In addition, children with clefts may exhibit language disorders. In this section, we discuss the presumed causes, assessment, and treatment of these communicative problems.

TABLE 11.5

Psychosocial concerns during the life span of a person
with a cleft palate

Developmental Stage	Areas of Concern
Prenatal/Perinatal Period	Parental adjustments to impending birth/birth of a child with cleft palate
Toddler Years	Parental attempts to protect the child from negative reactions of extended family and community members; stress of medical intervention
Preschool Years	Self-concept, peer relationships
Early School and Teen Years	Self-concept, peer relationships, school adjustment, negative judgments by teachers
Adults	Social interactions, life partners, and employment

Source: Adapted from Peterson-Falzone et al. (2001).

An SLP who specializes in craniofacial disorders probably has fewer adolescents and adult patients with cleft palate than once was the case. Persons with cleft palate now receive effective treatments earlier in their life and generally speak normally by the time they are adolescents (Peterson-Falzone et al., 2001). Thus, this section of the text will focus on communicative problems that are likely to be diagnosed and treated during childhood.

VOICE DISORDERS

In Chapter 9, we reported that approximately 3 to 6 percent of noncleft children and 3 to 9 percent of noncleft adults exhibit some form of voice disorder. Clinical research indicates that phonatory disorders are much more common in people with clefts, possibly involving over 80 percent of the cleft population. The most common vocal fold pathology is bilateral vocal nodules, which produce a hoarse, breathy vocal quality. The high incidence of individuals with vocal nodules among the cleft palate population is likely related to vocal hyperfunction (Peterson-Falzone, et al., 2001). Vocal hyperfunction is also the presumed cause of vocal nodules in noncleft children. In noncleft children, however, vocal hyperfunction is usually associated with excessive yelling and screaming.

Vocal hyperfunction among children with cleft palate appears to be compensatory behavior related to VPI. Children with VPI are unable to increase their vocal intensity in a normal fashion owing to the loss of energy into the nasal cavity. To compensate for this inability, these children position their larynx high in the neck during speaking, and this behavior exerts unusually high tension on the vocal folds, causing the vocal nodules.

Another voice disorder that occurs in children with cleft palates is called **soft-voice syndrome.** Soft-voice syndrome is also a compensatory behavior by which the child purposely reduces vocal intensity to prevent air escape through the nose and reduce hypernasality. Soft-voice syndrome is frequently accompanied by a monotone voice characterized by little variation in pitch.

ASSESSMENT OF VOICE DISORDERS

Four general steps have been recommended for the assessment of suspected voice disorders associated with clefts (McWilliams et al., 1990). First, a case history should be taken to determine whether the vocal symptoms are of recent origin or longstanding. If the symptoms have been present for a long time, patterns of potential vocal misuse need to be explored in detail.

The second step should explore the individual's personality. Vocal hyperfunction is commonly associated with people who are tense, loud, and/or aggressive. These personality characteristics are not typical of individuals with clefts, but the possibility of such a personality factor contributing to vocal hyperfunction needs to be explored.

A detailed phonation examination to determine the nature of the voice disorder is the third general step. Of interest is the appropriateness of the vocal pitch range, loudness, and vocal quality. Specific techniques and instruments for such assessments have been discussed in numerous texts on voice disorders and in Chapter 9.

The fourth step is to determine whether the person can modify his or her voice. A straightforward procedure to determine an individual's ability to change the voice is to have him or her "sigh" or produce an "um-hum." People who exhibit vocal hyperfunction during connected speech may demonstrate unconsciously the ability to change vocal quality when producing these easy, natural phonations.

As with any suspected disorder of voice, the individual needs to be examined by a physician before commencing therapy. When a hoarse voice quality accompanies a cleft, there is a strong possibility that bilateral vocal nodules exist. Voice therapy is usually the initial treatment of choice with the goal of reducing vocal hyperfunction.

TREATMENT OF VOICE DISORDERS

Therapeutic reduction of vocal hyperfunction is divided generally into three phases: auditory discrimination, establishing a new voice production, and habituating the new voice (Aronson, 1990; McWilliams et al., 1990).

During the auditory discrimination phase, the individual learns to differentiate his or her voice from the voices of people who do not have vocal nodules. A second step in the auditory discrimination phase is to train the individual to recognize differences in quality between their best and poorest vocalizations. This can be accomplished by contrasting connected speech with relaxed production of "um-hum."

A primary goal toward establishing a new voice regards the elimination of **hard glottal attacks.** A hard glottal attack occurs when one initiates speech using hypertensive vocal fold adduction.

T H O U G H T   Q U E S T I O N

Can you mimic a hard glottal attack? Try this. Inhale deeply and, with your mouth open, trap air in your lungs by approximating your vocal folds. Now say the vowel /a/. What does your voice sound like?

To eliminate hard glottal attacks, the individual is trained to initiate words beginning with vowels using a gentle glottal attack. This strategy is taught by having the individual begin by producing a prolonged /h/ and then gradually moving into the initial vowel in the word. This breathy, relaxed voicing onset can be felt and heard, and the individual is taught to sense the relaxed phonation. Initiating words with the /h/ is gradually phased out, and therapy progresses into two-word combinations, sentences, and finally conversational speech.

Habituating the new voice is divided into two phases: (a) limited habituation; and (b) overall habituation (McWilliams et al., 1990). Limited habituation involves having the individual use his or her new voice only in the presence of the SLP and then in highly controlled situations outside the clinic. Overall habituation involves using the new voice during the entire therapy session, then in specific classes in school, and during certain hours at home. The times and situations are gradually extended. Therapy is terminated when the individual and his or her significant others report a consistent use of the new voice.

RESONANCE DISORDERS

People with VPI are said to have a hypernasal voice quality. Hypernasality is not a problem associated with phonation; rather, it is the result of not partitioning the oral and nasal cavities by actions of the velopharyngeal mechanism. Hypernasality is a resonance problem created by the nasal cavity acting inappropriately as a second "filter" coupled to the oral cavity. Addition of this second filter alters the vocal tract's output in such a way that it sounds as though the individual is talking through his or her nose. In a sense, people with VPI are talking through their noses.

T H O U G H T   Q U E S T I O N

Have you ever used the frequency equalizer on your stereo? Frequency equalizers are filters of a sort. What happens to the sound coming from your speakers when you change the settings on your frequency equalizer?

Some degree of nasal resonance is present in the speech of people who have velopharyngeal competence; some nasal resonance is normal. To illustrate this point, say the sentence "Where were you last year?" aloud. Now pinch your nostrils shut and listen to the difference in your voice quality. Pinching your nostrils shut while speaking reduces normal nasal resonance, and as a result your voice sounds unnatural. This lack of nasal resonance is called **hyponasality.** Your voice may have a hyponasal quality when you experience a bad head cold.

Individuals with VPI exhibit increased nasal resonance and decreased oral resonance, and the voice quality is abnormally nasal sounding, or hypernasal. Hypernasality is associated mainly with vowels. High vowels such as /i/ tend to be perceived as more nasal than low vowels such as /a/, and perceived hypernasality may be greater in connected speech than during the production of isolated words.

ASSESSMENT OF RESONANCE DISORDERS

There are a number of standardized rating scales for assessing vocal resonance. Rating scales permit the assignment of numbers to express increasing severity of the disorder. In general, such rating scales are reliable and valid. Two such rating scales are presented in Table 11.6.

Specially designed instruments are also available to assess resonance disorders. One such instrument, manufactured by Kay Elemetrics, is called a **nasometer.** The nasometer measures simultaneously the relative amplitude of acoustic energy being emitted through the nose

Several different instruments are commercially available that will obtain nasalance scores. The computation and interpretation of these scores varies according to the instrument.

TABLE 11.6

Two examples of scales used to rate the degree of resonance disorders: (a) a seven-point scale emphasizing hypernasality, and (b) an eight-point scale for rating nasal resonance

(a)

		Hypernasality				
Normal	Mild		Moderate		Severe	
1	2	3	4	5	6	7

(b)

			Hypernasality				
Hypo-nasality	Normal	Mild		Moderate		Severe	
−1	0	1	2	3	4	5	6

Source: Adapted from McWilliams, Morris, & Shelton (1990).

and mouth during phonation. A numerical value, the **nasalance score,** is computed that reflects the magnitude of hypernasality. Nasalance scores have been shown to correlate well with rating scales and with the actual degree of velopharyngeal opening (Dalston, 1995; Dalston & Seaver, 1990). Nasometry can also be used as an effective therapeutic feedback technique. Examples of nasometry can be seen on the book's CD-ROM.

The definitive procedure for assessing velopharyngeal function is **multiview videofluoroscopy.** Videofluoroscopy is motion picture X-rays recorded on videotape. Multiview videofluoroscopy permits the imaging of velopharyngeal function from three different perspectives: from the front, from the side, and from beneath. These images provide a complete picture of velopharyngeal closure or the lack thereof.

TREATMENT OF RESONANCE DISORDERS

Behavioral treatments designed to improve velopharyngeal functioning and reduce hypernasality have a fifty-year history in the United States.

During this time, professional opinion has varied as to the clinical efficacy of such treatments. Contemporary thought about behavioral management of VPI suggests that for some individuals velopharyngeal closure may be improved without additional surgery (Tomes, Kuehn, & Peterson-Falzone, 1995). Before discussing some of the behavioral management techniques that are used to treat VPI, we need to consider a serious caveat.

People who have anatomical limitations such as a velum that is too short to contact the posterior pharyngeal wall or a velum that is completely immobile will not benefit from behavioral treatments. Such individuals will require further surgery or a prosthesis to achieve velopharyngeal competence. The decision to try behavioral treatments to improve velopharyngeal function must be made through careful collaboration of the cleft palate team.

Once the cleft palate team has decided that behavioral management is a viable option for a given individual with VPI, the SLP can choose from several different treatment protocols that are designed to improve velopharyngeal function. Two procedures that show promise for improving velopharyngeal function are the Whistling-Blowing procedure and a relatively new procedure named Continuous Positive Airway Pressure.

The Whistling-Blowing technique (Shprintzen, McCall, & Skolnick, 1975) is a behavioral treatment based on X-ray observations that indicate that velopharyngeal closure patterns during whistling and blowing are similar to closure patterns achieved during normal speech production. This technique can be used with individuals who achieve velopharyngeal closure during whistling and/or blowing, but not during speech production. The general steps of this procedure are outlined in Table 11.7. See Box 11.1 on page 377 for an example of the use of whistling-blowing techniques to treat a boy who developed VPI following tonsil and adenoid surgery.

Continuous Positive Airway Pressure (CPAP) therapy is based on the exercise physiology principle of progressive resistance training. Progressive resistance training asserts that when muscles are subjected systematically to weights greater than those to which they are accustomed, they adapt by adding muscle tissue and strength is increased. To continue building muscle tissue, weights are increased systematically until the desired muscle strength is achieved.

T H O U G H T   Q U E S T I O N

Have you tried to increase muscle strength by lifting weights? Did you use progressive resistance training?

TABLE 11.7

The general treatment sequence for the Whistling-Blowing therapy designed to improve velopharyngeal functioning

1. Determine whether the individual can achieve closure during whistling or blowing.
2. Teach the individual to blow or whistle and phonate at the same time. Monitor and identify nasal air leakage with a scape-scope.* Reward productions that are free of nasal air emission.
3. Gradually discontinue the use of blowing and whistling during phonation. Reward correct productions and punish nasal air emission during vowel productions.
4. Remove the scape-scope for monitoring and replace with auditory monitoring.

*A scape-scope is a simple device that monitors air escaping from the nose. A small hose inserted into the nostrils is connected to a tube. A Styrofoam ball inside the tube moves up and down in association with nasal emission.
Source: Adapted from McWilliams, Morris, & Shelton (1990).

The CPAP procedure attempts to strengthen the muscles of the velopharyngeal mechanism by having the velar musculature work against systematic increases of weight. It would be quite impractical and probably impossible to use free weights such as miniature barbells to strengthen the velopharyngeal musculature. CPAP uses air pressure in the nasal cavity as a substitute. Air pressure in the nasal cavity can be increased or decreased using a commercially available device.

During therapy, the velum works against the increased air pressure in the nasal cavity during the production of syllables that contain nasal consonants /n/ or /m/, vowels, and nonnasal consonants. The velum is lowered during production of the nasal consonant and elevated during vowel and nonnasal consonant productions. Nasal air pressure is increased systematically during velar elevation associated with production of the nonnasal consonant. The heightened air pressure in the nasal cavity is the "weight" that the velopharyngeal mechanism works against (Tomes et al., 1995).

CPAP is an experimental treatment procedure for training the velopharyngeal mechanism. The fact that this technique has its roots in physiological principles that are solidly grounded suggests great promise for future development and success.

BOX 11.1

Personal Story of a Boy with Velopharyngeal Insufficiency

Marty, a 9-year-old boy, was brought to the University Hospital's Communication Disorders Unit by his parents with the concern that after tonsil and adenoid surgery, his speech had deteriorated. At birth, Marty presented with a cleft of the hard and soft palate. The cleft was repaired surgically when he was 11 months old, and the SLP evaluated him regularly for two years after the surgery. On the basis of the SLP's recommendation to the cleft palate team, Marty was enrolled in formal speech training when he was 3½ years old. Speech therapy continued for two years, at which time he was dismissed from the clinic with age-appropriate speech and language skills and normal nasal resonance.

Marty was troubled frequently by throat infections, which caused severe swelling of his tonsils and adenoids that interfered with swallowing. His pediatrician recommended removal of the tonsils and adenoids.

The speech-language evaluation of Marty revealed that his speech was markedly hypernasal with frequent nasal emission. The SLP recommended that Marty be evaluated by a radiologist with multiview videofluoroscopy to determine the underlying cause of the hypernasal speech and nasal emission.

The videofluoroscopy revealed that Marty's velum was not making adequate contact with the right and left aspects of the pharyngeal walls where the adenoid tissue had been removed. Although adequate velar contact was observed during swallowing, he could not partition the oral and nasal cavities during speech production. A pharyngeal flap operation was the team's recommendation.

After the pharyngeal flap surgery, Marty was evaluated by the SLP and the radiologist. They determined that he was capable of velopharyngeal closure during speech, but he was not achieving closure consistently during speech. The team recommended that Marty receive speech therapy twice weekly for two months. After five weeks of therapy utilizing whistling-blowing techniques, Marty's speech was no longer hypernasal, and there was no evidence of nasal emission.

ARTICULATION DISORDERS

Individuals with clefts are at high risk for disordered articulation (i.e., the formation and production of the sounds of English). Disordered articulation can be the result of VPI, structural deviations in the oral cavity, misaligned or missing teeth, faulty learning, or combinations of these factors. Sounds that tend to be produced incorrectly more than 60 percent of the time in the cleft population include /s/, /z/, /θ/, /ʧ/, and /ts/ (McWilliams et al., 1990). Vowels and some consonants are produced with a hypernasal quality, as discussed above.

Production of consonants that require an air pressure buildup in the oral cavity, such as the stop consonants /p/, /t/, and /k/ (**pressure consonants**), is frequently accompanied by air escaping inappropriately through the nose. Air escaping through the nose during speech production is called **nasal emission.** Nasal emission is not the same as hypernasal speech quality. Rather, nasal emission is an audible or inaudible leakage of air into the nasal cavity.

People with clefts may also exhibit **compensatory articulation errors.** This term describes errors of articulation that occur in people with VPI and are distinguished from the articulation errors discussed above. A compensatory articulation error is a gross sound substitution error that is an attempt to compensate for the physical inability to produce a given sound correctly. A common compensatory articulation error is known as a **glottal stop.**

Individuals with VPI are unable to build the requisite oral air pressure to produce stops such as /p/, /t/, and /k/ because of air escaping into the nasal cavity, as discussed above. Stop sounds require a brief stoppage of air flow and a buildup of oral air pressure followed by a sudden release of that pressure. The normal production of a /p/ sound, for example, requires a buildup of oral pressure that is accomplished by holding the upper and lower lips together briefly (the stop) followed by a sudden release of that built-up air pressure. The person with VPI is incapable of producing the /p/ in this fashion and compensates by stopping the air at the glottis, approximating the vocal folds. Air is stopped, and pressure is built up beneath the vocal folds instead of behind the lips.

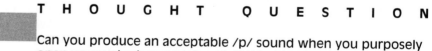

T H O U G H T   Q U E S T I O N

Can you produce an acceptable /p/ sound when you purposely open your velopharyngeal portal? What happens when you try?

Ten compensatory articulation substitutions have been identified in the speech of people with clefts and VPI (Witzel, 1995). Some of these compensatory behaviors may become strongly habituated and still be present after the structural deficit that caused them has been corrected. The SLP needs to make a careful inventory of such behaviors during the articulation assessment of people with clefts.

ASSESSMENT OF ARTICULATION DISORDERS

A number of widely used articulation tests can be used to assess the sound production skills of people with clefts. Some of these are the *Templin-Darley Test of Articulation,* the *Goldman-Fristoe Test of Ar-*

ticulation, and the *Fisher-Logemann Test of Articulation Competence.* The *Fisher-Logemann Test* is particularly useful for assessing individuals with clefts because it allows for an analysis of patterns of articulation errors regarding the place, manner, and voicing characteristics of sounds (McWilliams et al., 1990).

Specialized tests of articulation have been developed for use with people who are suspected of having VPI. The *Iowa Pressure Articulation Test* is a subtest embedded in the *Templin-Darley Test of Articulation.* This test is composed of forty-three sounds that have been identified as likely to be misarticulated by people with VPI. The test emphasizes sounds that require the buildup of oral pressure. Individuals who score poorly on this test because of VPI will produce a unique pattern of errors characterized by nasal emission, a lack of oral pressure, and gross compensatory substitutions (McWilliams et al., 1990).

The *Bzoch Error Pattern Diagnostic Articulation Test* is another specialized instrument designed for people with clefts and/or suspected VPI. The test is constructed to facilitate identification of error patterns in speech that are related more to VPI than to functional learning problems.

Phonological process analysis can also be used to assess the sound production skills of people with clefts. Because of the unique nature of articulation errors in the cleft population, several clinician-researchers have suggested that phonetic classification of voicing, manner of formation, and place of articulation allows for an easier identification of causation than the analysis of phonological process (McWilliams et al., 1990; Witzel, 1995). Sound formation difficulties caused by structural anomaly may lead to persistent phonological process simplifications. In this regard, phonological process analysis should not be ignored (Witzel, 1995).

MANAGEMENT OF ARTICULATION DISORDERS

The basic principles that underlie the treatment of deviant articulatory-phonological behaviors in the noncleft population also apply to the treatment of the cleft population. The use of longstanding speech-language pathology techniques for teaching individuals to produce sounds in syllables and words and then to establish the use of those sounds in conversation is recommended by many clinicians who are highly experienced in cleft palate speech management (McWilliams et al., 1990). Such techniques include the use of auditory and visual models for imitation, practice, and reinforcement of responses that are appropriate for the individual's capabilities.

Treatment of preschool-age children with repaired clefts should emphasize the development of stop consonant and fricative production. Establishing stopping and frication in a few sounds will contribute to generalization of those features to other sounds. Emphasis is also placed on instructing the child how to direct the air stream in an oral direction rather than a nasal direction.

Articulation-phonology therapy can help many individuals with repaired clefts to achieve normal speech. In some individuals, however, the prognosis for improvement is poor, and therapy must be terminated. The SLP "must have the courage and knowledge to make this decision" (McWilliams et al., 1990, p. 397).

LANGUAGE DISORDERS

In contrast to the communicative problems associated with clefts discussed above, very little attention has been paid to language development and language disorders with this population (Witzel, 1995). Research studies generally have found evidence of mild language delays in children with clefts, particularly children with clefts of the palate only. However, these studies are not in agreement regarding the nature and extent of language delays, and the origins of language delays within the cleft population have not been specified (McWilliams et al., 1990).

More research is needed on the relationship among potential contributing factors such as otitis media, learning disabilities, and specific syndromes and language delays in the cleft palate population. SLPs need to be aware of the potential for language disabilities among children with clefts. The SLP must also be aware that language disorders are not an invariable consequence of clefting and recognize those children "who are better served if we do not intervene" (McWilliams et al., 1990, p. 244).

ASSESSMENT OF LANGUAGE DISORDERS

Children born with clefts should be routinely examined for potential delays in language development and specific language impairments. Language evaluations should include information about environmental factors, motor and mental development, and hearing acuity. Language assessment of children with clefts is the same as language assessment of other children (McWilliams et al., 1990). Standard tests of receptive and expressive language like those discussed in Chapter 6 can be used effectively with the cleft palate population.

TREATMENT OF LANGUAGE DISORDERS

As with language assessment, treating language disorders for children with clefts does not differ substantively from treating language disorders in the noncleft population. In fact, it has been shown that delayed language development can in large part be prevented in this population. Early and repeated family counseling regarding receptive and ex-

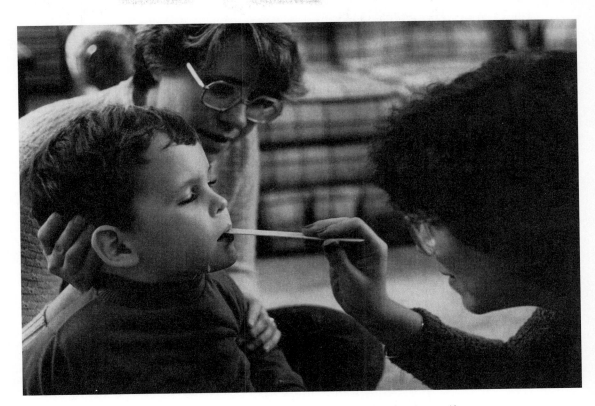

During the oral peripheral examination, the SLP checks muscle strength.

pressive language development, aggressive treatment of middle ear disease, and language enrichment programs have been shown to prevent language difficulties (Bzoch, 1997).

One last issue regarding language development in children with clefts should be noted. Mothers of cleft children may engage in significantly less verbal play with their child than mothers of noncleft children. The SLP should be mindful of this possibility and counsel new parents about how important early verbal play is to good language development. As the child matures, parents should be encouraged to read to the child and talk about daily events and experiences. Perhaps most important, parents should provide a good language model for their child. The SLP can be invaluable in helping parents to achieve this goal.

SUMMARY

Children with cleft palate face a myriad of problems from early infancy through adulthood. These problems can be treated effectively only when a team of professionals works cooperatively toward their resolution. The speech-language pathologist is an integral member of the cleft palate team who will work in conjunction with surgeons, orthodontists, and other professionals to facilitate the development of normal speech and language for the child with a cleft. Surgical correction of the cleft by reconstruction of the palate and velopharyngeal mechanism must in many cases be followed by long-term therapy to remediate voice, resonance, and articulation disorders.

REFLECTIONS

- Describe the embryological development of the face and palate.
- Describe how clefts of the lip and palate form.
- Describe the clinical features of a cleft of the lip.
- Describe the clinical features of a unilateral cleft of the lip and palate.
- Describe the clinical features of a bilateral cleft of the lip and palate.
- Explain the Veau classification system of cleft types.
- Discuss some of the possible causes of clefts.
- Discuss some of the medical and dental management concerns associated with clefts.
- Explain middle ear disorders associated with clefts.
- Describe some of the communicative problems associated with clefts.

SUGGESTED READINGS

Charkins, H. (1996). *Children with facial differences*. Bethesda, MD: Woodbine House.

Shprintzen, R. J. (1997). *Genetics, syndromes, and communication disorders*. San Diego: Singular.

ON-LINE RESOURCES

http://www.cleft.com/   American Cleft Palate-Craniofacial Association.

http://www.widesmiles.org/   Wide Smiles! Cleft Lip and Palate Resource.
Resources and networking for families of children with clefts.

http://www.cleft.org/   Smiles.
Stories by families with children born with cleft lip and/or cleft palate, with links to related information.

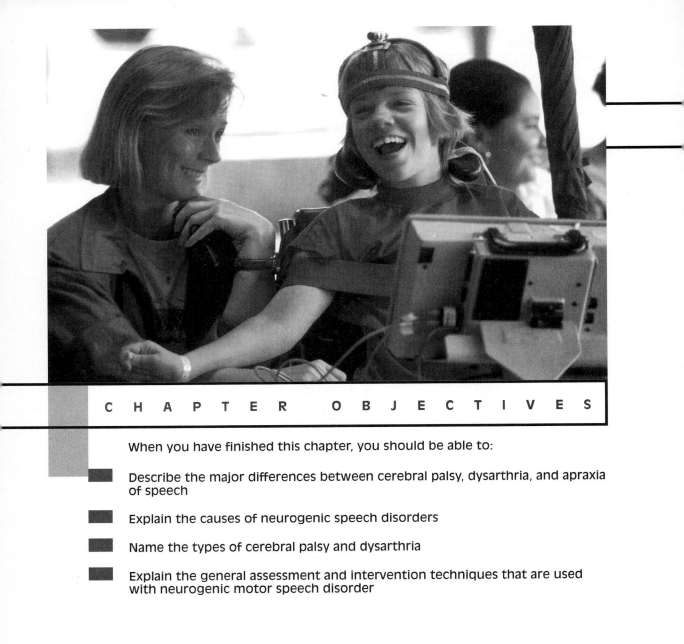

When you have finished this chapter, you should be able to:

Describe the major differences between cerebral palsy, dysarthria, and apraxia of speech

Explain the causes of neurogenic speech disorders

Name the types of cerebral palsy and dysarthria

Explain the general assessment and intervention techniques that are used with neurogenic motor speech disorder

Neurogenic Speech Disorders

Neurogenic speech disorders are speech difficulties that are related to problems of movement as a result of some neurological disorder or injury. They are sometimes referred to as motor speech disorders. The term "motor" refers to movement.

Neurogenic speech disorders are a heterogeneous group of neurological impairments that affect the planning, coordination, timing, and execution of the movement patterns that are used to produce speech in both children and adults. Any or all of the processes of respiration, phonation, resonation, and articulation, described in previous chapters, may be affected. Although voice and fluency are involved, these are addressed in other chapters. In addition, language disorders often co-occur with neurogenic speech disorders. These are described in Chapter 7, "Adult Language Impairments."

That brief explanation does not begin to hint at the complexity of the disorders that fall within the boundaries of neurogenic speech disorders. So finite and particular are the movements needed for speech that more area in the brain is devoted to control of the vocal folds, tongue, lips, and other articulators than to any other bodily movement, even walking. Given this complexity, it is amazing that the process of producing speech becomes almost automatic and little thought is given to it by most speakers. In fact, we rarely consider the process unless something is wrong.

Do you ever think about producing speech as you're doing it? Have you ever bitten your tongue or choked while talking and eating? Suddenly, you become aware of the movement and the structures. Notice how your mouth moves when you say your name. Production has become automatic. You might never have noticed these movements before.

In this chapter, we limit our discussion to the production of speech. We discuss three types of neurogenic speech impairments: cerebral palsy, dysarthria, and apraxia of speech. In discussing characteristics, such a division is not so simple. Many individuals with cerebral palsy also exhibit dysarthria and apraxia of speech.

It might help you to remember these disorders if we make a somewhat artificial distinction. Because cerebral palsy occurs before, at, or shortly after birth, it is considered a *developmental* neuromotor deficit. In contrast, most dysarthrias and apraxia occur after the neuromotor system is fully mature and therefore are considered to be *acquired* disorders.

Suppose a school-aged child had a stroke that resulted in a motor speech problem. Would the disorder be developmental, acquired, or both? Classification is not always clear-cut.

CAUSES OF NEUROGENIC SPEECH DISORDERS

The major causes of neurogenic language and neurogenic speech disorders are similar.

Many conditions can result in disturbances in brain function. Stroke or cerebrovascular accident, discussed in Chapter 7, is the leading cause of neurogenic speech disorders. The third leading cause of death in the United States, strokes cost the economy approximately $30 billion annually (Alberts, Bennett, & Rutledge, 1996). Certain racial/ethnic and gender differences exist in the incidence of strokes. African Americans are more susceptible to strokes and hypertension than are individuals from other ethnic backgrounds (Singh, Cohen, & Krupp, 1996). Although men of all backgrounds have more strokes than women, women seem particularly vulnerable to aneurysms (Leblanc, 1996). Such hemorrhaging is one of the leading causes of cerebral palsy.

Traumatic brain injury (TBI), also discussed in Chapter 7, is another leading cause of neurogenic speech disorders. Males who experience TBI far outnumber females, and nearly 70 percent of injuries resulting in TBI occur in the under-35 age group.

Brain injury also may result from deprivation of oxygen as in a drowning accident. Greatly reduced oxygen, or **anoxia,** is a more common cause of prenatal, natal, and neonatal brain injury than of adult injury.

THOUGHT QUESTION

Why are fetuses and newborns more susceptible to anoxia than adults?

Brain tumors, or neoplasms, can also lead to neurogenic speech disorders, destroying healthy brain tissue by taking nutrition, impinging on healthy cells, or increasing the pressure within the brain cavity. At any given time, over 60,000 individuals in the United States have tumors of the nervous system. Not all of these affect speech. Some individuals may experience a slow degeneration of their cognitive abilities, while others have a steep decline. Shortly before her death, a friend was reduced to eye blinks and finger squeezes to communicate. Six months earlier, she had little impaired functioning. Some, but not all, tumors are operable or treatable with chemotherapy.

Infections and toxins may also cause trauma to the CNS, although the incidence of these causes is changing. Infections such as meningitis and viral and fungal inflammations that once threatened healthy brains are now usually treatable by antibiotics if intervention begins in the early stages. The developing embryo is especially susceptible to infections. Some neural infections, such as those associated with new drug-resistant microbes and the human immunodeficiency virus (HIV), the virus that causes AIDS, offer a challenge to our pharmacological methods of treatment.

The list of brain-injuring toxins is lengthy, and new products are being introduced daily. Obvious neurotoxins are lead, mercury, certain pesticides, and pollution, but the most prevalent culprits are alcohol and drug abuse. Some toxins can pass the placental barrier between the mother and her infant.

Diseases, either inherited or acquired, can also affect the nervous system. Many are slow, degenerative diseases that gradually rob their victims of muscular control. A "Who's Who" of this rogues' gallery includes, but is not limited to, multiple sclerosis, amyotrophic lateral sclerosis (ALS), Parkinson's disease, Huntington's disease, and myasthenia gravis. Muhammed Ali, former world heavyweight champion boxer, Janet Reno, Attorney General of the United States in the Clinton administration, and actor Michael J. Fox all have Parkinson's disease. Each of the authors of this text has been touched in some way by a friend or relative with a neurological disease.

Whatever the cause, the speech of affected individuals may vary widely. Even individuals with the same etiology may have very different speech problems, depending on the severity of the disorder, the age of the client, the time since the incident, and the extent of the affected area. To the untrained ear, two very different clients may sound the same and be classified as having speech that is slurred, sloppy, thick, or unclear. Although a client's speech may in fact fit such descriptors, they do little to differentiate between the various etiologies.

CEREBRAL PALSY

The term "cerebral palsy" describes a heterogeneous group of neurological difficulties resulting from brain injury that occurs very early in fetal or infant development. The disorder is nonprogressive, meaning that the condition does not worsen over time. Affected areas include motor movement, communication, growth and development, locomotion, learning, and sensation. Physical manifestations may range from extreme rigidity and immobility to being ambulatory, or capable of moving about relatively freely. Cerebral palsy may affect one or more limbs and might or might not be accompanied by speech difficulties. The cognitive abilities of people with cerebral palsy range from mental retardation through superior intelligence.

Movement patterns are learned from many, many repetitions. Therefore, faulty movement results in faulty patterns being learned. If you have typical motor patterns, you can probably pick up an object without looking at it.

Although the reported incidence is low—1.5 to 3 per thousand births—the data may reflect poor reporting, misdiagnosis, or assignment of other labels, such as mental retardation, because the person has greater disorders in other areas. At present, more than 500,000 individuals in the United States have cerebral palsy; most are under 21 years of age. Approximately 30 to 90 percent of these have some dysarthria (Yorkston, Beukelman, & Bell, 1988).

Three characteristics distinguish cerebral palsy from some of the other neurogenic speech disorders that are discussed. First, it is a developmental neurogenic disorder. Most neurogenic speech disorders are considered to be acquired; that is, typical speech patterns were established before the disorder occurred. The insult to the neurological system with cerebral palsy occurs before the neuromotor system has fully matured. As a result, the child must learn motor movements for which no patterns have been established. Given the neuromotor difficulties of individuals with cerebral palsy, these movements may be learned in an atypical way.

Second, cerebral palsy is not a disease. It is a nonprogressive, noninfectious injury occurring before, at, or shortly after birth. Some children may improve with maturity, especially in the first few years of life as the brain matures rapidly.

Finally, the motor patterns in cerebral palsy are much more predictable than those in acquired neurogenic impairments. Although a person who has suffered a stroke may have severe impairment in an arm and a mild impairment in a leg on the same side, a person with cerebral palsy is more likely to have similar severity in all affected limbs. These may include involvement of the legs (*paraplegia*), all four extremities (*quadriplegia*), one side (*hemiplegia*), or one limb (*monoplegia*).

TYPES OF CEREBRAL PALSY

Not everyone with cerebral palsy is alike. Clients vary in age, culture, education, and type and severity of cerebral palsy. The type of cerebral palsy varies with the areas of the CNS that are affected. Injury may occur in the motor cortex, the pyramidal or extrapyramidal tracts, and the cerebellum.

Most types of cerebral palsy can be classified in one of three ways: spastic, athetoid, or ataxic. Although some infants with cerebral palsy exhibit poor muscle tone and weakness, a condition called **hypotonia,** muscle movement and control almost always evolve during infancy into one of the three predominant types discussed here. *Spasticity,* or **hypertonia,** is a condition in which there is too much muscle tone, especially in the muscles that oppose the bending of joints and that help us to stand erect. Tone increases as muscles are stretched. *Athetosis,* or **dyskinesia,** is a slow, involuntary movement of the body. With a change in an individual's emotional state, such as being under stress, excited, angry, or amused, there may be an accompanying increase in muscle tone. **Ataxia** is uncoordinated movement.

SPASTIC CEREBRAL PALSY

For approximately 60 percent of individuals with cerebral palsy, the prominent characteristic is spasticity, or increased muscle tone. When a muscle of someone with **spastic cerebral palsy** contracts, the opposing muscle may react abnormally to stretch by increasing muscle tone too much. Rigid opposing muscle groups make movement extremely difficult. Described as "exaggerated stretch reflex," movement is characterized by increased muscle tone in the muscles opposing the movement that is attempted. The tone increases as these muscles are stretched, resulting in muscle movements described as jerky, labored, and slow. Individuals with spastic cerebral palsy may also exhibit infantile reflex patterns, such as rooting—that is, the movement of the lips, tongue, and jaw in the direction of stimulation. In nonaffected children, these reflexes typically disappear within a few months of birth.

Individuals with cerebral palsy are a very heterogeneous group, varying in severity, type, and portion of the body affected. Like all individuals, they also differ in personality, interests, and maturity.

Why would movements in spastic cerebral palsy be jerky? Reach for your pen while trying to pull your arm back. Notice how your arm shakes as it moves.

Spasticity results from damage to the motor cortex and/or the pyramidal tract. Unable to direct and control the basal nuclei and other lower structures, higher centers of functioning cannot block signals to increase muscle tone or rigidity; the result is hypertonicity.

In severe cases, the limbs may be rotated inward with the arms drawn upward and the head drawn to one side. Walking or even standing may be extremely difficult. Figure 12.1a shows the posture of an individual with severe spastic cerebral palsy.

ATHETOID CEREBRAL PALSY

Accounting for approximately 30 percent of individuals with cerebral palsy, athetoid cerebral palsy is characterized by athetosis, a slow, involuntary writhing. Athetosis is most pronounced when the individual attempts volitional movement. The resultant behavior may be disorganized and uncoordinated. Individuals with athetoid cerebral palsy may also exhibit infantile reflex patterns throughout their lives. In nonaffected children, these typically disappear within a few months of birth.

Athetosis is caused by injury to the extrapyramidal tract, especially in the basal nuclei. Recall that the basal nuclei help to plan motor patterns and modify motor cortex impulses. When damage to the basal nuclei occurs, cortical impulses cannot be moderated. Inhibitor mechanisms in the extrapyramidal tract cannot appropriately monitor the excitation mechanisms of the motor cortex. The result is too much muscle activity.

In its most severe form, athetosis causes the individual's feet to turn inward, the back and neck to arch, and the arms and hands to be overex-

FIGURE 12.1   Characteristic posture of severe spastic and athetoid cerebral palsy

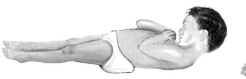

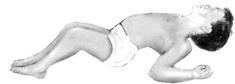

(a) Spastic cerebral palsy   (b) Athetoid cerebral palsy

tended above the head. The mouth may be open, resulting in drooling. Breathing may also be affected. Figure 12.1b shows the posture of an individual with severe athetoid cerebral palsy.

The severity of athetoid cerebral palsy varies between individuals. In a given person, the moment-to-moment strength of the athetosis varies with the situation. When the individual is quiet or at rest, athetosis might not be evident. Athetoid movements occur or are exaggerated when purposeful movement is attempted and when the individual is excited or emotionally upset.

ATAXIC CEREBRAL PALSY

Ataxic cerebral palsy, accounting for approximately 10 percent of the population with cerebral palsy, is characterized by uncoordinated movement and disturbed balance. The individual with ataxia seems clumsy and awkward. Movements lack direction, and hypotonic muscles lack adequate force and rate and have poor direction control. Walking is particularly difficult for the individual with ataxia and, in the most extreme cases, may be characterized by a wide stance with the head pushed forward and the arms back in an almost birdlike appearance. Even those who are less affected may have a gait resembling that of someone who is intoxicated; this can cause occasional social problems.

Ataxia results from injury to the cerebellum. Injury to this part of the brain impairs the monitoring of balance information from the inner ears and of proprioceptive information from the muscles regarding the rate, force, and direction of movements. Coordination of muscle movement is difficult without accurate feedback. It is easy to see why walking would be especially problematic.

It may be difficult to keep the types of cerebral palsy clear in your mind. The major features of each are presented on Table 12.1.

MOTOR SPEECH PROBLEMS ASSOCIATED WITH CEREBRAL PALSY

Not everyone with cerebral palsy has motor speech difficulties. For example, a few individuals have spastic cerebral palsy that involves primarily their legs (paraplegia) with no oral musculature involvement. Nearly all people with athetoid cerebral palsy exhibit an accompanying motor speech disorder that affects all aspects of production. Ataxic speech difficulties may be related to cognitive impairment and phonological processing problems (Love, 1992).

The different types of cerebral palsy result in differing speech characteristics.

Some professionals term the disordered speech of people with cerebral palsy *developmental dysarthria* because it is largely a disorder of motor speech control (Hardy, 1983; Love, 1992). However, adults with acquired motor speech disorders once had typical speech, but

TABLE 12.1

Characteristics of cerebral palsy

Type of Cerebral Palsy	Characteristics	Area of Brain Affected
Spastic	Spasticity, increased muscle tone in opposing muscle groups	Motor cortex and/or pyramidal tract
	Rigidity and exaggerated stretch reflex	
	Jerky, labored, and slow movements	
	Infantile reflex patterns	
Athetoid	Slow, involuntary writhing	Extrapyramidal tract, basal ganglia
	Disorganized and uncoordinated volitional movement	
	Movements occur accompanying volitional movement	
Ataxic	Uncoordinated movement	Cerebellum
	Poor balance	
	Movements lack direction, force, and control	

the developing child did not and consequently may develop atypical motor patterns of production in the process of learning speech using a faulty motor system. In working with individuals with cerebral palsy, the SLP considers both the dysarthric or control dysfunction and the overlaid learning problem.

All aspects of speech production—respiration, phonation, resonation, and articulation, plus prosody—may be affected. Speech may be slow and labored. In severe cases, it may be unintelligible. Swallowing may also be affected, and individuals may exhibit dysphagia (see Chapter 13).

Many individuals with cerebral palsy have breathing difficulties, which, in turn, may affect speech. Breathing may be rapid and shallow. Vital capacity or the total amount of air expelled after a deep inhalation may be decreased, making it difficult for an individual to exhale sufficiently to produce speech. A client's speech may be limited to a word or short phrase.

Inconsistent or inadequate airflow and involvement of the laryngeal muscles will affect phonation. Voice quality may demonstrate hypertonia in several ways, from a breathy voice with puffs of air to a strained voice with hard glottal attack. A breathy voice may indicate a compensatory movement to force air from the lungs.

Resonance difficulties may be characterized by hypernasality resulting from dysfunction of the velopharyngeal mechanism. Inability to seal off the nasal cavity results in loss of air pressure, a critical component for good consonant production.

THOUGHT QUESTION

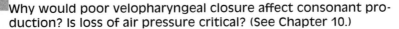

Why would poor velopharyngeal closure affect consonant production? Is loss of air pressure critical? (See Chapter 10.)

Articulation may be extremely difficult if there is involvement of the tongue, lips, and/or jaw. The tongue of an individual with cerebral palsy may move as one unit with limited ability to differentiate its parts. Consequently, consonants, especially those made with the aid of the tip of the tongue—/s/, /z/, /l/, and /r/—will offer a particular challenge. Lip movement may be slow and restricted. As in the motor behavior of typical infants, jaw and tongue movements may be unspecified, and they may move together. Articulation problems in athetoid cerebral palsy seem to result from excessive jaw movement, limited tongue mobility, and velopharyngeal insufficency.

The prosodic aspects of speech—pitch, loudness, and duration—may be very monotonous. The client may be unable to perform the subtle oral movements that are necessary to convey shades of meaning or mark grammatical structures or morphological changes. Poor muscle control can make it difficult to initiate phonation and sustain it. The resultant speech may be choppy with short phrases or words and frequent interruptions. Speech may be characterized as nonrhythmic or nonfluent.

Other factors may also complicate the production of meaningful speech. These include intellectual, auditory, information-processing, and language impairments. Although many individuals with cerebral palsy have average or above-average intelligence, approximately half have some significant cognitive deficits (Bottenberg & Hanks, 1986). Hearing and speech sound discrimination may also be problematic, especially for individuals with athetoid cerebral palsy. Attentional disorders may also be exhibited.

All of these factors plus injury to adjacent areas of the brain account for the language impairment that is found in many individuals with cerebral palsy. This impairment may include delayed language development and immature linguistic structures and use.

In the absence of established motor speech patterns, the child with cerebral palsy may develop abnormal movement patterns, further complicating intervention.

ETIOLOGY

It would be impossible to catalogue all the possible prenatal, natal, and neonatal conditions that could result in brain damage for an embryo, fetus, or child. In general, the younger the developing being, the more rapidly the brain is maturing, and the more susceptible his or her brain is to damage. The incidence of cerebral palsy is higher for extremely high-birthweight infants, extremely low-birthweight infants, nonwhite babies in the United States, children born to older mothers, multiple births, and males.

The two most common causes of cerebral palsy are anoxia and hemorrhages in the brain. Anoxia, especially to the neuromotor areas of the brain, which are high oxygen users, can kill neurons in the CNS. Any interruption in the blood supply, as occurs in a hemorrhage in the vascular system, a not uncommon event *in utero*, can cause damage to a developing brain.

Premature infants account for only 2 percent of all live births but represent a substantially larger percentage of the population of individuals with disability. In some cases, the premature birth is related to prenatal difficulties, including malformation of the CNS. Premature infants are also more susceptible to neonatal complications, including respiratory dysfunction, that can lead to anoxia.

Infections and toxins may also disrupt brain development. Bacterial and viral infections, such as HIV, may infiltrate the brain from other bodily organs or be transported within the blood supply. During the first few months of pregnancy, before the development of a placental barrier, the embryo is especially susceptible to infections of the mother, such as influenza, rubella, and mumps, that can damage the developing brain. Toxic agents, such as heavy metals, mercury, and lead, may lodge in the brain and disrupt development. In recent years, the increasing use of alcohol and illicit drugs by pregnant women has resulted in more children born with brain dysfunction.

Finally, accidents during pregnancy and in the neonatal period can result in fetal brain injury. The incidence of fetal injury due to automobile accidents has risen in recent years. Sadly, some infants are also physically abused or involved in automobile accidents.

LIFE SPAN ISSUES

Initial parental reactions on learning that their infant has cerebral palsy vary and may include guilt, grief, anger, and denial. One reaction may evolve into another. Typically, parents adjust well to their child but may exhibit *chronic grief*, or the continuing desire for their child to be "normal." The parent-child bonding process may be strained as the child fails to respond in predictable ways. In addition, the care of a child with cerebral palsy may tax the family and introduce stress into the familial relationship.

It may take up to two years to confirm a diagnosis of cerebral palsy among infants with mild involvement. The type of cerebral palsy may change within the first few years, and it is important for the child and family to be in contact with medical and educational professionals. Motor delays associated with cerebral palsy are often the first sign.

Children with cerebral palsy usually begin school or receive intervention services early in life. Training emphasis is on physical movement and communication. Communication training may focus on both speech and language, and augmentative/alternative communication methods, discussed in Chapter 15, may be introduced.

Variables such as severity, associated disorders, parental involvement, and school system flexibility are important in determining the appropriate educational environment. In general, children with average or better intelligence and mild cerebral palsy are more likely to have a more typical educational experience. It is extremely important to assess appropriately the cognitive abilities of people with severe motor disabilities, because a physical handicap may obscure intellectual functioning.

Many individuals, especially those with mild physical and cognitive difficulties, obtain higher education and/or go into competitive employment. Often, physical adaptations are made to improve performance. Other individuals may work and learn in centers run by United Cerebral Palsy, another agency, or the state. Sheltered workshops and day treatment programs also provide training in daily living and vocational skills for individuals with severe involvment and/or cognitive impairment. Box 12.1 presents the story of a young man with cerebral palsy.

ASSESSMENT

As with many other disorders discussed in this text, assessment and rehabilitation for people with cerebral palsy is a team effort. The team usually includes a pediatrician who often first identifies a disorder; a neurologist who confirms the diagnosis and describes the child's disability; a physical therapist who, along with an orthopedic surgeon, identifies motor patterns and implements muscle training and exercise to increase muscle tone, strength, and timing, and movement accuracy; an otolaryngologist who investigates and makes recommendations about the ear, nose, and throat; and a speech-language pathologist. Over the individual's life span, other professionals, including an occupational therapist, special education teacher, clinical psychologist, audiologist, ophthalmologist, rehabilitation engineer, and/or social worker, may also be involved. It is essential that professionals and parents become involved in the intervention process together as soon as possible.

Intervention team membership changes in response to the changing life span challenges of the individual with cerebral palsy.

BOX 12.1

Personal Story of a Boy with Cerebral Palsy

Tony was born three months prematurely in a small rural hospital. The delivering obstetrician was concerned about possible oxygen deprivation at the time of birth, although Tony was placed in an incubator shortly after he was born.

Because of their son's prematurity, Tony's parents were counseled to expect developmental delays. They reported that he was irritable and seemed to have difficulty ingesting milk. At 4 months, his pediatrician expressed concern because of the continued presence of some reflexive behaviors, such as the whole-body response to startle, and the lack of motor responding, such as eye-hand coordination. She referred Tony to a developmental team in a large urban hospital.

The interdisciplinary team consisted of a pediatrician, neurologist, physical therapist, occupational therapist, developmental specialist, and speech-language pathologist. They determined that Tony had cognitive and motor delays and moderate dyskinesia or athetoid cerebral palsy.

As a result of the evaluation, it was recommended that Tony participate in a home-based interdisciplinary program with periodic reevaluation at the hospital. During the evaluation and subsequent consultation, Tony's parents heard the term "cerebral palsy" used to describe their child for the first time. The team recommended that the parents receive counseling and participate in a parents' group as a portion of their son's intervention plan.

By age 3, Tony was able to self-feed handheld food with some difficulty. Dressing was limited to completing tasks, such as pulling down a shirt that had been fitted over his arms and head. He could walk with great difficulty and usually needed support to steady himself. His speech consisted of a few words and phrases that were often unintelligible to people other than family. When unsure of his meaning, the family often used the immediate situation for interpretation.

At this time, Tony was enrolled in a special preschool for children with disabilities. On the advice of the school's speech-language pathologist, he began training with AAC. At first, this involved pointing to pictures on a communication board. Although his pointing response was somewhat imprecise, he continued to use the communication board until he entered elementary school. In first grade, Tony began to use a direct selection method of communicating using a computer and a joystick interface. Pictures evolved into words, then to individual letters. Now in third grade, Tony is communicating using a combination of his own speech and selection of pictures, words, and simple spelling on a computer, which he accesses by using the joystick control. He has a computer at home and in school for his use.

Early symptoms of cerebral palsy may include irritability, weak crying and sucking, excessive sleeping, little interest in surroundings, and persistence of primitive reflexes beyond the newborn stage. When necessary, the SLP will be involved beginning in the child's infancy.

Speech and language problems differ with the type and severity of cerebral palsy and with the age and functioning level of the individual. In addition to the procedures outlined in Chapter 5, the SLP will want to make a more thorough evaluation of the oral mechanism and, in many cases, to assess potential client success with an augmentative/alternative form of communication. Within the oral peripheral examination, the SLP will note the following with particular interest:

> Symmetry, configuration, color, and general appearance of the
>   tongue, palate, lips, teeth, and jaw
> Movement of the tongue, soft palate, lips, and jaw
> Swallowing (see Chapter 13 for details)
> Valving
>   Lung capacity and control
>   Phonatory initiation, maintenance, and cessation
>   Pitch and volitional pitch variations
>   Loudness and volitional loudness variations
>   Volitional pitch-loudness variations
>   Velophayngeal adequacy
>   Range, velocity, and direction of tongue, lip, and jaw movement

The specific tasks will be modified for young children, who may be unable to follow directions.

Oral motor abilities will be very important in determining the appropriateness of augmentative/alternative communication (AAC). As the individual matures and develops, the AAC system must be continually reevaluated to determine whether it still maximizes the client's potential for communication (see Chapter 15).

It is extremely important that the AAC systems evolve with the client's abilities and needs.

The long-term nature of cerebral palsy necessitates the establishment of realistic long-term goals. Limits to motor function improvement exist and must be considered. Once set, goals must be continually reevaluated. Team members can often help each other to set achievable goals.

INTERVENTION

Speech and language training is essential for many individuals with cerebral palsy to correct or compensate for faulty motor speech patterns. Efficient motor patterns are strengthened, and inefficient ones are modified.

Because one motor pattern, such as breathing, may affect another, such as phonation, most SLPs now believe that it is best to target motor movement within the ongoing process of speech production. A systems approach—one that targets efficient use of the entire speech production system, rather than one that focuses exclusively on one organ or structure—is generally accepted. For example, a systems approach might consider poor lung capacity to be adequate for speech if the client can be taught to use shorter units of production, thus negating the need to strain the breathing system by increasing the demand. In other words, speech production may be possible within the physiological limitations of the individual. In contrast, a focused approach might target lung capacity and efficient breathing alone. In a second example, a clinician using a systems approach might train rate control or the slowing of speech rate to increase overall speech intelligibility. A focused approach might target speech sound production exclusively.

Prosthetic devices and/or intraoral surgery may help to decrease hypernasality. However, these procedures alone will be insufficient, and the client must be trained with the new or repaired structure (see Chapter 10).

Exercises to improve nonspeech movement are usually minimized. Little carryover exists from nonspeech to speech movement patterns (Love, 1992). Likewise, exercising specific muscle groups, such as those for respiration or articulation, does little to improve speech.

Specific sounds will be targeted on the basis of the ease of production. For the child with accompanying language deficits, these sounds and the child's interests will be important in the selection of initial words to be trained. The child's interests and the demands of the environment will also be important in content selection with augmentative/alternative communication.

Motor performance of individuals with cerebral palsy can often be improved by consideration of positioning and placement of the trunk, neck, and head for maximum facilitation.

The SLP often works closely with the physical therapist to maximize and facilitate movement patterns. Some employ the *Bobath method*, a procedure using head, body, and limb postures that inhibit reflexive and uncontrolled movements. The child is placed in positions that prohibit certain reflexive movements. For example, the child with athetoid cerebral palsy may be seated with her or his legs bent or flexed and feet firmly supported to inhibit extensor patterns. Once the child can perform desired movements within a reflex-inhibiting posture, the posture is gradually changed to a more functional one while attempting to maintain the desired movement. Even SLPs who do not subscribe to this method of intervention generally accept the notion of using either postural supports or seating systems to improve movement.

Parents must be counseled by the SLP and other professionals regarding their expectations for their child. It is important that parents be realistic about their child's functioning level and the prognosis for change. SLPs must be careful not to mislead parents who have a natural desire for their child to improve. Attempts to reach unattainable goals result in the placing of unrealistic demands on children. Interaction between the family, child, and professionals is essential, and the family should be involved as a fully participating member of the intervention team.

For many individuals with severe cerebral palsy, unaided augmentative and alternative communication (AAC) systems, such as sign, are inappropriate. However, neuromuscular involvement of the arms and hands makes signing difficult. For these individuals, aided electronic AAC can greatly enhance communication abilities. Recent technological advances have improved intelligible synthetic speech, flexibility of access through increasing variability in devices, and portability. In general, systems with individualized vocabulary and with letter encoding rather than icon or symbol encoding work best and provide optimal flexibility, although individual assessment is needed to determine the optimal system, including the client-device interface or input mode (Angelo, 1992; Light & Lindsay, 1991; Silverman, 1995; Yorkston, Smith, & Beukelman, 1990). See examples on the accompanying CD-ROM.

Much research needs to be done on the effects of AAC on language acquisition in children with cerebral palsy. Research findings suggest that making the process more typical facilitates acquisition (Rhea, 1997). Emphasis on the communication environment of these children is particularly important (Calculator, 1997; Light, 1997). AAC devices may be integrated into a client's technology system. For example, a keyboard that is used for functional communication may also serve as an alternative keyboard for the client's desktop computer.

It is not enough that the client learn symbols—pictures, pictographs, or letters—to be used in communication. Successful use of AAC requires operational, linguistic, social, and strategic competence (Light, 1989). Operational competence enables a client to make maximal use of the device. Linguistic and social competence is needed for the give and take of conversation. Finally, strategic competence includes individual strategies that each client uses to maximize the communication process and make it as typical as possible. These topics are discussed in more detail in Chapter 15.

To be maximally effective, AAC must be integrated into the user's everyday routine, and conversational partners must be trained in its use.

THE DYSARTHRIAS

As was mentioned previously, dysarthria is a group of neuromuscular impairments that may affect the speed, range, direction, strength, and timing of motor movement as the result of paralysis, weakness, or discoordination of the muscles. Motor movements that were previously established may have been lost or modified in some way, though the pattern for that movement still exists. The processes of respiration, phonation, resonation, and articulation all may be affected. Motor function may be excessively slow or rapid, decrease in range or strength, and have poor directionality and timing. It may be more appropriate to

It might seen strange that movement would be altered but the pattern remain. Have you ever broken a bone? Although movement is altered, you still remember how to make that movement.

speak of *the dysarthrias,* given the wide variety of impairments included under this name.

Speech may be slowed or, in some disorders, be excessively fast or contain involuntary movements. The range of movements may decrease until only tiny, barely discernible ones are possible. Direction may become imprecise and nonrepeatable. Strength may decrease, and timing may become either erratic—fluctuating wildly—or monotonous. Unlike apraxia, a problem of motor planning and coordination, which we discuss later in this chapter, the dysarthrias represent difficulties in motor speech control.

Speech intelligibility is most affected by motoric impairment of the tongue, lips, jaw, and soft palate. A variety of speech features may be affected, and describing them may overwhelm even a seasoned speech-language pathologist. Features that affect articulation, voicing, prosody, and respiration may be intertwined. Accurate description requires the SLP to unweave each speech parameter. The speech pattern presented by a client depends on the location and extent of the neural damage as well as on the etiology. Table 12.2 presents possible speech dimensions that may be observed in clients with dysarthria. Note that several parameters of voice, mentioned in Chapter 9, are present.

Dysarthria is not a language disorder. The individual with dysarthria but no other complications exhibits good language structure and vocabulary, has good reading comprehension, can participate in the give and take of conversation as well as her or his physical limitations permit, and is able to convey by other means, such as a computer, sentences that she or he seems unable to produce freely through speech. Audio and video speech samples of persons with dysarthia are presented on the accompanying CD-ROM.

TYPES OF DYSARTHRIA AND ASSOCIATED ETIOLOGIES

The muscular disorders that are found in dysarthria represent a variety of neurological diseases. Although individuals with dysarthria share some common symptoms, distinct clusters of neurological and speech characteristics exist that describe particular variations of the disorder.

Different types of dysarthria are the result of lesions to different parts of the CNS and PNS. Certain commonalities exist, as noted in Table 12.3. These include inadequate breath supply; voice deviations, such as pitch variations and breaks and voice quality anomalies; prosodic problems of slow, rapid, or varying speed; nasality; and articulation errors.

Five distinct types of dysarthria can be identified by their speech characteristics and the impaired neuromuscular processes (Bloom &

TABLE 12.2

Possible speech dimensions of dysarthria

Respiration
    Forced expirations and/or
    inspirations
    Grunt at end of expiration
    Audible inspiration

Voice
    Pitch
        Inappropriate pitch level
        Monopitch
        Pitch breaks
        Voice tremor
    Loudness
        Inappropriate loudness level
        Alternating loudness
        Excess loudness variation
        Monoloudness
        Loudness decay
    Quality
        Harsh, strained/strangled, or
        continuous or transient breathy
        voice
        Hyponasality or hypernasality
        Nasal emissions
        Voice stoppages

Prosody
    Inappropriate rate
        Increased overall or in segments
        or variable
        Prolonged intervals
        Short rushes of speech
        Short pauses
        Inappropriate silences
        Stress
            Reduced or excess and equal

Articulation
    Imprecise consonants
    Phonemes repeated or prolonged
    Vowels distorted

Source: Adapted from Darley et al. (1975).

Ferrand, 1997; Darley, Aronson, & Brown, 1975; Rosenbek & LaPointe, 1985). These include **flaccid, spastic, ataxic, hyperkinetic,** and **hypokinetic dysarthria.** Disorders affecting multiple motor systems may yield a mixed dysarthria, as is found in ALS, multiple sclerosis, and Wilson's disease, to name a few. Each type of dysarthria and etiology is discussed briefly below.

Dysarthria is a group of related motor disorders with a variety of etiologies and sites of lesion.

TABLE 12.3

Characteristics of the dysarthrias

Type of Dysarthria	Voice Quality	Speech Rate	Articulation
Flaccid dysarthria Weak, soft, flabby muscle tone; lesions in the lower motor neurons (cranial and spinal nerves) or in the muscle unit itself	Breathy voice, monopitch/tone, hypernasality, reduced pitch/loudness	Short phrases	Imprecise consonants
Spastic dysarthria Stiff and rigid muscles; lesions in the upper motor neurons and the pyramidal tract	Monopitch/loudness, reduced stress, harsh voice, hypernasality, strained/strangled voice	Slow	Imprecise consonants
Ataxic dysarthria Damage to the cerebellum; muscle weakness and coordination problems involving accuracy, timing, and direction	Excessive and equal stress, harsh voice	Prolonged pauses and rate	Imprecise consonants, irregular articulatory breakdown
Hyperkinetic dysarthria Increased movement from lesions of the extrapyramidal tract and basal nuclei	Monopitch, harsh voice, excess loudness	Variable rate, silences, prolonged intervals	Imprecise consonants, distorted vowels
Hypokinetic dysarthria Decrease or lack of appropriate movement from lesions of the extrapyramidal tract and basal nuclei; muscles rigid and stiff	Monopitch/loudness, reduced stress, harsh/breathy voice	Variable rate, silences, prolonged intervals	Imprecise consonants
Mixed dysarthrias Severe muscle weakness from diffuse brain damage	Hypernasality, harsh voice, low pitch, monopitch/loudness, excess and equal stress	Slow rate, prolonged intervals	Imprecise consonants, distorted vowels

Source: Adapted from Darley et al. (1975).

FLACCID DYSARTHRIA

Flaccid muscles possess a weak, soft, flabby tone, called *hypotonia*, resulting in weakness or paralysis of the affected muscle. Dysarthria of this type usually results from lesions in the lower motor neurons (cranial and spinal nerves) or in the muscle unit itself. Weak muscles tire quickly. Affected muscles may cause reduced vital capacity and shallow breathing, breathy voice and aphonia, reduced pitch and loudness levels, monotone, hypernasality, and imprecise articulation. Bell's palsy, a facial nerve disorder; bulbar palsy; myasthenia gravis; and muscular dystrophy are characterized by flaccid paralysis.

BULBAR PALSY A flaccid dysarthria, **bulbar palsy** results from involvement at the synaptic or neuron level. Most likely, the neurons or synapses fail or are slow in chemically resetting after nerve firing. In addition, bulbar palsy is characterized by muscle atrophy and by random and irregular contractions (**vasiculation**) of nerve bundles. These rapid, minute contractions have been described by individuals with bulbar palsy as feeling like a bubbling under the skin. Tremors may be obvious in the tongue when it is extended. In general, the speech of these individuals is weak, hypernasal, and monopitched with articulation difficulties. A sample of the speech of a person with bulbar palsy is presented on the accompanying CD-ROM.

MYASTHENIA GRAVIS A common disorder, **myasthenia gravis** affects the neuromuscular juncture. The disorder is characterized by a rapid weakening of the muscle due to the inadequate transmission of the nerve impulse. Muscles tire quickly but regain their strength after a short interval of rest. Velar and laryngeal muscles are often affected.

MUSCULAR DYSTROPHY In **muscular dystrophy,** the muscles themselves are affected. Muscles may be unable either to contract or to relax. A progressive degenerative disease, muscular dystrophy may eventually affect all aspects of speech.

SPASTIC DYSARTHRIA

Spastic paralysis—stiff and rigid muscles—is the result of lesions in the upper motor neurons and the pyramidal tract. The most common cause is stroke, and the results may be temporary or permenent. Lesions in the left hemisphere may be accompanied by aphasia and result in mild spasticity (see Chapter 7). More severe spastic dysarthria is bilateral, with the site of lesion in areas such as the brain stem where left and right innervation are in close proximity. Hypertonia makes movement difficult, and speech is characterized as slow with jerky, imprecise articulation and reduction of the rapidly alternating movements of speech.

PSEUDOBULBAR PALSY **Pseudobulbar palsy** is an example of spastic paralysis. Although individuals with pseudobulbar palsy exhibit the muscle weakness and loss of movement that are found in bulbar palsy, muscle atrophy and vasiculation do not seem to be present. Movement is characterized by hyperflexia, a combination of overreaction and over-reach. The voice of individuals with pseudobulbar palsy is strained and strangled-sounding, resulting from intermittent spasticity. The rate is slow, and articulation is imprecise.

ATAXIC DYSARTHRIA

Damage to the cerebellum can result in a combination of muscle weakness or reduced tone or hypotonia and problems with muscle coordination, called **ataxia** (Kent et al., 2001). Ataxic dysarthria is the result of breakdown in motor organization and control (Duffy, 1995). Little or no paralysis exists, and the problem is one involving the accuracy, timing, and direction of movement. Movements overshoot. The signal to start a movement is received, and the accompanying inhibition is impaired. As a result, movements are jerky and imprecise. Congenital ataxia is a form of cerebral palsy that is seen in children.

Speech is characterized by a shift in fundamental frequency and variability in the slow rate of moving between different speech sounds (diadochokinesis)(Kent, Kent, et al., 2000). Energy varies across repeated syllables, respiration is poorly coordinated, and voicing and articulation are inadequate and imprecise.

HYPERKINETIC DYSARTHRIA

Hyperkinesia, or increased movement, called tremors and tics, results from lesions of the extrapyramidal tract and basal nuclei. *Tremors* are involuntary, nonpurposeful, rhythmic movements caused by contractions of antagonistic muscles. Several types of tremors exist. **Tics** are involuntary, rapid and repetitive, stereotypic movements. Unlike tremors, tics can be suppressed for short periods of time. One characteristic of hyperkinetic dysarthria is inaccurate articulation. Two disorders, dystonia and chorea, are forms of hyperkinetic dysarthria.

DYSTONIA **Dystonia** is characterized by a slow increase and decrease of hyperkinesia involving either the entire body or localized sets of muscles. Excessive movement is slow and sustained, often writhing in nature. Like chorea, dystonia may involve the entire motor system or be localized. As a result, there are excessive pitch and loudness variations, irregular articulation breakdown, and vowel distortions.

CHOREA Unlike dystonia, **chorea** is characterized by rapid or continual hyperkinesia. Chorea movements are characterized as random, irregular, and/or abrupt, usually lasting less than one second (Rosenfield,

1991). Movement may involve the entire body or a particular segment. Hyperkinesia impairs control and reduces coordination, especially in rapid successive movements such as speech. Speech, when affected, may be characterized by inappropriate silences caused by voice stoppage; intermittent breathiness, strained harsh voice, and hypernasality; imprecise articulation with prolonged pauses; and forced inspiration and expiration resulting in excessive loudness variations (Duffy, 1995).

Huntington's Chorea. An inherited progressive disease that is also known as Huntington's disease, Huntington's chorea results from a genetic defect on chromosome 4 (American Psychiatric Association, 1994). Initial symptoms include involuntary movements and behavior change. As the disease progresses, movements become rigid with reduced speed and difficulty with coordination. Jerky, irregular movements affect the diaphragm, laryngeal muscles, tongue, and lips. In addition to the speech difficulties, language may be affected as a result of cognitive and memory changes. In general, individuals with Huntington's chorea have the same verbal output as their non-Huntington peers, but they are less informative with their language (Murray, 2000). Their language is characterized by a smaller proportion of grammatical utterances and a larger proportion of simple sentences than both non-Huntington individuals and those with Parkinson's disease. Accompanying personality changes may include depression, paranoia, delusional thoughts, and intellectual decline (Greenamyre & Shoulson, 1994).

HYPOKINETIC DYSARTHRIA

Like hyperkinetic dysarthria, hypokinetic dysarthria is caused by lesions of the extrapyramidal tract and basal nuclei, though the result is just the opposite: a decrease or lack of appropriate movement. Muscles become rigid and stiff, resulting in restricted motor movement. One form of hypokinetic dysarthria is found in many people with Parkinson's disease.

PARKINSON'S DISEASE   In **Parkinson's disease,** the individual's muscles become rigid as opposing pairs of muscles contract simultaneously. Motor movements become increasingly reduced, a condition called **hypokinesia.** Other characteristics include involuntary shaking or tremors when at rest, slowness of movement, and difficulty initiating voluntary movements. Symptoms reflect the reduced supply of dopamine, a neurotransmitter found in the extrapyramidal tract, a result of loss of dopaminergic neurons in the basal nuclei. Tremors may be controlled by different neural systems rather than one central tremor generator

(Gurd, Bessell, Watson, & Coleman, 1998). Comments by a professional with Parkinson's disease are presented in Box 12.2

The resultant speech is characterized by a rapid rate, a breathy voice, less speech per breath, difficulty initiating motor movement, and reduced loudness, pitch range, and stress. Although speech rate increases, it may be perceived to be even faster that it actually is (Tjaden, 2000). Although voice changes may occur early in the course of the disease, articulation deficits typically do not. Dysarthria is a symptom in the more advanced stages of Parkinson's disease. Speech may become extremely rapid, accompanied by imprecise consonant formation as a result of weak tongue strength and endurance (Solomon, Robin, &

BOX 12.2

Comments of a Speech-Language Pathologist with Parkinson's Disease

My medication is as helpful as the oil Dorothy used with the Tin Woodsman so that he could move and speak. My oil, pharmacological treatment, temporarily increases the level of dopamine that is reduced by Parkinson's. Unfortunately, the medication does not ensure relief or even last throughout the day. This, coupled with the fact that my schedule as a university professor varies from day to day, makes it challenging to time the medications so that they are at their peak when I need fluid, wide-ranging movement . . . . I live by the clock and I am never without my meds . . . .

One thing that I have learned since I've had Parkinson's is that when we discuss neurological disorders in our class, we so emphasize the effects of these impairments on communication that we underemphasize their broader effects on general health status. As a result, we may inadvertently lead some students to think that Parkinson's is "just" a movement disorder. There are other aspects of this problem that affect health, non-speech physiological function, and state of mind . . . .

Interestingly, the reactions of people to my speech and other movements, particularly when I'm having a bad day, have allowed me to relate better to some of my clients who have told me how hard they concentrate on their speech production in an attempt to monitor for maximum intelligibility. Speech has become a more demanding task for me. I am keenly aware of the changes in my speech and work at a high level of consciousness to make online adjustments to preserve normal-sounding articulation.

Source: From Caruso, A. J. (2001, July 24). Parkinson's disease and me. *The ASHA Leader,* 6(13), 7. © American Speech-Language-Hearing Association, reprinted by permission.

Luschei, 2000). Speech deficits may be accompanied by a decrease in nonlinguistic communication, such as gestures and facial expression.

Although individuals with Parkinson's have a similar verbal output to their non-Parkinson peers, they are less informative with their language (Murray, 2000). Individuals with Parkinson's disease also have a smaller proportion of grammatical sentences.

The most common form of Parkinson's disease occurs in 1 percent of the population over age 50 (Duvoisin, 1991). In real numbers, approximately half a million individuals have Parkinson's disease in the United States, and about 40,000 new cases occur annually (McDowell & Cederbaum, 1988). A sample of the speech of a person with Parkinson's disease is presented on accompanying CD-ROM.

MIXED DYSARTHRIAS

Some dysarthrias are not easily classified within the above system. Called **mixed dysarthrias,** these disorders are characterized by symptoms or areas of brain injury that cross several dysarthrias. Diffuse brain damage may result from degenerative disorders, toxins, metabolic disorders, stroke, trauma, tumors, and infectious diseases. Amyotrophic lateral sclerosis is one example of this category.

AMYOTROPHIC LATERAL SCLEROSIS   Commonly called Lou Gehrig's disease for the baseball player who was afflicted with it in the early twentieth century, **amyotrophic lateral sclerosis (ALS)** is a rapidly progressive degenerative disease that involves both the upper and lower motor neurons and spinal cord. Males are affected more frequently than females, the first symptoms typically appearing between 40 and 70 years of age. Death usually occurs within five years after the initial diagnosis.

Mental capacity is not affected, but the individual gradually loses control of her or his musculature. ALS is characterized by fatigue, muscle atrophy (loss of bulk), involuntary contractions, and reduced muscle tone. Speech deficits are common in the later stages of the disorder (Yorkston, Strand, Miller, Hillel, & Smith, 1993). These include a labored, slow rate; short phrasing, long pauses, hypernasality, and severely impaired articulation (Duffy, 1995). The slow rate influences the timing of elements within each sound, distorting its production (Tjaden & Turner, 2000).

ALS combines both flaccid and spastic dysarthria. Dysarthria increases as the disease progresses, approximately 75 percent of affected people being unable to speak at the time of death. Age of onset is usually in the mid-fifties. Incidence figures vary but may be as high as 2 per 100,000 individuals. A sample of the speech of a person with ALS is presented on the accompanying CD-ROM.

Can you imagine the terror of losing motor control while being fully cognizant of the process? Have you ever broken an arm or a leg? If so, you know a little of the frustration faced by those with physical disabilities.

LIFE SPAN ISSUES

Most acquired dysarthria occurs in adults. Even the individual with mild dysarthria may be reluctant to speak, leading to assumptions by others that the person is frightened, tense, shy, or unfriendly. For some individuals, even a slight speech imperfection can be cause for embarassment or depression. In the more advanced dysarthrias, individuals may be frustrated as loved ones and acquaintances attempt to communicate for them by finishing sentences or ordering for them in restaurants. In turn, the individual may communicate and socialize less. Difficulty communicating may limit the opportunities to participate in social, occupational, and educational activities, leading to feelings of isolation.

Neuromotor problems are not limited to speech production and may have a profound effect on many aspects of an individual's life.

Some individuals with dysarthria are unable to live independently and may need daily living assistance or institutional care. The social, physical, psychological, and familial adjustments in this situation can be enormous.

In the later stages of progressive degenerative disorders, the individual may be unable to care for herself or himself. Movement may be very difficult, and the person may be unable to speak. AAC devices may be helpful even for the most severely affected individuals.

ASSESSMENT

The SLP is an important member of the diagnostic team. By identifying differing speech patterns characteristic of specific neurological conditions, the SLP provides valuable information on localized neurological conditions to other team members.

The purposes of evaluation for dysarthria are many and include the following:

To determine whether a significant long-term problem exists

To describe the nature of impaired functions, specifically, the types of problems, their extent/severity, and the effect of these impairments on everyday, functional communication

To identify functions that are not impaired

To establish appropriate goals and decide where to begin intervention

To form a well-reasoned prognosis based on the nature of the disorder, the client's age, the age or stage of injury or disease, the presence of other accompanying conditions, client motivation, and family support

As described in Chapter 5, the speech-language pathologist will want to thoroughly evaluate oral peripheral function, conversational speech, and speech in special tasks.

The oral-motor mechanism is evaluated as outlined in the section on cerebral palsy. Of particular importance in assessment of dysarthria are the range, speed, and direction of oral movement.

Although very few commercially available test procedures are available, most SLPs working in hospitals or outpatient clinics have a standard assessment protocol that they use for motor speech evaluations. These procedures might or might not rely on the use of instrumental approaches and computerized analysis.

INTERVENTION

Some basic principles underlie intervention for acquired motor speech disorders (Darley et al., 1975):

Compensatory strategies: Maximize individual strengths while working to bypass physical limitations.

Automatic to volitional shift: Foster more purposeful control over automatic and overlearned behaviors.

Behavior change monitoring: Maintain precise records and foster self-monitoring by the client.

An early start: Early intervention forestalls formation of bad habits.

Motivation: Provide information and support.

The SLP begins with this basic foundation.

The type of intervention, its course, and the prognosis will vary with the underlying cause of the dysarthria. Some diseases, such as Parkinson's or Wilson's, are *progressive,* the client's condition degenerating gradually over time. As severity increases or a client becomes less motivated, the prognosis becomes less optimistic. In cases of irreversible disease, therapy goals become holding actions in which the client and the SLP attempt to hold the client's performance at a certain plateau, maintaining the client's speech abilities even as the client's overall function decreases (Yorkston, Miller, & Strand, 1995). Other goals might include teaching compensatory skills, such as the use of an augmentative/alternative form of communication. One young man we know used a keyboard to communicate through his computer. When this became too difficult, he used a joystick to navigate the

Just as the AAC system of the child with cerebral palsy must change as the child matures, so that of the individual with a degenerative disorder must change as the disorder progresses.

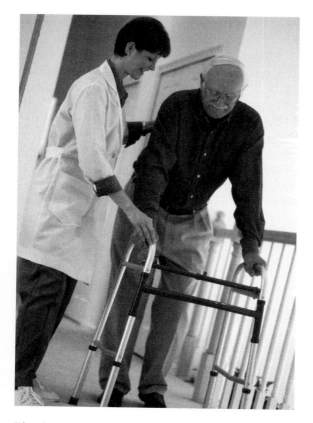

Physical and occupational therapists coordinate their interventions with those of speech-language pathologists.

keyboard. Spelling became too arduous, and electronic picture communication using the joystick was substituted. After several modifications, he now communicates with a combination of eye gazes and hand squeezes.

Because dysarthria affects all aspects of speech production, intervention must address the client's difficulties in respiration, phonation, resonance, and articulation, as well as prosody. Of concern within each area are muscle timing, strength, and tone. Therapy might focus on sustaining phonation, production of nasal and nonnasal words (*met-pet, neat-beat, king-kid*), and speech-sound production in meaningful words.

Intervention is best when it occurs within a meaningful speech context but may include drill, progressively more complex tasks, and feedback. The SLP works with the physical and occupational therapists to coordinate exercises to increase muscle functioning or to decrease hypertonia through relaxation techniques.

Respiratory exercises emphasize efficient breath control and sustained exhalation. These exercises inevitably lead into sustained phonation. Either vocal fold exercises or relaxation techniques accompanied by easy phonation may also be a part of the intervention regime. Intervention for voice disorders is discussed in Chapter 9. Likewise hypernasality, the primary disorder of resonance, is treated through exercise. In addition, prosthetic devices similar to those discussed with cleft palate (see Chapter 11) may be fitted; the client is then trained to use them properly to achieve either velopharyngeal closure or approximation. Although progress in all these areas will improve articulation, such improvement does not preclude working directly with the client's articulation abilities. Exercises will focus on auditory and proprioceptive feedback and placement of the articulators.

Many individuals with severe dysarthria never regain enough intelligible speech to communicate even simple conversational messages. These clients may benefit from the use of AAC as a substitution for or a complement to oral forms of communication. Even something as seemingly simple as alphabet cues in the form of pointing to the first letter of each word being spoken can greatly increase the intelligibility for severely dysarthric speech (Hustad & Beukelman, 2001). Most of the considerations mentioned in the discussion of cerebral palsy are also applicable.

Unaided AAC systems such as sign may be taught if the client does not have accompanying severe aphasia or severe involvement of the hands. Gestures may aid mildly impaired individuals, but involuntary limb movements, such as those found in Parkinson's disease, may interfere with communication (Garcia, Cannito, & Dagenais, 2000). People who have a language disorder in addition to a speech disorder may have some difficulty. Remember that signing is another mode of communication, but language encoding and decoding may still be impaired.

Aided systems, such as communication boards or electronic devices, have been used successfully, although the most common augmentative devices for speakers with dysarthria are speech amplifiers. Communication boards, discussed in detail in Chapter 15, consist of flat, durable surfaces, often attached to a wheelchair. Clients select symbols by touching or looking at them.

Mechanical and electronic devices differ widely in their cost, portability, ease of use, symbol systems, and input and output modes. The most common devices are simple, relatively inexpensive handheld printers with keys for each letter. More complex devices may translate pictures or pictographs into simple messages. Only very careful evaluation can help the SLP to determine the appropriate device and symbol system for a client. Chapter 15 discusses augmentative/alternative communication in detail.

> As long as there is no accompanying cognitive or language impairment, adults may find spelling of words on an AAC device to be an acceptable substitute for, or accompaniment to, speech.

Neurosurgical, genetic, and pharmacological interventions hold great promise for individuals with some forms of dysarthria. For example, surgical placement of an electronic stimulator on the globus pallidus of individuals with Parkinson's disease modifies abnormal neural activity in the basal ganglia (Solomon, McKee, et al., 2000). As a result, oral tremors decrease and the amount of voluntary responding increases. Unfortunately, the separately affected centers for speech and nonspeech movement respond differently to intervention (Camicioli, Oken, Sexton, Kaye, & Nutt, 1998).

APRAXIA OF SPEECH

Apraxia is a disorder in volitional or voluntary motor placement and sequencing that is unrelated to muscle weakness, slowness, or paralysis. It is the result of an acquired neurological impairment of the ability to program—organize and plan—and execute movement of the speech muscles for the production of volitional speech. Because apraxia can affect any muscle group, apraxia that affects the initiation and execution of the movement patterns particular to speech is more correctly called *apraxia of speech* or *verbal apraxia*. Apraxia of the mouth area is termed **oral apraxia** and is often, but not always, observed in association with apraxia of speech.

Apraxia of speech is a problem of speech-sound articulation and prosody or rhythm caused by a neurologically based movement disorder (Darley et al., 1975; Haynes, 1985; Kearns & Simmons, 1988; Kent & Rosenbek, 1983; Wertz, 1985; Yorkston et al., 1988). Difficulties are not the result of muscle or linguistic processing deficits, although these disorders may co-occur with apraxia of speech. Individuals with apraxia have difficulty planning and executing the movements to position the articulators for correct sound production.

The speech of individuals with apraxia is characterized by groping attempts to find the correct articulatory position, with great variability on repeated attempts. There are frequent speech-sound substitutions and omissions with sound-sequencing difficulties. Distortions and additions also occur. Unlike the person with dysarthria, who makes predominantly distortions and related substitutions, the person with apraxia makes unrelated substitutions, repetitions, and additions.

Recognizing the errors, the individual with apraxia of speech will make repeated attempts to correct them. As she or he tries to produce the correct sound, there are inordinately frequent pauses and reinitiations of words and sentences (Wertz, LaPoint, & Rosenbek, 1991). Unlike the person with dysarthria, who repeats the same error, the individual with apraxia of speech often produces widely varying productions on repeated attempts. A sample of speech from a person with apraxia follows:

> O-o-on . . . on . . . on our cavation, cavation, cacation . . . oh darn . . . vavation, oh, you know, to Ca-ca-caciporenia . . . no, Lacifacnia, vafacnia to Lacifacnion. . . . On our vacation to Vacafornia, no darn it . . . to Ca-caliborneo . . . not bornia . . . fornia, Bornifornia . . . no, Balliforneo, Ballifornee, Balifornee, Californee, California. Phew, it was hard to say Cacaforneo. Oh darn.

T H O U G H T   Q U E S T I O N

How do you know when you pronounce a word incorrectly? Does it sound wrong? Does it also feel wrong in your mouth?

Consonants and consonant clusters and blends offer a particular challenge, although more frequently used phonemes and words are produced with more accuracy. As you might expect, complex, long, or unfamiliar words are more difficult to produce, although few of the errors that are produced appear to be attempts to simplify the word.

Individuals with apraxia of speech may have no difficulty producing words on one occasion that they struggled to produce on another. In fact, clients may exhibit periods of error-free speech during automatic or emotional utterances. It is not uncommon to have a client struggle with volitional production of a word such as "vacation" only to hear the client easily say later, "Boy, I sure had a lot of trouble with *vacation*!" A sample of the speech of a person with apraxia of speech is presented on the accompanying CD-ROM.

The speaker with apraxia is typically aware of her or his errors and may even anticipate them but is unable to correct them. Monitoring of speech in anticipation of these errors results in a slowed, almost cautious rate with even stress and spacing.

Clients with apraxia of speech frequently report that they know what they want to say but can't initiate the sequence or keep it going. Faced with a naming task, these individuals frequently respond, "I know it, but I can't say it."

THOUGHT QUESTION

Can you imagine how frustrating it would be to be unable to say what you're thinking? Delay even a few seconds when someone speaks to you and note how it disrupts the conversation.

Although apraxia and aphasia often co-occur in an individual, the two are not the same. Aphasia is a language disorder; apraxia is a motor speech problem. The individual with aphasia will have difficulty with word recall in all modalities, while the person with apraxia of speech can recall the word easily when writing but is unable to say it. In addition, the individual with apraxia of speech has no difficulties with the structure of language. Box 12.3 presents the story of a woman with apraxia.

At this point, no doubt, your head is swimming with seemingly overlapping characteristics of the dysarthrias and apraxia of speech. Table 12.4 on page 415 presents the major differences between the two disorders. As with any attempt to simplify data, individual variations may become lost when presented in a table. The SLP provides the missing data through a thorough diagnostic evaluation adequately describing each person's observable behaviors in detail.

Although we have defined apraxia as a disorder of the mature nervous system, some experts insist that children can also exhibit apraxia of speech, termed *developmental apraxia of speech* (Hall et al., 1993). (see Chapter 10). Data are complicated by causal factors such as TBI and

Personal Story of a Woman with Dysarthria and Apraxia of Speech

Ruth is a 75-year-old female who suffered a stroke in the frontal lobe of the left cerebral hemisphere after surgery. On release from the hospital following her stroke, Ruth began receiving services twice weekly at a rehabilitation center for her speech and for other motor difficulties.

Six months after the incident, her speech is characterized by moderate dysarthria, which is evidenced in poor breath control, decreased loudness, and decreased articulatory precision. In addition, she exhibits apraxia in her ability to initiate and complete functional communication. Her speech is characterized by cluster reduction and inconsistent omission, substitution, and distortion of speech sound and consists primarily of single words. In reading samples, intelligibility decreases with increasingly complex material. Ruth

has difficulty begining speech initiation and with sound and syllable sequencing. Her speech seems to improve with preformulation of the message, word-by-word attack, and gesturing.

Auditory comprehension of both conversation and directions and silent reading comprehension of directions are good. Although she reads the newspaper, she seems uninterested in the more substantial pleasure reading that occupied much of her time previously. Ruth's memory and attention seem unaffected.

A retired schoolteacher and widow, Ruth lives alone. She has six children. Her two oldest daughters are attempting to supplement the home health care she receives. Ruth's diet consists primarily of soft foods and semiliquids, which require more time for ingestion than was previously allotted for meals.

disagreements over the exact characteristics (Thompson, 1988). Most frequently, children who are diagnosed as having developmental apraxia of speech exhibit multiple articulation errors, including addition of speech sounds, sound and syllable repetitions, and sound prolongations.

ETIOLOGY

In apraxia of speech, it is not the nerves or muscles that are defective but the part of the brain that coordinates and activates them.

In most clients, apraxia of speech is the result of a lesion in the central programming area for speech: Broca's area in the left frontal lobe (Kent, et al., 2001) (see Figure 3.13). Recall that Broca's area details and plans the coordination of sequenced motor movements for speech, much as an assembly line computer would organize the various aspects of car production. Breakdown in Broca's area makes speech difficult, just as a glitch in a factory computer might cause a chassis to arrive after the component

TABLE 12.4

Differences between dysarthria and apraxia

Dysarthria	Apraxia of Speech
Speech sound distortions	Speech sound substitutions
Substitution errors related to target phoneme	Substitution errors often not related to target phoneme
Highly consistent speech sound errors	Inconsistent speech sound substitution
Consonant clusters simplified	Schwa (/ə/) often inserted between consonants in a cluster
Little audible or silent groping for a target speech sound	Audible or silent groping for a target speech sound
Rapid or slow rate	Slow rate characterized by repetitions, prolongations, and additions
No periods of unaffected speech	Islands of fluency
Little difference between reactive or automatic speech and volitional speech; both affected	Often very fluent reactive or automatic speech, nonfluent volitional speech

parts to be installed have already moved on or painting to occur before completion of the body. Without a plan, the person with apraxia of speech has difficulty placing the articulators and sequencing his or her movement. Chewing, sucking, and swallowing may be possible, but speech is inconsistent. The language message is sent from Wernicke's area in the left temporal lobe, but production through speech is difficult.

ASSESSMENT

Because of the nature of apraxia of speech, the SLP must pay special attention to additional aspects of assessments. These include the following:

Imitation of single words of varying lengths
Sentence imitation
Reading aloud
Spontaneous speech
Rapid repetition of "puh," "tuh," "kuh," and "puh-tuh-kuh"

Note that a number of the tasks are repetitive or imitative in nature. Recall that in apraxia, performance may vary with repeated performance. Modes of stimulus presentation are also important because the person with apraxia performs better to auditory-visual stimuli than to either auditory or visual stimuli alone.

INTERVENTION

In conjunction with other health professionals, the SLP attempts to increase muscle tone and strength, especially those of the speech mechanism. Increased tone in the body may be accomplished with the use of braces and girdling or by postural adjustments. Prosthetic devices such as slings should be used only with the concurrence of the client's physician. The sequenced production of speech sounds and motor planning that are needed to accomplish this may begin with practice of nonspeech movements

Intervention often begins with sensory bombardment, in which the client hears the correct sound or word repeatedly and sees it in print. Gradually, the client moves to imitation, followed by simultaneous production and finally spontaneous speech. The SLP and the client discuss how the sound or word felt when the articulators were moved. More difficult sounds, consonant clusters, and words are gradually introduced. For clients with severe apraxia of speech, AAC may be introduced (see Chapter 15).

Some individuals will need additional input to be successful. The SLP may provide visual and physical cues and/or aid with physical manipulation. Electromagnetic articulography (EMA), which tracks oral movement, can remediate some articulatory deficits by providing visually guided biofeedback for tongue tip position improvement (Katz, Bharadwaj, & Carstens, 1999).

A decreased rate of production may also improve production. Some clients benefit from the use of carrier phrases that are repeated with each word, such as "I like _____" or "I want _____." Frequently used phrases such as "How are you?" are also practiced and incorporated into the client's verbal repertoire to help the client's speech to sound more

SUMMARY

The major types of neurogenic motor speech disorders are cerebral palsy, dysarthria, and apraxia of speech. Cerebral palsy is characterized as a group of developmental, nonprogressive neurological difficulties resulting from brain injury that occurs very early in fetal or infant development and affects motor movement, communication, growth and development, locomotion, learning, and sensation. The three main types of cerebral palsy—spastic, athetoid, and ataxic—result in very different motor patterns and speech difficulties.

Dysarthria is a group of acquired impairments that affect the speed, range, direction, strength, and timing of motor movement as the result of paralysis, weakness, or discoordination of the speech muscles. Unlike apraxia of speech, the dysarthrias represent difficulties in motor speech control. Five distinct types include flaccid, spastic, ataxic, hyperkinetic, and hypokinetic dysarthria. Disorders affecting multiple motor systems may yield a mixed dysarthria.

In contrast, apraxia is an acquired disorder in voluntary motor placement and sequencing that is unrelated to muscle weakness, slowness, or paralysis and results from a lesion in the central programming area for speech in the left frontal lobe. Called Broca's area, it details and plans the coordination of sequenced motor movements for speech.

Neurogenic motor speech disorders, both developmental and acquired, offer a special challenge to the affected individual, family, friends, and the speech-language pathologist. Many clients are in the very frustrating position of being able to formulate the message but unable to produce it intelligibly.

Intervention methods differ greatly. The child with cerebral palsy may be learning to communicate and to acquire language using an augmentative/alternative communication device. Meanwhile, the older adult with a motor speech problem may be relearning or retrieving older speech patterns. Finally, the individual with a progressive degenerative disease, such as Parkinson's disease or ALS may be attempting to cling to the level of effective communication that was previously possible or exploring additional methods of communication. Changing intervention techniques and promising new surgical procedures and drugs will continue to offer hope to individuals with neurogenic speech disorders.

REFLECTIONS

- What are the major differences between cerebral palsy, dysarthria, and apraxia?
- Name some of the causes of neurogenic speech disorders.
- Describe the main types of cerebral palsy.

- Describe the major types of dysarthria.
- What are the differences between dysarthria and apraxia of speech?
- How do the assessment and intervention techniques used with each neurogenic motor speech disorder differ? How are they similar?

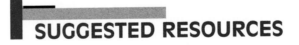

SUGGESTED RESOURCES

Brookshire, R. H. (1997). *Introduction to neurogenic communication disorders* (5th ed.). St. Louis, MO: Mosby.
My Left Foot. (1989). Miramax Pictures.

ON-LINE RESOURCES

http://www.alsa.org/   Amyotrophic Lateral Sclerosis Association.
  Official Web site contains consumer information.
http://www.apple.com/education/k12/disability/
  Apple K–12 resources contains downloadable Mac compatible files for adapting computers for persons with disabilities.
http://www.asel.udel.edu/at-online/
  Contains links and pointers to a variety of AAC topics including Web sites.
http://www.asha.org/professionals/multicultural/fact_14.htm
  Neurological/Fluency/Voice Disorders in Multicultural Populations.
http://www.at-center.com/
  Virtual Assistive Technology Center home page provides access to lists of freeware/shareware for AAC use.
http://www.healthtouch.com/level1/leaflets/ASLHA/ASLHA032.htm
  ASHA factsheet on developmental verbal apraxia.
http://www.irsc.org/cerebral.htm
  Links to online information concerning cerebral palsy.
http://www.ninds.nih.gov/healinfo/nindspub.htm
  National Institute of Neurological Disorders and Stroke Web site containing fact sheets and bibliographies on neurological conditions related to speech problems.

http://www.parkinson.org/

National Parkinson Foundation site contains information and a library with free and on-line publications.

http://www.ucpa.org/

United Cerebral Palsy site with search capability and information on advocacy and disability issues.

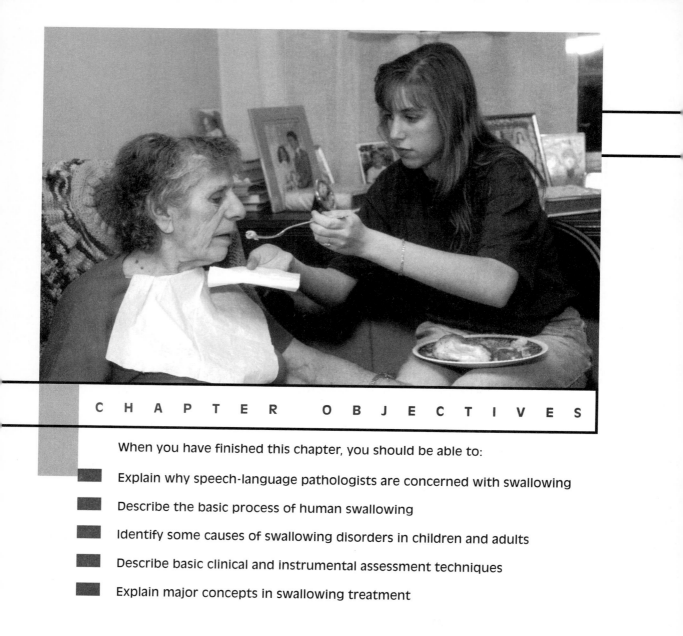

C H A P T E R   O B J E C T I V E S

When you have finished this chapter, you should be able to:

■ Explain why speech-language pathologists are concerned with swallowing

■ Describe the basic process of human swallowing

■ Identify some causes of swallowing disorders in children and adults

■ Describe basic clinical and instrumental assessment techniques

■ Explain major concepts in swallowing treatment

13

Disorders of Swallowing

You might be puzzled to see a chapter about swallowing in a textbook devoted to communication disorders. In fact, the assessment and management of *dysphagia* (swallowing disorders) has been of growing interest to speech-language pathologists, and about 50 percent of SLPs who work in hospitals and extended care facilities do some dysphagia assessment or intervention (Logemann, 1994). SLPs also often take a leadership position in coordinating services for an individual with swallowing difficulties. This degree of involvement depends on strong training and experience with the anatomy and physiology of the oral, pharyngeal, and laryngeal mechanisms (ASHA, 1992). In addition, the vast majority of individuals with dysphagia also have communication disabilities (Martin & Corlew, 1990). The SLP is typically responsible for identifying, evaluating, and treating people from infancy to old age who are experiencing problems with the ingesting and swallowing of food (ASHA, 1990).

The term "dysphagia" comes from the Greek and literally means difficulty with eating. It is pronounced both as "dis-FAH-gia" and as "dis-FAY-gia." The former pronunciation helps to differentiate it from "dysphasia" or "aphasia," which is a language impairment.

As with much of the work that speech-language pathologists do, they do not function alone. SLPs who treat patients with swallowing problems are generally part of a team consisting of a physician, nurse, nutritionist, radiologist, gastroenterologist, dentist, otolaryngologist, neurologist, occupational therapist, physical therapist, and respiratory therapist and family members. The role of each of these specialists will become clear when we discuss evaluation and treatment later in this chapter.

Swallowing and the efficient intake of food have both medical and psychosocial implications. Eating is essential to physical health. Without proper nourishment, one cannot grow, develop, or survive. Swallowing disorders increase the risk of choking and may lead to *aspiration* of food into the lungs and respiratory illnesses such as pneumonia (Langmore, Terpenning, Schork, et al., 1998). Inadequate swallowing may result in **gastroesophageal reflux (GER),** the movement of food or acid from the stomach back into the esophagus. Eating is also one of our major social activities. Feeding difficulties in children may stress the parent-child relationship. Among older people, dysphagia may lead to isolation, depression, frustration, and diminished quality of life.

T H O U G H T   Q U E S T I O N

What connections can you think of between swallowing, speech, and communication?

In this chapter, we describe the basics of swallowing, characteristics and correlates of disordered swallowing, evaluation, and treatment.

THE SWALLOWING PROCESS

Most of us don't typically think about how we swallow food. We know very generally that we put something edible in our mouth, chew for a while, and then swallow. Sometimes, however, we experience difficulty that calls attention to the process. For example, we might eat and cough or feel that the food has "gone down the wrong pipe." Occasionally while drinking, we might laugh and find that fluid comes out of our nose. Once in a while, we feel "all choked up" for an emotional reason and feel unable to eat and swallow. Perhaps you can recall a recent illness in which food that you've eaten was regurgitated; you "threw up" in what felt like a reverse swallow. Before we can understand disorders of swallowing, we need to examine the basics of nonproblematic swallowing. Normal swallowing can be described in four phases: anticipatory, oral, pharyngeal, and esophageal. Normal swallowing is presented on the accompanying CD-ROM.

ANTICIPATORY PHASE

Do you occasionally salivate as you pass a candy shop? How about when you're selecting ice cream at your local grocery store? When you do, you are preparing your mouth to take in food. You probably position yourself to eat by sitting down. A pleasant aroma and an attractive presentation stimulate your hunger, and you become physiologically ready to take in food. Many individuals have a ritual that they perform before a meal, such as hand washing, silent or spoken grace, or a sip of water or other beverage that helps to set the stage for eating. Without this premeal interlude, eating might feel rushed and less satisfying.

ORAL PHASE

The oral phase is sometimes considered in two stages: oral preparatory and oral transport.

ORAL PREPARATORY

When you are ready to eat, you put food or beverage into your mouth and close your lips. In the oral preparatory stage of drinking, the tongue forms a cupped position and holds the fluid in a liquid **bolus,** the substance that is to be ingested, against the front portion of the hard palate. In preparation for swallowing solid foods, the tongue and cheeks move the food to the teeth for chewing and mixing with saliva to form a solid bolus. The prepared liquid or solid bolus is held in the mouth by the soft palate, which moves forward and down to touch the back of the tongue and close the passage to the pharynx or throat.

ORAL TRANSPORT

Once the bolus is formed, oral transport begins. This stage consists of the movement of the bolus from the front to the back of the mouth. When the substance reaches the anterior faucial arch at the rear of the mouth, the pharyngeal swallow reflex is triggered. Oral transport typically takes about 1 second.

PHARYNGEAL PHASE

The soft palate now moves up to meet the rear wall of the pharynx and to prevent the bolus from going into the nasal cavity. The base of the tongue and the pharyngeal wall move toward one another to create the pressure that is needed to project the bolus into the pharynx. While this is occurring, the hyoid bone rises, bringing the larynx up and forward. The larynx prevents the bolus from entering the trachea, or windpipe, by closing the true and false vocal folds and lowering the epiglottis. The pharyngeal phase is complete when the cricopharyn-

The oral and pharyngeal phases of swallowing involve much of the same anatomy that is used in speaking. There is wisdom to the traditional advice "Don't eat and talk at the same time."

geal sphincter opens and the food or liquid moves into the esophagus. The pharyngeal phase usually lasts about 1 second.

ESOPHAGEAL PHASE

The last stage of the swallowing process occurs when the muscles of the esophagus move the bolus in peristaltic or rhythmic, wavelike contractions from the top of the esophagus into the stomach. This typically takes 8 to 10 seconds in an unimpaired individual.

DISORDERED SWALLOWING

Problems in swallowing can occur in any or all phases of the process. A person may lack appetite or be unable to form a bolus and transport it to the rear of the mouth. In addition, difficulties may arise later if the bolus moves inadequately or is blocked as it passes through the pharynx and esophagus to the stomach.

ANTICIPATORY PHASE

Lack of interest in food may be the result of depression or limited alertness. Sensory impairments involving vision and scent may interfere with a person's readiness to accept food. Some individuals, because of neuromuscular difficulties, cannot position themselves appropriately to take in food or liquid. Infants might not be guided to breast-feed adequately, and their lack of success may lead to a downward spiral culminating in termination of attempts to nurse.

ORAL PHASE

If the lips do not seal properly, drooling can occur. Chewing may be impaired because of poor muscle tone or paralysis involving the mouth or because of missing teeth. Insufficient saliva will impede adequate bolus formation. The muscles of the tongue might not function purposefully or efficiently enough to move the food to the teeth for chewing and to transport the bolus from the front to the rear of the mouth to prepare for the pharyngeal phase.

PHARYNGEAL PHASE

Several serious problems are associated with limitations during the pharyngeal phase. If the swallow is not triggered or is delayed, material may be *aspirated,* or fall into the airway, eventually ending in the lungs. Failure to close the velopharyngeal port, the passageway to the nose, can lead to substances going into and out of the nose. Poor tongue mobility may result in insufficient pressure in the pharynx, which is needed to drive the bolus into the esophagus. Aspiration is presented on the accompanying CD-ROM.

ESOPHAGEAL PHASE

If peristalsis is slow or absent, the complete bolus might not be transported from the pharynx to the stomach. Residue might be left on the esophageal walls, resulting in infection and nutritional problems.

T H O U G H T   Q U E S T I O N S

Have you or anyone you know ever experienced a swallowing difficulty? How would you describe it? What was the cause?

LIFE SPAN PERSPECTIVES

Feeding and swallowing problems exist in both children and adults. They may occur at any point in the life span. Newborns may be unable to suckle and/or ingest nutriment. As they age, they may refuse food and develop unhealthy food preferences. Neuromotor problems and structural anomalies that are congenital or acquired at any age can interfere with feeding, as can a host of psychosocial factors. Dysphagia may be related to many diverse conditions; therefore, we will describe only some of the more common ones. The correlates of swallowing disorders are not mutually exclusive; for example, an individual may be impaired in swallowing because of mental retardation as well as laryngeal cancer. Whatever the etiology, the outcomes of a swallowing disorder at any age include malnutrition, ill health, weight loss, fatigue, frustration, respiratory infection, aspiration and even death. Table 13.1 lists common correlates of swallowing disorders in children and adults.

PEDIATRIC DYSPHAGIA

Infants and children with swallowing disorders may experience inadequate growth, ill health, fatigue, difficulty learning, and poor parent-child relationships. Their development may be complicated by a broad spectrum of neurodevelopmental impairments (Rogers, 1996). The dysphagia may occur at any phase and may range from mild to severe. Some of the more prevalent correlates of pediatric dysphagia are described below.

TABLE 13.1

Correlates of swallowing problems in children and adults

Congenital Difficulties	Acquired Conditions
Cerebral palsy	Stroke
Spina bifida	Mouth, throat, laryngeal, or esophageal cancer
Mental retardation/developmental delay	HIV/AIDS
Pervasive developmental disability/autism	Multiple sclerosis
	Amyotrophic lateral sclerosis
HIV/AIDS	Parkinson's disease
Cleft lip or palate	Spinal cord injury
Pierre Robin syndrome	Medications and drugs
Treacher Collins syndrome	Dementia
Pyloric stenosis	Depression and social isolation

CEREBRAL PALSY

Cerebral palsy (CP) is the term for several disorders of motor function that are caused by a defect or lesion in the brain. When CP occurs, it is present at birth or soon thereafter. Cerebral palsy is a permanent, non-progressive condition. This means that although the individual generally does not recover from CP, the disorder should not get worse over time. Cerebral palsy is described in greater detail in Chapter 12, "Neurogenic Speech Disorders." A child with spastic cerebral palsy will have excessive muscle tension, exhibit abnormal postures and movements, and might have an exaggerated gag reflex. As an infant, this youngster may not respond well to breast-feeding. The child may be difficult to hold because of increased muscle tone and an arched posture. Once the nipple is in place, the infant may gag and be unable to rhythmically move the tongue to suckle. Gastroesophageal reflux may make ingestion of food painful. The combined unpleasantness of the feeding situation might make the mother not wish to nurse and might result in an infant who refuses to take food (Prontnicki, 1995).

Although you might expect that the type of cerebral palsy would relate to the presence of dysphagia, individual differences appear to be of greater importance.

About 25 percent of older children with CP have dysphagia. These youngsters may exhibit infantile bite reflexes, drool, have poor trunk control, be on anticonvulsant medication, and cough or choke during meals. Neither the cause and type of cerebral palsy nor the child's age appears to be related to whether a child with CP has a swallowing disorder (Waterman, Koltai, Downey, & Cacace, 1992). In addition, difficulty with sucking in infancy does not appear to be a predictor of swallowing problems later in childhood (Selley, Parrott, Lethbridge, et al., 2001).

SPINA BIFIDA

Approximately 1 in 1,000 infants is born with **spina bifida,** a congenital malformation of the spinal column typically involving associated neural damage, resulting in limited sensation and motor control difficulties. A child with spina bifida may experience feeding difficulties in all phases of the process. Sucking and intake of food are often disturbed, owing to sensory impairments and frequently exhibited dyspraxia (difficulty coordinating movement). The pharyngeal and esophageal stages of swallowing may be affected by cranial nerve damage due to the disorder (Prontnicki, 1995).

MENTAL RETARDATION AND DEVELOPMENTAL DELAY

About 2 of every 100 individuals are considered to have intellectual functioning that is enough below average to be labeled as mental retardation. Children with mental retardation are also delayed in mastering motor coordination, and the delay may interfere with self-feeding and the oral phase of swallowing. Communication disorders are common in this population, and children may be limited in their ability to express food desires and preferences, thereby causing disturbances in the anticipatory phase of swallowing. Many people with mental retardation have associated pathologies such as **Down syndrome** or **Prader-Willi syndrome** or a chronic disease such as **AIDS.** These disturbances further compound the dysphagia (Prontnicki, 1995; Rosenfeld-Johnson & Manning, 1997; Sheppard, 1991).

PERVASIVE DEVELOPMENTAL DISORDER AND AUTISM

Pervasive developmental disorder (PDD) includes a number of difficulties that impair social interaction in children. **Autism** is a severe form of PDD that is characterized by social withdrawal, communicative deficits, and repetitive and stereotypic behaviors. Many children with PDD also have disturbances of body posture and muscle tone. They may be hypersensitive to sound, light, pain, smell, and touch. This pattern of symptoms often contributes to eating difficulties. The social withdrawal and communication difficulties may negatively affect the anticipatory phase of swallowing. Infants do not readily snuggle for nursing; older children do not express their food desires. Impaired body posture and tone may interfere with positioning for eating. Hypersensitivity to smell may cause infants to recoil from food. Hypersensitivity to touch and taste may interfere with the oral phase of swallowing.

Children with PDD often lick, smell, or attempt to eat nonfood items (Prontnicki, 1995).

HIV/AIDS

HIV (human immunodeficiency virus) causes the illness known as **AIDS (acquired immunodeficiency syndrome).** The white blood cells, the brain, and other parts of the body are affected. In children, HIV/AIDS may have been transmitted while the developing infant was *in utero* and/or through the breast milk of an infected mother. Approximately 14 percent of children with HIV/AIDS have serious feeding problems (Grosz, 1989). These may be largely due to lowered immunity to infections such as oral herpes, which occur with some frequency in this population. These lesions in the mouth may result in pain during eating. Children with AIDS may also exhibit mental retardation, language deficits, and attention deficit disorder resulting in anticipatory swallowing problems (Prontnicki, 1995).

STRUCTURAL AND PHYSIOLOGICAL ABNORMALITIES

Children born with cleft palate or lip will be impaired in the oral phase of swallowing. Congenital abnormalities of the jaw, as in **Pierre Robin syndrome,** or of the face, as in **Treacher Collins syndrome,** will also negatively affect the ability to use the mouth for intake of food and swallowing. **Esophageal atresia,** which occurs when the esophagus does not have an open connection to the stomach, prevents normal esophageal swallowing and results in choking. This is a life-threatening condition for newborns and must be surgically treated immediately (Prontnicki, 1995).

Similarly life threatening is **pyloric stenosis,** in which the pyloric sphincter at the outlet of the stomach narrows and prevents food from passing to the small intestine. When this is a congenital condition, the infant vomits and cannot ingest milk or water. Prompt surgical intervention usually successfully corrects this difficulty. Pyloric stenosis may also be acquired later in life; it is caused by peptic ulceration or carcinoma.

Infants who are born today do not spend much time in a hospital. Rapid diagnosis of and attention to congenital defects are essential for the welfare of the child.

DYSPHAGIA IN ADULTS

While most Americans are concerned with excessive weight gain, many aged individuals are at risk for extreme weight loss. Poor nutrition and loss of weight may result in a failure to thrive, which has been termed "the dwindles" (Egbert, 1996). This situation may be the result of physical ailments, muscle weakness or incoordination, medications, psychological factors such as dementia and depression, and/or social isolation. Although most people as they age experience some reduction in swallowing efficiency and lung function, severe dysphagic problems are only likely in the presence of some other disorder such as stroke or the other correlates described in the following paragraphs (Colodny, 2001).

T H O U G H T   Q U E S T I O N S

Why do you think some people in their later years experience eating and swallowing problems? Do you know any older individuals with eating disorders? Have you ever visited a nursing home or adult care facility?

STROKE

In Chapters 7 and 12 we discussed the language and speech implications for someone who has had a cerebrovascular accident or stroke. Persistent dysphagia is also a serious problem for 5 to 10 percent of these individuals, and about twice that number may experience swallowing problems during the first six months after the stroke. Facial paresis (muscle weakness) appears to be the primary factor associated with dysphagia due to stroke. All phases of ingestion are likely to be slowed and impaired. Swallowing and breathing are poorly coordinated, putting the patient at risk for aspiration pneumonia (Nilsson, Ekberg, Olsson, & Hindfelt, 1998). Pneumonia is the cause for about one-third of deaths following stroke (Odderson, Keaton, & McKenna, 1995).

CANCER OF THE MOUTH, THROAT, OR LARYNX

Surgery, radiation, and chemotherapy are used to treat tumors of the mouth, throat, and larynx. Swallowing problems are likely after any type or combination of treatments. Surgery requires removal of the tumor and closing of the wound. For larger lesions, tissue from another area may be excised and used to help patch the deficit. The degree of swallowing impairment is closely related to the size and location of the original tumor and the surgical procedure that is used to close or reconstruct the area. For example, if a relatively small area of the tongue has been removed, a short-term swallowing problem is likely owing to the swelling following surgery. In more radical surgical procedures in which the tongue is sewn into the mandible to close the floor of the mouth, oral swallow will be severely affected (Logemann, 1998).

A visit to the dentist often makes the oral phase of swallowing difficult. Imagine how much more impaired a person is after oral surgery or radiation.

Radiation therapy may result in diminished salivation, swelling, and sometimes mouth sores. The swallowing reflex may be reduced. These interferences with normal swallowing may occur during, soon after, or even a year or two after oral radiation therapy. Chemotherapy may cause nausea, vomiting, and loss of appetite, which will interfere with the eating process (Tierney, 1993).

HIV/AIDS

Individuals with AIDS are susceptible to numerous opportunistic infections because of the immune deficiency nature of the disease. A recent situation was reported in which a 61-year-old man with AIDS complained of swallowing difficulties. The results of the clinical evaluation revealed perforations and growths in the esophagus, which were attributable to Hodgkin's disease, a form of cancer (Gelb, Medeiros, Chen, Weiss, & Weidner, 1997). Esophageal ulcers and esophagitis, or inflammation of the esophagus, were reported in about 16 percent of a group of heterosexual men with AIDS (Yang, Ko, Cheng, et al., 1996).

MULTIPLE SCLEROSIS

Numbness or a "pins-and-needles" sensation in the extremities or on one side of the face may be an early sign of MS.

Multiple sclerosis (MS), a central nervous system disorder, may affect one or several cranial nerves. Multiple sclerosis is of unknown cause and is typically characterized by periods of both relapse and remission. The major general symptoms are poor coordination, muscle weakness, and often speech and visual disturbances. Delayed swallowing reflex and reduced pharyngeal peristaltic action are the primary forms of dysphagia that are associated with multiple sclerosis (Logemann, 1998).

AMYOTROPHIC LATERAL SCLEROSIS (LOU GEHRIG'S DISEASE)

Amyotrophic lateral sclerosis (ALS) is a progressive disease that may begin in middle age. It is characterized by muscle atrophy due to degeneration of motor neurons. Poor tongue movement is sometimes an early sign. ALS may interfere with swallowing in several ways. Reduced tongue mobility may result in spillage into the airway before the pharyngeal swallow has been triggered. The larynx might not elevate and close adequately during the pharyngeal phase. Pharyngeal peristalsis is frequently reduced, causing material to remain in the pharynx. Any of these difficulties could result in aspiration of food or liquid (Hardy & Robinson, 1993; Logemann, 1998).

PARKINSON'S DISEASE

Tremors and rigidity that are visible in a person's extremities may also occur within the body, resulting in swallowing and other difficulties.

Parkinson's disease (PD) is a progressive disorder that typically has its onset in midlife. Its characteristics are slowness of movement, muscle rigidity, and tremor. PD is caused by an inadequate dopamine supply (a natural chemical) to a portion of the brain (the substantia nigra). About 30 percent of individuals with PD have been reported to exhibit dysphagia; however, this is not related to the severity or duration of the disease (Castell, Johnston, Colcher, et al., 2001).

Any or all phases of the swallowing process may be impaired, although in a recent study, only 10 percent of people with PD were found to need dietary advice, and none needed **gastrostomy** (a surgical opening through the abdomen into the stomach through which a feeding tube is inserted) or **tracheostomy** (an opening through the neck into the trachea through which a tube is placed to reduce risk of aspiration) (Clarke, Gullaksen, Macdonald, et al., 1998). When dysphagia occurs, the bolus is usually formed normally in the oral preparatory stage. However, oral transport may be impaired by a front-to-back to front-to-back rolling pattern until the back of the tongue finally lowers sufficiently to permit the bolus to pass to the pharynx. Pharyngeal swallow may be delayed and laryngeal closure may be impaired in advanced cases of PD. Aspiration sometimes occurs when the patient inhales after a swallow, and material remaining in the pharynx falls into the airway (Logemann, 1998). Esophageal motor abnormalities that impede swallowing may occur in PD even in early stages of the disease (Bassotti, Germani, Pagliaricci, et al., 1998; Johnston, Colcher, Li, et al., 2001).

SPINAL CORD INJURY

Individuals who have injured their spinal cords because of accidents have a higher incidence of esophageal dysphagia than noninjured people do. Among the problems that they experience are heartburn, chest pain while swallowing, and slow, abnormal peristaltic contractions of the esophagus (Stinneford, Keshavarzian, Nemchausky, Doria, & Durkin, 1993).

Surgery to the front portion of the upper (anterior cervical) spine may result in dysphagia. These swallowing problems may affect any phase of swallowing. Oral preparatory and transport stages are impaired in some postsurgical patients; others experience weakness in the pharyngeal phase or suffer upper esophageal sphincter malfunctioning (Martin, Neary, & Diamant, 1997).

T H O U G H T   Q U E S T I O N

Why might damage to the spinal cord impair swallowing?

MEDICATIONS AND NONFOOD SUBSTANCES

While medications are used to cure and manage disease, they may also have negative side effects. Some medications, including decongestants, cough suppressants, and muscle relaxants, might make the patient feel drowsy and/or confused. This condition can interfere with anticipation and the oral phase of swallowing. A dry mouth, or insufficient saliva, has been reported to be a side effect of more than 300 medications (Toner, 1997). High doses of steroids may impede pharyngeal swallowing. Antipsychotic drugs may result in **tardive dyskinesia** (involuntary, repetitive facial, tongue, or limb movements) after a year or more of use. At the extreme, tardive dyskinesia may result in the inability to chew and swallow (Feinberg, 1997).

Behaviors such as smoking and ingesting excessive amounts of caffeine and alcohol may also interfere with normal swallowing. Appetite may be depressed and sensations dulled, resulting in anticipatory phase impairment. Alcohol abuse has been implicated in pharyngeal phase dysphasia (Feinberg, 1997).

THOUGHT QUESTIONS

Did you need another reason to stop or not to start smoking? Have you ever experienced the effects of alcohol, caffeine, or smoking on food intake?

DEMENTIA

Unlike mental retardation, dementia is an acquired disorder. Although found in some older people, diminution of intellectual function is not an imperative of aging. We all know people in their eighties and nineties whose minds are sharp and capable. As we learned in Chapter 7, dementia is associated with Alzheimer's disease, several small strokes, Parkinson's disease, multiple sclerosis, and other ailments that may occur among older people. The cognitive deficits of dementia may impede attention and orientation to food. Oral preparatory tongue and jaw movements may be lacking in purpose, resulting in poor bolus formation and drooling. Transport of the bolus may be prolonged. Pharyngeal swallow may be delayed and laryngeal elevation reduced, resulting in possible aspiration (Cherney, 1994; Hardy & Robinson, 1993).

DEPRESSION AND SOCIAL ISOLATION

Life circumstances among the elderly may interfere with several phases of swallowing. Taking a meal is traditionally a social event. We eat with family and friends. As people enter old age, they may find themselves alone and lonely. Spouses and friends have died. Children have moved away. Some may have no experience preparing food and so do not have adequate meals. Others are not motivated to cook just for themselves. Communal meals in retirement homes or long-term care facilities may feature unfamiliar foods and be served in a noisy, hurried environment. Mealtime difficulties in one home for the aged were documented in 87 percent of the residents (Steele, Greenwood, Ens, et al., 1997). Feelings of depression among elderly people are common. Depression is associated with diminished interest in food, restlessness, and fatigue. The throat may feel tight, making swallowing uncomfortable. Some indi-

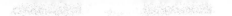

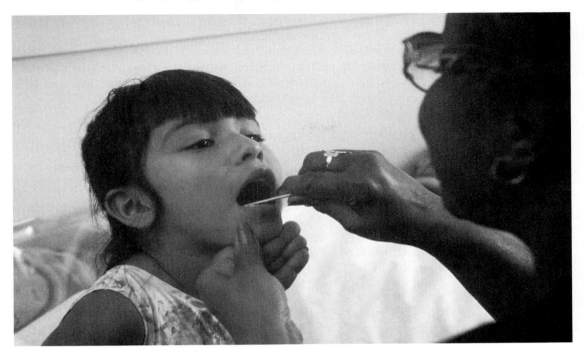

The clinician evaluates the oral mechanism for health, structure, and function.

viduals may feel too tired to eat and then are exhausted after they do eat. This may prompt a cycle of inadequate food intake, weight loss, and malnutrition (Toner, 1997).

EVALUATION FOR SWALLOWING

Not everyone with cerebral palsy, spina bifida, AIDS, multiple sclerosis, stroke, or any of the possible correlates described in the previous sections will have a swallowing disorder. Furthermore, swallowing problems are not always readily apparent. Patients may not report difficulties, and some may experience **silent aspiration** (lack of cough when food or liquid enters the airway) (Logemann, 1996). Therefore, the first step in evaluation is to identify the individuals who are at risk for dysphagia. Following this screening (refer to Chapter 5, "Assessment and Intervention," for a discussion of screening), the speech-language pathologist will serve on a team to obtain background information and to use clinical and instrumental techniques to assess swallowing. A determination is made about appropriate intervention, and treatment strategies are developed and implemented in coordination with other professionals. Speech-language pathologists are advocates for their clients and help to provide education and counseling to them, their families, and related others (ASHA, 1990).

SCREENING FOR DYSPHAGIA IN NEWBORNS AND THE ELDERLY

Some birthing centers have lactation consultants who encourage and assist mothers and infants in the nursing process.

A primary indication of dysphagia in infants is **failure to thrive.** Infants in a neonatal intensive care unit are carefully monitored for weight gain and development. Full-term infants who are not accepting breast or bottle are signaling feeding problems. The *Non-Instrumental Clinical Evaluation (NICE)* is a systematic way of obtaining clinical and family history and observing the child being fed by a caregiver (Scott, 1998). The child's breathing and physical coordination are evaluated. The child's ability to form a seal and suck are assessed by direct observation and by techniques that enable quantification of nutritive and nonnutritive sucking skill (Lau & Kusnierczyk, 2001). Caregivers will be counseled and instrumental evaluation will be recommended when warranted.

Checklists to screen for dysphagia in older individuals are also available. The *Burke Dysphagia Screening Test* is a relatively quick way to screen patients who have had a stroke (DePippo, Holas, & Reding, 1994) (see Table 13.2). The 3-ounce water swallow test used in the *Burke* has been found to identify 80 percent of patients who were aspirating as later confirmed by more elaborate tests (DePippo et al., 1992). Table 13.3 outlines this procedure. If oxygen saturation levels in the blood are measured and assessed before and after swallowing water, the accuracy of the water swallow test approaches 100 percent (Lim, Lieu, Phua, et al., 2001)

Additional screening instruments include the *Examine Ability to Swallow (EATS;* Wood & Emick-Herring, 1997) and the *ROSS (Repetitive Oral Suction Swallow),* which screens swallowing function as individuals sip water through a straw (Nilsson et al., 1998). Stroke patients who, at bedside, exhibit a delay in moving food from the front to the rear of the mouth and incomplete oral clearance signal the likelihood of dysphagic complications (Mann & Hankey, 2001).

For mentally retarded adults and others, inappropriate weight for the person's size may be an indication of nutritional problems that could be due to dysphagia (Sheppard, 1991). All of these measures and indicators have been reported to be useful in identifying serious swallowing difficulties and the need for more complete clinical and instrumental assessment.

TABLE 13.2

The Burke Dysphagia Screening Test

Patient Name: _____

ID Number: _____

Date of Evaluation: _____

	Present	Absent
1. Bilateral stroke	_____	_____
2. Brain stem stroke	_____	_____
3. History of pneumonia acute stroke phase	_____	_____
4. Coughing associated with feeding or during a 3-ounce water swallow test	_____	_____
5. Failure to consume one half of meals	_____	_____
6. Prolonged time required for feeding	_____	_____
7. Nonoral feeding program in progress	_____	_____

Presence of one or more of these features is scored as failing the Burke Dysphagia Screening Test.

Results: Pass   Fail

Source: Used with permission from *Archives of Physical Medicine and Rehabilitation* by W. B. Saunders Co.

TABLE 13.3

Three-ounce water swallow test

Task: Patient drinks three ounces of water from a cup without interruption.

Outcome:

1. No problems.
2. Coughing during swallow.
3. Coughing after swallow.
4. Wet-hoarse voice quality after swallow.

Pass: Outcome 1   *Fail:* Outcome 2, 3, or 4.

Source: Adapted from DePippo, Holas, & Reding (1992).

CASE HISTORY AND BACKGROUND INFORMATION REGARDING DYSPHAGIA

A parent, caregiver, physician, nurse, or professional from an early intervention program or adult day treatment center may make a referral to a dysphagia team, typically based on three general areas of concern:

- Difficulties have been observed related to feeding and ingestion of food or liquid.
- The client appears to be at risk for aspirating food or liquid into the lungs.
- The client appears not to be receiving adequate nourishment. (Rosenthal, Sheppard, & Lotze, 1995).

The swallowing therapist (often an SLP) will then seek answers to questions such as those presented in Table 13.4. The answers to these questions will give the swallowing therapist preliminary information about

---

TABLE 13.4

Important questions pertaining to swallowing

Does the infant accept breast or bottle?	When was the problem first observed?
Does the individual refuse certain foods? Which ones?	Did it worsen slowly or rapidly?
Does the individual appear to chew food?	What exactly happens when the person tries to swallow?
Has drooling been observed?	Does material seem to stop somewhere? Where?
Does the child or adult eat excessively slowly?	What medical diagnoses or conditions may affect the swallow?
Does the child or adult eat excessively rapidly?	Has the person had surgery that may relate to swallowing?
Does coughing or choking occur at meal times?	Is the individual using any medications?
Is food or liquid expelled from the nose?	How is the client's respiratory health?
Is food or liquid regurgitated?	How attentive is the client?
Is the child gaining weight?	Is the client able to follow directions?
Is the adult maintaining weight?	

Source: Adapted from Hardy & Robinson (1993).

---

the location of the swallowing problem (oral, pharyngeal, or both), the kinds of food substances that are easiest and hardest to swallow, and the nature and severity of the disorder (Logemann, 1998).

CLINICAL ASSESSMENT

CAREGIVER AND ENVIRONMENTAL FACTORS

The swallowing therapist will want to observe feeding as it occurs normally between caregiver and client. The therapist will pay special attention to the following:

- Is the caregiver patient and attentive?
- Does feeding take place in a reasonably quiet environment that is free from distractions?
- What position is the individual in when eating or drinking?
- How does the client express feeding preferences?

The parent or caregiver is an important part of the swallowing team. Careful observation and communication will help the swallowing therapist to assess how best to improve this person's contributions. This is also the opportunity for the SLP to learn about the client's position within the family and cultural and individual factors that may influence therapy. For example, certain foods and spices may be preferred to others. When possible, personal and cultural desires should be respected and accommodated (Logemann, 1998). Box 13.1 describes portions of the assessment of a 51-year-old man who was referred for a swallowing evaluation.

COGNITIVE AND COMMUNICATIVE FUNCTIONING

Is the client alert and awake during feeding? Can he or she follow directions? What is the client's general level of functioning? Answers to these questions will influence the type of intervention that is most suitable for the client.

HEAD AND BODY POSTURE

The swallowing therapist will observe whether the patient can hold his or her head erect. Does it lean to one side or the other? Does it tend to tilt forward or back? Can the client position the head when asked to do so? The SLP will also note general body posture and tone. Swallowing and ingestion of food and drink involve more than the head, so a complete picture of the individual is important.

ORAL-MOTOR SYSTEM

The swallowing therapist needs to assess the integrity of the anatomy and health of the mouth. Abnormalities of structure of the lips, teeth,

BOX 13.1

The Personal Story of a Man with Dysphagia

Mr. M. was 51 years of age when he was referred as an outpatient by the Director of Neurology and Rehabilitative Medicine at Municipal Hospital to Ms. R., the staff SLP in charge of swallowing disorders. The referral note read "myotonic dystrophy, dysarthria, dysphagia for solids." Ms. R. recognized her role in ensuring the patient's safety. Difficulty in swallowing foods could result in choking and/or aspiration pneumonia. Ms. R. was also concerned about the dysarthria and wondered to what degree this affected Mr. M.'s communication.

Myotonic dystrophy is a rare, slowly progressive hereditary disease. It is also called Steinert's disease and is characterized initially by poor muscle relaxation following contraction and later by muscle atrophy, especially of the face and neck.

At their first meeting, Ms. R. learned that Mr. M., a recent immigrant from Colombia, had limited English proficiency. Once again, Ms. R. was grateful for her own Spanish language skills; the summer she had spent in Spain after her third year of college had been worthwhile in a multitude of ways. Many of the patients and staff at this inner-city hospital had Spanish as their primary language. Although Mr. M. was mildly dysarthric, his speech was readily intelligible. His responses during the interview were appropriate in form (Spanish) and content. Mr. M. reported that he choked on rice and that this was a staple of his diet. Other foods and liquids did not appear to be a problem.

Mr. M. reported that he smoked "a little, just at the Saturday evening dances." A cursory evaluation of the oral mechanism revealed adequate strength and motion of the lips, tongue, velum, and mandible. Although coughing, choking, and gurgling were not observed during trial feeding, an apparent delay in the pharyngeal swallow reflex was noted with both liquids and solids. Ms. R. recommended a modified barium swallow study to confirm and document dysphagia.

Several types of foods were mixed with barium in preparation for the X-ray procedure. Mr. M. ate a spoonful of applesauce and then pudding as the radiologist and Ms. R. watched the X-ray monitor. No difficulties were noted in the oral phase. However, they observed food lingering in the esophagus and building up with each successive swallow. Although the larynx elevated for swallowing, the bolus did not clear, and residue remained on the right **aryepiglottic fold**. Mr. M. was instructed to produce an abdominal cough, but he was unsuccessful, and the food remained on the fold.

Ms. R. made the following recommendations: Mr. M. should not eat alone. He should avoid clear liquids and take only a small amount of food before swallowing. He should try to cough deeply when he feels food stuck in his mouth. At the next appointment, in two weeks, Mr. M. would be instructed in the supraglottic and hard swallow techniques. Because myotonic dystrophy is a progressive disease, Mr. M. requires regular monitoring.

tongue, palate, and velum will be noted. The SLP will look for facial symmetry and will note sagging and imbalances. Motor difficulties such as tremor, flaccidity, excessive muscle tone, and poor coordination will be observed. Oral reflexes will be examined. Certain reflexes such as sucking and rooting (turning in the direction of a stroke to the cheek) are expected in infants but should disappear as the child matures. The SLP will observe any drooling, which may signal neuromuscular deficits, gum and tooth infections, or upper airway obstruction (Sheppard, 1995). The SLP will also note the client's response to sensation. Does the client accept touch such as face washing? If the client is an older child or adult, is she or he aware of food residue or saliva on the face? (Cherney, 1994).

LARYNGEAL FUNCTION

The SLP cannot directly observe the larynx in the way that he or she can look at the oral mechanism. So the SLP will look for indirect signs of difficulty. In older children and adults, a hoarse, gurgly, or breathy voice quality before, during, or after a swallow may signal laryngeal dysfunction. Other indications of laryngeal problems include the following

- Inability to rapidly repeat the syllable /ha/ with a clear voiced vowel sound
- Inability to produce vocal tones up and down the musical scale
- An s/z ratio greater than 1.3 (See Chapter 9, "The Voice and Voice Disorders")
- Inability to produce a strong cough (Hardy & Robinson, 1993; Logemann, 1998)

If any difficulties are observed, it is essential that the swallowing therapist refer the client to an otolaryngologist for a thorough laryngeal evaluation.

T H O U G H T   Q U E S T I O N

Why is it important for a medical specialist to evaluate a person who may show signs of laryngeal dysfunction?

THE SWALLOWING EXAMINATION

If the client is alert and does not have a history of aspiration, the swallowing therapist will evaluate the client's ability to swallow. Usually, food or beverage is used, although some SLPs prefer to make the assessment with a piece of gauze that has been soaked in water or juice to prevent aspiration. If real food substances are used, anticipation and the oral phase of swallow can be observed. Pharyngeal phase swallowing efficiency can be judged in part by noting specific behaviors during food or drink intake.

The SLP should observe swallowing on more than one occasion. The nature of the food that is presented and the client's comfort level and hunger will influence the acceptance of foods.

The SLP evaluates the client's reaction to the appearance of food or drink and the associated utensils, observing whether the client's activity level changes and the person appears eager to receive food. A small amount (a quarter of a teaspoon) of thin or thick liquid may be placed in the mouth, and the client is then encouraged to swallow. Oral mechanism function is observed throughout the swallow.

The SLP examines the client's lips to see whether they are together before the taking in of food. The SLP is interested in answering questions such as the following:

- Do the lips open and then close around the nipple, cup, or spoon?
- Is there sucking activity on the nipple?
- Is food successfully removed from the spoon?
- Is liquid or food dribbled out of the sides of the mouth?

The SLP also observes tongue movement. Again, answers to certain questions are vital:

- When the mouth opens to take in food, does the tongue cup in anticipation?
- Does the client move the tongue to one side of the mouth if food is presented laterally?
- Does the client move the tongue adequately to form a bolus?
- Is the bolus transported efficiently from the front to the back of the mouth?
- Is the tongue used to remove food substances from the lips?

In addition, the SLP notes movements of the jaw and chewing patterns when solid foods are presented:

- Does the client bite food efficiently?
- Does the client isolate tongue and jaw movement?
- Does chewing continue for an adequate period of time?
- Is the jaw clenched?

Several observations pertaining to the adequacy of pharyngeal swallow are performed. If the client is unable to cough, this may suggest difficulty closing the larynx to protect the airway. Nasal regurgitation points to possibly inadequate velopharyngeal closure. The SLP observes the movement of the hyoid bone and thyroid cartilage in the neck by watching and possibly placing a finger gently on this area. These should move up during pharyngeal swallow. The SLP records the number of times the client swallows while ingesting each amount of food or drink. Multiple swallows may suggest inadequate pharyngeal contraction. If vocal quality changes after swallowing this may indicate pooling of liquid (Cherney, 1994).

Of importance to the SLP are which food consistencies appear to cause difficulties and which seem to be swallowed efficiently. Similarly, the SLP notices whether there is a preferential placement in the mouth for food or liquid.

MANAGING A TRACHEOSTOMY TUBE

Some clients will have a **tracheostomy tube** in place to facilitate breathing. A swallowing evaluation can still be conducted in most of these cases with the physician's approval. The SLP or nurse deflates the cuff of the tube before assessment and suctions secretions from the mouth and above the cuff. The swallowing evaluation is similar to the one outlined above; however, the patient is instructed to cover the tube with a gauze pad or gloved finger before each swallow to normalize tracheal pressure (Logemann, 1998).

See On-line Resource *Aaron's Tracheostomy Page*, referenced at the end of this chapter, for more information.

INSTRUMENTATION

Complete, accurate assessment of the swallowing procedure requires the use of instrumentation. The SLP collaborates with other team members such as the physician, radiologist, and X-ray technologist in the use of diagnostic technology. Some of the more commonly used instrumental procedures are described in the following paragraphs.

MODIFIED BARIUM SWALLOW STUDY

The **modified barium swallow study,** also referred to as **videofluoroscopy,** is an X-ray procedure that has been considered "the gold standard" in dysphagia diagnosis in children or adults (Sonies & Frattalli, 1997). This procedure is used when clinical evaluation or screening suggests dysphagia and/or aspiration. Barium, a substance that can be seen on X-rays, is coated onto or mixed into the food or beverage to be ingested. The SLP typically determines the size, texture, and consistency of the food or beverage to be presented and the head and body position of the patient during the study. A radiologist and an X-ray technologist use fluoroscopic (X-ray) equipment to observe the movement of the barium throughout the swallow. These views are videorecorded for later analysis by the physician and SLP. The study provides real-time visualization of the swallowing process and is highly useful in determining whether the client should be fed orally or nonorally, what food textures are safest, and what types of therapy are appropriate (Hardy & Robinson, 1993; Rogers, Arvedson, Buck, et al., 1994).

Solid knowledge of anatomy and physiology is essential in order to accurately interpret videofluoroscopic swallowing studies (Wooi, Scott, & Perry, 2001).

FIBER-OPTIC ENDOSCOPIC EVALUATION OF SWALLOWING

Fiber-optic endoscopic evaluation of swallowing (FEES) may be used with adult patients who are too ill to be brought to a radiology department for the modified barium swallow study. FEES is not an X-ray

The FEES procedure is increasingly used because of its convenience and portability.

procedure. Instead, following topical or localized anesthesia, an otolaryngologist inserts a flexible fiber-optic laryngoscope through the patient's nose and down into the pharynx. A specially trained SLP can also perform this procedure in consultation with a physician. When the scope is in place, the patient may be asked to cough, hold his or her breath, and swallow foods of different textures and thickness that have been dyed for better visualization. The views may be videotaped. FEES may reveal bolus spilling into the pharynx before swallowing and closing of the airway during swallow. Oral and esophageal phases of swallowing are not visible with FEES. Nevertheless, observations with FEES can be performed at the bedside and provide valuable information about desirable body and head posture during feeding, preferred food types, and aspiration. FEES may also be more cost effective than videofluoroscopy, particularly for patients with head and neck cancer (ASHA, 1992; Aviv, Sataloff, Cohen, et al., 2001; Leder, Sasaki, & Burrell, 1998; Sonies, 1997).

SCINTIGRAPHY

Scintigraphy is a computerized technique that is sometimes used with adults for measuring the amount of aspiration during or after a swallow. A specialized physician such as a radiologist, gastroenterologist, or otolaryngologist performs scintigraphy; however, the SLP plays a role in positioning the patient, suggesting swallowing procedures, and interpreting test results. A radioactive tracer is mixed with the food or liquid to be ingested. Radioactive markers may be placed externally on the chin, lip, thyroid notch, and other anatomical landmarks to facilitate measurement. A specialized gamma scintillation camera is used. When scintigraphy is used, it is generally to supplement information obtained from other tests. Scintigraphy provides insight regarding esophageal function and may help in the determination of the safety of oral feedings (ASHA, 1992; Sonies, 1997).

ULTRASOUND

Ultrasound, or **ultrasonography,** is an imaging technique that uses sound waves at a frequency that is inaudible to human ears, over 20,000 Hz. It is a noninvasive procedure that is safe to use with infants and children as well as adults. A transducer that generates and receives sound waves is placed below the chin for views of the oral cavity and on the thyroid notch for visualizing the laryngeal area. The acoustic images are videotaped. Ultrasonographic real-time measures are particularly helpful in assessing the duration of the oral phases of swallowing as well the structure and movement of the tongue and hyoid bone. One drawback is that ultrasound does not permit visualization of the pharyngeal stage of swallow (ASHA, 1992; Logemann, 1998; Sonies, 1997).

Ultrasound is used in various types of medical assessment. Can you name some? Why is ultrasound used in these situations?

DYSPHAGIA INTERVENTION AND TREATMENT

Disorders of swallowing present medical, nutritional, psychological, social, and communicative problems, so many individuals are involved in working toward their resolution. As was mentioned earlier, the speech-language pathologist is usually the coordinator of services and the professional who is most likely to implement dysphagia therapy. Nevertheless, input from other team members is essential to a satisfactory outcome.

FEEDING ENVIRONMENT

Whether the patient is an infant, a young child, or an adult, the environment for feeding sets the stage for a satisfactory experience. It is especially important for people with swallowing problems to have their meals in an environment that is conducive to success. Visual and auditory distractions should be minimized. This means that the eating area should not contain nonrelevant objects. Lighting should be comfortable, neither too bright nor too dark. Noise should be reduced and replaced with pleasant familiar music.

Whereas children who have excess muscle tone (hypertonia) benefit from low lighting, soft music, and minimal stimulation, children with insufficient muscle tone (hypotonia) often respond better to bright lights, peppy music, and physical stimulation.

The caregiver should have a relaxed, unhurried manner. He or she must be tuned in to the patient's signals regarding feeding speed, food choices, and quantity. When necessary, these communication strategies may be developed and trained. The caregiver should indicate an interest in the person being fed and reinforce his or her healthy, effective eating behaviors. When possible, the goal is the development of self-feeding skills.

Utensils for feeding need to be appropriate to the patient's functioning. For infants, a slow-flow nipple may be helpful in controlling the amount of liquid taken at a time. A Teflon- or latex-covered spoon may be used for children with infantile tonic bite reflex, who will bite hard on any object that is placed on the teeth or gums. Children and adults with motor coordination difficulties may benefit from the use of a shallow-bowled spoon. Special cutout cups may help to improve tongue positioning in drinking (Jelm, 1994; Sheppard, 1995).

BODY AND HEAD POSITIONING

Body posture and stability have a strong influence on oral-pharyngeal movements. The basic premise is that controlled mobility stems from a solid base (Woods, 1995). An upright, 90° hip angle, symmetrical position with sufficient postural support to provide stability is generally needed. The individual's head and neck must be positioned and prevented from making extraneous movement.

T H O U G H T   Q U E S T I O N S

Have you ever observed a parent trying to feed a child who was slumped over in a chair? Why would this interfere with effective feeding?

Occasionally, a child or adult may benefit from a hip angle other than 90°. For example, some infants with severe respiratory and swallowing problems may feed better when placed on their stomach. Some older individuals who have a considerable amount of pharyngeal residue may eat more safely at a bent-over 45° angle to prevent regurgitation of food from the esophagus into the airway (B. J. Martin, 1994; Woods, 1995).

The SLP works closely with the physical therapist and occupational therapist in obtaining optimum positioning for feeding. The **chin tuck** posture is often recommended for patients with delayed pharyngeal swallow. This position will help to prevent food and liquid from entering the airway. The chin tuck posture is presented on the accompanying CD-ROM. The **head-back position** has been found useful for patients with poor tongue mobility if they have excellent airway closure. **Head tilt** and **head rotation** postures are used when an individual has impairment on one side. In these positions, the head may be moved in the direction of (rotation) or away from (tilt) the impairment. Clients who have been found during videofluoroscopy to have residue in the pharynx may be advised to lie on one side while eating (Logemann, 1998; B. J. Martin, 1994).

MODIFICATION OF FOODS AND BEVERAGES

TEXTURES, QUANTITIES, AND TEMPERATURES

During the assessment, liquids and foods of varying consistencies, amounts, and possibly temperatures will have been presented to the patient. On the basis of the findings of these tests, appropriate recommendations will be made.

Certain foods that are hard to chew, are small or slick when wet, or are thick and sticky are not recommended for children under age 5 who exhibit neuromotor difficulties. Specific foods for these infants and young children to avoid are listed in Table 13.5.

TABLE 13.5

Specific foods that should be avoided for children under age 5 with neuromotor problems

Frankfurters	Nuts	Chewing gum
Grapes	Seeds	Raw carrots
Popcorn	Hard candy	

Source: Adapted from Lotze (1995).

Clients may exhibit a range of food consistency requirements. They might not tolerate any food by mouth, accept only thin or thick liquids, require a pureed consistency, or be able to ingest the range of normal foods. Table 13.6 lists possible food consistencies.

The amount of food that a client can manage in her or his mouth at a time may be determined by the modified barium swallow study. In general, the goal is to reduce the amount that is presented. Drinking through a straw typically causes too much fluid to enter the mouth, so straws are usually not advised. Spoons with a shallow bowl are helpful in limiting food amounts. Caregivers and patients must avoid placing food in the mouth until the previous bolus has been swallowed. Finally, patients may be encouraged to swallow twice per bite or sip.

Providing foods of varying temperatures may increase the client's sensory awareness of the food and improve swallowing. Cold food or drink sometimes improves tongue movement during the oral transport phase and helps to stimulate pharyngeal swallow, although some patients with respiratory problems prefer all substances to be ingested at room temperature (B. J. Martin, 1994).

PLACEMENT

The swallowing therapist places food or drink in the mouth where the patient has intact sensation and adequate muscle strength. For example, an individual who has had oral cancer will have diminished sensation in the region where surgery occurred. Similarly, the ability to feel may be reduced after radiation therapy. Neurological disease and damage may also impair a person's full awareness of foods that are placed in the mouth. Surgery and neurological problems may also compromise muscle tone and make the person less able to move parts of the tongue, lips, or cheeks. Appropriate placement along with the adjustments in texture, quantity, and temperature is critical to successful dysphagia intervention (B. J. Martin, 1994).

TABLE 13.6

Dietary consistencies

NPO	From the Latin, *non per os*, meaning nothing by mouth. If an individual aspirates more than 10 percent of all foods or is unable to swallow one bolus of food within 10 seconds, alternative means of feeding must be used.
No Liquid by Mouth	Liquids will need to be provided via a nasogastric tube or intravenously for patients who can tolerate pureed or more solid food but are at risk for aspiration of liquids.
Thin Liquid Consistency	This includes foods such as gelatin desserts, which are tolerated by some patients better than thicker consistencies.
Thick Liquid Consistency	Beverages are thickened to the consistency of fruit nectar or tomato juice. A variety of commercial thickeners are available.
Pureed Consistency	Foods are blended to the consistency of mashed potatoes or pudding. This may be recommended for individuals with oral preparatory or oral transport stage difficulties.
Crushed Medication	Pills and capsules are often difficult to swallow, and crushing may facilitate the process. Some medications are time-released, however, and lose effectiveness when crushed. The physician must be consulted before using this approach.
Mechanical Soft Consistency	This consistency is sometimes referred to as *dental soft*. It includes soft foods such as cooked vegetables, fruits, and pasta and may be easier than firmer foods for patients with oral or pharyngeal phase dysphagia to tolerate.
Regular Dietary Consistency	A patient with mild dysphagia may tolerate regular food textures but may need to adjust body or head posture, amount per mouthful, rate of eating, and so on.

Source: Adapted from Hardy, E., & Robinson, N. H. (1993). *Swallowing disorder treatment manual.* Bisbee, AZ: Imaginart. Reprinted by permission.

ORAL-MOTOR EXERCISES AND SWALLOWING TECHNIQUES

Each of the procedures described below is used only after clinical and instrumental assessment has demonstrated its safety and appropriateness. Clients will also need to be able to follow instructions. All of the techniques may be practiced without food. However, the swallowing techniques are specific to improving the actual swallowing process and are described with the use of food or drink.

MUSCLE EXERCISES

The motor system that is used in swallowing may be improved through exercise. Clients with impaired swallowing may have restricted mouth opening, tongue or lip movement, and laryngeal elevation. **Range of motion** may be improved by practicing specific exercises. Bite blocks of differing sizes may be used to encourage lowering the mandible. Flavored gauze or a toothette may be placed in various places around the mouth to stimulate tongue and lip movement. A licorice stick or a candy LifeSaver on a string may also be used to improve tongue movement. The client may be instructed in moving her or his lips from pucker to smile and back again. Exercises to facilitate awareness of laryngeal movement may involve placement of the hand on the neck at the level of the hyoid bone. A mirror is often used to provide visual feedback to the patient.

Lip strength and seal may be improved by having the client attempt to hold a tongue depressor with the lips. Pushing the tongue against a tongue depressor is a technique for strengthening that muscle. Improved coordination is taught by asking the client to follow instructions such as moving the tongue to explore the outside, then inside of the upper and lower front teeth.

HARD AND DOUBLE SWALLOWS

A hard or effortful swallow may be helpful for patients whose tongues do not retract enough to trigger pharyngeal swallow. In these cases, the client is instructed to swallow forcefully and try to feel the tongue moving backward. This technique is helpful as swallowing practice with or without food or drink (Logemann, 1997; B. J. Martin, 1994).

Double or multiple swallows are advised for individuals who, for whatever reason, retain some food in the oral cavity after a single swallow. Very simply, the client is instructed to swallow two or more times for each bolus (B. J. Martin, 1994).

SUPRAGLOTTIC SWALLOW

In the normal swallow, the vocal folds are closed to prevent food from entering the airway. The supraglottic swallow may be used for individuals who do not fully close the glottis during swallowing. This technique teaches voluntary closure of the glottal area, and reduces the depth of misdirected swallows (Bulow, Olsen, & Ekberg, 2001). The client is instructed to do the following:

1. Breathe in and hold your breath.
2. Put a small amount of food or liquid in your mouth.
3. Swallow.
4. Cough or clear your throat while exhaling.
5. Swallow again (Hardy & Robinson, 1993; B. J. Martin, 1994).

MENDELSOHN MANEUVER

The Mendelsohn maneuver is useful for clients who do not have adequate laryngeal elevation during swallowing. The patient is taught to manually hold the larynx at its highest point during the swallow (see Figure 13.1). The instructions are as follows (Hardy & Robinson, 1993; B. J. Martin, 1994):

1. Place a small amount of food or liquid in your mouth.
2. Chew if necessary.
3. Swallow while placing your thumb and forefinger on either side of your larynx.
4. Manually hold the larynx for 3 to 5 seconds during and after swallowing in the highest position it reached during swallowing.
5. Let go of your larynx and let it drop.

During the assessment process, the SLP determines which of the above exercises and techniques are appropriate for a particular client. Evaluation continues, however, and modifications in treatment approaches are often made as therapy proceeds.

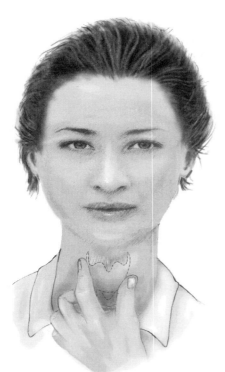

FIGURE 13.1 In the Mendelsohn maneuver, the client manually holds the larynx at its highest position to facilitate swallowing. (Adapted from Hardy, E., & Robinson, N. M. (1993). *Swallowing Disorders Treatment Manual*. Bisbee, AZ: Imaginart, p. 94. Reprinted by permission.)

A current reference book describing prescription drugs is an essential part of the personal library of the well-informed SLP.

MEDICAL AND PHARMACOLOGICAL APPROACHES

DRUG TREATMENTS

Neurological patients, such as those with Parkinson's disease and multiple sclerosis, who are taking medications to improve their condition benefit from being medicated with these drugs before eating. In addition, the medication atropine has been reported to control drooling (Logemann, 1998), and nifedipine may be useful in managing dysphagia in individuals who have had a stroke (Perez, Smithard, Davies, & Kaira, 1998). Injections of botulinum toxin have been shown to improve swallowing in individuals with spasticity and hypertonicity of the cricopharyngeal muscle (Shaw & Searl, 2001). As was discussed earlier in this chapter, some medications actually cause or contribute to swallowing disorders. In these cases, the swallowing therapist needs to work with the physician to determine whether alternatives can be used (Feinberg, 1997).

PROSTHESES AND SURGICAL PROCEDURES

Patients who lack an intact swallowing mechanism because of malformation, surgery, or another cause may benefit from a prosthetic device. For example, individuals who had oral cancer and have had a significant portion of the soft palate excised may have a **palatal obturator,** a permanent or removable plate, that helps to close this area during speaking or eating (Logemann, 1998). In addition, children with cerebral palsy who exhibit dysphagia have been shown to improve their feeding skills and growth significantly when using an appropriately designed intraoral appliance (Haberfellner, Schwartz, & Gisel, 2001).

If less invasive approaches have been unsuccessful, surgery to improve swallowing and prevent aspiration is sometimes needed. Some techniques attempt to correct organic defects. For example, if the patient has bony growths on the cervical vertebrae that displace the rear pharyngeal wall, these may be reduced surgically. Other surgical procedures are used to increase the dimensions of the vocal folds or elevate the larynx. In severe cases of aspiration, the true or false vocal folds may be sutured closed, and breathing will have to occur through a tracheostomy (Logemann, 1998). For patients with esophageal dysphasia, injection of botulinum toxin is sometimes effective (Sonies, 1997).

NONORAL FEEDING

Clients who require more than 10 seconds to swallow a liquid or food bolus or who aspirate more than 10 percent of either will likely require at least some nonoral feeding (Logemann, 1998). Several approaches are used.

Nasogastric tube (NG tube) feeding requires that a tube be placed from the nose to the pharynx, the esophagus, and finally the stomach. Liquefied food and water are inserted through this opening. Unlike the more long-term procedures described below, NG tubes are typically not used for periods of more than five or six months.

In **pharyngostomy,** a feeding tube is inserted into a **stoma,** or hole in the external neck region skin, which extends into the pharynx. **Esophagostomy** is a similar procedure; however, a hole is made into the esophagus from the chest area, and a food tube is inserted through it.

In gastrostomy, a hole is surgically made from the abdomen to the stomach. A soft tube is placed through this, and blended regular food can be inserted into the tube. This procedure is used in cases of severe dysphagia.

PROGNOSES AND OUTCOMES FOR SWALLOWING DISORDERS

The overriding objectives of swallowing therapy are to improve the intake of food and drink and to prevent aspiration of these materials into the lungs. The potential for success of swallowing therapy is determined largely by the cause of the disorder, the severity of aspiration, and the onset of treatment (Denk, Swoboda, Schima, & Eibenberger, 1997). In young children with developmental disabilities, treatment that is based on a careful diagnosis of the feeding disorder results in improved nutrition and generally better health (Schwarz, Corredor, Fisher-Medina, et al., 2001). Early identification and successful intervention for swallowing disorders reduces the risk of aspiration and death following stroke, shortens the length of time patients need to stay in hospital, and improves quality of life (Odderson et al., 1995). While the original causes of swallowing problems may not be remediable, treatment for dysphagia has been reported to be beneficial in at least 80 percent of cases (Johns Hopkins, 2000).

Swallowing specialists have sometimes been successful in preventing dysphagia. Caregivers of youngsters who are at risk are instructed in feeding techniques soon after the child's birth. Well-placed information for the older population is also valuable. Among the elderly, swallowing disorders are sometimes related to poor dentition, which might be corrected by appropriate dental care. Advice to avoid alcohol, caffeine, spicy products, and foods that are extremely hot or cold and may improve swallowing and prevent dysphagia (Toner, 1997).

SUMMARY

Speech-language pathologists who are specially trained often serve as swallowing therapists. They work with infants who are unable to nurse adequately, children with feeding problems, and older people who have dysphagia. The anticipatory, oral, pharyngeal, and/or esophageal phases of swallowing may be impaired. Causes include congenital or acquired neurological problems, stroke, cancer, developmental disability, dementia, and accident. Swallowing affects not only nutrition and health, but also social and personal aspects of life. A team approach is used for both assessment and intervention. Evaluation includes a careful history and direct observation of the client while he or she is feeding. The modified barium swallow study uses videofluoroscopic equipment and is considered the "gold standard" in dysphagia evaluation. Treatment procedures address the feeding environment, the client's body and facial posture, food textures and temperatures, oral-motor mobility, and specific swallowing techniques. Medical, prosthetic, and surgical approaches are used when necessary. Nonoral feeding may be required in severe cases.

REFLECTIONS

- What special skills and knowledge does the speech-language pathologist bring to swallowing therapy?
- Describe the phases of the swallowing process.
- What are some causes of swallowing difficulties in infants and children?
- What are some causes of swallowing problems in older individuals?
- Describe noninstrumental dysphagia assessment.
- Compare the modified barium swallow study and fiber-optic endoscopic evaluation of swallowing.
- What techniques are used to address disorders of swallowing?

SUGGESTED READINGS

Hall, K. (2000). *Pediatric dysphagia resource guide.* San Diego: Singular.

Logemann, J. A. (1998). *Evaluation and treatment of swallowing disorders* (2nd ed.). Austin, TX: Pro-Ed.

Mills, R. H. (2000) *A clinician's guide to the expanded evaluation of dysphagia in adults.* Austin, TX: Pro-Ed.

ON-LINE RESOURCES

http:///www.dysphagia.com   Dysphagia Resource Center.

Links to information about swallowing and swallowing disorders; includes anatomy and physiology, tutorials, research references.

http://www.tracheostomy.com   Aaron's Tracheostomy Page.

Personal insights from the mother of a child with a tracheostomy tube. Helpful suggestions regarding eating with a tracheostomy and other issues.

When you have finished this chapter, you should be able to:

- Define audiology and the role of the audiologist in various employment settings

- Describe the mechanics of sound propagation and demonstrate a basic understanding of the anatomy and physiology of the auditory system

- Identify the three types of hearing loss and some causes of each

- Name the components of the basic audiological test battery and explain the purpose and method used in each test

- Define aural rehabilitation and describe the basic techniques that are used to mitigate the effects of hearing loss on communication

14

Audiology and Hearing Loss

Some speech, language, and communication disorders have their etiology based partially or wholly in temporary or permanent hearing loss. While speech-language pathologists are able, under their scope of practice, to conduct basic hearing screenings, the detailed information that can be provided by a thorough audiological evaluation can be extremely useful in the development and implementation of a comprehensive plan of therapy. Additionally, the complementary nature of rehabilitative services provided by each of these professional disciplines requires speech-language pathologists and audiologists to work closely together to maximize client success. It is appropriate, therefore, that we consider hearing and auditory processing disorders and the discipline of audiology.

WHAT IS AUDIOLOGY?

The move to doctoral level entry into the field does not prohibit master's-level individuals from practice. Anyone certified by ASHA prior to the 2012 changeover will continued to be eligible to hold the CCC-A. While many audiologists have currently the Au.D. degree, there is no requirement for existing professionals with an M.S. degree to do so.

Audiology is defined as "the discipline involved in the prevention, identification, and evaluation of hearing disorders, the selection and evaluation of hearing aids, and the habilitation/rehabilitation of individuals with hearing impairment" (Bess & Humes, 1995, p. 6). The beauty of this definition is that it dismisses the notion that an audiologist is simply a person who sits in a booth, turning dials and pushing buttons. In their professional capacity, audiologists must be able to assume the role of diagnostician, therapist, and/or scientist. Obviously, this necessitates a great deal of preparation. Becoming an audiologist currently requires a master's degree as well as a year of postgraduate supervised work experience. Only on completion of this course of study can a person obtain a Certificate of Clinical Competence from the American Speech-Language-Hearing Association and begin to practice professionally. Recently, it was determined that the rapid advances in knowledge and technology within the field demanded even more preparation on the part of candidates for certification. As of 2012, the entry-level requirement for ASHA CCC in Audiology will be a doctoral degree. While a traditional, research-based doctorate (Ph.D.) will be appropriate, it is likely that most new practitioners will complete the newly developed Doctor of Audiology (Au.D.). The Au.D. is a four-year post-baccalaureate professional degree program.

The emphasis on proper preparation gives the audiologist the advantage of being able to choose from among a number of available employment settings. Most audiologists are employed in private practice. These are the people who specialize in diagnosing hearing loss and dispensing hearing aids. *Rehabilitative audiologists* work in hospitals, clinics, and rehabilitation centers to provide counseling and auditory training to those who have sustained hearing loss. *Educational audiologists* work in schools to provide services to hearing-impaired students in special education and regular education settings. *Medical audiologists* work in hospitals and clinics to provide diagnostic testing and neonatal hearing screenings. Recently, these audiologists have become members of surgical teams to provide intraoperative monitoring of auditory nerve function during head surgery. There are *industrial audiologists* whose primary concern is prevention of hearing loss due to excessive noise exposure in the workplace. They do so by monitoring employee hearing levels and by oversight of specialized hearing conservation programs. Finally, audiologists in college and university settings are engaged in teaching and research. In short, audiologists work in a multitude of settings with populations ranging from infants to the elderly.

To have developed such diversity, one would imagine that audiology as a profession has been around for many decades. Actually, it did not emerge as a formal profession until shortly after World War II.

Raymond Carhart, a speech-language pathologist working at a veterans' hospital, began to investigate ways to address the communication needs of the veterans who were returning home from the war. He observed that a number of the soldiers had hearing loss resulting from noise exposure and trauma during the fighting. Because standard methods of testing hearing did not really exist, Carhart and other scientists began to study the hearing mechanism and developed equipment and methodology that allowed for formal hearing evaluation. For his work, Raymond Carhart is considered the father of audiology, and his method of hearing evaluation, the Carhart method, is still in use today.

Improved research procedures and rapid developments in technology have done much to change the field of audiology since Carhart's time. We can now identify hearing losses in newborns through auditory brain stem response testing and otoacoustic emissions. We can help a hearing-impaired student succeed in school through the use of FM systems and other assistive listening devices. We can use computer software to program the smaller, state-of-the-art hearing aids that are now available, and through the advent of real ear measurements, we can measure and adjust the performance of the hearing aid while it is being worn. Audiology is an exciting, ever-changing profession that demands a constant effort from its practitioners to keep up to date. An audiologist who simply stays in the booth and turns the dials is going to be quickly left behind.

FUNDAMENTALS OF SOUND

All sound consists of a series of vibrations traveling through a medium such as air. A **vibration** is a series of rapid, rhythmic, back-and-forth movements within a space. An increase in pressure (compression) occurs when air molecules get closer together. The air molecules then rebound creating a decrease in pressure (rarefaction). Sound is a series of compressions and rarefactions moving outward from a vibrating source. When a sound source begins to vibrate, it sets in motion the air molecules adjacent to it. Each air molecule then begins to vibrate within its own space and as it does so, it "bumps" into neighboring air molecules. The next molecules begin to vibrate in synchrony with the sound source and set more molecules into motion, and so forth. The series of vibrations is passed from molecule to molecule until they reach the air molecules around your ear. It is important to note that it is the vibrations that are passed from molecule to molecule. The molecules themselves do not travel out of their original location.

Air molecules are in constant random motion. If one's hearing at birth were any more sensitive, this random motion would be heard.

Because the molecules move around a fixed point in space, their motion takes on some special qualities. First, the molecule travels a measurable distance in either direction from the original position. This is considered the amplitude or **intensity** of the vibration. The amplitude of the vibration is perceived as the *loudness* of the sound. Sound vibrations that have a small amplitude are identified as quiet sounds; sound vibrations with a greater amplitude are identified as louder sounds.

Second, this back-and-forth movement regularly repeats itself, creating cycles of movement. It is possible, then, to count the number of cycles that are completed within a specific time period. This is referred to as the **frequency** of the vibration. The frequency of the vibration is what is perceived as the *pitch* of the sound. Sound vibrations that complete few cycles within a specific time are considered to be low-pitched sounds; sound vibrations that complete many cycles within the same time are considered to be high-pitched sounds.

T H O U G H T   Q U E S T I O N

Why do sounds get softer (less loud) as you get farther away from the source?

Each sound, then, has a characteristic intensity and frequency, which are deciphered by the auditory system and identified by the brain. This is how you are able to tell the difference between a car horn and a doorbell, a dog barking and a bird singing, or the word "sun" and the word "fun" or the word "sum."

THE ANATOMY OF THE EAR

In discussing sound waves, we are speaking of vibrations that are of an infinitesimal size, such as a whisper or the slightest rustle of leaves. Luckily, the human ear is beautifully designed to make the most of these tiny fragments of sound.

The anatomy of the auditory system can be divided into six basic areas: the **outer ear**, the **middle ear**, the **inner ear**, the **auditory nerve**, the **auditory brain stem**, and the **auditory cortex** of the brain. The first four areas (Figure 14.1) are the peripheral structures of hearing. The last two areas are considered to be central structures. Damage to the peripheral structures results in hearing loss. Damage to the central (discussed in more detail later in the chapter) results in a variety of listening problems unrelated to hearing sensitivity.

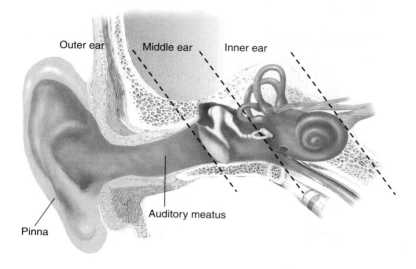

Outer ear   Middle ear   Inner ear

Auditory meatus

Pinna

FIGURE 14.1 The outer, middle, and inner ear

THE OUTER EAR

The outer ear is made up of the **pinna,** which is the outermost part of the ear, and the **external auditory meatus,** or *ear canal.* A deceivingly simple-looking structure, the pinna performs several important functions. Its funnel shape serves to collect the sound waves and channel them into the ear. The shape of the pinna also creates resonance characteristics that help to enhance and amplify some of the weaker, high-frequency sounds. Finally, in addition to frequency and intensity information, the position of the pinnae at opposite sides of the head provides the temporal cues that the brain uses to help localize sounds. Sound reaches each pinna at slightly different time intervals, and the brain is able to analyze the decrepancy to determine the direction from which the sound is coming.

The external auditory meatus, or ear canal, is a tubular structure that is approximately 1 inch long in adults. The diameter of the ear canal narrows somewhat as it progresses into the skull, continuing the funneling action of the pinna. Thus, one of the purposes of the ear canal is to increase the intensity of the sound waves by concentrating them over a progressively smaller area. The other important function of the ear canal is to resonate a specific range of middle to high frequencies that don't have much acoustic energy but provide critical information for the understanding of speech. The ear canal acts much like a musical instrument with its specific diameter and length creating a tuning effect so that certain frequencies are enhanced as they pass through.

THE MIDDLE EAR

The ear canal transfers these enriched and somewhat amplified sound vibrations to the middle ear beginning at the **tympanic membrane,** or **eardrum.** The eardrum is a cone-shaped structure composed of three layers of tissue that completely closes off one end of the ear canal so that all of the incoming sound vibrations strike its surface. The cone shape continues the funneling action of the outer ear, concentrating the acoustic energy of the sound to its center. Beyond the eardrum is the **middle ear space.** The middle ear space is a roughly cube-shaped area that is lined with a mucous membrane and filled with air. In the bottom wall of the middle ear space is an opening that leads to a structure called the **eustachian tube** or **auditory tube.** The eustachian tube connects the middle ear space with the upper portion of the pharynx and provides a passageway for air to move in and out, maintaining equality of air pressure on either side of the eardrum. This equalization of air pressure ensures the maximum mobility of the eardrum, which is essential for the transmission of sound vibrations.

Stretched across the middle ear space much like a suspension bridge are the **ossicles,** a chain of three small bones (see Figure 14.2). The **malleus,** the largest of the ossicles, rests against the eardrum. It articulates with the **incus,** the next bone in the chain. At the bottom of the

FIGURE 14.2   The middle ear structures

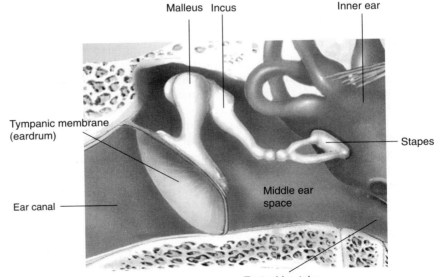

Malleus Incus

Inner ear

Tympanic membrane
(eardrum)

Stapes

Middle ear
space

Ear canal

Eustachian tube

incus is a projection that is joined to the smallest of the ossicles, the **stapes.** The stapes is oriented perpendicular to the side wall of the middle ear space. The structure of the stapes closely resembles a stirrup with two curved arms projecting from a center point to end in a flat piece of bone called the *footplate.* The sound vibrations are passed from the eardrum to the malleus, through the rest of the ossicular chain, to the footplate of the stapes.

THE INNER EAR

The inner ear is a complicated structure that performs two very important tasks. Primarily, it is responsible for supplying information to the brain regarding balance and spatial orientation. Surprisingly, hearing is only a secondary function of the inner ear. Audiologists also study and conduct testing related to balance, but that specialty area is beyond the scope of this chapter. Consequently, we'll focus specifically on hearing.

The footplate of the stapes rests against a thin membrane in the wall of a structure called the **cochlea.** The cochlea is the portion of the inner ear that contains the sensory cells for the auditory system. It is composed of two concentric labyrinths, the outer one made of bone and the inner one of membrane.

The bony labyrinth is filled with a thin, watery fluid called **perilymph,** which surrounds the outside of the membraneous labyrinth. Inside the membraneous labyrinth is another fluid called **endolymph.** Endolymph is a much more gelatinous fluid compared to perilymph and has a different chemical composition. Running along the center of the membraneous labyrinth, surrounded by endolymph, is the **organ of Corti** (see Figure 14.3).

The organ of Corti is an intricate structure that contains the auditory sensory receptors. The minute size and fragile nature of the organ of Corti have made it difficult to study its anatomy and physiology; however, several components have been identified. The bottom surface is formed by the **basilar membrane.** The structure of the basilar membrane is unique in that it is not of uniform width and thickness; rather, it is narrower and thinner at the base and wider and thicker at the apex. This allows it to respond differently to different frequencies of sound. It is said to be **tonotopically arranged;** that is, the end of the basilar membrane closest to the stapes responds best to higher-frequency sounds while the end nearest the apex of the cochlea responds best to lower-frequency sounds. Forming the roof of the organ of Corti is a gelatinous, tongue-shaped structure called the **tectorial membrane.** The tectorial membrane is fixed at one end, while the opposite end is free to move. This is an important point, for it allows the tectorial membrane to move up and down in response to the movement of the endolymph.

Each of the ossicles is progressively smaller in size, so the sound vibrations are further concentrated at the point of the stapes footplate. In total, the funneling action of the outer ear and middle ear creates an increase in the pressure exerted by the sound vibrations by a factor of 22:1. Without this increase in sound pressure, the sound vibrations could not pass to their final destination, the fluid-filled inner ear.

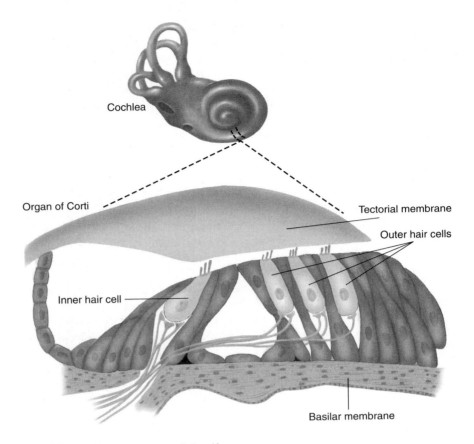

Cochlea

Organ of Corti

Tectorial membrane

Outer hair cells

Inner hair cell

Basilar membrane

FIGURE 14.3   The organ of Corti

Sitting on the basilar membrane are thousands of **hair cells,** which are the receptor cells for the auditory system. They are called hair cells because on the top of each cell are small, hairlike projections called **stereocilia.** Because of differences in their cell structure and orientation, the hair cells are separated into groups of *outer hair cells* and *inner hair cells.* The hair cells are responsible for encoding the auditory information for the brain. At the bottom of both outer and inner hair cells are nerve endings, which collectively become the **acoustic portion of the (VIIIth cranial) nerve.** The auditory nerve runs out of the base of the cochlea and enters the brain stem. From there, it projects upward and ends at the auditory cortex in the temporal lobe of the brain.

The progression of sound as it travels through the peripheral auditory system is as follows:

1. A sound source produces vibrations, which are passed as pressure fluctuations through the air molecules to the outer ear.
2. The pinna collects these vibrations and channels them into the ear canal. The shape of the outer ear allows for some amplification and enhancement of the vibrations.
3. The vibrations pass through the outer ear to strike the eardrum and are passed into the middle ear system. The vibration of the eardrum and ossicles significantly increases the sound pressure exerted by the vibrations.
4. The vibrations cause the stapes to move back and forth, much like a piston in an engine, to push against the wall of the cochlea.
5. This movement of the stapes causes pressure changes in both fluids in the cochlea to move.
6. The pressure changes in the fluids causes the basilar membrane and the tectorial membrane to rise and fall in a synchronous motion. The greatest displacement of these membranes will occur at a point corresponding to the frequency of the sound.
7. Because the stereocilia of the inner hair cells are embedded in the tectorial membrane, the movement of the fluid causes the stereocilia to be bent or sheared against the tectorial membrane.
8. This shearing begins a neurochemical reaction that generates neural impulses that are carried along the auditory nerve to the brain.

Thus, the sound vibrations go through a series of energy transformations as they pass through the auditory system. At the sound source and as they pass through the outer ear, they are acoustic energy. Going through the middle ear, the acoustic energy is transformed into mechanical energy. This mechanical energy is changed into hydraulic energy through the motion of the stapes footplate against the cochlea and the resulting vibrations in the perilymph and endolymph. Finally, the shearing action of the stereocilia in the organ of Corti changes the hydraulic energy into electrochemical energy, which is transmitted via the auditory nerve to the brain.

The vestibular system that monitors the body's balance is also located in the inner ear.

TYPES OF HEARING LOSS

The previous section described the ear from an anatomical standpoint. It is also helpful to discuss the ear functionally. In this regard, the outer and middle ears serve to collect sound, amplify it, and direct—or *conduct*—it to the cochlea. The outer and middle ear, therefore, are referred to as the **conductive system.** The cochlea is the actual *sensory* organ of hearing and the auditory nerve is responsible for transmitting a *neural* signal the brain can use. The cochlea and auditory nerve make up the **sensorineural system.** In describing peripheral hearing loss, it is most common to describe the loss from a functional perspective— conductive versus sensorineural— rather than anatomically.

CONDUCTIVE HEARING LOSS

A *conductive hearing loss* occurs when there is a malfunction or obstruction of the outer and middle ears. Problems in these areas impair or eliminate the amplification function of these structures and block sound from getting to the inner ear. The result is that the intensity of sound getting to the inner ear is reduced. This prevents sounds of low intensity from being heard and makes more intense sounds seem to be much softer. It is important to remember that the primary problem introduced by conductive problems is a loss of loudness. Because the sensorineural system remains intact, if sound is loud enough, it will be heard.

While conductive hearing losses can have a significant impact on hearing, they are never total. Luckily, most conductive losses are not permanent. Some resolve spontaneously. If not, the problem is usually medically treatable. In some instances, the conductive loss may not be treatable, or the treatment of the underlying disease does not completely remove the hearing loss. In these instances hearing aid use is a good option.

T H O U G H T   Q U E S T I O N S

Find out what it's like to have a mild conductive hearing loss. Purchase a set of inexpensive foam earplugs from a grocery or drugstore and insert them in your ears. Leave them in for at least four hours and go about your daily routine (within reason—don't wear the earplugs where it is unsafe to do so, such as while driving). Don't tell anyone about your experiment. What effect does it have on your communication? Your activities? How do others react to you? How does it affect you psychologically or emotionally?

Starting with the outer ear, two conditions can occur owing to the malformation of the structures during embryonic development. The first, **microtia,** refers to a small, malformed pinna or ear canal. **Atresia** is a similar disorder in which there is complete closure of the ear canal, either at the pinna or farther within the ear canal itself. These conditions most frequently occur in conjunction with other craniofacial disorders (see Chapter 11), as in the case of Down syndrome or Treacher Collins syndrome, and can create difficulties in localization of sounds as well as a significant hearing loss.

It is important to note that, because the structures of the external ear develop during the same gestational period as the cochlea, whenever a congenital malformation of the pinna or the external ear canal is present, a full hearing evaluation should be completed to rule out hidden sensorineural loss.

A much more common cause of conductive hearing loss in the outer ear is due to impacted **cerumen (earwax)** or foreign objects. Cerumen is a substance that is produced by the sebaceous glands in the ear canal. Cerumen serves useful purposes: It provides some lubrication for the ear canal to prevent the skin from drying out, and because of its sticky consistency, bad smell, and taste, it protects the ear from the invasion of insects (believe it or not!) and other foreign bodies. The sticky nature of cerumen also helps trap and clean dead skin cells from the ear canal. However, if the ear canal is particularly small, as in children, or convoluted or if there is an overproduction of cerumen, the ear canal can become blocked to the point that sound cannot pass through to the eardrum. This can create a significant hearing loss and may require medical intervention to remove the cerumen plug. Of course, blockage of the ear canal can be brought about by factors other than cerumen. Particularly when working with children, an audiologist is bound to come across cases in which small objects of every description (e.g., pieces of toys, food, crayons, paper, cotton swabs) can be found lodged in the ear canal. If an audiologist discovers such a case, the person is referred for medical examination.

There are many causes of conductive hearing loss that affect the middle ear, far more than can be discussed within the scope of this chapter. Generally speaking, they can involve the perforation or absence of the eardrum; the absence, malformation, or breakage of the ossicles (*ossicular disarticulation*); or the presence of various types of growths, benign or malignant, on the eardrum or within the middle ear space (*cholesteatoma*) or on the ossicles (*otosclerosis*). In lieu of addressing these pathologies in detail, the remaining discussion of conductive hearing loss will focus on the most common cause involving the middle ear: *otitis media.*

Otitis media is an inflammation of the middle ear, with or without infection. There are two primary causes of otitis media. The first is a eustachian tube blockage; the second is direct infection of the middle ear.

Eustachian tube blockage prevents ventilation of the middle ear. A vacuum forms in the middle ear as the oxygen in that area is absorbed.

This first stage of otitis media is referred to as **atelectasis.** This vacuum begins to pull on the eardrum and draw it inward. As a result, the eardrum is stiffened, and its ability to vibrate freely is diminished. If the function of the eustachian tube is not restored, the retraction of the eardrum continues, and it may subsequently become inflamed. At this point, the person may experience a sensation that his or her ear has become plugged or begin to experience some ear pain.

T H O U G H T   Q U E S T I O N S

Have you ever had difficulty hearing on an airplane flight or felt your ears "pop" when in an elevator? What do you think causes these temporary problems?

While pulling on the eardrum, the force of the vacuum also begins to draw the moisture out of the mucous membrane, which lines the middle ear space. This fluid begins to fill the space, further stiffening the eardrum and changing completely the medium through which the sound waves must travel to the inner ear. Consequently, the amplitude of the sound vibrations is diminished, and sounds become muffled if not inaudible altogether. This second stage of otitis media is termed **otitis media with effusion (OME),** "effusion" being another term for "fluid." It does not present a health hazard per se, as the fluid is sterile, but the presence of the fluid usually produces a noticeable hearing loss. This condition may last anywhere from a few days to several months, depending on the status of the eustachian tube. Treatment often consists of simply monitoring the situation to see whether it will be resolved on its own. If the fluid remains for six months or more, a more aggressive approach involving the insertion of **pressure equalization (PE) tubes** into the eardrums may be recommended. These tiny PE tubes take over the function of the eustachian tube to allow air back into the middle ear space. Under some conditions, the sterile fluid that forms following a eustachian tube blockage may become infected. This requires medical treatment of the infection.

The second common cause of otitis media is inflammation of the middle ear lining due to infection that has migrated up the eustachian tube from the nasopharynx. Under these conditions the cells of the middle ear lining discharge pus (**suppurative fluid**) into the middle ear. At this stage, called **purulent otitis media,** medical intervention should be obtained to treat the infection. It is important to realize that while antibiotics will stop the infection, they usually will do nothing to open the eustachian tube or dissipate middle ear fluid. Consequently, the three-stage cycle of otitis media without effusion, otitis media with effusion, and purulent otitis media may be repeated several times and may bring periods of time when hearing is significantly reduced.

The significance of this last point becomes apparent when one considers the fact that otitis media is the most frequently diagnosed disorder in the United States in children under 15 years of age (Skoner, 1998). It is most prevalent in children from birth to 2 years. In young children, the structure and function of the eustachian tube are immature and do not achieve adult form until 5 years of age. Very likely, this is the reason why as many as 75 percent of children have one or more episodes of otitis media by the time they are 6 years old (Teele, Klein, & Rosner, 1989, as cited by Lanphear, Byrd, Auinger, & Hall, 1997). However, evidence exists that the number of children who experience multiple episodes (i.e., five or more) during a single year is growing. A study of National Health Interview Survey data from 1981 and 1988 by Lanphear and colleagues (1997) reports a dramatic increase in the prevalence of recurrent otitis media among preschool children: from 18.7 percent in 1981 to 26.9 percent in 1988. Children who are placed in public day care have also been found to be at increased risk for ear infections. Why are certain children prone to recurrent otitis media and why are their numbers on the rise? Many studies have been published looking at factors that may predispose children to recurrent otitis media, such as gender, geographic location, socioeconomic status, and race. Unfortunately, these studies have yielded inconsistent information, so otitis media remains difficult to predict.

Whatever the reason for the increase, it is still an alarming statistic, especially for those professionals who are concerned with communication disorders. The numbers certainly suggest that there is an ever-growing group of children who are experiencing fluctuating hearing acuity and middle ear function during the time that is most crucial for them in developing speech and language. Dozens of studies have been conducted to examine the long-range effect of recurrent otitis media on the acquisition of speech-language skills, cognitive development, and academic performance. Although these studies have failed to demonstrate an absolute cause-and-effect relationship between recurrent otitis media and future learning problems, they certainly present evidence that such children are at great risk educationally (Gravel & Ellis, 1995; Roberts & Schuele, 1990). Consequently, it is the responsibility of speech-language pathologists and audiologists to educate parents about otitis media and to assist them in the early identification of the condition and obtaining of appropriate medical intervention.

The societal proliferation of antibiotic drug use may also contribute to the increase of otitis media cases as certain strains of bacteria that cause the disorder become resistant to the drugs used in its treatment.

SENSORINEURAL HEARING LOSS

The second type of hearing loss, *sensorineural hearing loss*, involves the absence or malformation of or damage to the structures of the inner

If a hearing loss goes undetected until a child is 4 or 5 years old, the hearing loss will have a far more adverse effect on communication. If the hearing loss is discovered while the child is still an infant and intervention is readily obtained, the prognosis for development of good communication skills is much more positive. The critical issue of the need for early intervention, combined with recent technological advances, has led to the development of universal newborn hearing screening programs in many states.

ear. It is, in many aspects, the direct opposite of conductive hearing loss. Sensorineural hearing losses are generally permanent hearing losses for which medical treatment is unavailable. While sensorineural losses may affect any frequency to any extent, most people with sensorineural hearing losses predominantly have difficulty hearing higher frequency sounds, while the ability to hear lower frequencies remains intact. Unlike conductive hearing losses, in which the problem stems from sounds not being loud enough, sensorineural hearing losses create a problem with clarity of sound. Not only are some sounds not heard, even those sounds that are heard may be distorted.

A useful analogy to illustrate the difference between the two types of pathologies is to think about a radio. When the radio is tuned to a station but is playing at a very low volume level, it simulates a conductive hearing loss. If the volume level is increased (i.e., the conductive pathology is overcome), the radio signal becomes clear and can be easily understood by the listener. Now take the same radio, but this time move the tuner slightly so that it is no longer centered on the desired station. The signal is still audible, but it becomes distorted and harder to understand. Altering the volume does little to improve the situation; indeed, increasing the volume may further garble the signal. This best represents what is experienced by a person who has a sensorineural hearing loss. It is not a problem of audibility but of intelligibility.

Because of its permanency and its corrupting effect on the auditory signal, a sensorineural hearing loss can be expected to have a definite impact on speech-language and cognitive development. To what degree this will affect the person depends on three factors: what caused the hearing loss, when the hearing loss occurred (age of onset), and when it was discovered. Causes of sensorineural hearing losses are **genetic** (hereditary) or *acquired* (nonhereditary). Age of onset is described in terms of being **congenital** (present at birth) or **adventitious** (occurring sometime after birth). Another way of looking at age of onset is to consider whether the hearing loss occurred **prelingually,** that is, before the person developed speech, or **postlingually,** after the person had the opportunity to experience speech and language.

Let's take a look, then, at some common causes of sensorineural hearing loss, starting with those that are congenital and hereditary. When the hearing loss is due to the absence or malformation of the inner ear structures during embryonic development, it is called **aplasia.** There are several types of aplasias, depending on which part of the inner ear (i.e., the hair cells, the organ of Corti, or the entire cochlea itself) is affected. Very often, congenital hereditary sensorineural hearing impairment is a main component of a group of symptoms that make up an entire syndrome. **Usher's syndrome** is found in approximately 3 to 6 percent of profoundly deaf children (Northern & Downs, 1991). The person with Usher's syndrome not only experiences a severe to profound hearing loss, but is subject to a progressive blindness as well. People with **Waardenburg's syndrome** are distinguished by pigmentary discoloration, particularly in the irises and hair, craniofacial malformation of the nasal area, and a severe to profound hearing impairment. Congenital sensorineural hearing loss can also occur as a secondary feature to other neurological disorders such as cerebral palsy (see Chapter 12) or neurofibromatosis ("Elephant Man" disease). The amount of hearing loss in these cases can range from very mild to severe.

Sensorineural hearing loss can be present at birth, but not because of genetic factors. It may be due to some illness or toxic agent experienced by the mother during pregnancy. The most notorious example of these congenital but acquired causes of hearing losses is **maternal rubella.** During the 1960s and 1970s, an outbreak of maternal rubella (German measles) resulted in an estimated 10,000–20,000 children being born with handicapping conditions. Over 50 percent of these children had severe to profound hearing losses.

Damage to a child's inner ear structures can also result from other diseases contracted by the mother during pregnancy. Sexually transmitted diseases such as syphilis can cause various degrees of central nervous system disorders, mental retardation, and hearing loss in the developing fetus. Aside from disease, complications during pregnancy, such as Rh incompatibility or anoxia (oxygen deprivation), can create a host of problems for the developing fetus, including hearing loss.

Sensorineural hearing loss can occur because of factors that a person may encounter at any point during his or her lifetime. Most adventitiously acquired hearing losses are due to illnesses, such as meningitis. **Meningitis** is an inflamation of the meninges, the layers of tissue covering the brain, and is frequently a cause of severe to profound hearing loss in young children as well as adults. The structures of the inner ear are very susceptible to damage either from the bacteria that cause the disease or from the high fever that is an accompanying symptom. Moreover, because bacterial meningitis can be a life-threatening disease, it requires treatment with high doses of very powerful antibiotics, which themselves can be toxic to the inner ear structures. In this case, it might not be the disease but the cure that results in the hearing loss. Whether through the disease or the cure, the person is often left with a severe to profound hearing loss. In addition to certain antibiotics, particularly the mycin family, there are other drugs that are known to be **ototoxic,** or destructive to inner ear structures. Many of the chemotherapy treatments fall into this category, as does aspirin in extremely large quantities and certain drugs in the medications used to treat HIV and AIDs.

Occasionally, an **acoustic neuroma** or tumor on the auditory nerve may develop. These tumors are typically benign and usually grow at the point where the auditory nerve exits the bony labyrinth of the cochlea.

Sadly, in recent years, there has been a marked increase in the number of children born with significant disabilities due to abuse of alcohol by mothers during pregnancy. Fetal alcohol syndrome is estimated to occur at a rate of 1 in every 750 births and is now a leading cause of mental retardation in the United States. The alcohol severely impairs the neurological and physical development of the fetus, resulting in growth deficiencies, sensorineural hearing loss, and limited cognitive development.

Symptoms of acoustic neuromas include vertigo, tinnitus (a ringing in the ear), and hearing loss. Treatment is surgical removal of the tumor, which often necessitates severing of part or all of the auditory nerve, creating a permanent hearing loss.

Noise-induced hearing loss is the leading type of acquired sensorineural hearing loss in young and middle-aged adults. Exposure to high noise levels puts considerable stress on the delicate structures of the inner ear. This results in swelling of the hair cells. That, in turn, causes them to be unable to fire until the swelling goes down. The result is called **noise-induced temporary threshold shift (NITTS).** Most people are familiar with this effect. After being at a very loud party or a rock concert most people experience a reduction in hearing (things sound muffled) and often there is a ringing sensation, called **tinnitus.** After several hours the ringing stops and hearing returns to normal.

Some noise exposures are intense enough to cause some of the hair cells to swell enough to rupture. These hair cells are gone for good. The person has now sustained **noise-induced permanent threshold shift (NIPTS).** Initially, no sustained hearing loss may be noticed. The NIPTS may be quite small compared to the accompanying temporary shift. Once the temporary shift has dissipated, the noise-exposed individual may not recognize that a permanent change has taken place. Over time, repeated noise exposure damage accumulates to produce a significant hearing loss.

Exposure to loud noise is an occupational hazard that is not limited to the industrial sector. Farmers are often at risk because of the machinery used in modern agriculture, and both classical and rock musicians have routine exposure to hazardous levels. Additionally, over the past few decades there has been a significant increase in daily nonoccupational noise exposure. Personal power tools, noisy appliances and amplified music—especially delivered directly into the ear through personal stereo headphone use—have significantly increased the incidence of NIPTS in industrialized countries around the world.

Of critical importance with regard to NIPTS is that this type of hearing loss is almost completely preventable. Noise exposure is a function of how long a person is exposed compared to the intensity of the sound—a time-intensity tradeoff. There is also some degree of variability in the individual sensitivity. For instance, sounds less than 80 decibels sound pressure level (using a special filter that mimics hearing sensitivity; dBA) are considered generally safe regardless of the exposure duration. It's estimated that between 20 and 30 percent of workers exposed to 90 dBA during a typical work day will, over the course of a working career, develop significant amounts of hearing loss. Sound levels in excess of 115 dBA can cause significant damage from a single exposure of only a few minutes. Current regulations for industrial settings limit daily eight-hour noise exposure to no more than 90 dBA. For every 5 decibel increase, the time of exposure must be cut in half, so that at 95 dBA the worker should only be exposed for four hours, and at 100 dBA exposure should be limited to two hours. Workers who will exceed those time limits must wear hearing protection (acoustic ear plugs or ear muffs). Additionally, all workers with noise exposure over 85 dBA must have annual hearing tests to monitor for relatively small changes in hearing. This monitoring process is designed to identify workers who are susceptible to noise damage and take more stringent steps to protect their hearing before a significant hearing loss develops.

Finally, the reality of sensorineural hearing loss is that everyone will eventually experience it to some degree, and we have little control over it. Hearing loss induced through the aging process is called **presbycusis.** Created through the slow deterioration of the hair cells and acoustic nerve, it affects an estimated 30 percent of noninstitutionalized people over 65 years of age and 70 to 80 percent of residents of nursing facilities (Schow & Nerbonne, 1980, as cited by Weinstein, 1994). Consequently, it is a factor that the speech-language pathologist or audiologist who works with a geriatric population must take into consideration when developing any kind of communication treatment plan.

T H O U G H T   Q U E S T I O N

Do you have a family member with a hearing loss? How does it affect his or her life or the lives of other family members?

MIXED HEARING LOSS

The third type of hearing loss, *mixed hearing loss,* is a combination of a sensorineural hearing loss with a conductive component. For example, a person with a sensorineural hearing loss from meningitis may also experience an ear infection, which could further depress hearing acuity.

CENTRAL AUDITORY PROCESSING DISORDERS

The three types of hearing loss described in the preceding section refer to damage sustained by the peripheral auditory system, that is, the structures from the pinna to the auditory nerve. However, audiologists are also concerned with problems affecting the **auditory nervous system,** which includes the brain stem pathways and the auditory cortex of the brain (see Figure 14.4). Problems along these pathways do not typically result in a hearing loss per se, but in an inability to efficiently

How can people tell if they are being exposed to sounds that are too loud in the general environment? Three simple rules, while not perfect, can help: (1) The background noise is potentially hazardous if you need to raise your voice to converse with someone standing three feet away from you. (2) If you feel any discomfort, the sound is too loud. (3) If things sound muffled or you have ringing in your ears after you leave a noisy place, that noise was too loud and you should avoid that type of exposure in the future.

How can you protect your hearing from loud noise? (1) Avoid situations such as those described above. (2) If you must be in a high-noise environment, wear acoustical ear plugs and try to keep your exposure time as short as possible.

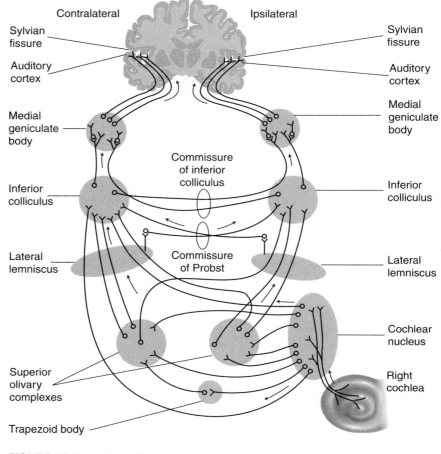

FIGURE 14.4 Schematic representation of auditory nervous system

use and interpret auditory information. Such a deficiency is what is referred to as a *central auditory processing disorder (CAPD)*.

Defining central auditory processing disorders (CAPD) has been a controversial issue. Problems of the central auditory system manifest in a variety of ways, with the signs and symptoms being similar to disorders such as language learning delay (LLD) or attention deficit hyperactivity disorder (ADHD). Typically, children eventually diagnosed with CAPD first present as children who have difficulty learning in a typical classroom environment. The behavioral signs usually present as problems listening during instruction. A "simple" diagnosis of CAPD is too broad to be practical. It may be helpful to consider some of the processing capabilities of the central system under normal conditions, as described by the ASHA Task Force on Central Auditory Processing (1995d) and compare those capabilities to a model of CAPD such as that proposed by Katz, Stecker, and Henderson (1994). (Please note that this is not the only model of CAPD and that, given the nature of this text, not all proposed areas of CAPD are discussed in the following section.)

The normal auditory system is able to localize sounds in space. It can tell what direction a sound comes from. Additionally, experience with sound allows for prediction of how far away the sound source is from the listener. Related to the localization is the ability to lateralize sounds when listening through headphones. All these abilities are the result of neurological comparisons of sounds coming from each ear, with those comparisons beginning in the brainstem. Related to the ability to localize/lateralize is the ability to "squelch" background noise and key in on a specific signal with the clutter of other events. In a group situation, when there are several conversations occurring simultaneously, most people are able to focus on one talker and ignore the rest. They are also able to rapidly switch and listen in on a different conversation even as the original conversation continues (of course, in doing so they lose track of what the first talker was saying). This is squelch in action. It is likely the result of complex activity in both the afferent and efferent nervous system. The inability to squelch can lead to significant listening difficulty in group situations or in the presence of general background noise. This type of intolerance for competing signals is one type of central auditory processing problem.

The normal auditory system is able to discriminate fine detail in the auditory signal. From the simple ability to tell whether two sounds are the same or different, it is also able to rapidly recognize patterns (i.e., words). From a "knowledge base" of the way the sounds and words of the language work, it is therefore able to deal with degradation of the signal due to competing (masking) noise, rapid speech, or speech that is in other ways altered from the norm. Persons who are not able to process speech rapidly, have difficulty with degraded speech, or who have not developed an innate understanding of the phonetic sound system of language are said to have a problem with decoding.

The normal system is able to store a short-term echoic memory trace what has been heard. This is necessary in order to process long utterances, or even to hold short bits of speech long enough to act an what has been said, such as when writing down a number left as part of a phone mail message. Some individuals with CAPD appear to have an inordinately short, or rapidly fading, auditory memory.

Another aspect of auditory processing is the ability to resolve and maintain the timing, or temporal, aspects of an auditory signal. Temporal resolution is important in processing the sounds of speech. The ability to maintain temporal order also, for instance, keeps the digits in the phone number referred to above in the correct order. Persons with breakdown in temporal processing may have a CAPD problem in the area of auditory organization.

Some central auditory capabilities are likely ingrained, or hardwired, into the auditory nervous system and others appear be the result of learning. The hardwired aspects also appear to be related to maturational processes.

Assessing CAPD requires the administration of special tests by either an audiologist, a speech-language pathologist, or the school psychologist. These tests usually involve digit sequences, sounds, words or sentences that are presented **diotically,** that is, to both ears simultaneously, or **dichotically,** to each ear independently. An example of a diotic task is asking the child to point to pictures in a book while a competing message (e.g., a story) is presented simultaneously. This task assesses the child's ability to attend to one set of auditory stimuli and ignore the presence of a competing signal. A dichotic task may entail the presentation of one word or sentence to the right ear while a different word or sentence is presented to the left ear. The child is then required to repeat both sentences. This assesses memory skills and the ability to integrate auditory information. Other tests involve the presentation of isolated speech sounds, which the child is asked to combine into a meaningful word. For example, the stimulus item may be "/m/,/ɪ/,/l/,/k/," which the child must identify as "milk."

Because of the maturational nature of central auditory processes and the contribution of learning, tests of CAPD are scored based on age-based norms. Also, it is critical that the CAPD test data be interpreted in conjunction with test results from other specialists such as speech-language pathologists and psychologists.

The treatment of CAPD often involves at least one of three approaches and often a combination of all three. Modification of the listening environment may be undertaken to reduce noise and to provide an enhanced speech signal to the student. Specific therapies may be used to develop listening abilities such as decoding speech or increasing auditory memory. Finally, the child may be taught strategies that allow the student to work around or compensate for the processing problem. Therapeutic and strategic intervention is often the role of the speech-language pathologist.

DEGREES OF HEARING LOSS

When describing a hearing loss, audiologists use terminology such as *conductive, sensorineural,* and *mixed* to identify the portion of the auditory system that has been affected. Another important set of terms has been developed to describe the amount, or **degree of hearing loss.** Degree of hearing loss is expressed in units called *decibels (dB).* A decibel is a mathematically derived unit based on the pressure exerted by a particular sound vibration. Each degree of hearing loss refers to a specific decibel range. This system was invented to replace the idea of "percentage of hearing loss" commonly used by the medical profession. In an effort to use more precise language, audiologists have adopted the terms presented in Table 14.1.

In very general terms, individuals with degrees of hearing loss that fall within the mild to moderately severe categories are referred to as **hard of hearing.** These individuals will usually depend as much as possible on their hearing for communication and learning of new concepts. For people with a severe to profound hearing loss, however, the auditory system provides little or no access to the world. These individuals are usually referred to as **deaf.** As one can imagine, their experiences are radically different from those of people who are born with normal hearing or even people who are hard of hearing. But rather than look on their deafness as a disability, many deaf individuals celebrate the uniqueness of their lifestyle in a movement known as **Deaf culture.**

For many individuals in the Deaf community, the term "Deaf" is preferred regardless of the degree of hearing loss. The term "hard of hearing" is used by those not affiliated with the Deaf culture.

TABLE 14.1

Degrees of hearing loss

Decibel Range	Degree of Loss	Description
0 dB–20 dB	Normal hearing	
21 dB–40 dB	Mild	Difficulty with distant or faint speech.
41 dB–55 dB	Moderate	Difficulty following conversational level speech.
56 dB–70 dB	Moderately severe	Can hear only loud speech.
71 dB–90 dB	Severe	Difficulty understanding even loud speech; may require alternative communication system.
91 dB +	Profound	Usually considered "deaf"; cannot depend on auditory system alone to obtain information.

DEAFNESS AND DEAF CULTURE

A culture is created when a group of people share in a common background of language, traditions, and values. There is an important distinction to be made between individuals who are "deaf" (with a lowercase "d," reflecting the presence of a common physiological condition) and those among them who consider themselves "Deaf" (with an uppercase "D," reflecting their membership in an identifiable group). The primary method by which a deaf individual becomes part of the Deaf culture is through the use of what is considered its native language, **American Sign Language (ASL).** One's fluency in ASL, not the presence of a hearing loss, is often the factor that determines whether a person is considered Deaf. Consequently, not every individual with a hearing loss, even a severe to profound hearing loss, is automatically included in the Deaf culture.

It is interesting to note that American Sign Language has its linguistic roots in the French language.

T H O U G H T   Q U E S T I O N S

Do you know a few ASL signs? This is similar to knowing a few English words but no grammar. Like English, ASL has its own separate grammar. Do you think a hearing person who learns ASL as an adult might sign with a "hearing accent"?

The continued existence of any culture depends on the perpetuation of its native language and traditions. Among the Deaf, this is accomplished through education and marriage. Residential schools for the deaf provide the means for deaf children to interact with each other and to be able to communicate freely. Through their socialization, pride in their identity as Deaf individuals is encouraged. Hearing loss is not seen as an impairment, but as something that gives them the opportunity to share in something unique. On reaching adulthood, very often members of the Deaf community marry others who share the same cultural ideals. Moreover, Deaf parents are delighted to have deaf children to whom they may pass on their traditions.

Maintaining the Deaf culture is not without its struggles, however. A deaf person faces many challenges in trying to coexist with the hearing world. Because ASL is considered the primary language of the Deaf, they are faced with learning English as a second language and thus encounter many of the same limitations as do other nonnative speakers. It is well documented that many Deaf individuals cannot read English past the third- or fourth-grade level. Their skills in written English are also delayed. Since most hearing people cannot sign, this limited knowledge of English leaves the deaf person with an inability to communicate with the majority of people with whom they come into contact. Certainly, for a young person, this can lead to extreme loneliness and isolation. For an adult, poor English skills and the presence of the hearing loss significantly limit employment opportunities. Many must settle for lower-paying jobs. However, overcoming adversity creates further unity among Deaf individuals and is something in which they are encouraged to take great pride. Rather than surrendering their culture and being assimilated into the hearing world, it is the goal of Deaf persons to increase awareness among hearing people regarding Deaf issues, especially pertaining to language, and to have equal access to the same opportunities as the hearing majority.

This is not to suggest that all deaf individuals accept the idea of a Deaf culture. In fact, it is a hotly debated topic with passionate feelings on both sides. Some Deaf individuals have very little tolerance for what is referred to as the "hearing world" or even for hard-of-hearing people. Someone who is considering entering the fields of speech pathology or audiology should be aware that among some Deaf individuals, such professionals are treated with disdain. By emphasizing the need for spoken language or for use of amplification, speech-language pathologists and audiologists are seen as trying to label deaf individuals as "abnormal" or in need of "treatment" to help them become more like hearing people. On the other hand, some deaf individuals, usually those with hearing parents and/or those who are products of mainstream education with hearing peers, are more comfortable with the idea that they are part of the hearing world. Obviously, there is no right or wrong answer here, but it is important to be aware of the issue. The direction and success of any therapy will depend greatly on which philosophy the deaf person espouses.

AUDIOLOGICAL TESTING PROCEDURES

Having described the basic principles of sound, the anatomy and physiology of the auditory system, and type and degree of hearing loss, we are ready to take a look at how the audiologist uses all of this information clinically.

REFERRAL AND CASE HISTORY

Referral for audiological testing may originate from a variety of sources such as a physician, school nurse, speech-language pathologist, psychologist, teacher, family members or through self-referral.

Before beginning the testing, the audiologist will spend some time interviewing the client and collecting case history information. It is important to know whether there is a family history of hearing loss, whether the person has sustained any recent injury or is taking medication, whether he or she has been exposed to noise, and so on. The audiologist will have the client describe the situations in which he or she is having difficulty or any symptoms that may be present, such as tinnitus, earache, or dizziness. A complete case history can often provide the audiologist with a strong indication of what the problem is even before any testing is administered. An audiologic interview can be seen on the book's CD-ROM.

TESTING INFANTS AND CHILDREN

As was indicated in the discussion of sensorineural hearing loss, the importance of early identification of hearing loss cannot be stressed enough. In testing infants and young children, the special skills of the audiologist are particularly valuable, since obtaining reliable information from this population can be challenging. Obviously, an infant will not be able to respond in the traditional manner of raising a hand when he or she hears a sound. Like speech and language, auditory behavior is developmental, and if audiologists are familiar with the different stages of auditory development, they should be able to elicit from the child a response that is appropriate for his or her age.

PHYSIOLOGICAL TESTS

In the past twenty to thirty years advances in technology and advances in our understanding of hearing have led to the development of physiological tests of the auditory system. These tests evaluate the integrity of the peripheral auditory system and do not require cooperation from the person being tested. While they are not true "hearing" tests—hearing requires the person to be able to recognize and use sound—they represent a major step forward in the early diagnosis of hearing loss and in the thorough evaluation of the auditory system.

One such test is the test of **otoacoustic emissions (OAEs).** Otoacoustic emissions are low-level sounds produced by the cochlea either spontaneously or in response to stimulation. Essentially, in the latter situation, when a brief sound of moderate intensity is presented to a healthy cochlea, the outer hair cells contract slightly. After the sound stops the hair cells expand back to their original size and shape. This results in a pressure wave within the fluid of the cochlea that pushes back against the ossicles, in turn, vibrating the eardrum. The eardrum then acts like a tiny loudspeaker creating a slight sound (an OAE) in the ear canal. Results are interpreted by analyzing the amplitude of the resultant waveform relative to the frequency of the stimulus as in Figure 14.5. Research has shown these emissions to be present in most normal cochleae and to be particularly robust in young children. This

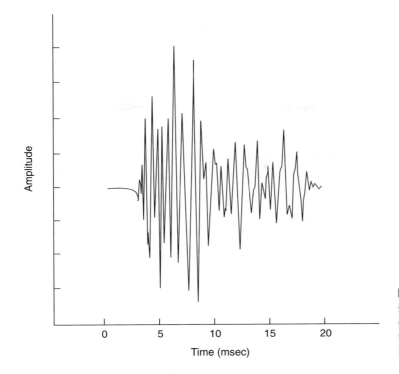

FIGURE 14.5 A typical transient-evoked otoacoustic emission generated by presenting a click stimulus to a normal ear

makes them a very powerful tool for use in screening the hearing of newborns and infants. In terms of the sensitivity of the technique, it appears that OAEs are absent in people with a hearing loss greater than 40 dB (Norton & Stover, 1994).

Because of the demonstrable utility of OAEs as a screening tool in infants, many states now have laws that require the screening of all newborns. It is hoped that by using OAE screening most children born with significant hearing losses will be identified and begin to receive intervention services very early in the critical developmental period for language and speech.

Other physiological tests of the auditory system are available. Two of these tests are **electrocochleography (ECoG)** and **auditory brain stem evoked response (ABER) audiometry.** Electrocochleography measures the electrical activity of the auditory nerve, while ABER measures the electrical activity of the auditory nerve and the brainstem. These tests use computerized equipment to measure involuntary responses to sound within the auditory nervous system and therefore do not depend on the patient's cooperation. The most common of these procedures is auditory brain stem evoked response (ABER) audiometry. In this

ABER testing is particularly useful for children with a cleft palate. Because of the high risk of otitis media and associated hearing loss, these children need to be monitored carefully very early in life.

method, a click or a tone pip stimulus is introduced to the patient's auditory system through earphones. Electrodes are placed at various points on the scalp to gather and record the neural responses generated as the stimulus progresses from the auditory nerve to designated points along the brain stem. The result is a waveform known as a **Jewett wave,** named after the scientist who first described it.

Although they vary somewhat from person to person, Jewett waves have a typical form with regard to amplitude and latency or time interval that allows them to be used for diagnostic purposes (see Figure 14.6). Depending on the amplitude of the wave and the time lag between peaks, an audiologist can identify the degree and type of hearing loss.

Auditory brain stem evoked response audiometry is the most common electrophysiological procedure and is a very useful follow-up tool to OAEs when diagnosing hearing loss in infants because it can provide at least some degree of frequency specific information about the auditory system.

BEHAVIORAL TESTING

A limitation of electrophysiological tests is that, while they yield information about sensitivity of the peripheral structures, they do not provide information about how the client responds to sound. Behavioral data are necessary to fully define a hearing loss and to appropriately fit hearing aids. The pediatric audiologist must, therefore, be skilled at **behavioral observation audiometry.**

As the term implies, the audiologist presents different stimuli to the child through speakers and watches for the child's reaction. The basic response that the audiologist will look for is the **startle reflex,** which can be obtained in newborn children who are presented with a sound of 90 dB. An audiologist may also present a soothing stimulus, such as speech or music, and try to observe a quieting behavior on the part of the child. As the child becomes older, the ability to localize a sound emerges, and an audiologist may employ a technique called **visual reinforcement audiometry.** In this method, the child is rewarded for looking for a sound by the use of moving toys and/or flashing

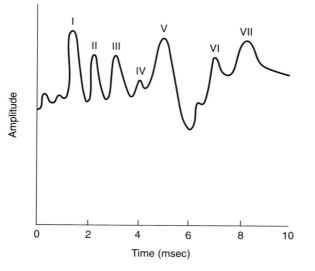

FIGURE 14.6 Schematic drawing of typical Jewett wave pattern from auditory brain stem evoked response (ABER) testing of a normal ear

lights. This method can be attempted with children as young as 3 to 4 months of age, who should be able to turn their head from side to side in the general direction of a moderate level of sound. By 24 months, a child should be able to directly locate a quiet sound of 25 dB presented at any angle (Northern & Downs, 1991).

By 2½ to 3 years of age, a child should be able to engage in testing procedures that approximate those used with an adult. The child should be able to wear earphones and can be taught to respond to frequency-specific sounds and speech using a technique called **play audiometry.** Using items such as blocks, tokens, or puzzle pieces, children are told that they are going to play a game. They are instructed to put the block in a basket, the peg in a board, or the like whenever they hear a sound. Most children, after a few demonstrations, are able to comply with the task and, by playing the game, provide the audiologist with the desired information.

TESTING OLDER CHILDREN AND ADULTS

The procedure for testing older children and adults includes three basic components: **pure tone audiometry, speech audiometry,** and **immittance testing.** The pure tone and speech testing is administered by using a specialized piece of equipment called an **audiometer.** An audiometer has controls that allow for the manipulation of the intensity and frequency of a stimulus. Immittance testing is conducted by using a different piece of equipment called an **immittance bridge** or *tympanometer.* This equipment will be described in a later section.

PURE TONE TESTING

Most of the critical information about a person's hearing is obtained through pure tone tests. Therefore, if time is of the essence or test equipment is limited (as it is in on-site testing at a school or a factory), it is possible to determine both the type and degree of hearing loss by conducting a pure tone test only.

Pure tone stimuli are sounds that contain only one individual frequency. Those that are typically used in testing begin at a very low frequency of 125 Hz and increase by octaves to 250 Hz, 500 Hz, 1000 Hz, 2,000 Hz, 4,000 Hz, and 8,000 Hz. By following this progression of frequencies, the integrity of the entire basilar membrane, from apex to base, is tested.

The purpose of pure tone testing is to discover the person's threshold for each frequency. A **threshold** is defined as the quietest presentation level (in decibels) at which a person can detect a stimulus 50 percent of the time. The audiologist establishes the client's threshold by presenting a single pure tone (e.g., 1,000 Hz) while raising and lowering the intensity level. At each presentation of the tone, the audiologist looks for a response from the client to indicate whether it was heard. This process continues until the audiologist determines the presentation level at which the client is just barely able to detect the tone. Once the threshold is established for 1,000 Hz, the audiologist repeats the procedure at 2,000 Hz, then 4,000 Hz, and so forth until all of the frequencies are tested. Results are recorded on a graph called an **audiogram.** An example of an audiogram is shown in Figure 14.7. The decibel range in which the thresholds fall determines the degree of the hearing loss.

Pure tone thresholds are established in two ways: through **air conduction** and **bone conduction.** Air conduction testing is administered while the person is wearing earphones, the method with which most people are familiar. The purpose of this technique is to assess the function of the entire auditory system from the outer ear through the inner ear. Once testing under earphones is completed, the process is repeated

During pure tone threshold testing, the subject is asked to raise her hand when she hears a tone.

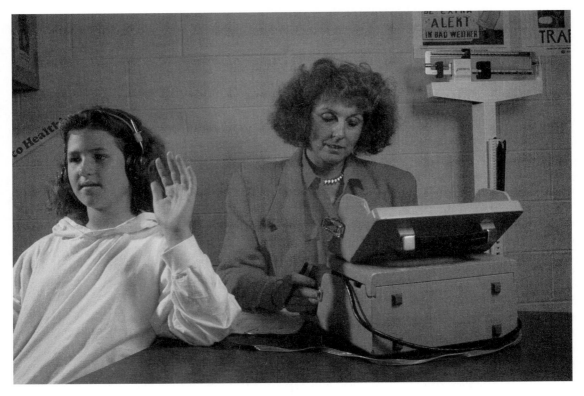

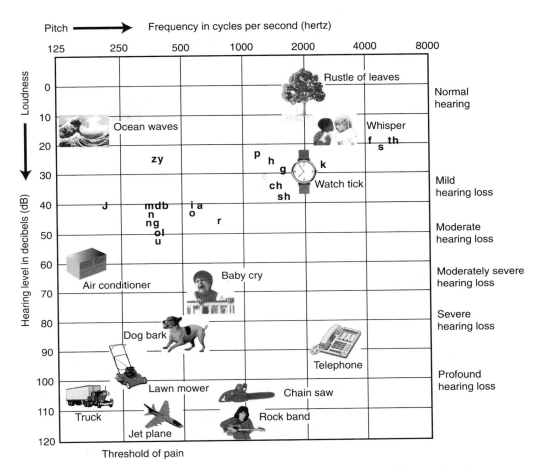

FIGURE 14.7 Audiogram showing typical frequency range and intensity of common environmental and speech sounds. (Adapted from: J. Northern & M. Downs (1976). *Hearing in Children* (2nd ed.). Baltimore, MD: Williams and Wilkins.)

by using an apparatus called a **bone oscillator,** a small, vibrating device that is positioned against the skull behind the pinna. When the stimulus is presented through a bone oscillator, the bones of the skull are vibrated at the same frequency. This vibration of the skull causes the fluids in the inner ear to move, which, in turn, activates the hair cells. Consequently, the person is able to hear the sound even though it has not passed through the outer or middle ears but is processed through direct stimulation of the cochlea. A demonstration of pure tone screening exam can be viewed on the CD-ROM.

Have you ever listened to your voice when it has been recorded on an audiotape? Does it sound different to you in comparison to your normal speaking voice? What might explain this difference?

By comparing the results from the air conduction testing to the bone conduction results, it is possible to identify the type of hearing loss. Consider the audiograms in Figures 14.8 and 14.9. In Figure 14.8, the right ear air conduction thresholds (represented by the circles) fall within the moderate hearing loss range. However, the bone conduction thresholds (represented by the brackets) fall within the normal range of hearing. From this, the audiologist can infer that the client has difficulty hearing sound when it is introduced into the entire auditory system; however, the client has no difficulty hearing sound if the outer and middle ears are bypassed and the cochlea is stimulated

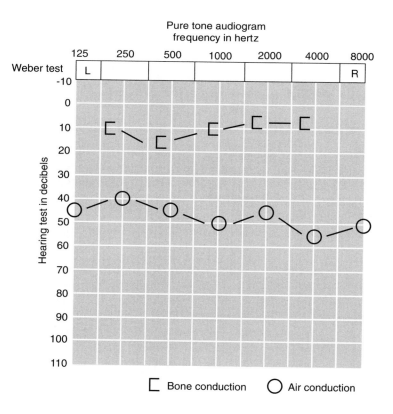

FIGURE 14.8 Audiogram representing moderate conductive hearing loss in the right ear. (Note: The symbol used to denote bone conduction is dependent on the method used to assess it.)

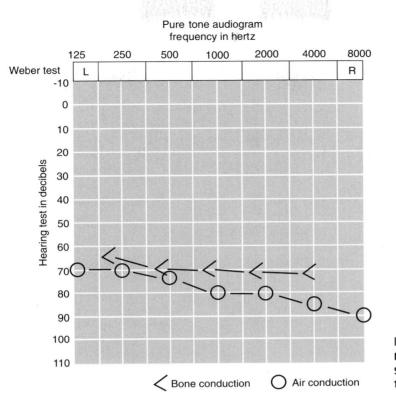

Pure tone audiogram frequency in hertz

	125	250	500	1000	2000	4000	8000
Weber test	L						R

Hearing test in decibels: -10, 0, 10, 20, 30, 40, 50, 60, 70, 80, 90, 100, 110

< Bone conduction   ○ Air conduction

FIGURE 14.9 Audiogram representing severe sensorineural hearing loss in the right ear

directly. Therefore, the conclusion can be drawn that the client is suffering from a *conductive* hearing loss. In Figure 14.9, both the air and bone conduction thresholds fall outside normal limits to within the severe hearing loss range. Since the client's hearing did not improve when the inner ear was stimulated directly, the audiologist can conclude that the inner ear itself must be damaged. Therefore, this client is probably suffering from a *sensorineural* hearing loss.

In Figure 14.10, again both the air and bone conduction thresholds fall outside the normal range. However, the degree of hearing loss represented by the air conduction thresholds is greater than the degree of hearing loss represented by the bone conduction thresholds. In this case, the audiologist concludes that while there is obvious damage to the inner ear, the person has the potential to hear better if the outer and middle ears are bypassed. Consequently, there is evidence that both a sensorineural and a conductive hearing loss exist here; in other words, the client is suffering from a *mixed* hearing loss.

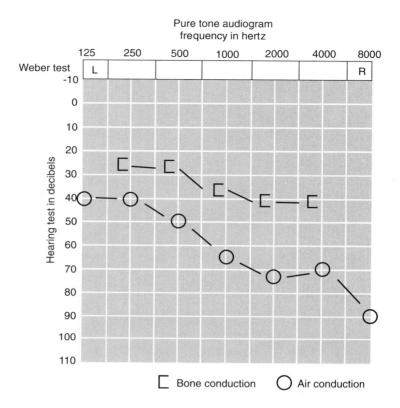

Pure tone audiogram
frequency in hertz

FIGURE 14.10 Audiogram
representing moderately
severe mixed hearing loss in
the right ear

SPEECH AUDIOMETRY

While quite a bit of information is obtained from the pure tone testing, it is also useful to evaluate how well a person can hear and understand a complex stimulus such as speech. After all, the spoken word is much more relevant to us as humans than are individual frequencies. Two basic tests make up the speech audiometry battery. The first is the **speech reception threshold (SRT) test.** The SRT is a measure of the quietest level of speech a person can hear and understand 50 percent of the time. The speech stimuli that are used for this test are a special group of words called **spondees.** Spondees are two-syllable compound words, such as "hotdog" or "cowboy," that are spoken with equal emphasis on both syllables. As the words are presented, the intensity level is raised and lowered until the patient is able to repeat approximately half of the words correctly. This final intensity level is recorded as the SRT. The SRT should agree with pure tone sensitivity in the range between 500 Hz and 1,000 Hz. It is important to perform additional testing when there is not agreement between the pure tone data and the SRT data. The SRT may also be used as an estimate of overall hearing sensitivity when pure tome results cannot be obtained, such as with younger children and adults who, for whatever reason, are unable to comply with the pure tone test. A demonstration of SRT testing can be viewed on the book's CD-ROM.

The second test procedure is speech audiometry is called the **word recognition test (WRT)**. The WRT is quite different from the other procedures discussed thus far. The WRT is not a measure of sensitivity, per se. Instead, this is a test of how well the auditory system is able to *understand* words. The speech stimuli that are used in the WRT are different from those used to assess thresholds in that they are taken from lists of one-syllable, **phonetically balanced (PB)** words. The term "phonetically balanced" simply means that each speech sound is included in the list in the same proportion in which it appears in everyday language. For persons with normal hearing, the WRT is administered at an intensity approximating conversational speech. For persons with hearing loss, the WRT is administered at an intensity designed to compensate for the degree of hearing loss. The purpose of this test is to examine how well, given optimal listening conditions, a person can identify all of the individual speech sounds that give a word its meaning. For example, a stimulus word might be "sled." In turn, the client might repeat "sled" or might say "fled." As you can see, missing that one high-frequency consonant sound /s/ at the beginning of the word changes the meaning entirely. The audiologist counts the number of words the patient repeats correctly and computes a score. This score gives a strong indication of the impact the hearing loss is having on the patient's communication.

THOUGHT QUESTION

Are there characteristics of speech sounds that make them more complex than other sounds, such as a car horn or a hand clap?

IMMITTANCE TESTING

Audiograms provide only limited information. What cannot be ascertained from the information on the audiogram is the possible cause of the hearing loss. To determine what type of pathology is present, the audiologist must perform specialty tests. The electrophysiological testing that was previously described is one example of specialty testing that can help to distinguish cochlear from auditory nerve pathology. Immittance testing is another example of specialty testing. The purpose of immittance testing is to assist in the differential diagnosis of conductive pathology.

As was mentioned at the beginning of this section, immittance testing is performed by using an immittance bridge or tympanometer. The tympanometer consists of a handheld probe that contains a microphone, air pressure pump, and sound generator connected to a recording instrument. The probe is placed against the pinna so that an airtight seal is created between the probe and the ear. During testing, the air pressure pump alters the air pressure in the canal, which in turn changes the mobility of the eardrum. As the test progresses, the tympanometer measures and records these changes.

From the recorded data, the tympanometer generates a graph that compares changes in air pressure to compliance of the eardrum. This is called a **tympanogram;** an example is shown in Figure 14.11. The results of the testing and the shape of the tympanogram will suggest whether the conductive hearing loss is due to **otosclerosis** (a stiffening of the ossicular chain), **ossicular discontinuity** (a break in the ossicular chain), otitis media, otitis media with effusion, or a perforation of the eardrum. This is very important information to have if a medical referral is to be made. A demonstration of immittance testing can be seen on the book's CD-ROM.

ELECTROPHYSIOLOGICAL TESTS

Electrophysiological tests such as the auditory brain stem evoked response (ABER) can provide valuable information about the auditory system beyond providing an estimate of hearing sensitivity and type of hearing loss, as discussed earlier in this chapter. Because there are ties between the various peaks in the Jewett wave sequence and locations

FIGURE 14.11 Schematic of three common tympanogram patterns: (a) normal middle ear function, (b) somewhat reduced eardrum compliance due to otosclerosis, (c) no eardrum compliance due to otitis media with effusion

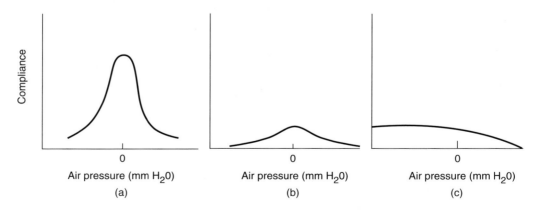

in the auditory nervous system, it is possible to establish general site of lesion information when there is a problem such as an acoustic tumor.

AURAL HABILITATION/REHABILITATION

Aural habilitation/rehabilitation refers to a variety of services and procedures that are designed to help a person cope with the difficulties presented by a hearing loss (Schow & Nerbonne, 1996). The term "aural habilitation" alludes to therapies that are used primarily with children who are hearing impaired from an early age. Because they essentially have had no time to develop communication, the focus of aural habilitation is to teach the missing skills. "Aural rehabilitation" is the term used for services that are provided to clients who lose their hearing later in life, after communication skills have been established. The focus of rehabilitation is to help the person recover these skills or to learn compensatory strategies. For the sake of convenience, the single term "aural rehabilitation" will be used for the remainder of this section and understood to include both aspects of therapy.

Once the diagnosis of the hearing loss is made, it is the audiologist's responsibility to advise the patient—or, in the case of a child with hearing loss, the parents—of the implications of the hearing loss and to provide recommendations for follow-up. These may include medical examination, a recommendation for amplification, speech-language therapy, services of a special education teacher or teacher of the deaf and hard of hearing, and psychological or vocational counseling, depending on factors such as the causes and severity of the hearing loss or the age of the client. Audiologists may find themselves working with many of these other professionals to provide a comprehensive therapy program.

The important idea to remember is that the goal of any aural rehabilitation program is to improve communication. Typical issues that are considered in creating an aural rehabilitation program are **amplification,** *auditory training,* and **oral/manual communication methods.** Depending on the degree to which the hearing loss affects communication, the clinician will develop goals pertaining to one or more of these areas.

AMPLIFICATION

The first step in most aural rehabilitation programs is to obtain appropriate amplification for the patient. **Personal hearing aids** come in a multitude of styles from tiny, in-the-ear models to those worn behind the ear or on the body. Whatever the case, every hearing aid contains three basic components: the microphone, the amplifier, and the receiver. The microphone picks up the sounds in the environment and converts the acoustic signal to an electrical signal, which is channeled to the amplifier. The *amplifier* increases the amplitude of the electrical signal and sends it to the receiver. The *receiver* converts the amplified electrical signal back into acoustic energy and routes it to the ear canal.

The purpose of a hearing aid is to amplify a speech signal and deliver it at an appropriate level above threshold in the impaired range (Ross, 1994). Unlike eyeglasses, which can restore a person's sight to 20/20, a hearing aid does not return hearing to normal. When a person is fitted with a hearing aid, it is critical that he or she understand this point so as not to develop unrealistic expectations. It takes some training and much practice before the patient can become a successful hearing aid user. Often, a formal aural rehabilitation program will include several goals that center on teaching the client the care and maintenance of the hearing aid, how to properly adjust the controls for different listening situations, and how to practice using the amplified signal to improve the understanding of speech. If an audiologist does not take the time to teach the client these skills, more than likely the hearing aids will end up stuffed in a dresser drawer. Box 14.1 is a letter from a mother whose young son is benefiting greatly from his hearing aid. A demonstration of hearing aid counseling can be seen on the book's CD-ROM.

Most people who have sensorineural hearing losses or those who have non-medically correctable conductive hearing losses can benefit from some hearing aid use. However, people who have the most severe and profound hearing losses may find that traditional hearing aids fail to perform with enough amplification to make sound audible to them. For this select group, consideration of a *cochlear implant* (Figure 14.12) may be warranted. There are several components to a cochlear implant. The microphone, speech processor, and an external transmitter are worn outside the skull. Traditionally, the microphone has been located at the ear and been connected by a wire to a body-worn processor. The signal from the processor has then been sent to a transmitting coil magnetically coupled to the head in the area behind the pinna. Current options include speech processors that are worn at the ear much like a behind-the-ear hearing aid. A short wire connects the processor to the external transmitting coil. The components that are surgically implanted in the skull include an internal receiver and an electrode array, the latter of which is inserted in to the bony spiral of the cochlea. In most cochlear implants the electrode array allows for many sites in the cochlea to be stimulated by electrical current. Once the user has healed following surgery, the functionality of each of these sites must be assessed to determine the sensitivity of each location within the cochlear and the most comfortable level of stimulation for that loca-

Digital signal-processing advances have led to the development of digital hearing aids that are in many ways far superior to analog hearing aids.

Letter from a Parent Whose 3-Year-Old Son Was Fitted with Hearing Aids

Dear Dr. Lauffer:

It's been six months since we moved away and last saw you. David is doing great! He has adjusted perfectly to his hearing aids. He knows they are important and they have to either be in his ears or in his "special" case. He's already learned how to turn them off, take them out, and put them away. Whenever he puts on a shirt or something, it's so cute because he checks really quickly to make sure they're in place. He *likes* having them because he says he can hear better. Something classic happened a few days after he got them. David and I were standing on the front porch and he asked me, "Mom, what is that? What is that noise?" I didn't know what he was talking about so David imitated it, and Dr. Lauffer, he was talking about the birds. So I told him it was the birds and he said, "Wow, Mommy, birds are really noisy!" Isn't that cute? He's doing better with his speech and language already. It's amazing the difference it has made for him, really. Thanks for all of your help with David. We appreciate it.

Sincerely,
Julie Brown

---

tion. This "mapping" or "tune-up" process helps determine what sites will receive stimulation from the implant.

The processor of the cochlear implant is a very sophisticated computerized device. It is designed to only send certain aspects of the sound signal to electrode array. These are defined by the speech-processing scheme that has been incorporated by each manufacturer based on research on speech acoustics and the experiences of adult cochlear implant users. The intent is to send the impaired ear only those features of the speech signal that are most critically important for speech intelligibility. Extensive follow-up therapy is often needed for the cochlear implant user to obtain maximum benefit from the device, although some adults do very well with a relative minimum of rehabilitation. Routine adjustment of the device is also needed, especially with children (Chute & Nevins, 2000).

Assistive listening devices (ALDs) make up another type of amplifying equipment that may be utilized as part of an aural rehabilitation program. While traditional hearing aids work well in many situations, it is common for hearing aid users to have difficulty in situations where

Cochlear implants are quite controversial, especially when it comes to the implantation of young children. At least some individuals in the Deaf community feel that implants represent the hearing community's inability to accept deafness and Deaf culture. They see implants as an attempt to "fix" something that does not need to be fixed.

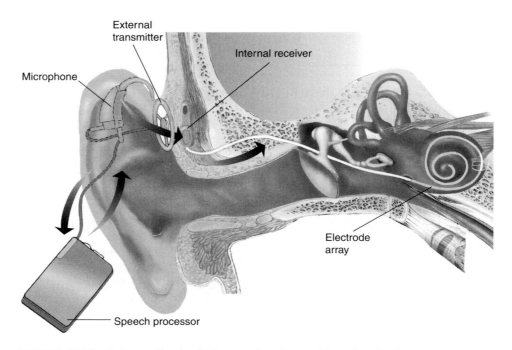

External transmitter

Internal receiver

Microphone

Electrode array

Speech processor

FIGURE 14.12 Schematic depicting parts of a cochlear implant

there is a lot of background noise or when they are more than a few feet from the person with whom they are talking. Trying to hear well can be difficult, for instance, in a classroom, restaurant, meeting room, or auditorium. Assistive listening devices can be helpful in these settings.

The primary principle behind most ALDs is to eliminate distance problems by locating the input microphone as close as possible to the talker. This, in turn, increases the intensity and clarity of the talker's voice compared to any background noise in the room.

One style of ALD that is quite popular is the personal FM system. In personal FM systems the talker wears a radio-transmitting microphone, with either a clip-on lapel microphone or a headworn boom microphone similar to those on hands-free cellular telephones. The listener wears a receiver tuned to the radio frequency of the microphone. The signal from the receiver may be sent to personal headphones, to the listener's personal hearing aid via **direct audio input (DAI)** or to the hearing aid by magnetic induction through a special pick-up in the hearing aid called a **telecoil.**

A few manufacturers have recently introduced personal hearing aid with built-in FM receivers, eliminating the need for a separate receiver unit. A variety of other ALD styles are available, as well as equipment to help the person with a hearing loss better communicate via the telephone. There are also specialized alerting systems for individuals who are deaf or hard-of-hearing.

AUDITORY TRAINING

Once the appropriate amplification device has been obtained, patients may need to be taught (or retaught) how to use their residual or remaining hearing. This process is known as *auditory training*. The goal of auditory training is to maximize a person's use of speech and non-speech cues (Schow & Nerbonne, 1996). In developing an approach to auditory training, it is important that the clinician consider the amount of hearing that the client has. For clients with aided hearing levels in the mild to moderately severe hearing loss range, it would be appropriate to work on sound discrimination skills (e.g., distinguishing the word "mouse" from the word "mouth"). For clients for whom even aided thresholds fall within the severe to profound hearing loss range, it is unreasonable to expect that they have sufficient residual hearing to allow for comprehension of speech. Instead, an appropriate goal would be to improve the detection of sounds, particularly environmental sounds, so that the person may develop at least a functional use of his or her hearing (to be able to detect warning sounds such as smoke detectors, fire alarms, etc.).

There is no single recommended approach to auditory training. For children, the emphasis is on teaching the auditory skills that may be delayed or missing altogether. One example is Raymond Carhart's four-step approach based on the normal developmental stages of auditory development (Schow & Nerbonne, 1996). The procedure is presented in Table 14.2.

In working with adults, auditory training usually focuses on refining skills that are essential to everyday life. Training may include teaching the person how to optimize the listening environment by minimizing background noise and decreasing her or his distance from the speaker. The client may be taught strategies to use when there is a breakdown in communication, such as asking the speaker to rephrase or restate what was said. Depending on the client's needs, the clinician may do some structured practice of speech discrimination skills.

For most adults with hearing impairment, auditory training involves practice in using the telephone. Understanding speech over the telephone is one of the most difficult communication situations they will likely encounter, yet it is a critical skill for both vocational and social purposes. Clients who don't understand what is being said can be taught to help facilitate communication. If the person does not have sufficient residual hearing to use a telephone, the clinician may spend

TABLE 14.2

Carhart approach to auditory training

Step 1: Develop an awareness of sound. The clinician presents various sounds until the child can detect the presence of sound, understand that sounds have meaning, and pay attention to sound.

Step 2: Gross or general sound discrimination. The child is taught that different sources generate different sounds, to distinguish between very dissimilar sounds (such as a car horn versus a doorbell), and to discriminate between the suprasegmental aspects of sound, such as loud versus soft intensity, high versus low pitch, long versus short duration.

Step 3: Broad discrimination among simple speech patterns. The child is now ready to apply knowledge gained from the first two steps to speech sounds. Usually, the clinician begins with vowel discrimination (e.g., /i/ vs /a/) or discrimination of meaningful familiar phrases, such as "good morning" or "how are you?"

Step 4: Development of finer discrimination of speech. The child practices distinguishing all of the different speech sounds that are available to him or her, depending upon the type and degree of hearing loss.

Source: Adapted from: J. Northern & M. Downs (1976). *Hearing in children* (2nd ed.). Baltimore, MD: Williams and Wilkins.

time teaching the client to use a **teletypewriter** (**TTY**), as well as the relay services that are available through the telephone company.

COMMUNICATION METHODS

Communication methods for people with hearing impairments may be broken into two primary categories: spoken (oral) communication and manual communication. The decision to utilize either or both is somewhat based on the degree of loss, but there are also complex personal and philosophical issues that must be considered, especially for individuals with severe and profound hearing losses. It is beyond the scope of this chapter to discuss these issues with the depth required to do them justice. Rather, a brief overview of the nature of oral and manual communication will be provided in this section.

One of the most difficult issues facing a speech-language pathologist working with individuals, especially children, who are hearing impaired is how to determine which mode of communication is best for the client. Many factors are to be considered, such as the amount of residual hearing, language and cognitive abilities, manual dexterity, and client preference. The preference of the family is especially important. Remember, for a deaf child of Deaf parents, language is not just a means of communication, but a cultural issue, and there is no other choice but the use of ASL. On the other hand, some parents don't want their children to appear different from their hearing peers and will allow only an aural/oral approach without any use of sign. Since family support is critical to the success of either approach, the speech-language pathologist might need to educate the family on the benefits of various modes of communication. Consequently, the SLP must be sensitive to all aspects surrounding the communication issue and be prepared, if necessary, to negotiate in the best interests of the child.

AURAL/ORAL APPROACH

The vast majority of people who have hearing losses will communicate through spoken (oral) language. This is not so much an indication of a better modality as it is a recognition that the majority of hearing losses are no worse than moderately severe and most of the people who have these losses have sufficient residual hearing to be able to use spoken language both receptively and expressively.

The best candidates for an aural/oral apprach are those who are consistent users of their hearing aids, since amplification is essential for this approach to work. *Speechreading* (lipreading) skills are also taken into consideration. There are differing opinions on this issue as well. Some professionals believe that speechreading ability is an inherent skill that someone either has or doesn't have; therefore, it should not be a determining factor in choosing a communication mode. Others believe that speechreading can be taught through formal instruction, and therefore speechreading training is incorporated into the goals of an aural/oral program.

The key to an aural/oral approach is practice. The child must be immersed in a speech-intensive environment both at home and at school. The method of instruction may vary somewhat in terms of the amount of structure. A *pure oralism* approach strongly emphasizes the importance of sound; there is absolutely no signing, and visual or tactile stimuli are limited. The use of appropriate amplification is rigidly enforced, and speech is the only acceptable means of response. Strong commitment to the principles of the aural/oral approach by both educators and family members is essential to the success of the method. Without this commitment, carryover of the necessary skills will be difficult at best or might not take place at all.

Total reliance on spoken communication becomes more difficult as the degree of hearing loss becomes more severe. As indicated above, speechreading may provide access to some of the information that cannot be heard due to the hearing loss. Another method that has been

The debate over "best" communication modality for a young child with a severe or profound hearing loss is one of the most heated issues facing professionals who work with these children. Regardless of the targeted end result, it is critical that the issues of communication, language development, and speech development be kept separate. It may be necessary to incorporate a **"total communication"** philosophy in which several different methods are utilized to achieve different aspects of the final goal.

gaining popularity is Cued Speech. Many speech sounds are visually similar (e.g., in words, /b/, /p/, and /m/ all look the same when spoken). For a person relying on speechreading to decode the message, this can lead to confusion. Cued Speech uses a series of hand shapes and positions near the face and neck to visually distinguish the sounds being spoken. Cued Speech is a way to provide full access to spoken communication through the visual code.

MANUAL COMMUNICATION

Some form of manual communication is preferable for individuals whose residual hearing is insufficient to be able to make use of the speech signal. This usually includes those with severe to profound hearing impairments; however, it may also apply to people with lesser degrees of hearing loss if the hearing loss occurred prelingually but was discovered after the critical period for speech development or if the client simply prefers to use sign. Use of amplification is encouraged, but not required. Speechreading skills are also beneficial but, again, not necessarily emphasized.

Depending on the background and communication goals of the client, a continuum of signing methods exists from which to choose (see Table 14.3). At one end of the continuum is the signing system of **signed exact English (SEE).** SEE is referred to as a signing "system" because it is a visual method of representing the English language, not a language unto itself. Signing exact English requires the breaking down of English words into syllables and representing each syllable through a specific sign. SEE is the method that is used primarily when the goal is to teach English vocabulary and sentence structure.

On the opposite end of the continuum is American Sign Language (ASL). As was mentioned in a previous section, ASL is considered the "natural" language of the deaf. It was developed in France in 1750 and brought to the United States by Thomas Gallaudet in 1815. Unlike the signing systems of SEE and PSE, ASL is a signed language with its own vocabulary, grammar, and sentence structure. ASL is very much a conceptual language, and one sign may convey an entire thought. ASL does not have specific signs for pronouns or modifiers but depends on the use of space, facial expression, body orientation, and repetition to express these ideas. Even the speed at which something is signed has significance to the overall meaning. Considering all of this, then, the difficulties of translating ASL into English and vice versa begin to become apparent. That is why many advocates in the Deaf community encourage the use of both languages in teaching deaf children.

In the middle of the continuum is a signing system that is referred to as **pidgin signed English (PSE).** PSE incorporates more ASL-like signs but maintains English word order. Facial expression, body position, and gestures are also incorporated.

TABLE 14.3

Sign-language continuum

Signing Systems ————————————→ Sign Language

Signed Exact English (SEE)	Pidgin Signed English (PSE)	American Sign Language (ASL)
Word meaning is NOT considered (e.g., the word "right" will have the same sign regardless of context).	Signs used are more conceptual. One word may have many signs depending upon meaning.	Has its own vocabulary, grammar, and sentence structure. One sign may represent an entire thought.
All grammatical markers (articles, auxiliary verbs, plurals, etc.) are signed.	Grammatical markers may or may not be signed.	Does not have specific signs for grammatical markers.
	Facial expression and gestures are incorporated.	Facial expression, body position, space, and repetition are used extensively.

T H O U G H T   Q U E S T I O N S

Why is knowledge of ASL useful for both audiologists and SLPs? Does your college offer courses in ASL? Do you think they should fulfill foreign language requirements? Why or why not?

▌SUMMARY

The profession of audiology is a richly diverse field that offers the opportunity to work with many populations in many different employment settings. The audiologist has the responsibility for measuring hearing and hearing loss. A hearing loss is caused by an interruption at one or more points along the auditory pathway. The three types of hearing loss are conductive, sensorineural, and mixed. Audiologists are also concerned with problems affecting the auditory nervous system, including the brain stem and the auditory cortex of the brain. Problems along these pathways result in an inability to efficiently use and interpret auditory information, referred to as a central auditory processing disorder.

When describing a hearing loss, audiologists use terminology such as conductive, sensorineural, and mixed to identify the portion of the auditory system that has been affected. Another important set of terms describe the amount or degree of hearing loss in units called decibels. Each degree of hearing loss refers to a specific decibel range. Individuals with degrees of hearing loss in the mild to moderately severe categories are referred to as hard of hearing and depend as much as possible upon their hearing for communication. For people with a severe to profound hearing loss, referred to as deaf, the auditory system provides little or no access to the world.

When testing children, audiologists rely on behavioral observation audiometry and electrophysiological testing, including auditory brain stem evoked response audiometry. The procedure for testing adults includes pure tone audiometry, speech audiometry, and immittance testing.

Aural habilitation/rehabilitation refers to the services and procedures that are designed to help a person cope with the difficulties presented by a hearing loss. Aural habilitation alludes to therapies that are used primarily with children to teach missing communication skills. Aural rehabilitation refers to services provided to those who lose their hearing later in life after communication skills have been established. The focus of rehabilitation is to help the person recover these skills or to learn compensatory strategies. Typical issues that are considered in creating an aural rehabilitation program are amplification, auditory training, and oral/manual communication methods.

REFLECTIONS

- In what settings are audiologists employed?
- What are the main functions of the outer, middle, and inner ear?
- Explain the differences between conductive, sensorineural, and mixed hearing loss.

- What are some causes of different types of hearing loss?
- Identify the methods used in hearing testing in children. How do these compare with methods used for adults?
- What are the goals of aural habilitation and aural rehabilitation?

SUGGESTED READINGS

Bess, F., & Humes, L. (1995). *Audiology: The fundamentals* (2nd ed.). Baltimore, MD: Williams and Wilkins.

Katz, J., Stecker, N., & Henderson, D. (1992). *Central auditory processing: A transdisciplinary view.* St. Louis, MO: Mosby-Year Book.

Martin, F. N. (1994). *Introduction to audiology* (5th ed.). Englewood Cliffs, NJ: Prentice Hall.

Ross, M. (1994). Overview of aural rehabilitation. In J. Katz (Ed.), *Handbook of clinical audiology* (4th ed., pp. 587–595). Baltimore, MD: Williams and Wilkins.

Tye-Murray, N. (1998). *Foundations of aural rehabilitation.* San Diego, CA: Singular Publishing Group.

ON-LINE RESOURCES

http://ww.acoustics.org/press/133rd/2paaa2.html   Simulated hearing loss.

http://asha.org   General information about audiology.

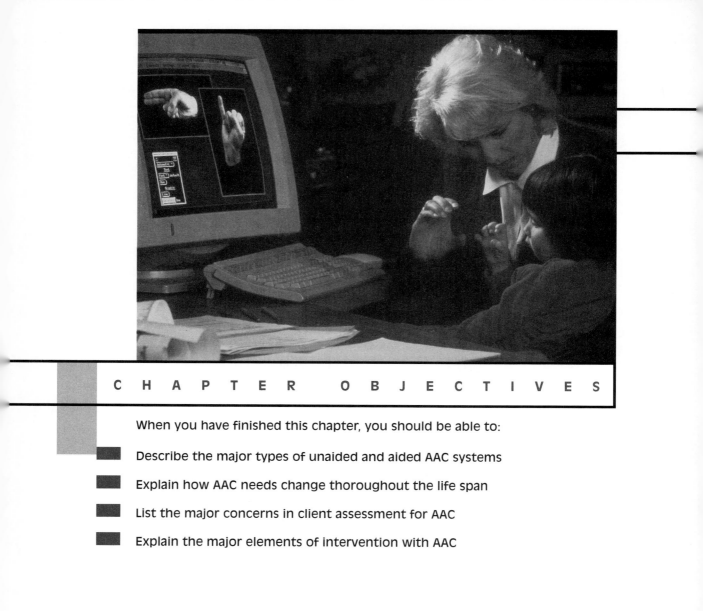

C H A P T E R   O B J E C T I V E S

When you have finished this chapter, you should be able to:

Describe the major types of unaided and aided AAC systems

Explain how AAC needs change thoroughout the life span

List the major concerns in client assessment for AAC

Explain the major elements of intervention with AAC

Augmentative and Alternative Communication

Throughout this text, we've mentioned individuals with severe speech and language impairments who might need either additional support or a nontraditional method of communication. These forms of communication, called **augmentative/ alternative communication (AAC)**, include gestures, signing, pictures systems, print, computerized communication, and voice production (Glennen & DeCoste, 1997). More correctly, AAC includes these forms of communication and the strategies and methods to assist individuals in using them to meet their communication needs.

Using other means of communication in addition to speech is not totally new. As communicators, we augment our speech all the time with facial expressions, body language, and gestures. AAC does the same thing. Similarly, the use of AAC with individuals with communication impairments is not new. In the United States, the Deaf population has been using sign for about 200 years.

In a clinical setting, we may enhance or augment an individual's speech with AAC or we may explore AAC's becoming the primary means of communication. It is in recognition of these possibilities that ASHA has chosen to use the somewhat awkward, but inclusive term augmentative/alternative communication.

Individuals who might benefit from AAC include, but are not limited to, those

All typical communicators augment speech with other means of communication, such as gestures and facial expression.

with deafness, mental retardation (MR), autism spectrum disorder (ASD), aphasia, traumatic brain injury (TBI), motor speech problems, cerebral palsy (CP), glossectomy, laryngectomy, dysarthria, and apraxia of speech, to name a few. More than at any time in human history, people with disabilities are meeting new challenges, participating in life to the fullest, and demanding that their voices be heard. As mentioned in Chapter 2, legislation, adaptations, and technology are helping to ensure this participation. Individuals are overcoming what were considered only a few years ago to be insurmountable barriers to independence.

In this chapter we shall explore AAC, first describing what it is and how it works, then exploring the assessment and intervention considerations. We recognize that this chapter may seem odd in a text in which most chapters discuss different types of communication disorders, but it is an important area of intervention that is of benefit to people with many disorders.

The goals for AAC intervention vary. Although the specific goals vary with each individual user, in general treatment aims to:

1. Assist individuals with their daily communication needs.
2. Help facilitate the development of speech and language.
3. Help facilitate the return of speech and language. (Blackstone, 1989)

Only careful and ongoing evaluation of a client's abilities, his or her needs, and the environment can ensure that these goals will be met effectively and efficiently.

TYPES OF AAC

AAC systems can be roughly divided into those requiring no external devices and those that do. The former are called unaided methods and the latter are called aided.

UNAIDED AAC

All of us use gestures to communicate. We shake our head, shrug our shoulders, point, and reach. Gesturing is a form of unaided AAC as are signing, fingerspelling, Cued Speech, and writing.

Signing is a highly developed form of communication, as is speech. Because signing is other than speech, it is considered to be a form of AAC. The sign system is the code or the language. As noted in Chapter 14, "Audiology and Disorders of Hearing," American Sign Language or ASL, the language of the Deaf culture in the United States, is a language with its own vocabulary and syntax. Other sign systems in use in the United States are translations of English into sign and include

American Sign Language is a language, just as Spanish is a language.

Signed English, Signing Essential English (SEE-I), and Signing Exact English (SEE-II). Signed English is the most frequently taught sign system in the United States.

American Indian gestural or hand communication, called AmerInd, is a gestural system used with some nonspeaking individuals. It is a relatively grammar-free, nonsign system of 250 concept signals. Almost all gestures in AmerInd can be made with one hand, making it easier for those with hemiplegia, paralysis on one side of the body, or hemiparesis, weakness on one side.

Individual signs can be classified based on their ease of production or comprehension. In general, it's easier to produce signs that touch the body and that use both hands, and, when two hands are used, that are symmetrical.

Some signs are easy to comprehend because they look like their meaning. These signs are called *iconic*. For example, the sign for "drink" in most systems is made by miming drinking. Unfortunately, few signs are of this type. Signs that are easily guessable, explainable, and memorable are called *transparent*. In most sign systems "America" is made by interlocking the fingers, palms in, and moving them in a circle. Definitely not iconic, but consider the explanation. When the early Europeans came to the Western Hemisphere they were impressed by the abundance of timber; so much that it could be stacked to make fences that resemble the hand shape for "America." Whether this is the derivation of the sign or not, it makes sense, thus the sign is easy to remember. Many signs are transparent. AmerInd has a high proportion of transparent signs. Signs, such as "apple," that are difficult to interpret are called *opaque*. Examples of iconic, transparent, and opaque signs are presented in Figure 15.1.

T H O U G H T Q U E S T I O N S

Might the degree of sign transparency differ across individuals, cultures, and ability levels? "Milk" is signed by miming milking a cow. Does every child know where milk comes from?

Sign systems differ in their grammar as well. Because ASL is a language, it has its own grammar. Signed English, SEE-I, and SEE-II mirror English, thus they are not separate languages. AmerInd has a very flexible grammar but is limited by the limited number of signs.

For most Deaf signers, fingerspelling is mixed with signs and used for new words or names. Fingerspelling, or the manual alphabet, is inappropriate for severely retarded or very young clients and for those with poor fine motor skills, but may be good for older clients with both good

ICONIC 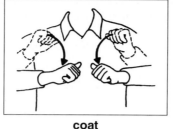	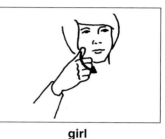
coat A shape both hands. Trace shape of lapels with thumbs	**cold** *(adj.)* S shape both hands. Draw hands close to body and "shiver."
TRANSPARENT 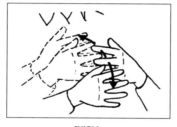	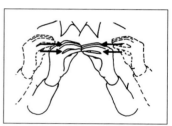
boy Snap flat O at forehead twice, indicating brim of cap.	**girl** A shape RH. Place thumb on right cheek and move down jaw line.
OPAQUE	
gray Five shape both hands, palms in tips facing. Move right fingers back and forth between left fingers, (Sometimes made like sign for *black*, using right G shape instead of index finger.)	**more** Flat O shape both hands, palms and tips facing. Tap tips together twice.

FIGURE 15.1 Examples of iconic, transparent, and opaque signed English signs

cognitive and fine motor abilities. The client has ultimate flexibility because any word in the language can be spelled for transmission.

Cued Speech consists of eight handshapes made in four locations in combination with the natural mouth movements that enable the partner to interpret the speech sounds of the user. Hand configurations represent various articulatory postures used in the production of speech sounds. Figure 15.2 presents examples of Cued Speech hand shapes. As with fingerspelling, Cued Speech is inappropriate for severely retarded or very young clients and for those with poor fine motor skills.

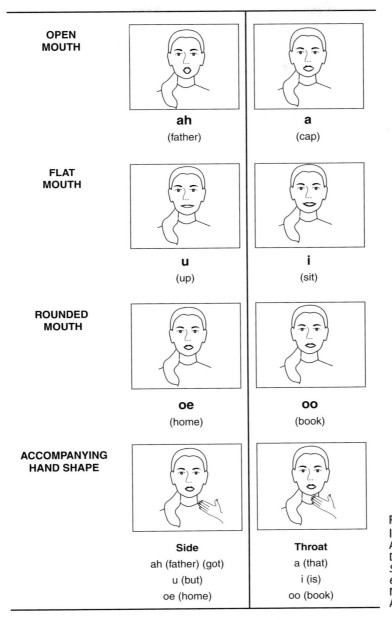

OPEN MOUTH

ah (father)

a (cap)

FLAT MOUTH

u (up)

i (sit)

ROUNDED MOUTH

oe (home)

oo (book)

ACCOMPANYING HAND SHAPE

Side
ah (father) (got)
u (but)
oe (home)

Throat
a (that)
i (is)
oo (book)

FIGURE 15.2 Examples of selected Cued Speech vowels. Adapted from Carnett, R. O., & Daisey, M. E. (1992). *The Cued Speech resource book for parents of deaf children.* Raleigh, NC: National Cued Speech Association.

AIDED AAC

Unaided systems are not appropriate for every individual who needs either to enhance or replace his or her current method of communicating. For example, an individual with severe motor involvement in the limbs as in some forms of CP may be unable to make the fine motor adjustments necessary for many signs. For these individuals, a communication board or an electronic mode of communication may be more appropriate. These devices are collectively called **assistive technologies,** a broad term that includes aids for daily living, communication aids, environmental controls, prosthetic and orthotic devices, sensory aids, seating and positioning systems, and mobility/transportation aids.

Aided systems differ in the type of system, the graphic means of representation, and the input and output modes. Selection of each is determined by ongoing careful assessment.

AIDED AAC SYSTEMS

Systems vary from very "low-tech," such as the communication board, through the latest in computer technology. In between are other electronic devices such as hand-held printers and computers, as well as laser pointers.

GRAPHIC MEANS OF REPRESENTATION

Whether on a communication board or an electronic device, graphic symbols are just as important to aided AAC as words are to speech or signs to signing. Symbols may include pictures, various representational systems, and/or printed words, grouped together to form symbol systems. Some symbol systems have been specifically designed for AAC use.

Graphic symbol systems include highly pictographic representations, such as Picture Communication Symbols (PCS) and some Rebus Symbols, less pictographic representations, such as Picsyms and Pictogram Ideogram Communication (PIC), and symbol systems, such as Blissymbolics. In general, less representational systems allow for more abstract meanings. In addition, symbolic systems are more rule-governed and generative, allowing for symbol combination and the creation of new symbols.

Graphic symbol systems may use a variety of means to express different referents. Rebus symbols are line drawings of both concrete and abstract concepts and of sound sequences, originally developed as an aid for teaching reading. Picsyms and PIC contain ideograms used to represent an idea rather than the way a referent, or the concept it refers to, appears in the real world. Ideograms and symbols, such as those used in Blissymbolics, can be used for abstract concepts just as words can. Blissymbols consist of 100 pictographic representations and arbitrary symbols that can be combined in creative ways to create words. Examples of graphic symbol systems are presented in Figure 15.3.

With very young children or more severely cognitively impaired individuals, SLPs may choose to use actual objects, product packaging, photographs, or drawings. These are very concrete and may not represent anything beyond the immediate referent. A system called Tangible Symbols (Rowland & Schweigert, 1989) attempts to bridge the gap between actual objects and graphic representations by using objects or pictures with a clear relationship to the referent. For example, a key or a shoelace might represent *car* or *shoe* respectively.

AIDED SYSTEM INPUT

Input is especially important and great care must be exercised in choosing the appropriate interface between the client and the device. The two primary means of symbol selection are direct selection and scanning. The client may select the symbol directly by pointing with a finger, hand, head pointer, or laser sensor or pointer, or by operating a joystick, much like a car gearshift. The client might point directly at the symbol or touch the keys on a keyboard. In cases of severe neuromuscular involvement, eye gaze may be used to select symbols. Most users of communication boards indicate their message by pointing. For individuals with inconsistent or inaccurate pointing, electronic devices can choose the symbol based on the client's most consistent movement.

Pointing may be aided by the use of either hand splints or pointing sticks that strengthen or enable the client's response. Light-emitting devices may be used with both communication boards and electronic devices, but light-sensing devices are limited to electronic means. Usually mounted on the head, light-emitting devices shine on the de-

Graphic symbols may be selected directly by the AAC user or scanned, when each symbol is highlighted in turn until the desired one is reached.

FIGURE 15.3   Comparison of graphic symbols

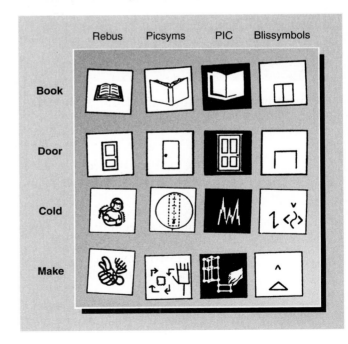

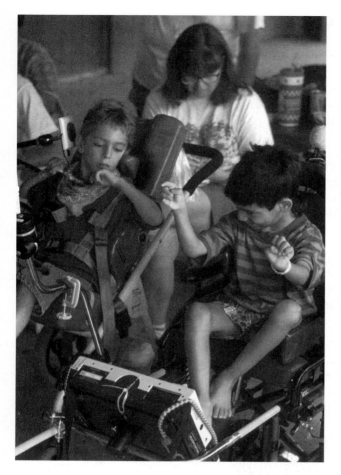

For many individuals with oral motor impairments, AAC provides a viable option.

sired symbol. The partner may see the light beam directly or an electronic AAC device may interpret the signal. Some electronic devices emit light and the head pointer senses the light from the display, which is transmitted back to the AAC device.

Individuals using eye gaze look at symbols on a clear acrylic board located between the user and the communication partner. The user gazes at desired symbols, which appear on both sides of the board.

Clients can also scan an electronic display and select the desired symbol. Possible choices are offered, and the client indicates when the desired symbol has been located. This is accomplished by starting and stopping the cursor until the symbol is highlighted. This action requires only the ability to use a two-position switch for start-stop. The cursor can be adjusted for the speed and accuracy of the client's movement.

Pressure switches can be used for this start-stop purpose and placed in any location in which the individual can obtain pressure. For example, the user pushes with her elbow to start the cursor's movement, then presses again to stop it. Other pressure switches may use eyebrow wrinkling, eye movement, or sip/puff to activate the switch. Obviously, this method will be slow and laborious. It requires extended concentration and has the potential to be very frustrating, especially when symbols are missed and the process must be repeated.

Efficiency can be obtained by the placement of symbols so that the most frequently used symbols are scanned most frequently. For example, if the cursor begins at the top of the display and returns there after each symbol selection, then the most frequently used symbols would be placed at the top. Obviously, such an arrangement requires constant monitoring by those in the user's environment to insure peak efficiency.

Various scanning methods can also increase efficiency (Venkatagiri, 2000). For example, in linear scanning each possible selection is presented in sequence. In contrast, both row-column and block scanning enable the user to scan larger areas, then refine the scan once the desired area has been highlighted. As an example, the user might press the switch to begin the display. Rows are lighted in sequence until the desired one is found. The user presses the switch again and individual symbols within that row are highlighted one at a time.

Obviously, the type of interface is as important as the symbol system used. In general, the SLP and client will determine the most efficient and accurate interface given the client's cognitive and physical abilities and the environmental demands. Several individuals are presented using AAC deviced on the accompaying CD-ROM.

AIDED SYSTEM OUTPUT

As in unaided AAC, with communication boards the partner interprets the message directly. With electronic AAC devices, a wide range of outputs are possible. Electronic output or transmission may be as simple as a light over or behind a symbol or as elaborate as a voice and printed message. SLPs help the client to find the appropriate output for his or her needs. Either printed symbol or written messages may be appropriate for some environments; speech would be appropriate for others. For example, in employment situations, the client may desire a more natural speech output, while at home, a graphic printout is all that is needed.

Speech transmission can be prerecorded, synthesized, or both. Prerecorded or digitized speech sounds more natural but is limited to only conveying messages stored in the device's memory. Synthesized speech has more flexibility but often sounds mechanical and unnatural. Instead of recording actual words or phrases, the synthesized speech program contains speech sounds and rules for combining them. Commands may be entered by typing the message alphabetically or phonetically or by entering a code. Combined systems may use prerecorded high usage words and phrases along with synthesis of less frequently used ones. Consonant blends and coarticulation can be added to increase the naturalness of the speech output.

T H O U G H T   Q U E S T I O N S

Computers sometimes use synthetic speech. When you have heard synthetic speech, did it seem artifical to you? Would you want this voice to be yours in communication?

Compared to natural speech, comprehension of synthesized speech requires increased focused attention by the partner. When attention is divided, partners comprehend significantly less synthesized speech

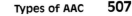

(Drager & Reichle, 2001). Partners tend to respond more slowly to synthesized speech (Reynolds & Jefferson, 2000).

Decisions on the appropriate type of AAC are made only after careful evaluation. As the user's abilities or needs change, that decision may need to be revisited. Users may also employ multiple types of AAC communication. Training of both the user and others in the user's environment is essential for maximum efficacy. Figure 15.4 presents some of the manual and graphic systems available.

SPEECH AND AAC

Obviously, AAC is not the same as speech. There are some important distinctions that may not be readily apparent. First, with the exception of expert signers, the typical AAC user is much slower than the typical speaker. This has implications for the user or producer as well as the audience or receiver. Receivers may feel compelled to complete the message for the user or take more responsibility for the communication than during speech. The untrained receiver may take control away from the AAC speaker unintentionally.

AAC use can change the communication process in ways that are not always predictable.

Second, some AAC communication will be less face to face. Both participants may be attending to the device in aided systems. In unaided systems, such as signing, it is easier to glance from hands to face and back but eye contact will still be less than in speaking situations. With less face-to-face communication, shades of meaning may be missed.

Caregivers sometimes worry that learning a different means of communication will adversely affect speech. In reality, the opposite is true. As you will see in the following section, learning to use AAC enhances all other aspects of communication.

THEORY AND REALITY

Use of AAC has been documented to increase conversational participation, speech intelligibility, and conversational initiations (Dattilo & Camarata, 1991; Glennen & Calculator, 1985; Hunter, Pring, & Martin, 1991; Spiegel, Benjamin, & Spiegel,1993). Training conversational partners as well as the client results in increased reciprocity in turn taking and initiations (Light, Dattilo, English, Gutierrez, & Hartz, 1992).

T H O U G H T   Q U E S T I O N S

Why is it important to train conversational partners to use AAC systems? How might your conversational behaviors be affected if your partner used an AAC device that was considerably slower than speech?

Unaided

Gestures

American Indian Sign System (AMERIND)

Signing

American Sign Language (AMESLAN or ASL)

Signed English, SEE$_1$, SEE$_2$

Finger spelling

Aided

Communication board

Objects

Photos

Black-and-white pictures

Line drawings

Picsyms

Rebus

Blissymbolics

Alphabet

Electronic

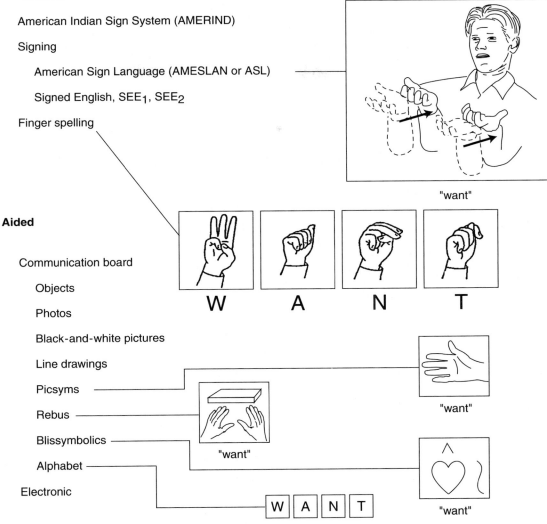

FIGURE 15.4 Graphic and manual systems

In short, AAC facilitates the development of both communication and language. None of these positive statements about AAC suggests that it is the great panacea for "curing" all communication ills, but, as with any good intervention method, AAC works very well with certain clients.

Several factors can explain the effects of AAC. These are presented in Table 15.1. When others in the user's environment also use AAC, they increase the user's comprehension by producing the symbols at a slower rate than speech, by reducing the number of symbols and grammatical structures used, and by eliminating many irrelevant or wordy comments that often accompany speech. For the user, production may

---

TABLE 15.1

Why AAC facilitates communication as compared to speech

Simplification of input
    Irrelevant and parenthetical comments eliminated.
    Slower rate permits more processing time.
Response production advantages
    Pressure to speak removed.
    Physical demands decreased compared to speech.
    Physical manipulation of client's hands or other parts of body by trainer is possible.
    Client observation of physical manipulation facilitated.
Advantages for individuals with severe cognitive impairment
    Limited and functional vocabulary.
    Individual's attention easier to maintain.
Receptive language/auditory processing advantages
    Structure of language is simplified.
    Auditory short-term memory and/or auditory processing problems minimized.
Simultaneous processing/stimulus association advantages
    Visual nature of the symbol makes it more obvious.
    Visual symbols have more consistency.
    Duration of symbol is greater than spoken word.
    Visual symbols more easily associated with visual referents.
Symbolic representation advantages
    Supplement speech symbols.
    Symbols visually represent referents.

Source: Adapted from Lloyd, L. L., & Kangas, K. A. (1994). Augmentative and alternative communication. In G. H Shames, E. H. Wiig, & W. A. Secord (Eds.), *Human communication disorders* (4th ed.). Boston: Allyn and Bacon.

be easier than speech because of reduced physical demands, removal of the pressure to speak, hand-over-hand shaping and modeling, and increased involvement of the right hemisphere.

The use of AAC does not relieve the SLP of his or her responsibilities to follow good clinical practice. Even the best of methods must be monitored for progress and use within the everyday environment of the client. Sometimes AAC methods fail, especially when they are not a good match for the client's abilities and needs and the needs of the environment. For example, if no one in the client's home or school is willing to learn sign, sign usage will not generalize to these situations. Several other factors may account for lack of progress or failure to generalize. These include the lack of functional client-centered content, the precedence of training over communication, nonuse in the environment, and inflexibility in the use of the means of communication. Inflexibility is an insistence by either the SLP or the client on the exclusive use of only one means of communication.

T H O U G H T   Q U E S T I O N

Why might a client decide to use one AAC method exclusively? Can you imagine a situation in which this might occur?

Generally, communication is best when multiple means can be used. For example, the client may have some usable speech, a few easily recognizable signs, and a communication board with symbols in various stages of maturity from photos through black and white drawings to Blissymbolics. Most SLPs would not recommend training with such a variety of AAC systems but clients with a history of AAC use may have acquired some symbols in a few different systems. Generally, the user has some vocalizations, some speech, nonlinguistic behaviors such as gestures and body language, and AAC. If the client has an easily comprehended verbal "no," it seems inflexible to ignore that word and insist on the sign or symbol equivalent.

LIFE SPAN ISSUES

Severe communication impairments, whether developmental or acquired, often affect many aspects of an individual's life. In addition, those with severe communication deficits also may have a wide array of other disabling conditions.

Children with evident syndromes or impairments, those at risk, or those failing infant measures, such as hearing screenings, will be candidates for early intervention (EI). For some of these children, especially

AAC users may have other needs that call for the use of additional assistive technologies.

those with CP or deafness, exposure to augmentative communication may begin within the first few months. Caregivers will talk to the infant, but supplement this input with sign or other visual input. AAC may or may not become the primary means of communication and the SLP will continue to work on oral motor skills and sound production. Box 15.1 presents the story of one young woman whose life was changed by AAC.

BOX 15.1

Jean's Story

Her parents eagerly anticipated Jean's birth. She was their first child. Although her motor behavior seemed rigid at birth, the pediatrician assured them that her behavior was typical reflexive behavior for an infant. They were saddened and confused when Jean was later diagnosed with spastic cerebral palsy.

Although her parents tried to give Jean a typical childhood, their task was complicated by her motor impairment. Jean was enrolled in a preschool, but her lack of speech and language inhibited her interactions with other children. She was later enrolled in a special preschool where she received speech and language services, daily living skills training, and academic preparation.

Unfortunately, Jean's SLP chose to emphasize speech intervention and AAC was not attempted. When she began first grade, Jean had only a few words that were understood by her immediate family, teacher, and the SLP. Her new SLP decided to use AAC with Jean but opted for signing primarily because other children in the school signed. Signing was not a good match for Jean because of the motor involvement of her hands.

Finally, after several frustrating years of less than adequate communica-tion, Jean's new SLP suggested combined use of an electronic communication board, plus some of Jean's easily recognizable signs and words. Using creative funding and a state grant, the SLP was able to purchase two electronic devices, one for home and one for school. The manual board was used when Jean was between these two sites or when she traveled in the car with her family. Although she used direct selection on her manual board, it was a slow, frustrating process. Her elctronic board was accessed through the use of a joystick that enabled Jean to go to the desired sign.

Now a young adult, Jean lives at home with her parents and attends vocational training at the local United Cerebral Palsy Association workshop. She continues to receive speech-language pathology services and has a large repertoire of graphic symbols at her disposal. She is able to request, to ask and answer questions, and to make conversational comments. Her life has become more fulfilling thanks to the many means she can use to communicate. It is hoped that soon she will be able to attempt an assistive living arrangement.

Just as a developmental continuum exists for speech, so it does for AAC (Cress, 2001). Communication begins with an infant prior to development of speech, language, and AAC use. Experiencing AAC signs and symbols prior to using them directly facilitates a child's understanding of their nature and function (Romski & Sevcik, 1996, Rowland & Schweigert, 2000).

Later, the child may begin to use AAC to produce language. If exposed to signs, children with deafness will begin to sign their first words at about 8 months. Unfortunately, some infants and toddlers with deafness live in nonsign environments and do not begin to learn sign until they attend a special preschool.

Some children may not be identified as having a communication impairment until later. As you will recall, children with autism spectrum disorder (ASD) are often identified as toddlers. AAC can provide initial communication and a motivation for learning language. For example, using behavior chain interruption, a technique in which the SLP stops a pleasurable activity and prompts the child to signal beginning again, the SLP can establish initial meaningful communication with the child. Communication can then be expanded as new desires by the child are identified.

Inevitably, some children and adolescents will experience acquired communication impairments because of accidents or illness. Many children and adolescents with TBI benefit from short-term or long-term use of AAC. In one case, a young man who had lost speech and language as the result of a gun-related suicide attempt was able to retrieve language and some speech by learning signs. His new communication system consists of vocalizations, verbalizations, gestures, and signs.

As AAC users mature, communication needs change. Approximately 20 percent enjoy full- or part-time employment (Balandin & Morgan, 2001). Adults with CP are less likely to marry and own a home, two factors that are important for continued independent living in old age. Nursing home staffs rarely are knowledgeable in AAC use. Changes in hearing and vision with age may also affect AAC use. Good communication skills can positively affect health, well-being, and safety (Straus, Cable, & Shavelle, 1999).

T H O U G H T   Q U E S T I O N

How might the potential changes in your life affect your communication needs? Suppose that you are an AAC user and think about this question again.

For both children and adults with degenerative disorders, aided AAC may provide continued communication when speech is no longer possible. For one young man, it was extremely important to his family that he be able to express his needs and thoughts for as long as possible. Although he became less able to control his body's movements, he continued to communicate. His computer was modified and modified again as his ability to interface changed. Typing letters gave way to touching pictures which in turn changed to scanning the same pictures. When he could no longer use his computer, a yes/no signal system and eye contact were used. Throughout this process, the SLP worked closely with the family and the visiting caretakers.

In the early stages of intervention with individuals with degenerative neuromuscular conditions, intervention focuses on maintaining natural communication (Doyle & Phillips, 2001). During the middle stages, as motor function deteriorates, the individual may begin to use AAC in specific situations. As motor control and speech become severely impaired, the individual may rely on AAC. The SLP continually monitors the progress of the disease and modifies the AAC system and/or the interface between the client and the AAC device.

Adults may also experience accidents and illness. As with children, they may benefit from AAC use. Those with apraxia of speech may have very good hand coordination and may be primary candidates for augmentative use. Individuals with aphasia may benefit from the use of graphic symbols or signs. Much visual information is interpreted in the right hemisphere. By tapping into this area of the brain, it is possible with some clients to build a "bridge" to the damaged areas of the left hemisphere and to improve access to language. It may be more difficult for an adult who once spoke typically to accept AAC. Embarrassment and shame may accompany the loss of speech or language. The SLP must stress the positive benefits of AAC use.

ASSESSMENT CONSIDERATIONS

As noted in other assessments of communication impairment, assessment for AAC use is a team effort.

As in other areas of speech-language pathology, careful thorough assessment of a client's abilities and needs is essential for determining the appropriate AAC system and the course of intervention services. Assessment should include not only the client's speech, language, and communication abilities and needs but also motor and perceptual skills, preferences, and the willingness of the environment to support AAC use. This data will be collected through the help of a team of professionals who will be identified as we discuss each element of the evaluation.

Speech considerations include the types of sounds and sound combinations produced, intelligibility, and connected speech. Spontaneous speech and imitative speech samples should be collected and analyzed. In addition, an oral peripheral examination with attention to different motor behaviors, swallowing, and oral movement imitation is essential.

Hearing is extremely important for speech production and feedback and should be assessed thoroughly by an audiologist. Seniors may have hearing loss that is unrelated or related to the acquired speech and/or language impairment. Individuals with developmental speech and/or language impairments may have hearing, perceptual, or central auditory processing impairments related to various syndromes or disorders.

Language and prelanguage skills, both receptive and expressive, will be important for programming content and selection of symbol systems, especially graphic. Although certain cognitive abilities seem to be needed for some types of symbol use, clients should not be excluded from AAC consideration because these abilities are still developing. Prelinguistic skills can be taught at the same time the client is learning to communicate with the AAC system.

Communication skills are very important. The desire to communicate or to communicate better forms the basis for AAC intervention and the motivation for learning. Although individuals with severe disabilities have great difficulty making clear and intentional signals, they often create their own individualistic gestures (Iacono, Carter, & Hook, 1998; Yoder & Munson, 1995). The multimodality nature of AAC necessitates a systematic exploration of the role these gestures play in communication (Hunt-Berg, 2001; Reichle, Halle, & Drasgow, 1998).

It is very difficult not to communicate. As best as possible, the SLP should determine the method of communication currently used by the client. Communication often is demonstrated by consistent behaviors exhibited in the same situations. Some clients with severe motor or perceptual impairments may have atypical ways of expressing needs and wants. The SLP should also attempt to determine the current and future communication needs of the client.

T H O U G H T   Q U E S T I O N S

Can you not communicate? Do some behaviors communicate information even when we do not intend them to do so?

An occupational (OT) and/or physical therapist (PT) can aid in motor assessment. Of interest is ambulation or the ability to move about, fine motor dexterity for signing or pointing, range of movement especially of the upper limbs, motor imitation skills, and the consistency and accuracy of motor responses. This data will be extremely important in deciding the appropriate aided or unaided system and the placement and size of graphic symbols.

Visual and auditory acuity and perception will be important for system selection and intervention. Vision, along with motor skills, will be used to decide the size of graphic symbols. An ophthalmologist will be an invaluable member of the team in assessing these abilities.

Occasionally, the environment will not support the use of AAC. Caregivers may be uncomfortable, feel inadequate, or just not want to be involved. The SLP may need to educate caregivers on the benefit of AAC to the client and to the home or school. Explaining the likely course of intervention may increase caregiver comfort levels.

Intervention will be maximally effective if caregivers also use AAC along with speech. Teaching caregivers a few simple signs or graphic symbols may relieve their natural anxieties when faced with a new mode of communication.

Caregivers are sometimes fearful that they will be expected to sign as if interpreting for a deaf audience. Nothing could be further from reality with most clients. Signs or graphic symbols can be used as gestures for important words in an utterance as the caregiver continues to speak.

Lastly, the SLP is interested in collecting a list of client preferences and of possible symbols to train. Likes and desires of the client will be important for intervention. This information can be gathered from client responses or choices, from caregiver suggestions, or through observation of the client. This portion of the assessment can be very positive with the focus on communication potential rather than on impairment and is especially important with acquired communication impairments (Klasner & Yorkston, 2001). With these impairments, such as dysarthria, the focus tends to be on loss rather than potential, so a positive shift is welcome.

It is not always clear whether a client will benefit from AAC use. If the SLP believes that AAC support may be beneficial in the future, the topic should be introduced early in the assessment and intervention process. Need becomes apparent if the client's communication abilities are being constrained by slowly recovering or developing speech. The following recommendations can help families accept AAC use (Zangari, 2001):

- Provide honest information
- Honor their concerns and provide information that addresses those concerns
- Recognize the emotional impact in realizing that a loved one may use AAC and try to address concerns that are stated and those that are not
- Address the client's strengths and the way in which AAC enhances them
- Provide specific rationales for your recommendations

The actual assessment is only a first step. The SLP, in coordination with the family and other professionals, such as the OT, PT, audiologist, ophthalmologist, psychologist, rehabilitation engineer, and/or classroom teacher, uses the data from the assessment to make decisions on the appropriate AAC method, AAC symbol system, and potential vocabulary. These decisions will be adjusted and modified as the client progresses.

AAC SYSTEM SELECTION

In deciding on the appropriate AAC system or method, the SLP will consider the client's motor and cognitive abilities, the potential size of the client's lexicon, the ease in learning and using the system, the acceptability of the system to the user and potential communication partners, and the flexibility and intelligibility of the system. For example, unaided systems are very portable and can be expanded easily without concern for limited storage or display space but allow for no permanent record, thus necessitating use of some graphic system for purposes such as homework. Many graphic symbols appear with the printed word, making them easy for communication partners to use, but these same symbols require the partner to concentrate on the graphic message to the exclusion of the user's face and can be confusing when combined to form new words.

AAC system selection is much more than merely matching the client and the system.

The potential user's motor abilities are very important in determining the best system to use. Those with severe motor impairment in the arms and hands may be poor candidates for unaided systems. Poor hand pointing need not deter the individual from using a communication board with head or eye pointing. Likewise, poor motor abilities may dictate the use of certain interfaces between the user and an electronic AAC device.

Those in the potential user's communication environment must find the AAC system acceptable. Lack of portability or embarrassment concerning use may lead to nonuse in certain situations or by some potential partners.

The selection of the AAC system can lead to further questions. For example, if the SLP decides to use a communication board, several considerations influence its final design. These include, but are not limited to, the construction material, overall size, arrangement and size of the symbols, placement and organization of the symbols, and the mounting of the board if necessary.

AAC SYMBOL SELECTION

Decisions on the appropriate symbol system will flow naturally from the method of communication chosen. If signing is deemed to be the appropriate method, the SLP must make decisions on the best gestural or sign system to use. In addition to the cognitive and motor abilities of the potential user, the SLP might consider the gestural or signing system used most frequently in the client's school or workplace and in the local community, the availability of teaching materials, and the ease in using these materials.

Selection of aided symbol systems may be guided by the potential user's cognitive abilities, the ease of learning different graphic AAC systems, and the willingness of potential communication partners. Aided symbols form a continuum from actual objects, which may represent only themselves, to letters that can be used to spell words. As we move from concrete objects to abstract symbols and letters, the client gains increased communication flexibility. Although not all clients can spell or use an encryption code, potential partners may be uneasy with interpretation of pictures, photographs, or other symbols. If we expect the client to use the system at home or in school, then partner concerns are important.

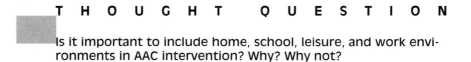

T H O U G H T   Q U E S T I O N

Is it important to include home, school, leisure, and work environments in AAC intervention? Why? Why not?

AAC VOCABULARY SELECTION

Vocabulary should reflect the client's current needs and communication potential.

The vocabulary chosen will have a great impact on future communication. Decisions about potential vocabulary will continue to be made as long as the client uses an AAC method of communication. The best guideline is to select vocabulary that reflects the user's needs, desires, likes, and preferences and is functional or useful based on observation of the client and the communication environment. The resultant vocabulary should be highly individualized.

Several lists of potential vocabulary are available and may serve as a guide when matched with the client's communication needs. These lists may also suggest various communication intentions and semantic categories of language that are important for early language development with presymbolic clients. Individuals with acquired speech and language impairments may have very different needs and rarely must relearn language.

Lists of the most frequently used words are of little use. For example, the top ten words used by adults in American English are *I, to, is, you, the, a, it, this, not,* and *yes.*

The order of teaching signs or symbols must also be guided by the client's immediate needs. In addition, the iconicity and transparency of different signs must be considered. With aided symbol systems such as Rebus, it might be wise to begin with more graphic icons before introducing sound sequencing symbols.

INTERVENTION CONSIDERATIONS

Although intervention will be a team effort, it is important for services not to become fragmented (Beukelman & Mirenda, 1992). Rather, a coherent, holistic approach is needed—one that includes the user's natural environment and communication partners. Family members, whether parents of a child with a developmental communication impairment or spouses and children of an adult with an acquired communication impairment, must be integral members of the intervention team.

The SLP must be concerned with linguistic and communicative competence as well as operational competence for the AAC system being trained. Intervention must include both the short-range and long-range needs of the client (Beukelman & Mirenda, 1992). The good intervention practices described in Chapter 5 will be just as important when working with individuals using AAC (Zangari & Kangas, 1997).

Some intervention considerations apply more specifically to AAC. These include but are not limited to the following:

- Establish an environment of AAC
- Use everyday experiences as the training context
- Individualize the content as discussed earlier
- Train others to modify their interactional style
- Consider positioning for those with severe motor impairments
- Make communication real

Each of these will be discussed in some detail.

An environment of augmentative communication is very important and highlights the need to have others, such as caregivers and teachers, involved. The AAC system should be used by others and aided systems should always be available for the user. We are reminded of one teacher who constructed a huge communication board on one wall of her classroom so that she could use it when addressing the entire class. Naturally, integration into the classroom requires a collaborative strategy involving both the classroom teacher and the SLP. AAC training for the entire educational team—teachers, instructional aides, SLPs, and parents—is a key element in success with children (Soto, Muller, Hunt, & Goetz, 2001).

As much as possible we want to program so that the client has multiple partners in multiple situations to increase social integration, especially among peers. In one classroom, we trained partners to

All members of the intervention team should use the AAC system to provide multiple partners and multiple situations.

interact with AAC users and reinforced them when they did. Educators can also organize clubs and experiences, such as an integrated dramatic arts program, to promote AAC use (McCarthy & Light, 2001).

In short, the SLP must identify opportunities for communication, create a need for communication, and maximize the instructional benefit of these opportunities (Sigafoos, 2000). Partners will need instructional support if they are to function as effective communication partners for AAC users.

Clients with acquired communication impairments may elect, if possible, to continue to work. Self-reports indicate that access to appropriate AAC systems is an important factor in facilitating continued employment (McNaughton, Light, & Groszyk, 2001).

Everyday events and routines provide *scripts* or personalized event sequences that enable each of us to participate. When circumstances are modified as in the use of AAC, we rely heavily on the script to help us. Use of the script frees "cognitive energy" to be applied to other aspects of the situation. In addition, the use of everyday events teaches the client to use AAC as the need arises. The SLP must use instructional strategies that integrate AAC into the different communication environments of the user (Ball, Marvin, Beukelman, Lasker, & Rupp, 2000; Rainforth, York, & MacDonald, 1992).

THOUGHT QUESTIONS

Are some communication situations easier than others for you? Are more familiar situations easier? Can you think of the script that helps you in these situations?

Acceptance of AAC is the degree to which the system is integrated into the life of the user (Lasker & Bedrosian, 2000). Optimal use occurs when AAC is used willingly and at every opportunity. Community-based training approaches in which the client becomes more comfortable and efficient using AAC in public may lead to optimal use (Lasker & Bedrosian, 2001). In these approaches, venues, such as the post office, grocery store, and fast food outlets, are identified. Training begins with scripted interactions that are modified gradually to more spontaneous communication.

Unless trained, well-meaning communication partners may assume too active a role in their interaction with the AAC user. Partners need to offer real choices, to acknowledge the user's communication attempts, and to allow time for the user to express the message. Because communication partners may be unfamiliar with AAC, it is important that systems and their purpose be explained carefully (Cress, 2001). Partners should also be trained to use AAC expressively, not because they need AAC to be understood, but because they can help the user acclimate to this new method of communication. Finally, partners should be consulted for their observations, suggestions, and ideas for intervention. As members of the intervention team, they become invested in the outcomes for the client.

For clients with severe motor impairments, such as CP, positioning is very important and can often be the determining factor in successful motor movement. Control of the head, shoulders, spine, and hips and alignment along the midline is essential.

Finally, the user of AAC must be involved in real communication with meaningful outcomes. It is all too easy for intervention to evolve into touching objects or pictures with no real outcome except a reinforcing word by the SLP or other partner. Training must include real communication choices not just performance of a sign or locating of a symbol. With meaningful communication, the grief and sense of loss that accompanies acquired communication impairments and laryngectomy and glossectomy can be replaced by a sense of empowerment (Fox & Rau, 2001).

Issues of efficacy or the effective use of AAC intervention methods must still be explored (Calculator, 2000). AAC is a relatively new area—only since the late 1970s for most methods—and much clinical research remains to be accomplished.

SUMMARY

Augmentative/alternative communication (AAC) includes many forms and the strategies and methods to assist individuals in using them to meet their communication needs. AAC may enhance or augment an individual's speech or may become the primary means of communication. Individuals who might benefit from AAC include those with deafness, MR, ASD, aphasia, TBI, motor speech problems, CP, glossectomy, laryngectomy, dysarthia, and apraxia of speech.

Although the specific goals of AAC intervention vary with each individual user, treatment aims include the following:

1. Assist individuals with their daily communication needs.
2. Help facilitate the development of speech and language.
3. Help facilitate the return of speech and language.

Caregivers sometimes worry that learning a different means of communication will adversely affect speech. In reality, learning to use AAC enhances all other aspects of communication.

AAC systems can be roughly divided into unaided, those requiring no external devices, and aided, those that do. Unaided AAC includes includes signing, gesturing, fingerspelling, cued speech, and writing. These systems are not appropriate for every individual, and an aided system, such as a communication board or an electronic mode of communication, may be more appropriate. Aided systems differ in the type of system, the graphic means of representation, and the input and output modes. Selection of each is determined by ongoing careful assessment.

Decisions on the appropriate type of AAC may need to be revised as the user's abilities or needs change. Users may also employ multiple types of AAC communication. Training of both the user and others in the user's environment is essential for maximum efficacy.

A careful, thorough assessment of a client's abilities and needs is essential for determining the appropriate AAC system and the course of intervention services. Assessment should include not only the client's speech, language, and communication abilities and needs but also motor and perceptual skills, preferences, and the willingness of the environment to support AAC use. The SLP, in coordination with the family and other professionals, uses the data from the assessment to make decisions on the appropriate AAC method, AAC symbol system, and potential vocabulary.

The SLP must be concerned with linguistic and communicative competence as well as operational competence for the AAC system being trained. Intervention must include both the short-range and long-range needs of the client. Intervention considerations include but are not limited to the following:

- Establish an environment of AAC.
- Use everyday experiences as the training context.
- Individualize the content as discussed earlier.
- Train others to modify their interactional style.
- Consider positioning for those with severe motor impairments.
- Make communication real.

REFLECTIONS

- What are the major types of unaided and aided AAC systems?
- How do AAC needs change throughout the lifespan?
- What are the major concerns in client assessment for AAC?
- What are the major elements of intervention with AAC?

SUGGESTED READINGS

Lloyd, L. L., Fuller, D. R., & Arvidson, H. H. (1997). *Augmentative and alternative communication: A handbook of principles and practices.* Boston: Allyn and Bacon.

Reichle, J., Halle, J. W., & Drasgow, E. (1998). Implementing augmentative communication systems. In A. Wetherby, S. Warren, & J. Reichle (Eds.), *Transitions in prelinguistic communication* (pp. 417–436). Baltimore: Brookes.

ON-LINE RESOURCES

http://www.aacintervention.com/   Julie Maro and Caroline Musselwhite of AAC Intervention offer ideas and products for teaching AAC.

http://apple.com/disability/language/   Apple Computer site. Contains downloadable files (Mac compatible) for adapting computers for use with persons with disabilities.

http://www.at-training.com/   University of Buffalo. Assistive technology training online.

http://www.augcominc.com   Augmentative Communication Inc. Newsletter site with on-line tutorials and article synopses.

http://www.closingthegap.com/   Delores and Budd Hagan founded this internationally recognized source of information on innovative applications of computer technology in special education.

http://www.creative-comm.com   Creative Communicating, Inc. Teaching ideas and materials.

http://www.mrtc.org/~duffy/yaack/   AAC Connecting Young Kids site. Useful information on how to get started, to assess, and to teach for AAC with references to professional articles.

http://www.trace.wisc.edu/   Trace Center, University of Wisconsin. AAC research site offering materials on research and products at the center.

http://www.unl.edu/   University of Nebraska-Lincoln. Device tutorials and resources.

An Afterword:
Future of the Professions

Speech-language and audiology are relatively new academic disciplines that trace their origins back to the late 1920s and a few enterprising individuals who had migrated from fields of study such as linguistics, speech communication, and other related areas. The disciplines have grown steadily since the 1920s, experiencing exponential growth beginning in the 1970s. The number of certified members of ASHA is projected to reach 100,000 by the millennium, but the U.S. Bureau of Labor Statistics estimates that there will be a need for at least 125,000 SLPs and audiologists by the year 2005. Given these figures, it should come as no surprise that when *Money* magazine ranked America's fifty hottest jobs, speech-language pathology and audiology ranked eleventh (Giles, Hube, & Wuorio, 1995). Additionally, speech-language pathology and audiology have been identified as among the fastest-growing professions in the United States (Brindley, Bennefield, Danyliw, Hetter, & Loftus, 1997).

The impressive growth rates of speech-language pathology and audiology can be attributed to increases in the scope of practice, many of which are associated with the aging of the U.S. population; increases in the knowledge base generated by clinical research; and greatly improved technology. Over the past few decades, the age range of the people we serve has extended to cover the complete life span. From neonatal hearing screenings to speech-language assessment and therapy with Alzheimer's patients, specialists in communication disorders are actively engaged.

The nature of our concerns has also been extended. Attention to the pragmatics of communication, the use of computers, assistive and augmentative technology, and evaluation and treatment of swallowing disorders are relatively new approaches and services. In addition, because our professions have become more sensitive to the multicultural nature of modern society, international opportunities have become increasingly available (Uffen, 1998).

It is likely that because of the expanding expectations of communication disorders specialists, career preparation will become more demanding. Already, many universities have increased the number of courses required in preparation for a degree. ASHA is moving toward competency-based certification, in which individuals will have to demonstrate not just that they have completed specific courses, but that they are capable and knowledgeable in relevant areas. Toward the end of the twentieth century, the issues of mandating clinical doctorates in audiology or speech-language pathology were raised, debated, and left unresolved. Similarly, specialty recognition has often been suggested, but it is not yet determined whether this is desirable. At the same time as higher-level education may be required for professional titles in communicative disorders, it is likely that a credential for speech-language pathology assistants (SLPAs) will be established for those working in support positions (Kimbarow, 1997). We know that continuing education will remain a priority, and it is likely that future professionals will have to document ongoing study to maintain certification. How we learn may also change. You may already be taking some courses through distance learning, and this type of study may increase.

A clinical doctorate in audiology (Au.D.) will be required in 2012. The specific requirements of this degree have not yet been established.

The future of any profession is based on research. It is through scientific study that advancement occurs. In speech-language pathology and audiology, research is of three types: basic, applied, and efficacy. Basic research seeks to raise and answer questions related to communication processes and disorders. For example, research in digital signal processing has led to better methods of studying disordered speech production and providing real-time meaningful feedback to clients during therapy. Applied research strives to make basic information available in clinical, educational, and rehabilitation settings. Applied research has recently shed light on the nature of developmental apraxia of speech, resulting in better assessment procedures and treatment of the disorder (Shriberg, Aram, & Kwiatkowski, 1997a, b). Finally, efficacy studies are directed at examining the outcome of treatment approaches and their cost effectiveness. The *Journal of Speech-Language-Hearing Research* devoted an entire section of one of its 1997 issues to treatment efficacy across a variety of communication disorders, underscoring the importance of this enterprise. Documenting the need and efficacy of professional services is a task that will engage all speech-language pathologists and audiologists, wherever they work (Seymour, 1997).

No matter what changes occur in the professions of communication disorders, a core concern will remain. Speech-language pathologists and audiologists are people who recognize the importance of communication. They value individuals in their full diversity, and they are committed to research and service that will improve the human condition.

SUGGESTED READINGS

Giles, D. K., Hube, K., & Wuorio, J. (1995). The fifty hottest jobs in America. *Money*, March, 115–117.

Seymour, C. M. (1997). Research, graduate education, and the future of our professions. *Asha, 39* (3), 7.

ON-LINE RESOURCES

http://www.nap.edu/readingroom/books/obas   On Being a Scientist: Responsible Conduct in Research.

National Academy of Sciences. Information on topics such as the social foundations of science, experimental technique, ethical standards, and the role of the scientist in society. Includes case histories.

Glossary

Acoustic immittance The sound that the eardrum reflects during tympanometric testing.

Acoustic nerve (VIIIth cranial nerve) The auditory nerve running from the base of the cochlea to the brain stem and upward to end at the auditory cortex in the temporal lobe of the brain.

Acoustic neuroma A tumor on the auditory nerve that may result in vertigo, tinnitus (ringing in the ear), and hearing loss.

Acquired Occurring after birth.

Acquired immunodeficiency syndrome (AIDS) A viral disease in which a person becomes susceptible to an assortment of other illnesses.

Acute laryngitis Temporary swelling of the vocal folds, resulting in a hoarse voice quality.

Addition In articulation, the insertion of a phoneme that is not part of the word.

Adventitious Occurring sometime after birth.

Affricate A combination of a stop and fricative phoneme.

Age-equivalent score The average score for people of a given age.

Agnosia Sensory deficit accompanying some aphasias that make it difficult to understand incoming sensory information.

Agrammatism Omission of spoken and written grammatical elements found in some aphasias in which individuals omit short unstressed words and morphological endings.

Agraphia Writing difficulty accompanying some aphasias and characterized by mistakes and poorly formed letters.

AIDS See *Acquired immunodeficiency syndrome.*

Air conduction A method of establishing pure tone thresholds by assessing the function of the entire auditory system.

Alexia Reading difficulties found in some aphasias in which the client may be unable to recognize even common words that he or she says.

Allophone A phonemic variation.

ALS See *Amyotrophic lateral sclerosis.*

Alveolar Refers to the alveolar or gum ridge of the mouth. In speech, alveolar consonants are those that are produced with the tongue on the alveolar ridge.

Alveolar processes Embryonic structures that will form the bony hard palate.

Alveolus Area of the mandible and maxilla that houses the teeth.

Alzheimer's disease A cortical pathology that affects primarily memory, language, or visuo-spatial skills as a result of diffuse brain atrophy; presenile dementia.

American Sign Language (ASL) A complex, nonvocal language containing elaborate syntax and semantics. The primary method by which a deaf individual becomes part of the American Deaf culture.

Amplification Personal hearing aids, cochlear implants, and FM assistive listening devices; often a first step in aural rehabilitation.

Amyotrophic lateral sclerosis (ALS) Commonly called Lou Gehrig's disease, ALS is a rapidly progressive degenerative disease in which the individual gradually loses control of her or his musculature. It is characterized by fatigue, muscle atrophy or loss of bulk, involuntary contractions, and reduced muscle tone. Speech in the later stages is labored and slow with short phrasing, long pauses, hypernasality, and severely impaired articulation.

Anatomy The study of the structures of the body and the relationship of these structures to one another.

Aneurysm A type of hemorrhagic stroke resulting from the rupture of a sac-like bulging in a weakened artery wall.

Angular gyrus The area of the brain that assists in integrating visual, auditory, and tactile information and linguistic representation.

Ankyloglossia Tongue-tie; a relatively short lingual frenum.

Anomia Difficulty naming entities.

Anomic aphasia A fluent aphasia characterized by naming difficulties and mild to moderate auditory comprehension problems.

Anoxia Deprivation of oxygen.

Aphasia An impairment due to localized brain injury and affecting understanding, retrieving, and formulating meaningful and sequential elements of language.

Aphemia Severe difficulty producing speech due to a stroke; marked apraxia.

Aphonia Persistent absence of voice that is perceived as whispering.

Aplasia Hearing loss due to the absence or malformation of the inner ear structures during embryonic development.

Approximant Sometimes called a semivowel; an oral consonant that is produced with less constriction than the obstruents, includes glides and liquids.

Apraxia or **verbal apraxia** A neurological impairment of the ability to program—organize and plan—and execute movement of the speech muscles, unrelated to muscle weakness, slowness, or paralysis.

Arcuate fasciculus A white fibrous tract below the cortex that connects Wernicke's and Broca's areas.

Arteriovenous malformation A poorly formed tangle of arteries and veins that may result in a rare type of stroke in which arterial walls are weak and give way under pressure.

Articulation Rapid and coordinated movement of the tongue, teeth, lips, and palate to produce speech sounds.

Articulatory/resonating system Structures used during sound production including the oral cavity, nasal cavity, tongue, and soft palate.

Aryepiglottic folds The membrane and muscle that connect the sides of the epiglottis to the arytenoid cartilages in the larynx.

Arytenoid cartilages Small cartilages on the posterior aspect of the cricoid cartilage that serve as the posterior attachments of the vocal folds.

ASHA The American Speech-Language-Hearing Association.

Aspiration Inhaling; used to mean the inhalation of fluid or food into the lungs; in phonology, a puff of air that is released in the production of various allophones.

Assessment of communication disorders The systematic process of obtaining information from many sources, through various means, and in different settings to verify and specify communication strengths and weaknesses, identify possible causes, and make plans to address them.

Assistive listening device (ALD) Any of several types of equipment, other than a conventional hearing aid, that amplifies or enhances hearing, for example, FM systems and telephone and television amplifiers.

Assistive technologies Aids for daily living, communication, environmental controls; prosthetic or orthotic devices; sensory aids; seating and positioning systems; and mobility/transportation aids.

Ataxia Disorder of muscle coordination.

Ataxic cerebral palsy A congenital disorder characterized by uncoordinated movement and disturbed balance. Movements lack direction, and hypotonic muscles lack adequate force and rate and have poor directional control.

Ataxic dysarthria A motor speech disorder involving a combination of muscle weakness or reduced tone or hypotonia and problems with muscle coordination. Little or no paralysis exists, and the problem is one involving the accuracy, timing, and direction of movement. Speech is characterized by excessive and equal stress and imprecise articulation, especially in repetitive movements.

Atelectasis First stage of otitis media.

Athetoid cerebral palsy A congenital disorder characterized by athetosis, a slow involuntary writhing that is most pronounced when the individual attempts volitional movement. The resultant behavior may be disorganized and uncoordinated.

Atresia Complete closure of the ear canal, either at the pinna or within the ear canal, that may result in a conductive hearing loss.

Atropine A medication that is used to control drooling.

Attention deficit hyperactivity disorder (ADHD) Hyperactivity and attentional difficulties in children who do not manifest other characteristics of learning disabilities.

Audiogram A graph on which results of pure tone audiometry are recorded.

Audiologist A professional whose distinguishing role is to identify, assess, manage, and prevent disorders of hearing and balance.

Audiology "The discipline involved in the prevention, identification, and evaluation of hearing disorders, the selection and evaluation of hearing aids, and the habilitation/rehabilitation of individuals with hearing impairment" (Bess & Humes, 1995, p. 6).

Audiometer A device used for pure tone and speech testing that allows for the manipulation of the intensity and the frequency of a stimulus.

Auditory bombardment In phonological therapy, the repeated presentation of target phonemes at a slightly amplified level.

Auditory brain stem Nuclei and colliculi located in the brain stem that are related to audition.

Auditory brain stem evoked response (ABER) audiometry A type of electrophysiologic testing in which electrodes placed at various points on the scalp gather and record neural responses generated as a "sound" progresses from the auditory nerve to designated points along the brain stem. The result is a waveform known as a Jewett wave.

Auditory cortex Hershl's gyri located in the temporal lobe concerned with the analysis and elaboration of speech.

Auditory nerve VIIIth cranial nerve or vestibuloacoustic nerve. See *Acoustic nerve.*

Auditory nervous system The brain stem pathways and the auditory cortex of the brain.

Auditory training Teaching a person with a hearing impairment how to use the residual or remaining hearing that is available to him or her with the goal of maximizing use of speech and nonspeech cues. The term also applies to intervention with people with phonological and articulatory disorders in which the client is trained to listen to particular sounds.

Auditory tube See *Eustachian tube.*

Augmentative and alternative communication (AAC) Gestures, signing, picture systems, print, computerized communication, and voice production used to complement or supplement speech for persons with severe communication impairments.

Aural habilitation/rehabilitation Services and procedures designed to help a person cope with difficulties presented by a hearing loss.

Authentic data Information about an individual that is based on real life.

Autism A severe form of pervasive developmental disorder characterized as an impairment in reciprocal social interaction with a severely limited behavior, interest, and activity repertoire that has its onset before thirty months of age (American Psychiatric Association, 1987).

Autism spectrum disorder (ASD) Term used to characterize individuals at the severe end of the pervasive developmental disorder (PDD) continuum. ASD is an impairment in reciprocal social interaction with a severely limited behavior, interest, and activity repertoire that has its onset before 30 months of age.

Automaticity The ease with which a person uses a particular skill without apparent thought.

Babbling Single-syllable nonpurposeful consonant-vowel (CV) or vowel-consonant (VC) vocalizations that begin at about 4 months of age.

Backing A phonological process in which a back phoneme is produced for a front one; for example, /k/ is produced for /t/.

Basal ganglia Nuclei deep in the cortex that are important regulators of motor function. See *Basal nuclei*.

Basal nuclei A cluster of neuron cell bodies, sometimes referred to as the basal ganglia, including the caudate, globus pallidus, and putamen. They regulate motor functioning and maintain posture and muscle tone.

Baseline data Information about client performance before intervention begins.

Basilar membrane The floor of the organ of Corti. It is nonuniform in width and thickness, allowing it to respond differentially to different frequencies of sound (tonotopically). The basilar membrane contains thousands of hair cells, the receptor cells for the auditory system.

Behavior modification A systematic method of changing behavior through careful target selection, stimulation, client response, and reinforcement.

Behavioral observation audiometry (BOA) The method of screening infant hearing by presentation of different stimuli and watching for the child's response.

Bernoulli effect The drop in pressure in the glottis during the open phase of vocal fold vibrations that assists in bringing the folds back to a closed state.

Bifid uvula A uvula that is split in half.

Bilabial Pertaining to two lips, as phonemes produced with both lips.

Bilateral Both sides.

Body-mass index Measure of relative fatness; ratio of weight to height.

Bolus A chewed lump of food ready for swallowing.

Bone conduction A method in which pure tone thresholds are established by using an apparatus called a bone oscillator to vibrate the bones of the skull causing the fluids in the inner ear to move, which, in turn, activates the hair cells, thus bypassing the outer or middle ears by direct stimulation of the cochlea.

Bone oscillator A small, vibrating device that is positioned against the skull behind the pinna in bone conduction testing.

Bony hard palate Anterior two-thirds of the roof of the mouth.

Booster treatment Additional therapy, based on retesting, offered after treatment has been terminated.

Bound morpheme A morpheme that must be attached to a free morpheme to communicate meaning; grammatical morpheme.

Brain stem A structure located below the cerebrum and consisting of three major structures: the midbrain, pons, and medulla. It is important for the regulation of respiration, chewing, swallowing, and automatic or autonomic activities of the body.

Breathiness Perception of audible air escaping through the glottis during phonation.

Broca's aphasia A nonfluent aphasia that is characterized by short sentences with agrammatism; anomia; problems with imitation of speech because of overall speech problems; slow, labored speech and writing; and articulation and phonological errors.

Broca's area The area of the cortex located in the frontal lobe that is responsible for detailing and coordinating the programming for verbalizing the message. Signals are then passed to the regions of the motor cortex.

Bulbar palsy A progressive neurological condition resulting in flaccid dysarthria characterized by muscle atrophy and by rapid, random, irregular, and minute contractions (vasiculation) of nerve bundles.

Carryover Transference or generalization; the use of the corrected form outside of the clinical setting.

Case history Background information on a client.

Caudate Portion of the basal nuclei.

Central auditory processing disorder (CAPD) Problems along the brain stem pathways and the auditory cortex of the brain resulting in an inability to efficiently utilize and interpret auditory information, although hearing is within the normal range.

Central nervous system (CNS) The brain and spinal cord.

Central sulcus Also known as the fissure of Rolando, this valley separates the frontal and parietal lobes of the brain.

Cerebellum A lower brain structure consisting of two hemispheres that smoothly regulates and coordinates the control of purposeful muscle movement, including very complex and fine motor activities. The cerebellum revises the transmission from the cortex's motor strip to produce accurate, precise movements.

Cerebral arteriosclerosis A type of ischemic stroke resulting from a thickening of the walls of cerebral arteries in which elasticity is lost or reduced, the walls become weakened, and blood flow is restricted.

Cerebral palsy (CP) A heterogeneous group of neurogenic disorders that result in difficulty with motor movement; were acquired before, during, or shortly after birth; and affect one or more limbs.

Cerebrovascular accident (CVA) Stroke, the most common cause of aphasia, results when the blood supply to the brain is blocked or when the brain is flooded with blood.

Cerebrum The upper brain, which is divided into two hemispheres. The outermost layer is called the cortex.

Cerumen (earwax) A substance produced by the sebaceous glands in the ear canal that provides some lubrication and protects the ear from the invasion of insects.

Cervical vertebrae Upper most region of the vertebral column consisting of seven individual vertebrae.

Chin tuck A posture with the chin down that is helpful with some patients who have a swallowing disability.

Chorea A form of hyperkinetic dysarthria characterized by rapid or continual, random, irregular, and/or abrupt hyperkinesia. Speech, when affected, may be characterized by inappropriate silences caused by voice stoppage; intermittent breathiness, strained harsh voice, and hypernasality; imprecise articulation with prolonged pauses; and forced inspiration and expiration resulting in excessive loudness variations.

Chronemics The study of the effect of time on communication.

Chronic laryngitis Vocal abuse during acute laryngitis that leads to vocal fold tissue damage.

Clavicle Collar bone.

Cleft An abnormal opening in an anatomical structure.

Cleft palate A congenital opening in the midline of the roof of the mouth that may extend through the hard palate, soft palate, and uvula.

Closed syllable A syllable, or basic acoustic unit of speech, that ends in one or more consonants.

Cluttering Disfluent speech that is characterized by overuse of fillers and circumlocutions associated with word-finding difficulties, rapid speech, and word and phrase repetitions. Cluttering does not seem to contain the fear of words or situations found in stuttering.

Coccygeal vertebrae Three fused vertebrae immediately below the sacral vertebrae.

Coccyx Fused structure comprised of three coccygeal vertebrae.

Cochlea The portion of the inner ear that contains the sensory cells for the auditory system. It is composed of two concentric labyrinths; the outer one is made of bone, the inner one of membrane.

Cochlear implant An amplifying device that is surgically implanted into the cochlea and temporal bone.

Code switching Process in which bilingual speakers transfer between two languages based on the listener, context, or topic.

Cognitive ability   The capacity to think and understand.

Cognitive rehabilitation   A treatment regimen for individuals with TBI that is designed to increase functional abilities for everyday life by improving the capacity to process incoming information.

Collaborative model   A model of intervention in which the classroom teacher and SLP plan and implement intervention in the classroom.

Columella   A strip of tissue connecting the tip of the nose to the base.

Communication   An exchange of ideas between sender(s) and receivers(s).

Communication disorder   An impairment in the ability to receive, send, process, or comprehend concepts of verbal, nonverbal, or graphic symbol systems.

Compensatory articulation error   Gross sound substitution errors that are an attempt to make up for the physical inability to produce a given sound correctly.

Complete cleft   A total separation of a normally fused structure.

Compliance   The mobility of the tympanic membrane.

Conduction aphasia   A fluent aphasia in which the individual's conversation is abundant and quick. Characterized by anomia, mildly impaired auditory comprehension if at all, extremely poor repetitive or imitative speech, and paraphasia.

Conductive hearing loss   A mild to moderate impairment in auditory acuity due to malformation or obstruction of the outer and/or middle ears.

Conductive auditory system   Outer and middle ear.

Congenital   Present at birth.

Congenital laryngeal webbing   Extraneous tissue on the anterior aspects of the vocal folds that can interfere with breathing; present at birth.

Consistent aphonia   Persistent absence of voice.

Consonant   A phoneme that is produced with some vocal tract constriction or occlusion.

Contact ulcer   A benign lesion that may develop on the posterior surface of the vocal folds.

Content   The substance or meaning of communication.

Contralateral   Organization of the nervous system that enables motor control to and sensory information from one side of the body to be processed in the opposite side of the brain.

Conversion aphonia   Psychologically based loss of voice.

Conversion disorder   Condition in which emotion is suppressed and transformed into a sensory or motor diability.

Correlate   Something that tends to exist in the presence of something else or be associated with it, but without a demonstrated causal relationship.

Cortex   The outer gray layer of cell bodies in the cerebrum, approximately one-quarter inch in thickness.

Costal   Pertaining to the ribs.

Cranial nerves   The twelve pairs of nerves emerging from the brain stem that carry impulses that are important for speech, hearing, vision, facial expression, and many other functions.

Craniofacial anomalies   Congenital malformations involving the head (cranio: above the upper eyelid) and face (facial: below the upper eyelid).

Craniosynostosis   Premature closing of the sutures of the skull, which greatly disfigures the forehead.

Cricoid cartilage   Signet ring-shaped cartilage at the base of the larynx.

Criterion referenced   An evaluation of an individual's strengths and weaknesses with regard to specific skills.

Cycles approach   A method of phonological therapy in which the same target processes are addressed in several training periods, or cycles.

DAI   Direct auditory input.

DAS   See *Developmental apraxia of speech.*

Deaf   A severe to profound hearing loss in which the auditory system provides little or no access to the world.

Deaf culture A celebration of the uniqueness of their lifestyle by individuals with deafness.

Decibel (dB) A mathematically derived unit based upon the pressure exerted by a particular sound vibration. Degrees of hearing loss refer to a specific decibel range.

Degree of hearing loss Amount of hearing loss expressed in units called decibels (dB).

Dementia An acquired pathological condition or syndrome that is characterized by intellectual decline, especially memory, due to neurogenic causes. Additional deficits include poor reasoning or judgment, impaired abstract thinking, inability to attend to relevant information, impaired communication, and personality changes.

Dentition The number, type, and arrangement of teeth.

Derived score A unit of measurement that compares an individual with others on the basis of the normal curve.

Developmental apraxia of speech (DAS) An impairment in programming the musculature for speech without apparent muscle weakness or paralysis. Apraxia of speech in children is characterized by multiple articulation errors including addition of speech sounds, sound and syllable repetitions, and sound prolongations.

Developmental disfluency or developmental stuttering Whole-word repetitions and other self-conscious nonfluency that is apparent in many young children.

Developmental verbal dyspraxia (DVD) See *Developmental apraxia of speech.*

Diadochokinetic syllable rate Rate of speed with which an individual can rapidly produce target syllables.

Diagnosis A statement distinguishing an individual's difficulties from the broad range of possibilities.

Diagnostic therapy Ongoing assessment and evaluation as intervention takes place.

Dialect A linguistic variation that is attributable primarily to geographical region or foreign language background. It includes features of form, content, and use.

Diaphragm Dome-shaped muscle separating the thorax and abdomen; primary muscle of inhalation.

Dichotically Different signals are applied either simultaneously or at different time intervals to each ear.

Diotically The same signal is applied to each ear simultaneously.

Diphthong Two vowels that are said in such close proximity that they are treated as a single phoneme.

Diplophonia The perception of two vocal frequencies.

Distinctive features The attributes of phonemes that differentiate one from another on the basis of a binary principle.

Distortion In articulation, a deviant production of a phoneme.

Double swallow A technique in which the patient swallows more than once per bolus.

Down syndrome A congenital condition that is characterized by multiple defects and varying degrees of intellectual deficit.

Dynamic Characterized by energy or effective energy, changing over time.

Dynamic assessment Probing during evaluation in an attempt to identify possibly effective intervention procedures.

Dysarthria One of several motor speech disorders that involve impaired articulation, respiration, phonation, or prosody as a result of paralysis, muscle weakness, or poor coordination. Motor function may be excessively slow or rapid, decreased in range or strength, and have poor directionality and timing.

Dysgraphia A disability that is characterized by difficulty producing written symbols.

Dyskinesia Impairment in the ability to control voluntary movement; sometimes due to prolonged use of certain medications.

Dyslexia A disability that is characterized by difficulty comprehending printed symbols and recognizing words. Children with dyslexia often exhibit delayed language development, listening comprehension problems, and poor phonological awareness.

Dysphagia   A disorder of swallowing.

Dysphonia   Any impairment of phonation.

Dystonia   A form of hyperkinetic dysarthria that is characterized by a slow, sustained increase and decrease of hyperkinesia involving either the entire body or localized sets of muscles. As a result, there are excessive pitch and loudness variations, irregular articulation breakdown, and vowel distortions.

Eardrum   See *Tympanic membrane.*

Ear training   The first stage in the Van Riper approach to articulation therapy. It involves identification, localization, stimulation, and discrimination of the target phoneme.

Early expressive language delay (EELD)   A characteristic of children who are late in their early language development and do not outgrow the delay but continue to have problems.

Echolalia   An immediate imitation of another speaker. Among children with ASD, it may represent the storage and production of unanalyzed whole units of language.

ECoG   Electrocochleography; measurement of responses arising from the cochlea to sound in the form of electrical potentials that occur within the first few milliseconds after signal presentation.

Edema   Swelling due to an accumulation of fluid.

Electrolarynx   Battery-powered device that sets air in the vocal tract into vibration.

Embolism   A blood clot, fatty materials, or an air bubble that may travel through the circulatory system until it blocks the flow of blood in a small artery. If it travels to the brain, it may cause a stroke.

Embryological period   The third week through the eighth week of gestation.

Endolymph   A gelatinous fluid that fills the membraneous labyrinth of the cochlea.

Endoscope   A lens coupled with a light source used for viewing internal bodily structures, including the vocal folds.

Epiglottis   Leaf-shaped cartilage attached to the thyroid cartilage that prevents food from entering the trachea during swallowing.

Episodic aphonia   Uncontrolled and unpredictable occasional loss of voice.

Esophageal atresia   The absence of a normal open passageway from the esophagus to the stomach.

Esophageal speech   Speech that is produced by using burping as a substitute for the laryngeal voice.

Esophagostomy   A surgical hole in the esophagus through which a feeding tube may be inserted.

Etiology   Cause or origin of a problem; also the study of cause.

Eustachian tube or **auditory tube**.   The tube that connects the middle ear space with the upper portion of the pharynx and provides a passageway for air to move in and out, maintaining equality of air pressure on either side of the eardrum and ensuring its maximum mobility.

Examination of the peripheral speech mechanism   Sometimes called *oral peripheral exam*; assessment of the structure and function of the visible speech system.

Expansion   The supplying of grammatical forms and/or additional words to complete a child's utterance or make it more syntactically correct. For example,

Child: Baby cry.

Adult: Yes, the baby is crying.

Explicit   Clearly defined.

Extension   A conversational reply that adds information beyond the child's assumed meaning. For example,

Child: Baby cry.

Adult: Yes, the baby is hungry.

External auditory meatus or **ear canal**   Tubular structure that continues the funneling action of the pinna to increase the intensity of the sound waves and to resonate a specific range of middle to high frequencies.

External error sound discrimination   Perceiving differences in the production of the target phoneme in another person's speech.

Extrapyramidal tract   The portion of the nervous system involving the brain stem, cerebellum, and basal nuclei, complementing the

pyramidal tract by smoothing and coordinating movement.

Extrinsic muscles (laryngeal) Muscles that have one point of attachment on the larynx and the other point of attachment on a structure external to the larynx.

Failure to thrive The absence of healthy growth and development.

False negative When an individual passes a screening test but in fact has a problem. Also known as Type II error.

False positive When an individual fails a test and is identified as having a disorder, but in fact has no problem. Also known as Type I error.

False ribs Three pairs of ribs attached indirectly to the sternum.

Fast mapping Process in which a child infers the meaning of a word from context and uses it in a similar context at a later time. A fuller definition evolves over time. Fast mapping enables preschool children to expand their vocabularies quickly by being able to use a word without fully understanding the meaning.

FEES See *Fiberoptic endoscopic evaluation of swallowing.*

Fetal alcohol syndrome Overuse of alcohol during pregnancy, which severely impairs the neurological and physical development of the fetus, resulting in growth deficiencies, craniofacial disorders, central nervous system dysfunction, limited cognitive development, and, in some cases, sensorineural hearing loss.

Fiberoptic endoscopic evaluation of swallowing (FEES) A laryngoscopic technique for viewing swallowing.

Figurative language Nonliteral phrases consisting of idioms, metaphors, similes, and proverbs.

Filler Utterances such as "er," "um," and "you know" that are used within productions. Sometimes characteristic of dysfluent speech and/or stuttering.

Fissure Little valleys within the wrinkled cortex.

Flaccid dysarthria Speech disorder caused by weak, soft, flabby muscle tone, called hypotonia. May result in hypernasality, breathiness, and imprecise articulation.

Fluency Smoothness of rhythm and rate.

Fluent Speech that is relatively smooth and free of disruptions.

Fluent aphasia Speech characterized by word substitutions, neologisms, and often verbose verbal output. Also called Wernicke's aphasia.

Follow-up testing Assessment after dismissal from therapy to ensure that skills have been maintained.

Form The perceivable aspect of language.

Free morpheme The portion of a word that can stand alone and designate meaning; root morpheme.

Frequency In acoustics the number of soundwave cycles that are completed within a specific time period; perceived as the pitch of the sound.

Fricative A consonant phoneme that is produced by exhaling air through a narrow passageway.

Fronting A phonological process in which a front phoneme is produced for a back one; for example, /t/ is produced for /k/.

Frontonasal process Embryonic structure that develops into the nasomedial processes and the lateral nasal processes during the fifth week of gestation.

Functional Having no known organic cause; perhaps psychogenic or learned.

Fundamental frequency The lowest-frequency component of a complex vibration.

Gastroesophageal reflux (GER) Movement of food or acid from the stomach back into the esophagus.

Gastrostomy A surgical opening through the abdomen into the stomach through which a feeding tube may be placed.

Genderlect Variations in language associated with males or females; gender-based dialect.

Generalization The extending of a skill learned in a clinical setting to other "natural" environments or skills; carryover or transference.

Generative Capable of being freshly created; refers to the infinite number of sentences that can be created through the application of grammatical rules.

Genetic   Hereditary.

Glide   Phonemes in which the articulatory posture changes from consonant to vowel.

Global or mixed aphasia   A profound language impairment in all modalities as a result of brain damage.

Glossectomy   The surgical removal of the tongue.

Glottal   Relating to, or produced in or by the glottis, the space between the vocal cords.

Glottal stop   A compensatory behavior where a stoppage of air occurs at the level of the glottis rather than in the oral cavity.

Grammar   The rules of a language.

Granuloma   A nodular lesion due to injury or infection. May occur on the vocal folds and be caused by a breathing tube placed through the glottis.

Gyri   Little hills within the wrinkled cortex.

Habitual pitch   The basic frequency level that an individual uses most of the time.

Hair cells   Auditory receptor cells found on the basilar membrane that are responsible for encoding the auditory information for the brain.

Hard glottal attacks   Abrupt initiation of voicing using hypertensive vocal fold adduction.

Hard of hearing   Mild to moderately severe hearing loss. Hard-of-hearing individuals usually depend as much as possible on their hearing for communication and learning of new concepts.

Harmonics   Frequencies in a complex sound that are integer multiples of the fundamental frequency.

Head-back position   A posture with the head held back that is useful for some clients with a swallowing disability.

Head rotation   A posture with the head turned toward the impairment, used for some clients with a swallowing disability.

Head tilt position   A posture with the head away from the impairment, used for some individuals with a swallowing disability.

Hematoma   Blood trapped in an organ or skin tissue owing to injury or surgery.

Hemianopsia   Blindness in the left or right visual field of both eyes caused by lesions on the temporal or lower parietal lobe.

Hemiparesis   Muscle weakness on one side of the body, resulting in reduced strength and control.

Hemiplegia   Paralysis on one side of the body.

Hemisensory impairment   Loss of the ability to perceive sensory information on one side of the body.

Hemorrhagic stroke   A type of stroke resulting from the weakening of arterial walls that burst under pressure.

Hertz (Hz)   Number of complete vibrations per second.

Heschl's gyrus   An area in each cerebral hemisphere that receives all incoming auditory stimuli and separates it into linguistic and paralinguistic information.

Hesitation   A pause before or between parts of utterances. If used excessively, it may be considered a sign of dysfluency or stuttering.

HIV/AIDS   See *Human immunodeficiency virus* and *Acquired immunodeficiency syndrome*.

Hoarseness   A voice quality that is characterized by a rough, usually low-pitched quality.

Holistic   Pertaining to the whole; multidimensional.

Human immunodeficiency virus   The organism responsible for AIDS.

Huntington's chorea   An inherited progressive disease also known as Huntington's disease, resulting from a genetic defect on chromosome 4.

Hyoid bone   Free floating bone above the larynx that anchors tongue and laryngeal muscles.

Hyperadduction   Excessive movement toward the midline, often resulting in a tense voice quality.

Hyperfluent speech   Very rapid speech found in people with fluent aphasia and characterized by few pauses, incoherence, inefficiency, and pragmatic inappropriateness.

Hyperkinetic dysarthria   A speech disorder characterized by increased movement, such as tremors and tics, and by inaccurate articulation.

Hyperlexia   A mild form of pervasive developmental disorder (PDD) characterized by an inordinate interest in letters and words and by early ability to read but with little comprehension.

Hypertonia   A condition in which there is too much muscle tone, especially in those muscles that oppose the bending of joints and that help us to stand erect. Also called spasticity.

Hypoadduction   Reduced movement toward the midline of the vocal folds, often resulting in a breathy voice quality.

Hypokinesia   Abnormally decreased motor function or activity.

Hypokinetic dysarthria   A speech disorder that is characterized by a decrease or lack of appropriate movement as muscles become rigid and stiff, resulting in monopitch and monoloudness and imprecise articulation.

Hyponasality   A lack of nasal resonance.

Hypotonia   Poor muscle tone and weakness.

Idiolect   An individual's unique way of speaking, a personal dialect.

Immittance bridge (tympanometer)   A handheld probe that is used in audiometric testing of the mobility of the eardrum as the air pressure in the canal is systematically modified. From the recorded data, the tympanometer generates a graph, or *tympanogram*, comparing changes in air pressure to compliance of the eardrum.

Immittance testing   A procedure for assessing mobility of the eardrum in the differential diagnosis of conductive pathology.

Implicit   Assumed but not directly expressed.

Inappropriate pitch   Pitch judged to be outside the normal range for age and/or sex.

Inaudible prolongations   Stuttering behavior characterized by a silent break before or within a word, such as "—girl."

Incidence   The number of new cases of a disorder at a particular point in time in a designated population.

Incidental language teaching   A child-directed strategy in which the caregiver utilizes unstructured or daily activities to enhance language learning.

Incidental teaching   Using a natural activity to train targets.

Incomplete cleft   A separation of a normally fused structure that involves only a portion of the structure.

Incus   The middle bone of the ossicles of the middle ear. It articulates with the malleus at the top and has a projection that is joined to the stapes at the bottom.

Infarction   Death of bodily tissue due to deprivation of the blood supply.

Inferior longitudinal muscle (tongue)   Intrinsic muscle of the tongue that shortens the tongue.

Inner ear   The interior section of the ear containing the cochlea. It supplies information to the brain regarding balance, spatial orientation, and hearing.

Intelligibility   The ease with which an individual's speech is understood.

Intensity   A measure of loudness generally expressed in decibels.

Intentionality   Goal directedness in interactions. It is first demonstrated at about eight months of age primarily through gestures.

Interarytenoid muscle   Intrinsic laryngeal muscle that adducts the vocal folds.

Interdental   Between the teeth; see *Linguadental*.

Internal error sound discrimination   Judging the accuracy of one's own phoneme production; intrapersonal error sound discrimination.

Internal intercostal muscles   Eleven pairs of muscles between the ribs that assist in exhalation.

Internal oblique muscle   Abdominal muscle that can contribute to forced exhalation.

Interpersonal error sound discrimination   See *External error sound discrimination*.

Intonation   Pitch movement within an utterance.

Intrapersonal error sound discrimination   See *Internal error sound discrimination*.

Intrinsic muscles (laryngeal)   Muscles that have both points of attachment on the larynx.

Ischemic stroke   A cerebrovascular accident resulting from a complete or partial blockage or occlusion of the arteries transporting blood to the brain.

Jargon In infancy, long strings of unintelligible sounds with adultlike intonation that develop at about 8 months of age and exhibit the pitch and intonational pattern of the language to which the child is exposed. Jargon may sound like questions, commands, and statements. In some aphasias, jargon refers to meaningless or irrelevant speech, characterized by typical intonational patterns and frequently correct syntax.

Jewett wave The waveform resulting from auditory brain stem evoked response (ABER) audiometry, which measures amplitude and latency or time interval and enables an audiologist to identify the degree and type of hearing loss present and to establish a general site of a lesion.

Kernahan's Striped Y A visual classification system for cleft lip and palate.

Kinesics The study of bodily movement and gesture. Also known as body language.

Labiodental Pertaining to lips and teeth; phonemes produced with lip and tooth contact.

Language A socially shared code for representing concepts through the use of arbitrary symbols and rule-governed combinations of those symbols.

Language impairment A heterogeneous group of deficits and/or immaturities in the comprehension and/or production of spoken or written language.

Language-learning disability Term used to describe the approximately 75 percent of children with learning disability (LD) who have difficulty primarily with learning and using symbols.

Language sample A systematic collection and analysis of a person's speech or writing. Sometimes called a corpus; used as a part of language assessment.

Laryngeal papillomas Wartlike growths on the vocal folds.

Laryngeal prominence The bulge produced by the thyroid cartilage of the larynx. Also known as the Adam's apple.

Laryngeal system Structures of the larynx used for sound production.

Larynx The superior termination of the trachea that protects the lower airways and is the primary sound source for speech production.

Lateral Pertaining to the side. In phonology, it refers to the phoneme /l/, which is produced with air released on both sides of the tongue.

Lateral nasal processes Primitive embryological tissue that gives rise to the nasal alae.

Lateral sulcus The valley separating the frontal and temporal lobes of the brain. Also known as the fissure of Sylvius.

Learning disability (LD) A heterogeneous group of disorders characterized by significant difficulties in the acquisition and use of listening, speaking, reading, writing, reasoning, or mathematical abilities thought to be due to central nervous system dysfunction.

Limited English proficiency (LEP) Language differences that are found in some individuals learning English as a second language. Differences do not in themselves constitute language impairments.

Linguadental Pertaining to tongue and teeth; phonemes produced with tongue and tooth contact.

Linguist A scientist who studies the nature and structure of language(s) and often child language acquisition.

Linguistic intuition A language user's underlying knowledge about the system of rules pertaining to his or her native language; linguistic competence.

Liquid Refers to the oral resonant consonants /r/ and /l/.

Lower motor neurons Cranial and spinal nerves that innervate the muscles.

Lumbar vertebrae Five individual vertebrae located immediately below the thoracic vertebrae.

Lungs Organs that exchange oxygen and carbon dioxide during breathing and generate air pressure for speech production.

Maintaining cause The perpetuating cause that keeps a problem from self-correcting; for example, parents of an 8-year-old considering a lisp "cute."

Malar hypoplasia Underdevelopment of the cheek bones.

Malleus The largest of the ossicles. It rests against the eardrum and articulates with the *incus*, the next bone in the chain.

Malocclusion Improper alignment of the maxillary (upper) and mandibular (lower) dental arches.

Mandible Lower jaw.

Mandibular processes Primitive embryological tissue that gives rise to the mandible.

Maternal rubella German measles during pregnancy; may result in various disorders in the developing fetus.

Maxilla Upper jaw.

Maxillary processes Primitive embryological tissue that gives rise to the lateral aspects of the maxilla and palatal shelves.

Maximal contrast A minimal pair in which the differing phonemes differ in more than one distinctive feature; for example, "say" (/se/) and "bay" (/be/).

Maximal opposition See *Maximal contrast*.

Mean length of utterance (MLU) The average length of utterances measured in morphemes. In English, this is an important measure of preschool development, because language becomes more complex as it becomes longer.

Medial Toward the midline.

Meningitis An inflammation of the meninges, or layers of tissue covering the brain, and frequently a cause of severe to profound hearing loss.

Mental retardation/developmental disabilities A disorder characterized by substantial limitations in intellectual functioning, concurrent related limitations in adaptive skill areas, and manifestation before age 18.

Metalinguistic skills Abilities that enable a child to consider language in the abstract, to make judgments about its correctness, and to create verbal contexts, such as in writing.

Metaphon An approach to phonological therapy that is based on the premise that phonological disorders in children are developmental language learning disorders.

Micrognathia Underdeveloped mandible.

Microtia A small, malformed pinna or ear canal that may result in a conductive hearing loss.

Midbrain A structure in the brain stem. Also known as the mesencephalon.

Middle ear A small cavity separated from the outer ear by the eardrum; transmits sound waves from the eardrum to the partition between the middle and inner ears through a chain of small bones.

Middle ear space A cubed-shaped area between the outer and inner ear containing the ossicles.

Minimal contrast A minimal pair in which the differing phonemes differ in a single distinctive feature; for example, "lope" (/lop/) and "lobe" (/lob/).

Minimal pair Two words that differ in a single phoneme; for example, "say" (/se/) and "bay" (/be/).

Mixed dysarthrias Symptoms or areas of brain injury that cross several dysarthrias as a result of degenerative disorders, toxins, metabolic disorders, stroke, trauma, tumors, and infectious diseases.

Mixed hearing loss Combination of a sensorineural hearing loss with a conductive component.

Modeling Demonstrating the desired response.

Modified barium swallow study An X-ray procedure that is used to visualize the swallowing process. Also known as *videofluoroscopy*.

Monoloudness Voice lacking normal variations of intensity that occur during speech.

Monopitch Voice that lacks normal inflection in tone.

Monotone Voice that is produced without varying the fundamental frequency.

Morpheme The smallest meaningful unit of language.

Morphology The study of word structure.

Morphophonemic contrasts   Changes in pronunciation as a result of morphological changes.

MS   See *Multiple sclerosis.*

Mucosal tissue   Pinkish tissue lining the inside of the mouth.

Multiple sclerosis (MS)   A progressive disease characterized by demyelinization of nerve fibers of the brain and spinal cord.

Multiview videofluoroscopy   Motion picture X-rays recorded from various angles.

Myasthenia gravis   A disorder characterized by fatigability and rapid weakening of muscles, a cause of flaccid dysarthria.

Myelination   Development of a protective myelin sheath or sleeve around the cranial nerves.

Myofunctional disorder   See *Tongue thrust.*

Myringotomy   A surgical procedure in which a small tube is placed in the tympanic membrane to drain fluid from the middle ear.

Nasal alae   Lateral flaring of the nostrils.

Nasal cavity   Cavity above the oral cavity related to the nose.

Nasal emission   Air escaping through the nose during speech production.

Nasalance score   A numerical score that reflects the magnitude of hypernasality when measured by a nasometer.

Nasals   Phonemes that are produced with nasal resonance.

Nasogastric tube (NG tube)   A tube placed into the nose then through the pharynx and esophagus by which liquefied food may be fed.

Nasomedian processes   Primitive embryological tissue that gives rise to the anterior portion of the upper lip and premaxilla.

Nasometer   A commercially available device that is used to measure nasality.

Neologism   A novel word that does not exist in the language. Neologisms are created and used quite confidently by some individuals with aphasia.

Neonate   Newborn.

Neurogenic stuttering   Disorder of fluency associated with some form of brain damage.

Neuron   The basic unit of the nervous system, consisting of the cell body, axon, and dendrites.

NIPTS   Noise-induced permanent threshold shift.

NITTS   Noise-induced temporary threshold shift.

Noise-induced hearing loss   Hearing impairment as a result of working around noisy equipment, listening to loud music, or a similar experience.

Nonfluent aphasia   A language disorder that is characterized by slow, labored speech and struggle to retrieve words and form sentences.

Nonresonant   In articulation refers to speech sounds that are produced with little vocal resonance (stops, fricatives, affricates); also called nonresonant phonemes.

Nonverbal   Without words.

Nonvocal   Without voice.

Norm referenced   A comparison that is usually based on others of the same gender and similar age.

NPO   No food by mouth.

Obstruent   In articulation refers to speech sounds that are produced with a significant amount of constriction in the vocal tract (stops, fricatives, affricates); also called nonresonant phonemes.

Obturator   A prosthetic device that forms an artificial palate. It is used to cover a cleft palate.

Occupational therapist   A professional who works with clients' small motor movements.

Olfactory pits   Depressions between the nasomedian and lateral nasal processes that will ultimately become the right and left nasal cavities.

Omission   In articulation, the absence of a phoneme that has not been produced or replaced.

Open syllable   A syllable, or basic acoustic unit of speech, that ends in a vowel.

Optimal pitch level   A particularly suitable pitch level for an individual largely determined by vocal fold structure.

Oral apraxia   A neurological impairment in programming and executing speech and non-speech movements of the mouth.

Oral cavity The mouth, housing the teeth and tongue.

Oral/manual communication method Aural habilitation procedure that combines speech and sign language.

Oral-motor training Exercises and activities that train volitional control over movements needed for speech. Also known as motor programming.

Oral peripheral exam See *Examination of the peripheral speech mechanism.*

Organ of Corti An intricate structure that runs along the center of the membraneous labyrinth of the cochlea and contains the auditory sensory receptors consisting of the basilar membrane and the tectorial membrane.

Organic Physiological.

Orthodontist A dental specialist who is concerned primarily with alignment of the teeth.

Ossicles Small bones within the middle ear, including the malleus, the incus, and the stapes.

Ossicular discontinuity A break in the chain of small bones in the middle ear.

Otitis media Inflammation of the middle ear, with or without infection.

Otitis media with effusion (OME) Inflammation of the middle ear with fluid, resulting in temporary hearing loss.

Otoacoustic emissions (OAEs) Measurable low-level sounds or echoes produced by the cochlea either spontaneously or in response to sound stimulation.

Otosclerosis A stiffening of the ossicular chain in the middle ear.

Ototoxic Refers to destructive drugs that may damage inner ear structures.

Outer ear The pinna and the external auditory meatus or ear canal.

Palatal Refers to the front area of the roof of the mouth. In speech, palatal consonants are produced with the tongue touching or approximating the hard palate.

Palatal obturator A plate that covers a portion of the soft palate. It is useful for individuals who have had palatal surgery.

Palatal shelves Wedge-shaped tissue masses that will become the bony hard palate.

Palatoplasty Surgical correction of a cleft palate.

Paralysis Inability to move a muscle.

Paraphasia Word substitutions that are found in some individuals with aphasia who may talk fluently and grammatically.

Paresis Muscle weakness, partial paralysis.

Parietal pleura Pleural membrane that lines the inner aspects of the thorax.

Parkinson's disease A progressive neurogenic disorder that is characterized by resting tremors, slowness of movement, and difficulty initiating voluntary movements. Speech may be rapid, breathy, and reduced in loudness, pitch range, and stress.

Passive recoil forces Nonmuscular forces that assist the exhalation process.

Pectoral girdle Clavicle and scapula bones.

Pedunculated polyp Polyp that appears to be attached to the vocal fold by a stalk.

Percentile rank A number that indicates the percentage of people who are below a particular level on a variable value such as height or a score on a test.

Perceptual training See *Ear training.*

Perilymph Watery fluid that fills the bony labyrinth of the cochlea and surrounds the outside of the membraneous labyrinth.

Peripheral nervous system (PNS) Located outside the CNS, it consists of twelve pairs of cranial nerves, thirty-one pairs of spinal nerves, and portions of the autonomic nerves that regulate smooth muscles and glands and helps the CNS to communicate with the body.

Perpetuating cause See *Maintaining cause.*

Personal hearing aids Amplification devices ranging from tiny, in-the-ear models to those worn behind the ear or on the body.

Pervasive developmental disability (PDD) Any of several disorders of childhood that are characterized by markedly atypical behaviors and severe impairment in the ability to relate to others, including infantile autism and childhood schizophrenia.

Pharyngeal cavity   The throat.

Pharyngeal flap   A secondary surgical procedure to correct velopharyngeal incompetence.

Pharyngostomy   A surgical hole in the pharynx through which a feeding tube may be placed.

Pharynx   The anatomical passageway connecting the nasal and oral cavities.

Phonation   Production of sound by vocal fold vibration.

Phoneme   A family of speech sounds that are phonetically similar. Phonemes combine with each other to form words, phrases, and sentences.

Phonetically balanced (PB)   Refers to word lists used in speech discrimination or word identification testing in which each speech sound is included in the list in the same proportion in which it appears in everyday language.

Phonetically consistent forms (PCFs)   Consistent vocal patterns that function as meaningful "words" for the infant. These are a transition to words.

Phonological process   A simplification of adult phonology; a system of describing children's articulatory patterns.

Phonology   The study of the sound systems of language.

Phonotactic   The study of the way in which phonemes are combined and arranged in syllables and words of a particular language or dialect.

Physiology   The branch of biology that is concerned with the process and function of parts of the body.

Pidgin signed English (PSE).   A sign system that incorporates ASL-like signs but maintains English word order.

Pierre Robin syndrome   A congenital condition resulting in a small mandible, cleft lip, cleft palate, and other facial abnormalities.

Pinna   The funnel-shape outermost part of the ear, which serves to collect the sound waves and channel them into the ear.

Pitch   The perceptual counterpart to fundamental frequency associated with the speed of vocal fold vibration.

Pitch breaks   Sudden uncontrolled upward or downward changes in pitch.

Play audiometry   A method of assessing the hearing of children ages 2½ to 3 years and older who are instructed to put a block in a basket, a peg in a board, or other action whenever they hear a sound.

Portfolio   A collection of information and material about an individual taken from various sources that may be used both for initial assessment and to measure progress.

Portfolio evaluation   Multiple samples of a variety of writing tasks used by SLPs and others to evaluate the proficiency and flexibility of a child's written language and to assess change over time.

Postlingually   Refers to hearing loss acquired after the person has had the opportunity to experience speech and language.

Posttherapy testing   Assessment following intervention.

Prader-Willi syndrome   A congenital condition characterized by obesity and intellectual deficit.

Pragmatics   The use, function, or purpose of communication; the study of communicative acts and contexts.

Precipitating cause   Factors that trigger a disorder; for example, a stroke.

Predisposing cause   Underlying factors that contribute to a problem; for example, a genetic basis.

Prelingually   Refers to hearing loss acquired before the person developed speech.

Premaxilla   The anterior portion of the hard palate to the incisive foramen.

Presbycusis   Hearing loss induced through the aging process caused by the slow deterioration of the hair cells and acoustic nerve.

Pressure consonant   A consonant sound that requires the build up of intra-oral air pressure like the sound /t/.

Pressure equalization (PE) tubes   Tiny tubes that are inserted surgically into the eardrums to take over the function of the eustachian tube and allow air back into the middle ear space.

Prevalence   The total number of cases of a disorder at a particular point in time in a designated population.

Primary motor cortex   A 2-centimeter-wide gyrus immediately in front of or anterior to the central sulcus that controls motor movements.

Production training   In the Van Riper approach to articulation, therapy that involves teaching the client to say the target phoneme in isolation, then syllables, words, phrases, and sentences.

Prognosis   An informed prediction of the outcome of a disorder.

Prolabium   Central prominence of the lip; also isolated soft tissue mass in unrepaired bilateral clefts.

Prolongation   In fluency analysis, the process of holding a phoneme longer than is typical; for example, "ssssso."

Prosody   The rate and rhythm of language; the melodic pattern of speech.

Prosthodontist   A dental specialist who is concerned with the replacement of missing teeth and other oral structures with various appliances.

Proxemics   The study of physical distance between people.

Pseudobulbar palsy   A condition that resembles progressive bulbar palsy, characterized by spastic dysarthria and dysphagia.

Psychogenic   Caused by psychological factors.

Pull-out therapy   Removing a child from a classroom so that she or he can participate in a therapy session.

Pure tone audiometry   A procedure that is used to measure hearing thresholds via air and bone conduction.

Pure tone stimuli   Sounds that contain a single frequency—usually 125 Hz, 250 Hz, 500 Hz, 1,000 Hz, 2,000 Hz, 4,000 Hz and 8,000 Hz—and are used in pure tone audiometry.

Purulent otitis media   A middle ear infection.

Push-in therapy   Communication intervention by a speech-language pathologist within a classroom.

Pyloric stenosis   A narrowing of the sphincter connecting the stomach to the small intestine, resulting in a blockage to the intestines.

Pyramidal tract   The primary voluntary motor control system or path, originating in the primary motor cortex.

Range of motion   The extent of movement of a joint from maximum extension to maximum flexion.

Rate   The speed at which something occurs. In speech this may be the number of words or syllables in a given period of time.

Raw score   The number of correct answers on a test or subtest.

Recurrent branch   Branch of the tenth cranial nerve that innervates muscles of the larynx.

Reduplicated babbling   Long strings of consonant-vowel syllable repetitions, such as "ma-ma-ma-ma-ma."

Reflexes   Automatic, involuntary motor patterns. Most disappear, but some, such as the gag reflex, remain for life.

Reinforcement   A procedure that follows a response with the intent of perpetuating or extinguishing it; used in conditioning.

Reliability   In tests, the likelihood that the instrument will yield comparable results if administered by someone else, at a later date, or under different conditions.

Repetition   In fluency analysis, the process of repeating a word or a part of a word, as in "the-the-the" or "b-b-ball."

Representation   Process of having one thing stand for another, such as a piece of paper used as a blanket for a doll.

Resonant   A consonant phoneme that is produced with resonance occurring throughout the vocal tract; refers to nasals, liquids, and glides.

Resonation   Modification of the vibratory pattern of the laryngeal tone through changes in the size and configuration of the vocal tract.

Respiratory system   Stuctures, including the lungs, bronchi, trachea, larynx, mouth, and nose, that are used in breathing for life and speech.

Response   The reaction to a stimulus.

Reverse swallow   See *Tongue thrust.*

Rhotic   Phonemes made with the tongue in either a bunched or turned back posture; the /r/ family of sounds.

Rib cage   Twelve pairs of ribs that constitute the major portion of the thorax.

Right hemisphere injury or syndrome (RHI)   A group of neuromuscular, perceptual, and/or linguistic deficits that result from damage to the right hemisphere of the brain and may include epilepsy, hemisensory impairment, and hemiparesis or hemiplegia.

Sacrum   Fused structure comprised of five sacral vertebrae.

Scintography   A computerized technique for measuring aspiration during or after a swallow.

Self-monitoring   The ability to recognize one's own errors and correct them.

Semantic features   The pieces of meaning that come together to define a particular word.

Semantic-pragmatic disorder   A mild form of pervasive developmental disorder characterized by limited vocabulary, concrete definitions, and poor conversational skills.

Semantics   The study of word and language meaning.

Sensorineural hearing loss   Permanent hearing loss as the result of the absence, malformation, or damage to the structures of the inner ear.

Sensorineural system   Cochlea and auditory nerve.

Sensory-motor training   An approach to articulation therapy in which the client is made aware of tactile and proprioceptive sensations associated with sound production.

Sessile polyp   Polyp with a broad-based attachment to the vocal fold.

Signed exact English (SEE)   A signing system for representing English that requires the breaking down of English words into syllables and representing each syllable through a specific sign.

Silent aspiration   Lack of coughing when food or liquid enters the airway.

SLP   See *Speech language pathologist.*

Sociolinguistics   The study of influences such as cultural identity, setting, and participants on communicative variables.

Soft-voice syndrome   Compensatory behavior in which a child with velopharyngeal incompetence purposely reduces vocal intensity to prevent air escape through the nose and reduce hypernasality.

Somatogenic   Coming from the body; organic or physiological.

Spastic cerebral palsy   A congenital disorder that is characterized by increased muscle tone, such that when a muscle contracts, the opposing muscle may react abnormally to stretch by increasing muscle tone too much. Muscle movements are described as jerky, labored, and slow.

Spastic dysarthria   Speech that is characterized as slow with jerky, imprecise articulation and reduction of the rapidly alternating movements of speech because of stiff and rigid muscles.

Spastic dysphonia   A voice disorder that is characterized by hyperadduction of the vocal folds resulting in a strained/strangled voice production with intermittent stoppages.

Spectrum   Representation of a sound in which amplitude is displayed as a function of frequency.

Specific language impairment (SLI)   Impairment of language that affects primarily preschoolers and cannot be attributed to deficits in hearing, oral structure and function, general intelligence, or perception; therefore, it is characterized primarily by the exclusion of other disorders. The major distinction between people with LLD and those with SLI is that those with SLI do not exhibit perceptual difficulties.

Speech audiometry   A procedure that is used to assess loudness levels at which words are understood, speech reception threshold (SRT), and speech discrimination or word identification.

Speech bulb   An obturator that fills the velopharyngeal space, closing the velopharyngeal portal.

Speech community   A group of people who share a common understanding of the rules and restrictions that govern communicative situations.

Speech-language pathologist (SLP)   A professional whose distinguishing role is to identify, assess, treat, and prevent speech, language, communication, and swallowing disorders.

Speech reception threshold (SRT) test   A test procedure in speech audiometry that measures the quietest level at which a person can hear and understand speech 50 percent of the time using a special group of words called *spondees*.

Speech sample   A systematic collection and analysis of a person's speech, a corpus; used in language assessment.

Spina bifida   A congenital malformation of the spinal column.

Spinal cord   A collection of neuron cell bodies protected within a fatty myelin sheath located within the bony spinal column.

Spondee   Two-syllable compound words that are spoken with equal emphasis on both syllables and used in speech reception threshold testing.

Spontaneous recovery   A natural recovery process that proceeds without professional intervention.

Stabilization   In the Van Riper approach to articulation therapy, reinforcement and maintenance of the corrected phoneme.

Standard score   A derived score that uses an arbitrary number, such as 10 or 100, as the numerical average and uses statistical formulae to compute scores above and below this average; for example, an IQ score.

Stapes   The smallest of the ossicles in the middle ear.

Startle reflex   A generalized response to a sudden stimulus, for example, a noise. It is present from birth; premature or impaired infants may lack this reflex.

Stereocilia   Small, hairlike projections on the top of each hair cell.

Sternum   Breast bone.

Stimulability   The ability to imitate a target phoneme when given focused auditory and visual cues.

Stimulus   Anything that is capable of eliciting a response.

Stoma   A small opening; for example, a surgical hole in the external neck region extending into the pharynx to permit breathing following laryngectomy.

Stopping of fricatives   The phonological process in which stop phonemes are used in place of fricatives.

Stops   Consonant phonemes produced by building air pressure behind the point of constriction.

Strain and struggle   Difficulty initiating and maintaining voice.

Stridor   Noisy breathing or involuntary sound that accompanies inspiration and expiration.

Stroke   Cerebrovascular accident (CVA), the most common cause of aphasia, resulting when the blood supply to the brain is blocked or when the brain is flooded with blood.

Stuttering   A disorder of speech fluency characterized by hesitations, repetitions, prolongations, tension, and avoidance behaviors.

Subglottal pressure   Pressure beneath the vocal folds that sets them into vibration.

Substitution   In articulation, the production of one phoneme in place of another.

Sulci   Little valleys within the wrinkled cortex.

Superior longitudinal muscle (tongue)   Intrinsic muscle of the tongue that elevates lateral tongue margins.

Supplemental muscles (laryngeal)   Muscles that have one point of attachment on the hyoid bone and the other point of attachment on some other structure.

Support group   Individuals with similar problems who meet together to share feelings, information, and ideas.

Suppurative fluid   Pussy discharge from the middle ear tissue into the middle ear.

Supramarginal gyrus   An area in the left temporal lobe of the brain that assists in integrating visual, auditory, and tactile information and linguistic representation.

Suprasegmental   Features such as loudness, rate, and intonation that affect more than a single phoneme and add meaning to an utterance.

Synapse   The minuscule space between the axon of one neuron and the dendrites of the next.

Syndactyly   Webbing of the fingers and toes.

Syndrome   A combination of symptoms that occur together in predictable and consistent combinations of traits.

Syntax   How words are arranged in sentences.

Tactiles   Touching behaviors.

Tardive dyskinesia   Involuntary, repetitive facial, tongue, or limb movements that sometimes occur as a side effect of certain medications.

TBI See *Traumatic brain injury.*

Tectorial membrane The gelatinous, tongue-shaped structure that forms the roof of the organ of Corti.

Telecoil Device in a hearing aid that picks up sound through magnetic induction.

Teletypewriter (TTY) A device connected to a telephone by a special adapter; allows communication between persons who are hearing impaired and those who are not.

Tensor veli palatini Muscle of the soft palate that opens the auditory tube.

Teratogens Chemical or environmental agents that produce congenital abnormalities.

Thalamus A pair of spherical neural structures, each acting as a receiving station for relaying information to areas of the brain or beyond. The thalamus may set the tone for the brain, alerting it to prepare to receive or to transmit information.

Thoracic vertebrae Twelve individual vertebrae located immediately beneath the cervical vertebrae.

Thorax The chest area between the neck and abdomen.

Threshold The quietest presentation level (in decibels) at which a person can detect a stimulus 50 percent of the time.

Thrombosis A blood clot within a blood vessel of the body. It may result in an ischemic stroke.

Thyrohyoid membrane Membrane extending from the hyoid bone to the thyroid cartilage.

Thyrohyoid muscle Extrinsic muscle of the larynx that pulls the larynx upward.

Thyroid cartilage "V" shaped largest cartilage of the larynx.

Tics Involuntary, rapid and repetitive, stereotypic movements.

Tidal breathing Breathing to sustain life.

Timing Accuracy of the beginning and ending of a muscle contraction and the duration of that contraction.

Tinnitus Ringing sensation in the ears.

TMJ Temporomandibular joint, articulation of the temporal bone and mandible.

Tone Resistance to stretch; the near constant state of a muscle.

Tongue thrust Swallowing with a forward movement of the tongue, resulting in misarticulation of various phonemes. Also known as *myofunctional disorder.*

Tonotopically arranged Refers to the basilar membrane in which different areas respond differently to different frequencies of sound.

Total communication The use of sign, amplification, and speech in the communication training of individuals with deafness.

Trachea Cartilaginous tube extending from the larynx to the lungs via the bronchi.

Tracheo-esophageal shunt (TEP) A device that directs air from the trachea to the esophagus for esophageal speech.

Tracheostomy An opening through the neck into the trachea through which a tube is placed to reduce the risk of aspiration.

Tracheostomy tube A tube that is inserted into the trachea to relieve a breathing obstruction.

Transcortical motor aphasia A nonfluent aphasia that is characterized by impaired conversational speech, good verbal imitative abilities, and mildly impaired auditory comprehension.

Transcortical sensory aphasia A rare fluent aphasia that is characterized by word substitutions, lack of nouns and severe anomia, and poor auditory comprehension, but ability to repeat or imitate words, phrases and sentences.

Traumatic brain injury (TBI) Damage to the brain resulting from bruising and laceration caused by forceful contact with the relatively rough inner surfaces of the skull or from secondary edema or swelling, infarction or death of tissue, and hematoma or focal bleeding.

Treacher Collins syndrome An inherited disorder that is characterized by excessive muscle tone in the face and jaw.

Treatment plan Recommendations for addressing the problem, including placement,

therapy approaches, counseling suggestions, and referrals.

Tremors Involuntary, rhythmic movements caused by contractions of antagonistic muscles.

Tympanic membrane or **eardrum.** A cone-shaped structure composed of three layers of tissue that completely closes off one end of the ear canal so that all of the incoming sound vibrations strike its surface.

Tympanogram The graph generated by a tympanometer during immittance testing that depicts compliance of the eardrum relative to changes in air pressure.

Tympanometer Audiometric equipment that is used to assess the compliance of the tympanic membrane.

Type I error See *False positive.*

Type II error See *False negative.*

Ultrasonography Ultrasound.

Ultrasound A technique that uses high frequency sound waves to visualize internal bodily organs.

Unilateral On one side.

Upper motor neurons A part of the central nervous system between the primary motor cortex and the lower motor neurons, responsible for relaying nerve impulses to the muscles.

Usher's syndrome A congenital hereditary syndrome. The main components are a profound sensorineural hearing impairment and progressive blindness.

Uvula Fleshy mass termination of the soft palate.

Validity In tests, the accuracy with which the instrument measures what it intends or claims to measure.

Variegated babbling Long strings of consonant-vowel syllables, in which adjacent and successive syllables in the string are not identical.

Vasiculation Rapid, random, irregular, and minute contractions of nerve bundles.

Veau system Roman numeral classification system for describing clefts of the lip and/or palate.

Velar Refers to the posterior area of the roof of the mouth. In speech, velar consonants are produced with the tongue touching or approximating the velum or soft palate.

Velopharyngeal competence Adequate closure of the velopharyngeal portal (soft palate and back of throat) during swallowing and speech production.

Velopharyngeal incompetence (VPI) Inability of the velopharyngeal mechanism to separate the oral and nasal cavities during swallowing and speech.

Velopharyngeal mechanism Velum (soft palate) and walls of pharynx (back of throat), used to close the velopharyngeal portal.

Velopharyngeal portal Opening or the conduit connecting the oral and nasal cavities.

Velum The soft palate, which constitutes the posterior one third of the palate.

Verbal stereotype An expression that is repeated over and over; characteristic of some individuals with aphasia.

Vermilion Pinkish to brown coloration of the lips.

Vertebral column The backbone comprised of thirty-two separate vertebrae.

Vibration A series of rapid, rhythmic, back-and-forth movements.

Videofluoroscopy See *Modified barium swallow study.*

Visual reinforcement audiometry (VRA) A method of hearing testing in which a child, often as young as 3 to 4 months, is rewarded for looking for a sound by the use of moving toys and/or flashing lights.

Vocal abuse Any of several behaviors, including smoking and yelling, that can result in damage to the laryngeal mechanism.

Vocal fold paralysis Immobilized vocal fold usually due to nerve damage.

Vocal hygiene Proper care of the voice.

Vocal nodules Localized growths on the vocal folds that are associated with vocal abuse.

Vocal polyp A fluid-filled lesion of the vocal fold that results from mechanical stress.

Vocal tremor   Variations in the pitch and loudness of the voice that are involuntary.

Voice   Vocal tone and resonance.

Voiced   Vocal fold vibration; phonemes that are produced with vocal fold (laryngeal) vibration.

Voiceless   Without vocal fold vibration; phonemes that are produced without vocal fold (laryngeal) vibration.

Vowel   Any of several voiced phonemes that are produced with a relatively open vocal tract.

Waardenburg's syndrome   A disorder characterized by pigmentary discoloration, particularly in the irises and hair; craniofacial malformation of the nasal area; and severe to profound hearing impairment.

Wernicke's aphasia   A fluent aphasia that is characterized by rapid-fire strings of sentences with little pause for acknowledgment or turn taking. Content may seem to be a jumble and may be incoherent or incomprehensible, though fluent and well articulated.

Wernicke's area   The section in the left temporal lobe of the brain in which incoming language is analyzed and the outgoing message is organized.

Word recognition test (WRT)   A procedure used in speech audiometry.

References

Air, D. H., Wood, A. S., & Neils, J. R. (1989).
Considerations for organic disorders. In
N. A. Creaghead, P. W. Newman, & W. A.
Secord (Eds.), *Assessment and remediation
of articulatory and phonological disorders*
(2nd ed.). Columbus, OH: Merrill.

Alberts, M. J., Bennett, C. A., & Rutledge,
V. R. (1996). Hospital charges for stroke
patients. *Stroke, 27,* 1825–1828.

Ambrose, N., Yairi, E., & Cox, N. (1993). Genetic aspects of early childhood stuttering.
*Journal of Speech and Hearing Research,
36,* 701–706.

American Association on Mental Retardation.
(1992). *Mental retardation: Definition,
classification, and systems of support* (9th
ed.). Washington, DC: Author.

American Medical Association Staff. (2001).
*CPT Plus! 2001: A comprehensive guide to
current procedural terminology.* Los Ange-
les, CA: Practice Management Information
Corporation.

American Psychiatric Association. (1987). *Diagnostic and statistical manual of mental
disorders* (3rd ed. rev.) Washington, DC:
Author.

American Psychiatric Association. (1994). *Diagnostic and statistical manual of mental
disorders* (4th ed.). Washington, DC:
Author.

American Speech-Language-Hearing Association. (2001, December 26). Code of ethics
(revised). *ASHA Leader, 6*(23), 2.

Andrews, G., Craig, A., Feyer, A. M., Hod-
dinott, S., Howie, P., & Neilson, M.
(1983). Stuttering: A review of research
findings and theories circa 1982. *Journal
of Speech and Hearing Disorders, 48,*
226–246.

Andrews, G., Guitar, B., & Howie, P. (1980).
Meta-analysis of the effects of stuttering
treatment. *Journal of Speech and Hearing
Disorders, 45,* 287–307.

Angelo, J. (1992). Comparison of three computer scanning modes as an interface
method for persons with cerebral palsy.
*American Journal of Occupational Ther-
apy, 46,* 217–222.

Aram, D. M. (1997). Hyperlexia: Reading without meaning in young children. *Topics in
Language Disorders, 17*(3), 1–13.

Aram, D. M., & Eisele, J. A. (1994). Limits to a
left hemisphere explanation of specific
language impairment. *Journal of Speech
and Learning Research, 37,* 824–830.

Aronson, A. E. (1990). *Clinical voice disorders.*
New York: Thieme.

ASHA (American Speech-Language-Hearing
Association). (1990). Skills needed by
speech-language pathologists providing

services to dysphagic patients/clients. *Asha, 32* (Suppl. 2) 7–12.

ASHA. (1992). Instrumental diagnostic procedures for swallowing. *Asha, 34* (March, Suppl. 7), 25–33.

ASHA. (1993). Definitions of communication disorders and variations. *Asha, 35* (Suppl. 10), pp. 40–41.

ASHA. (1995a). Characteristics of state licensure laws. *Asha, 37*(3), 84–94.

ASHA. (1995b). *Guidelines for the training, credentialing, use, and supervision of speech-language pathology assistants.* Rockville, MD: Author.

ASHA. (1995c). *Omnibus survey results: 1995 Edition.* Rockville, MD: ASHA.

ASHA. (1995d). *Task force on central auditory processing consensus development.* Washington, DC: Author.

ASHA. (1997). *Preferred practice patterns for the profession of speech-language pathology.* Rockville, MD: Author.

ASHA. (1999). "Code of Ethics," 1995. [On-line]. Available: http://www.asha.org/professionals/library/code_of_ethics.htm.

ASHA. (2000a). Council on Professional Standards. Background information for the standards and implementation for the certificate of clinical competence in speech-language pathology. (Effective date: January 1, 2005) [On-line] http://professional.asha.org/library/slp_standards.htm

ASHA. (2000b). Council on Professional Standards. Background information for the standards and implementation for the certificate of clinical competence in audiology. (Effective date: January 1, 2007) [On-line] http://professional.asha.org/library/audiology_standards.htm

ASHA. (2000c). Fact Sheet: Speech-Language Pathology. Online at http://professional.asha.org/students/careers/slp.htm

ASHA. (2000d). Speech-Language Disorders and the Speech-Language Pathologist. Online at http://professional.asha.org/students/careers/sld.htm

ASHA. (2001a). Council on Academic Accreditation. Standards for accreditation of graduate education programs in audiology and speech-language pathology. [On-line] http://professional.asha.org/students/caa_programs/standards.htm

ASHA. (2001b). Fact Sheet: Audiology. On line at http://professional.asha.org/students/careers/audiology.htm

ASHA. (2002). About ASHA: mission statement. Online at http://professional.asha.org/services/about_asha.cfm

Alexander, M. P., & Naeser, M. A. (1988). Cortical-subcortical differences in aphasia. In F. Plum (Ed.), *Language, communication and the brain.* New York: Raven Press.

Aviv, J. E., Sataloff, R. T., Cohen, M., et al. (2001). Cost effectiveness of two types of dysphagia care in head and neck cancer: A preliminary report. *Ear, Nose, and Throat Journal, 80,* 553–558.

Azuma, T., & Bayles, L. A. (1997). Memory impairments underlying language difficulties in dementia. *Topics in Language Disorders, 18*(1), 58–71.

Baken, R. J. (1987). *Clinical measurement of speech and voice.* Boston, MA: College Hill Press.

Baken, R. J., & Orlikoff, R. F. (2000). *Clinical measurement of speech and voice* (2nd ed.). San Diego, CA: Singular Thompson Learning.

Balandin, S., & Morgan, J. (2001). Preparing for the future: Aging and alternative and augmentative communication. *Augmentative and Alternative Communication, 17,* 99–108.

Ball, L. J., Marvin, C. A., Beukelman, D. R., Lasker, J., & Rupp, D. (2000). Generic talk use by preschool children. *Augmentative and Alternative Communication, 16,* 145–155.

Bankson, N. W., & Bernthal, J. E. (1990). *Bankson-Bernthal Test of Phonology.* Austin, TX: Pro-Ed.

Bankson, N. W., & Bernthal, J. E. (1998a). Factors related to phonologic disorders. In J. E. Bernthal & N. W. Bankson (Eds.), *Articulation and phonological disorders* (4th ed.). Boston: Allyn and Bacon.

Bankson, N. W., & Bernthal, J. E. (1998b). Phonological assessment procedures. In J. E. Bernthal & N. W. Bankson (Eds.), *Articulation and phonological disorders* (4th ed.). Boston: Allyn and Bacon.

Barron, S. (2001, September 25). A personal story. *The ASHA Leader, 6*(17), 5, 7, 17.

Bass, P. M. (1988, November). *Attention deficit disorder: Management in preschool, adolescent, and adult populations.* Paper presented at the Annual Convention of the American Speech-Language-Hearing Association, Boston.

Bassotti, G., Germani, U., Pagliaricci, S., Plesa, A., Giulietti, O., Mannarino, E., & Morelli, A. (1998). Esophageal manometric abnormalities in Parkinson's disease. *Dysphagia, 13*(1), 28–31.

Baumann-Waengler, J. (2000). *Articulatory and phonological impairments: A clinical focus.* Boston: Allyn and Bacon.

Bayles, K. A., & Kazniak, A. W. (1987). *Communication and cognition in normal aging and dementia.* Boston: Little, Brown.

Bedore, L. M., & Leonard, L. B. (2000). The effects of inflectional variation on fast mapping of verbs in English and Spanish. *Journal of Speech, Language, and Hearing Research, 43,* 21–33.

Bedore, L. M., & Leonard, L. B. (2001). Grammatical morphological deficits in Spanish-speaking children with specific language impairment. *Journal of Speech, Language, and Hearing Research, 44,* 905–924.

Beebe, S. A., Beebe, S. J., & Redmond, M. V. (1996). *Interpersonal communication: Relating to others.* Boston: Allyn and Bacon.

Behrman, A., & Orlikoff, R. F. (1997). Instrumentation in voice assessment and treatment: What's the use? *American Journal of Speech-Language Pathology, 6,* 9–16.

Bello, J. (1994). Prevalence of speech, voice, and language disorders in the United States. *Communication facts, 1994 ed.* Rockville, MD: American Speech-Language-Hearing Association.

Ben-Yishay, Y., & Diller, L. (1993). Cognitive remediation in traumatic brain injury: Update and issues. *Archives of Physical Medicine and Rehabilitation, 74,* 204–213.

Bernhardt, B. H., & Holdgrafer, G. (2001). Beyond the basics I: The need for strategic sampling from in-depth phonological analysis. *Language, Speech, and Hearing Services in Schools, 32,* 18–27.

Bess, F., & Humes, L. (1995). *Audiology: The fundamentals* (2nd ed.). Baltimore, MD: Williams and Wilkins.

Beukelman, D. R., & Mirenda, P. (1992). *Augmentative and alternative communication: Management of severe communication disorders in children and adults.* Baltimore: Brookes.

Bienemann, L. L. (1989). Psychological implications of right hemisphere injury. In P. A. Pimental & N. A. Kingsbury (Eds.), *Neuropsychological aspects of right brain injury* (pp. 65–72). Austin, TX: Pro-Ed.

Blackstone, S. (1989). Augmentative communication services in the schools. *Asha, 31*(1), 61–64.

Bloodstein, O. (1995). *A handbook on stuttering.* San Diego, CA: Singular Publishing Group.

Bloom, L. (1970). *Language development: Form and function of emerging grammars.* Cambridge, MA: MIT Press.

Bloom, R. L., & Ferrand, C. T. (1997). Neuromotor speech disorders. In C. T. Ferrand & R. L. Bloom (Eds.), *Introduction to organic and neurogenic disorders of communication: Current scope of practice.* Boston: Allyn and Bacon.

Boburg, E., & Kully, D. (1995). The comprehensive stuttering program. In C. W. Starkweather & H. F. M. Peters (Eds.), *Stuttering: Proceedings of the first world congress on fluency disorders* (pp. 305–308). Munich: International Fluency Association.

Bonita, R. (1992). Epidemiology of stroke. *Lancet, 339*–320.

Boone, D. R., & McFarlane, S. C. (2000). *The voice and voice therapy* (4th ed.). Boston: Allyn and Bacon.

Boshart, C. A. (1998, April). *Oral-motor techniques.* Short course presented at the New York State Speech-Language-Hearing Association Annual Convention, New York.

Bottenberg, D. E., & Hanks, J. M. (1986). Language and speech of physically handicapped children. In V. A. Reed (Ed.), *An introduction to children with language disorders* (pp. 201–219). New York: Macmillan.

Boudreau, D. M., & Chapman, R. (2000). The relationship between event representation and linguistic skills in narratives of children and adolescents with Down syndrome. *Journal of Speech, Language, and Hearing Research, 43,* 1146–1159.

Boudreau, D. M., & Hedberg, N. L. (1999). A comparison of early literacy skills in children with specific language impairment and their typically developing peers. *American Journal of Speech-Language Pathology, 8,* 249–260.

Bradley, D. P. (1997). Congenital and acquired velopharyngeal inadequacy. In K. R. Bzock (Ed.), *Communicative disorders related to cleft lip and palate* (4th ed., pp. 223–243). Austin, TX: Pro-Ed.

Bradshaw, M. L., Hoffman, P. R., & Norris, J. A. (1998). Efficacy of expansions and cloze procedures in the development of interpretations by preschool children exhibiting delayed language development. *Language, Speech, and Hearing Services in Schools, 29,* 85–95.

Brand Robertson, S., & Ellis Weismer, S. (1999). Effects of treatment on linguistic and social skills in toddlers with delayed language development. *Journal of Speech, Language, and Hearing Research, 42,* 1234–1248.

Brindley, D., Bennefield, R. M., Danyliw, N. G., Hetter, K., & Loftus, M. (1997). 20 hot job tracks: Best careers of '98 and beyond. *U.S. News Online.* Available: http://www.usnews.com/usnews/issue/971027/27core.htm

Brinton, B., Fujiki, M., & Powell, J. M. (1997). The ability of children with language impairment to manipulate topic in a structured task. *Language, Speech, and Hearing Services in Schools, 28,* 3–11.

Bryan, K. L. (1989). *The right hemisphere language battery.* Leicester, UK: Far Communications.

Bulow, M., Olsson, R., & Ekberg, O. (2001). Videomanometric analysis of supraglottic swallow, effortful swallow, and chin tuck in patients with pharyngeal dysfunction. *Dysphagia, 16,* 190–195.

Burns, M. M., Halper, A. S., & Mogil, S. I. (1985). *Clinical management of right hemisphere dysfunction.* Rockville, MD: Aspen.

Bzoch, K. R. (1997). Introduction to the study of communicative disorders in cleft palate and related craniofacial anomalies. In K. R. Bzoch (Ed.), *Communicative disorders related to cleft lip and palate* (4th ed., pp. 3–44). Austin, TX: Pro-Ed.

Calculator, S. (1997). Fostering early language acquisition and AAC use: Exploring reciprocal influences between children and their environments. *Augmentative and Alternative Communication, 13,* 149–157.

Calculator, S. N. (2000). AAC outcomes for children and youths with severe disabilities: When seeing is believing. *Augmentative and Alternative Communication, 16,* 4–12.

Calvert, D. (1982) Articulation and hearing impairments. In Lass, L., Northern, J., Yoder, D., & McReynolds, L. (Eds.), *Speech, language, and hearing* (Vol. 2). Philadelphia: Saunders.

Calvin, W. H., & Ojemann, G. A. (1980). *Inside the brain.* New York: New American Library.

Camicioli, R., Oken, B. S., Sexton, G., Kaye, J. A., & Nutt, J. G. (1998). Verbal fluency task affects gait in Parkinson's disease with motor freezing. *Journal of Geriatric Psychiatry and Neurology, 11,* 181–185.

Carlson, V., Cicchetti, D., Barnett, D., & Braunwald, K. B. (1989). The development of disorganized/disoriented attachment in maltreated infants. *Developmental Psychology, 25,* 525–531.

Carlsson, G. S., Svardsudd, K., & Welin, L. (1987). Long-term effects of head injuries sustained during life in three male populations. *Journal of Neuropsychology, 67,* 197–205.

Caruso, A. J. (2001, July 24). Parkinson's disease and me. *The ASHA Leader, 6*(13), 7.

Casby, M. W. (1997). Symbolic play of children with language impairment: A critical review. *Journal of Speech, Language, and Hearing Research, 40,* 468–479.

Castell, J. A., Johnston, B. T., Colcher, A., et al. (2001). Manometric abnormalities of the oesophagus in patients with Parkinson's disease. *Neurogastroenterology and Motility: The Official Journal of the European Gastrointestinal Motility Society, 13,* 361–364.

Castrogiovanni, A. (1999a). Incidence and prevalence of hearing impairment in the United States. *Communication facts, 1999 ed.* Rockville, MD: American Speech-Language-Hearing Association.

Castrogiovanni, A. (1999b). Incidence and prevalence of speech, voice, and language disorders in the United States. *Communication facts, 1999 ed.* Rockville, MD: American Speech-Language-Hearing Association.

Castrogiovanni, A. (1999c). Special populations: Dysphagia. *Communication facts, 1999 ed.* Rockville, MD: American Speech-Language-Hearing Association.

Catts, H. W. (1996). Defining dyslexia as a developmental language disorder: An expanded view. *Topics in Language Disorders, 16*(2), 14–29.

Catts, H. W., Fey, M. E., Zhang, X., & Tomblin, J. B. (2001). Estimating the risk of future reading difficulties in kindergarten children: A research-based model and its clinical implementation. *Language, Speech, and Hearing Services in Schools, 32*, 38–50.

Causino Lamar, M. A., Obler, L. K., Knoeful, J. E., & Albert, M. L. (1994). Communication patterns in end-stage Alzheimer's disease: Pragmatic analysis. In R. L. Bloom, L. K. Obler, S. DeSanti, & J. L. Ehrlich (Eds.), *Discourse analysis and application: Studies in adult clinical populations* (pp. 217–235). Hillsdale, NJ: Lawrence Erlbaum Associates.

Chapman, S. B. (1997). Cognitive-communication abilities in children with closed head injury. *American Journal of Speech-Language Pathology, 6*(2), 50–58.

Chapman, S. B., Watkins, R., Gustafson, C., Moore, S., Levin, H., & Kufera, J. A. (1997). Narrative discourse in children with closed head injury, children with language impairment, and typically developing children. *American Journal of Speech-Language Pathology, 6*(2), 66–76.

Cherney, L. R. (1994). Dysphagia in adults with neurologic disorders: An overview. In L. R. Cherney (Ed.), *Clinical management of dysphagia in adults and children.* Gaithersburg, MD: Aspen.

Chomsky, N. (1965). *Aspects of the theory of syntax.* Cambridge, MA: The M. I. T. Press.

Chomsky, N., & Halle, M. (1968). *The sound patterns of English.* New York: Harper & Row.

Chute, P. M., & Nevins, M. E. (2000). Cochlear implants in children. In M. Valente, H. Hisford-Dunn, & R. J. Roeser (Eds.), *Audiology treatment.* New York: Thieme.

Clarke, C. E., Gullaksen, E., Macdonald, S., et al. (1998). Referral criteria for speech and language therapy assessment of dysphagia caused by idiopathic Parkinson's disease. *Acta Neurologica Scandinavica, 97*(1), 27–35.

Clarke, L., & Witte, K. (1991). Nature and efficacy of communication management in Alzheimer's disease. In R. Lubinski (Ed.), *Dementia and communication* (pp. 238–256). Philadelphia: B. C. Decker.

Cleave, P. L., & Fey, M. E. (1997). Two approaches to the facilitation of grammar in children with language impairments: Rationale and description. *American Journal of Speech-Language Pathology, 6*(1), 22–32.

Coelho, C. A. (1997). Cognitive-communicative disorders following traumatic brain injury. In C. T. Ferrand & R. L. Bloom (Eds.), *Introduction to organic and neurogenic disorders of communication: Current scope of practice* (pp. 110–137). Boston: Allyn and Bacon.

Coelho, C. A., Liles, B. Z., & Duffy, R. J. (1995). Impairments of discourse abilities and executive functions in traumatically brain injured adults. *Brain Injury, 9*, 471–477.

Cole, K. N., Coggins, T. E., & Vanderstoep, C. (1999). The influence of language/cognitive profile on discourse intervention outcome. *Language, Speech, and Hearing Services in Schools, 30*, 61–67.

Colodny, N. (2001). Effects of age, gender, disease, and multisystem involvement on oxygen saturation levels in dysphagic persons. *Dysphagia, 16*, 48–57.

Colton, R. H., & Casper, J. K. (1990). *Understanding voice problems: A physiological perspective for diagnosis and treatment.* Baltimore, MD: Williams & Wilkins.

Colton, R. H., & Casper, J. K. (1996). *Understanding voice problems: A physiological perspective for diagnosis and treatment* (2nd ed.). Baltimore, MD: Williams & Wilkins.

Connell, P. J., & Stone, C. (1992). Morpheme learning of children with specific language impairments under controlled conditions. *Journal of Speech and Hearing Research, 35*, 844–852.

Conture, E. G. (1990a). Childhood stuttering: What is it and who does it? In J. Cooper (Ed.), *Research needs in stuttering: Roadblocks and future directions* (ASHA Reports 18, pp. 2–14). Rockville, MD: American Speech-Language-Hearing Association.

Conture, E. G. (1990b). *Stuttering* (2nd ed.). Englewood Cliffs, NJ: Prentice-Hall.

Conture, E. G. (1996). Treatment efficacy: Stuttering. *Journal of Speech and Hearing Research, 39*, S18–S26.

Conture, E. G., & Guitar, B. (1993). Evaluating efficacy of treatment of stuttering:

School-age children. *Journal of Fluency Disorders, 18,* 253–287.

Convit, A., deLeon, J. J., Tarshish, C., DeSanti, S., Tsui, W., Rusinek, H., & George, A. (1995). *Hippocampal volume in pre-clinical and early Alzheimer's dementia: Relationship to cognitive function.* Austin, TX: Pro-Ed.

Cooper, E. B. (1984). Personalized fluency control therapy: A status report. In M. Peins (Ed.), *Contemporary approaches to stuttering therapy* (pp. 1–38). Boston: Little, Brown.

Crago, M. B., Eriks-Brophy, A., Pesco, D., & McAlpine, L. (1997). Culturally based miscommunication in classroom interaction. *Language, Speech, and Hearing Services in Schools, 28,* 245–254.

Craig, A., & Calvert, P. (1991). Following up on treated stutterers: Studies of perception of fluency and job status. *Journal of Speech and Hearing Research, 34,* 279–284.

Crary, M. A. (1993). *Developmental motor speech disorders.* San Diego, CA: Singular.

Cress, C. J. (2001). Language and AAC intervention in young children: Never too early or too late to start. *American Speech-Language Hearing Association Special Interest Division 1, Language Learning and Education Newsletter, 8*(1), 3–4.

Crites, L. S., Fischer, K. L., McNeish-Stengel, M., & Siegel, C. J. (1992). Working with families of drug-exposed children: Three model programs. *Infant-Toddler Intervention: The Transdisciplinary Journal, 2*(1), 13–23.

Culatta, R., & Goldberg, S. A. (1995). *Stuttering therapy: An integrated approach to theory and practice.* Boston: Allyn and Bacon.

Cummings, J. L., & Benson, D. F. (1992). *Dementia: A clinical approach* (2nd ed.). Boston: Butterworth-Heinemann.

Curlee, R. (1993). Evaluating treatment efficacy for adults: Assessment of stuttering disability. *Journal of Fluency Disorders, 18,* 319–331.

Dalston, R. M. (1995). The use of nasometry in the assessment and remediation of velopharyngeal inadequacy. In K. R. Bzoch (Ed.), *Communicative disorders related to cleft lip and palate* (4th ed., pp. 331–346). Austin, TX: Pro-Ed.

Dalston, R. M., & Seaver, E. J. (1990). Nasometric and phototransductive measurements of reaction times in normal adult speakers. *Cleft Palate Journal, 27,* 61–67.

Daly, D., Simon, C., & Burnett-Stolnack, M. (1995). Helping adolescents who stutter focus on fluency. *Language, Speech, and Hearing Services in Schools, 26,* 162–168.

Damico, J. S. (1997, April). *Authentic classroom assessment for the speech-language pathologist.* Workshop presented at annual convention of the New York State Speech-Language-Hearing Association, Buffalo.

Damico, J. S., Oller, J. W., & Storey, M. E. (1983). The diagnosis of language disorders in bilingual children: Surface-oriented and pragmatic criteria. *Journal of Speech and Hearing Disorders, 48,* 385–394.

Darley, F., Aronson, A., & Brown, J. (1975). *Motor speech disorders.* Philadelphia: W. B. Saunders.

Dattilo, J., & Camarata, S. (1991). Facilitating conversation through self-initiated augmentative communication treatment. *Journal of Applied Behavior Analysis, 24,* 369–378.

Davis, A. (1993). *A survey of adult aphasia and related language disorders.* Englewood Cliffs, NJ: Prentice-Hall.

Denk, D. M., Swoboda, H., Schima, W., & Eibenberger, K. (1997). Prognostic factors for swallowing rehabilitation following head and neck cancer surgery. *Acta Otolaryngolica, 117*(5), 769–774.

Dennis, M. (1992). Word finding in children and adolescents with a history of brain injury. *Topics in Language Disorders, 13*(1), 66–82.

DePippo, K. L., Holas, M. A., & Reding, M. J. (1992). Validation of the 3-oz water swallow test for aspiration following stroke. *Archives of Neurology, 49*(12), 1259–1261.

DeSanti, S. (1997). Differentiating the dementias. In C. T. Ferrand & R. L. Bloom (Eds.), *Introduction to organic and neurogenic disorders of communication: Current scope of practice* (pp. 84–109). Boston: Allyn and Bacon.

Dollaghan, C. A., Campbell, T. F., Paradise, J. L., Feldman, H. M., Janosky, J. E., Pitcairn, D. N., & Kurs-Lasky, M. (1999). Maternal education and measures of early speech and language. *Journal of Speech, Language, and Hearing Research, 42,* 1432–1443.

Dore, J., Franklin, M., Miller, R., & Ramer, A. (1976). Transitional phenomena in early language acquisition. *Journal of Child Language, 3,* 13–28.

Downey, D. M., & Snyder, L. E. (2000). College students with LLD: The phonological core as risk for failure in foreign language classes. *Topics in Language Disorder, 21*(1), 82–92.

Doyle, M., & Phillips, B. (2001). Trends in augmentative and alternative communication use by individuals with amyotrophic lateral sclerosis. *Augmentative and Alternative Communication, 17,* 167–178.

Drager, K. D. R., & Reichle, J. E. (2001). Effects of age and divided attention on listeners' comprehension of synthesized speech. *Augmentative and Alternative Communication, 17,* 109–119.

Dromi, E., Leonard., L. B., Adam, G., & Zadunaisky-Ehrlich, S. (1999). Verb agreement morphology in Hebrew-speaking children with specific language impairment. *Journal of Speech, Language, and Hearing Research, 42,* 1414–1431.

Duffy, J. R. (1995). *Motor speech disorders; Substrates, differential diagnosis, and management.* St. Louis: Mosby Year Book.

Duvoisin, R. C. (1991). *Parkinson's disease: A guide for patient and family* (3rd ed.). New York: Raven Press.

Edwards, H. T. (1997). *Applied phonetics: The sounds of American English* (2nd ed.). San Diego, CA: Singular.

Edwards, M. L. (1983). Selection criteria for developing therapy goals. *Journal of Childhood Communication Disorders, 7,* 36–45.

Egbert, A. M. (1996). The dwindles: Failure to thrive in older patients. *Nutrition Review, 54* (1, Pt. 2), pp. S25–S30.

Ellis Weismer, S., Murray-Branch, J., & Miller, J. (1994). A prospective longitudinal study of language development in late talkers. *Journal of Speech, Language, and Hearing Research, 37,* 852–867.

Fagundes, D. D., Haynes, W. O., Haak, N.J., & Moran, M. J. (1998). Task variability effects on the language test performance of southern lower socioeconomic class African American and Caucasian 5-year-olds. *Language, Speech, and Hearing Services in Schools, 29,* 148–157.

Fairbanks, G., & Green, E. (1950). A study of minor organic deviations in "functional" disorders of articulation: 2. Dimension and relationships of the lips. *Journal of Speech and Hearing Disorders, 15,* 165–168.

Feinberg, M. (1997). The effects of medications on swallowing. In B. C. Sonies (Ed.), *Dysphagia: A continuum of care.* Gaithersburg, MD: Aspen.

Felsenfeld, S. (1997). Epidemiology and genetics of stuttering. In R. F. Curlee & G. M. Siegel (Eds.), *Nature and treatment of stuttering: New directions* (2nd ed., pp. 3–23). Boston: Allyn and Bacon.

Fleming, J., & Forester, B. (1997). Infusing language enhancement into reading curriculum for disadvantaged adolescents. *Language, Speech, and Hearing Services in Schools, 28,* 177–180.

Fluharty, N. B. (2000). *Fluharty Preschool Speech and Language Screening Test,* 2nd edition. Austin, TX: Pro-Ed.

Fosnot, S. (1993). Research design for examining treatment efficacy in fluency disorders. *Journal of Fluency Disorders, 18,* 221–251.

Fox, L. E., & Rau, M. T. (2001). Augmentative and alternative communication for adults following glossectomy and laryngectomy surgery. *Augmentative and Alternative Communication, 17,* 161–166.

Fox, R. J., Kasner, S. E., Chatterjee, A., et al. (2001). Aphemia: An isolated disorder of articulation. *Clinical Neurology and Neurosurgery, 103,* 123–126.

Frome Loeb, D., & Leonard, L. B. (1991). Subject case marking and verb morphology in normally developing and specifically language-impaired children. *Journal of Speech and Hearing Research, 34,* 340–346.

Fujiki, M., Brinton, B., Isaacson, T., & Summers, C. (2001). Social behaviours of children with language impairment on the playground: A pilot study. *Language, Speech, and Hearing Services in Schools, 32,* 101–113.

Fujiki, M., Brinton, B., Morgan, M., & Hart, C. H. (1999). Withdrawn and sociable behaviour of children with language impairment. *Language, Speech, and Hearing Services in Schools, 30,* 183–195.

Furia, C. L, Kowalski, L. P., Latorre, M. R., et al. (2001) Speech intelligibility after glossectomy and speech rehabilitation. *Archives of Otolaryngology—Head and Neck Surgery, 127,* 877–883.

Galaburda, A. M. (1989). Ordinary and extraordinary brain development: Anatomical variation in developmental dyslexia. *Annals of Dyslexia, 39,* 67–80.

Garcia, J. M., Cannito, M. P., & Dagenais, P. A. (2000). Hand gestures: Perspectives and preliminary implications for adults with acquired dysarthria. *American Journal of Speech-Language Pathology, 9,* 107–115.

Gelb, A. B., Medeiros, L. J., Chen, Y. Y., Weiss, L. M., & Weidner, N. (1997). Hodgkin's disease of the esophagus. *American Journal of Clinical Pathology, 108*(5), 593–598.

Gelfer, M. P. (1996). *Survey of communication disorders: A social and behavioral perspective.* New York: McGraw-Hill, Inc.

German, D. J. (1987). Spontaneous language profiles of children with word-finding problems. *Language, Speech, and Hearing Services in Schools, 18,* 3–230.

German, D. J., & Simon, E. (1991). Analysis of children's word-finding skills in discourse. *Journal of Speech and Hearing Research, 34,* 309–316.

Geschwind, N., & Galaburda, A. (1985). Cerebral lateralization, biological mechanisms, associations and pathology: I. A hypothesis and a program for research. *Archives of Neurology, 42,* 428–459.

Gibbs, D. P., & Cooper, E. B. (1989). Prevalence of communication disorders in students with learning disabilities. *Journal of Learning Disabilities, 22,* 60–63.

Gierut, J. A. (1989). Maximal opposition approach to phonological treatment. *Journal of Speech and Hearing Disorders, 54,* 9–19.

Gierut, J. A. (1998). Treatment efficacy: Functional phonological disorders in children. *Journal of Speech, Language, and Hearing Research, 41*(1), S85–S100.

Giles, D. K., Hube, K., & Wuorio, J. (1995, March). The fifty hottest jobs in America. *Money,* 115–117.

Gillam, R. B. (1999). Computer-assisted language intervention using Fast For Word: Theoretical and empirical considerations for clinical decision making. *Language, Speech, and Hearing Services in Schools, 30,* 363–370.

Girolametto, L., Hoaken, L., Weitzman, E., & van Lieshout, R. (2000). Patterns of adult-child linguistic interaction in integrated day care groups. *Language, Speech, and Hearing Services in Schools, 31,* 155–168.

Girolametto, L., Weitzman, E., van Lieshout, R., & Duff, D. (2000). Directiveness in teachers' language input to toddlers and preschoolers in day care. *Journal of Speech, Language, and Hearing Research, 43,* 1101–1114.

Girolametto, L., Weitzman, E., Wiigs, M., & Steig Pearce, P. (1999). The relationship between maternal language measures and language development in toddlers with expressive vocabulary delays. *American Journal of Speech-Language Pathology, 8,* 364–374.

Glennen, S., & Calculator, S. (1985). Training functional communication board use: A pragmatic approach. *Augmentative and Alternative Communication, 1,* 134–145.

Glennen, S. L., & DeCoste, C. (1997). *Handbook of augmentative communication.* San Diego, CA: Singular.

Golding-Kushner, K. (1995). Treatment of articulation and resonance disorders associated with cleft palate and VPI. In R. J. Shprintzen & J. Bardach (Eds.), *Cleft palate speech management: A multidisciplinary approach.* St. Louis, MO: Mosby.

Goldman, R., & Fristoe, M. (2000). *Goldman-Fristoe test of articulation-Second edition (GFTA-2).* Circle Pines, MN: American Guidance Service.

Goodglass, H., & Kaplan, E. (1983a). *The Boston diagnostic aphasia examination.* Philadelphia: Lea & Febiger.

Goodglass, H., & Kaplan, E. (1983b). *Boston naming test.* Philadelphia: Lea & Febiger.

Gottwald, S., & Starkweather, W. C. (1995). Fluency intervention for preschoolers and their families in the public schools. *Language, Speech, and Hearing Services in Schools, 26,* 117–126.

Grabb, W. C., Rosenstein, S. W., & Bzoch, K. R. (1971). *Cleft lip and palate: Surgical, dental, and speech aspects.* Boston: Little, Brown.

Gravel, J., & Ellis, M. A. (1995). The auditory consequences of otitis media with effusion: The audiogram and beyond. *Seminars in Hearing, 16*(1), 44–58.

Gray, S., Plante, E., Vance, R., & Henrichsen, M. (1999). The diagnostic accuracy of four vocabulary tests administered to preschool-age children. *Language, Speech, and Hearing Services in Schools, 30,* 196–206.

Gray, S. D., Titze, I. R., & Lusk, R. P. (1987). Electron microscopy of hyperphonated canine vocal cords. *Journal of Voice, 1,* 109–115.

Greenamyre, J. T., & Shoulson, I. (1994). Huntington's disease. In D. Calne (Ed.), *Neurodegenerative diseases* (pp. 685–704). Philadelphia: W. B. Saunders.

Greene, J. F. (1996). Psycholinguistic assessment: The clinical base for identity of dyslexia. *Topics in Language Disorders 16*(2), 45–72.

Greenhalgh, K. S., & Strong, C. J. (2001). Literate language features in spoken narratives of children with typical language and children with language impairments. *Language, Speech, and Hearing Services in Schools, 32,* 114–126.

Gregory, R. L. (1981). *Mind in science.* New York: Cambridge University Press.

Grice, H. (1975). Logic and conversation. In D. Davidson & G. Harmon (Eds.), *The logic of grammar.* Encino, CA: Dickenson Press.

Grosz, J. (1989). The development and family services unit. In P. B. Kozlowski, D. A. Snider, P. M. Victze, & H. M. Wisniewski (Eds.), *Proceedings of the Conference on Brain and Behavior in Pediatric HIV Infection* (pp. 115–125). New York: Karger.

Grunwell, P. (1985). *PACS: Phonological assessment of child speech.* San Diego, CA: College-Hill.

Grunwell, P. (1987). *Clinical phonology* (2nd ed.). London: Chapman & Hall.

Grunwell, P. (Ed.). (1993). *Analysing cleft palate speech.* London: Whurr.

Guitar, B. (1998). *Stuttering: An integrated approach to its nature and treatment.* (2nd ed.). Baltimore, MD: Williams and Wilkins.

Gummersall, D. M., & Strong, C. J. (1999). Assessment of complex sentence production in a narrative context. *Language, Speech, and Hearing Services in Schools, 30,* 152–164.

Gumperz, J. J. (1972) Introduction. In J. J. Gumperz & D. Hymes, *Directions in sociolinguistics: The ethnography of communication.* New York: Holt, Rinehart, & Winston.

Gumperz, J. J., & Hymes, D. (1972). *Directions in sociolinguistics: The ethnography of communication.* New York: Holt, Rinehart and Winston.

Gurd, J. M., Bessell, N., Watson, I., & Coleman, J. (1998). Motor speech vs. digit control in Parkinson's disease: A cognitive neuropsychology investigation. *Clinical Linguistics and Phonetics, 12,* 357–378.

Gutierrez-Clellan, V. F. (1999). Language choice in intervention with bilingual children. *American Journal of Speech-Language Pathology, 8,* 291–302.

Gutierrez-Clellan, V. F., Restrepo, M. A., Bedore, L., Peña, E., & Anderson, R. (2000). Language sample analysis in Spanish-speaking children: Methodological considerations. *Language, Speech, and Hearing Services in Schools, 31,* 88–98.

Haberfellner, H., Schwartz, S., & Gisel, E. G. (2001). Feeding skills and growth after one year of intraoral therapy in moderately dysphagic children with cerebral palsy. *Dysphagia, 16,* 83–96.

Hadley, P. A. (1998). Language sampling protocols for eliciting text-level discourse. *Language, Speech, and Hearing Services in Schools, 29,* 132–147.

Hagan, C., & Malkamus, D. (1979, November). *Interaction strategies for language disorders secondary to head trauma.* Paper presented at the annual convention of the American Speech-Language-Hearing Association, Atlanta.

Hall, E. T. (1966). *The hidden dimension.* New York: Doubleday.

Hall, P. K., Jordan, L. S., & Robin, D. A. (1993). *Developmental apraxia of speech: Theory and clinical practice.* Austin, TX: Pro-Ed.

Hanson, M. L. (1994). Oral myofunctional disorders and articulatory patterns. In J. Bernthal & N. Bankson (Eds.), *Child phonology: Characteristics, assessment, and intervention with special populations* (pp. 29–53). New York: Thieme Medical Publishers.

Hardy, E., & Robinson, N. M. (1993). *Swallowing disorders treatment manual.* Bisbee, AZ: Imaginart.

Hardy, J. C. (1983). *Cerebral palsy.* Englewood Cliffs, NJ: Prentice-Hall.

Haynes, S. (1985). Developmental apraxia of speech: Symptoms and treatment. In D. F. Johns (Ed.), *Clinical management of neurogenic communicative disorders* (2nd ed., pp. 259–266). Boston: Little, Brown.

Haynes, W. O., & Pindzola, R. H. (1998). *Diagnosis and evaluation in speech pathology* (5th ed.). Boston: Allyn and Bacon.

Hegde, M. N. (1993). *Treatment procedures in communicative disorders* (2nd ed.). Austin, TX: Pro-Ed.

Heiss, W. D., Kessler, J., Thiel, A., Ghaemi, M., & Karbe, H. (1999). Differential capacity of left and right hemisphere areas for compensation of partstroke aphasia. *Annals of Neurology, 45*, 430–438.

Helm-Estabrooks, N., & Albert, M. C. (1991). *Manual of aphasia therapy.* Austin, TX: Pro-Ed.

Helm-Estabrooks, N., Fitzpatrick, P. M., & Barresi, B. (1982). Visual action therapy for global aphasia. *Journal of Speech and Hearing Disorders, 47*, 385–389.

Hewlett, N. (1990). The processes of speech production and speech development. In P. Grunwell (Ed.), *Developmental speech disorders: Clinical issues and practical implications.* Edinburgh: Churchill Livingstone.

Hodson, B. (1985). *Computerized analysis of phonological processes: Version 1.0* (Apple II Series Computer Program). Danville, IL: Interstate.

Hodson, B. (1986). *The assessment of phonological processes—Revised.* Danville, IL: Interstate.

Hodson, B., & Paden, E. (1991). *Targeting intelligible speech: A phonological approach to remediation* (2nd ed.). Austin, TX: Pro-Ed.

Holland, A., & Fridriksson, J. (2001). Aphasia management during the early phases of recovery following stroke. *American Journal of Speech-Language Pathology, 10*(1), 19–28.

Holland, A. L. (1980). *Communication abilities in daily living: A test of functional communication for adults.* Baltimore: University Park Press.

Hollien, H. (1987). Old voices: What do we really know about them? *Journal of Voice, 1*, 2–17.

Howell, J., & Dean, E. (1994). *Treating phonological disorders in children: Metaphon—theory to practice* (2nd ed.). London: Whurr.

Huang, R., Hopkins, J., & Nippold, M. A. (1997). Satisfaction with standardized language testing: A survey of speech-language pathologists. *Language, Speech, and Hearing Services in Schools, 28*, 12–29.

Hunt-Berg, M. (2001). Gestures in development: Implications for early intervention in AAC. *American Speech-Language Hearing Association Special Interest Division 1, Language Learning and Education Newsletter, 8*(1), 5–8.

Hunter, L., Pring, T., & Martin, S. (1991). The use of strategies to increase speech intelligibility in cerebral palsy: An experimental evaluation. *British Journal of Disorders of Communication, 26*, 163–174.

Hurst, M., & Cooper, G. (1983). Employer attitudes towards stuttering. *Journal of Fluency Disorders, 8*, 1–12

Hustad, K. C., & Beukelman, D. R. (2001). Effects of linguistic cues and stimulus cohesion on intelligibility of severely dysarthric speech. *Journal of Speech, Language, and Hearing Research, 44*, 497–510.

Hutchinson, J., & Marquardt, T. P. (1997). Functional treatment approaches to memory impairment following brain injury. *Topics in Language Disorders, 18*(1), 45–57.

Hynd, G. W., Marshall, R., & Gonzalez, J. (1991). Learning disabilities and presumed central nervous system dysfunction. *Learning Disabilities Quarterly, 14*, 283–296.

Iacono, T., Carter, M., & Hook, J. (1998). Identification of intentional communication in students with severe and multiple disabilities. *Augmentative and Alternative Communication, 14*, 102–114.

Iglesias, A., & Goldstein, B. (1998). Language and dialectical variations. In J. E. Bernthal & N. W. Bankson (Eds.), *Articulation and phonological disorders* (4th ed.). Boston: Allyn and Bacon.

Ingham, R. J. (1990). Research on stuttering treatment for adults and adolescents who stutter: A perspective on how to overcome the malaise. In J. Cooper (Ed.), *Research needs in stuttering: Roadblocks and future directions* (ASHA Reports 18, pp. 91–97). Rockville, MD: American Speech-Language-Hearing Association.

Ingham, R. J., & Cordes, A. K. (1997). Self-measurement and evaluating stuttering treatment efficacy. In R. F. Curlee & G. M. Siegel (Eds.), *Nature and treatment of stuttering: New directions* (2nd ed., pp. 413–437). Boston: Allyn and Bacon.

Iskowitz, M. (1999). Coding conundrum. *Advance for Speech-Language Pathologists and Audiologists, 9* (46), 11, 13, 17.

Jacobs, B. J., & Thompson, C. K. (2000). Cross-modality generalization effects of training noncanonical sentence comprehension and production in agrammatic aphasia. *Journal* of Speech, Language, and Hearing Research, 43, 5–20.

Jelm, J. M. (1994). Treatment of feeding and swallowing disorders in children: An overview. In L. R. Cherney (Ed.), *Clinical management of dysphagia in adults and children*. Gaithersburg, MD: Aspen.

Johns Hopkins. (2000). Help when it's hard to swallow. *Johns Hopkins Medical Letter, Health after 50, 11*(12), 6–7.

Johnston, B. T., Colcher, A., Li, Q., et al. (2001). Repetitive proximal esophageal contractions: A new manometric finding and a possible link between Parkinson's disease and achalasia. *Dysphagia, 16*, 186–189.

Johnston, J. R. (2001). An alternative MLU calculation: Magnitude and variability of effects. *Journal of Speech, Language, and Hearing Research, 44*, 156–164.

Kaderavek, J. N., & Sulzby, E. (1998). Parent-child joint book reading: An observational protocol for young children. *American Journal of Speech-Language Pathology, 7*(1), 33–47.

Kagan, A., Black, S. E., Duchan, J. F., Simmons-Mackie, N., & Square, N. (2001). Training volunteers as conversation partners using "Supporting conversation for adults with aphasia" (SCA): A controlled trial. *Journal of Speech, Language, and Hearing Research, 44*, 624–638.

Kahane, J. (1982). Anatomy and physiology of the organs of the peripheral speech mechanism. In N. Lass, L. McReynolds, J. Northern, & D. Yoder (Eds.), *Speech, language and hearing* (Vol. I, pp. 109–155). Philadelphia, PA: Saunders.

Kamhi, A. G. (1998). Trying to make sense of developmental language disabilities. *Language, Speech, and Hearing Services in Schools, 29*, 35–44.

Kamhi, A. G., Gentry, B., Mauer, D., & Gholson, B. (1990). Analogical learning and transfer in language-impaired children. *Journal of Speech and Hearing Disorders, 55*, 140–148.

Karagiannis, A., Stainback, W., & Stainback, S. (1996). Historical overview of inclusion. In S. Stainback & W. Stainback (Eds.), *Inclusion: A guide for educators*. Baltimore: Paul H. Brooks.

Katz, J., Stecker, N., & Henderson, D. (1994). *Central auditory processing: A transdisciplinary view*. St. Louis, MO: Mosby Year Book.

Katz, R. C., & Wertz, R. T. (1997). The efficacy of computer-provided reading treatment for chronic aphasic adults. *Journal of Speech, Language, and Hearing Research, 40*, 493–507.

Katz, W. F., Bharadwaj, S. V., & Carstens, B. (1999). Electromagnetic articulography treatment for an adult with Broca's aphasia and apraxia of speech. *Journal of Speech, Language, and Hearing Research, 42*, 1355–1366.

Kay-Raining Bird, E., & Chapman, R. S. (1994). Sequential recall in individuals with Down syndrome. *Journal of Speech and Learning Research, 37*, 1369–1380.

Kearns, K. P., & Simmons, N. N. (1988). Motor speech disorders: The dysarthrias and apraxia of speech. In N. J. Lass, L. V. McReynolds, & D. E. Yoder (Eds.), *Handbook of speech-language pathology and audiology* (pp. 592–621). Burlington, Ontario, Canada: B. D. Decker.

Keith, R. W. (1995). Tests of central auditory processing. In R. Roeser & M. Downs (Eds.), *Auditory disorders in children* (3rd ed., pp. 101–116). New York: Thieme Medical Publishers.

Kemker, F. J. (1995). Audiologic management of patients with cleft palate and related disorders. In K. R. Bzoch (Ed.), *Communicative disorders related to cleft lip and palate* (4th ed., pp. 245–260). Austin, TX: Pro-Ed.

Kemper, T. (1984). Neuroanatomical and neuropathological changes in normal aging and in dementia. In M. L. Albert (Ed.), *Clinical neurology of aging*. New York: Oxford University Press.

Kent, R. D. (1997). *The speech sciences*. San Diego, CA: Singular Publishing Group.

Kent, R. D., Duffy, J. R., Slama, A., Kent, J. F., & Clift, A. (2001). Clinicoanatomic studies in dysarthria: Review, critique, and directions for research. *Journal of Speech, Language, and Hearing Research, 44*, 535–551.

Kent, R. D., Kent, J. F., Duffy, J. R., Thomas, J. E., Weismer, G., & Stuntebeck, S. (2000). Ataxic dysarthria. *Journal of Speech, Language, and Hearing Research, 43*, 1275–1289.

Kent, R. D., & Rosenbek, J. C. (1983). Acoustic patterns of apraxia of speech. *Journal of Speech and Hearing Research, 26*, 231–249.

Kertesz, A., & McCabe, P. (1982). *Western Aphasia Battery*. New York: Grune & Stratton.

Kertesz, A., & McCabe, P. (1997). Recovery patterns and prognosis in aphasia. *Brain, 100,* 100–118.

Khan, L. M., & Lewis, N. P. (2002). *Khan-Lewis Phonological Analysis-2* (KLPA-2). Circle Pines, MN: American Guidance Service.

Kidd, K. (1984). Stuttering as a genetic disorder. In R. F. Curlee & W. H. Perkins (Eds.), *Nature and treatment of stuttering: New directions* (pp. 149–169). Boston: Allyn and Bacon.

Kiernan, B., Snow, D., Swisher, L., & Vance, R. (1997). Another look at nonverbal rule induction in children with specific language impairment: Testing a flexible reconceptualization hypothesis. *Journal of Speech and Hearing Research, 40,* 75–82.

Kimbarow, M. L. (1997). Ahead of the curve: Improving service with speech-language pathology assistants. *Asha, 39*(4), 41–44.

Kirshner, H. S. (1995). *Handbook of neurological speech and language disorders.* New York: Marcel Dekker.

Klasner, E. R., & Yorkston, K. M. (2001). Linguistic and cognitive supplementation strategies as augmentative and alternative communication techniques in Huntington's disease: Case study. *Augmentative and Alternative Communication, 17,* 154–160.

Klee, T., Schaffer, M., May, S., Membrino, I., & Mougey, K. (1989). A comparison of the age-MLU relationship in normal and specifically language impaired preschool children. *Journal of Speech and Hearing Disorders, 54,* 226–233.

Klein, H. B. (1997). *Clinical implications of nonlinear phonological theory: An Introduction.* Paper presented at the New York State Speech-Language-Hearing Association Annual Convention, Buffalo.

Klein, K. (1995). *Aphasia community group manual.* New York: National Aphasia Association.

Koo, E., & Price, D. (1993). The neurobiology of dementia. In P. Whitehouse (Ed.), *Dementia* (pp. 55–91). Philadelphia: F. A. Davis.

Kratcoski, A. M. (1998). Guidelines for using portfolios in assessment and evaluation. *Language, Speech, and Hearing Services in Schools, 29,* 3–10.

Kraus, J. F. (1993). Epidemiologic features of head injury. In P. R. Cooper (Ed.), *Head injury* (3rd ed.). Baltimore: Williams and Wilkins.

Kummer, A. W. (2001). *Cleft palate and craniofacial anomalies: The effects on speech and resonance.* San Diego, CA: Singular Thompson Learning.

Laguaite, J. K. (1972). Adult voice screening. *Journal of Speech and Hearing Disorders, 37,* 147–151.

Lahey, M., & Edwards, J. (1995). Specific language impairment: Preliminary investigation of factors assessed with family history and with patterns of language performance. *Journal of Speech and Hearing Research, 38,* 643–657.

Langmore, S. E., Terpenning, M. S., Schork, A., Chen, Y., Murray, J. T., Lopatin, D., & Loesche, W. J. (1998). Predictors of aspiration pneumonia: How important is dysphagia? *Dysphagia, 13*(2), 69–81.

Lanphear, B., Byrd, R., Auinger, P., & Hall, C. (1997, March). Increasing prevalence of recurrent otitis media among children in the United States. *Pediatrics* [On-line], 99(3). Available: www.pediatrics.org/cgi/content/full/99/3/e1

Lapko, L., & Bankson, N. (1975). Relationship between auditory discrimination, articulation stimulability and consistency of misarticulation. *Perceptual and Motor Skills, 40,* 171–177.

Larson, V. L., & McKinley, N. L. (1998). Characteristics of adolescents' conversation: A longitudinal study. *Clinical Linguistics and Phonetics, 12,* 183–203.

Lasker, J. P., & Bedrosian, J. L. (2000). Acceptance of AAC by adults with acquired disorders. In D. Beukelman, K. Yorkston, & J. Reichle (Eds.), *Augmentative communication for adults with neurogenic and neuromuscular disabilities* (pp. 107–136). Baltimore, MD: Brookes.

Lasker, J. P., & Bedrosian, J. L. (2001). Promoting acceptance of augmentative and alternative communication by adults with acquired communication disorders. *Augmentative and Alternative Communication, 17,* 141–153.

Lau, C., & Kusnierczyk, I. (2001). Quantitative evaluation of infant's nonnutritive and nutritive sucking. *Dysphagia, 16,* 58–67.

Le Blanc, E. M., & Cisneros, G. J. (1995). The dynamics of speech and orthodontic management in cleft lip and palate. In R. J. Shprintzen & J. Bardach (Eds.), *Cleft palate speech management: A multidisciplinary approach.* St. Louis, MO: Mosby.

Leblanc, R. (1996). Familial cerebral aneurysms. *Stroke, 27,* 1050–1054.

Leder, S. B., Sasaki, C. T., & Burrell, M. I. (1998). Fiberoptic endoscopic evaluation of dysphagia to identify silent aspiration. *Dysphagia, 13*(1), 19–21.

Leonard, R. J. (1994). Characteristics of speech in speakers with oral/oral pharyngeal ablation. In J. Bernthal & N. Bankson (Eds.), *Child phonology: Characteristics, assessment, and intervention with special populations* (pp. 54–78). New York: Thieme Medical Publishers.

Lesar, S. (1992). Prenatal cocaine exposure: The challenge to education. *Infant-Toddler Intervention: The Transdisciplinary Journal, 2*(1), 37–52.

Levine, M. (1987). *Developmental variation and learning disorders.* Cambridge, MA: Educators Publishing Service.

Light, J. (1989). Toward a definition of communication competence for individuals using augmentative and alternative communication systems. *Augmentative and Alternative Communication, 5,* 137–144.

Light, J. (1997). "Let's go star fishing": Reflections on the contexts of language learning for children who use aided AAC. *Augmentative and Alternative Communication, 13,* 158–171.

Light, J., Dattilo, J., English, J., Gutierrez, L., & Hartz, J. (1992). Instructing facilitators to support the communication of people who use augmentative communication systems. *Journal of Speech and Hearing Research, 35,* 865–875.

Light, J., & Lindsay, P. (1991). Cognitive science and augmentative and alternative communication. *Augmentative and Alternative Communication, 7,* 186–203.

Lim, S. H., Lieu, P. K., Phua, S. Y., et al. (2001). Accuracy of bedside clinical methods compared with fiberoptic endoscopic examination of swallowing (FEES) in determining the risk of aspiration in acute stroke patients. *Dysphagia, 16,* 1–6.

Lincoln, M., & Onslow, M. (1997). Long-term outcome of early intervention for stuttering. *American Journal of Speech-Language Pathology, 6,* 51–58.

Lippke, B. A., Dickey, S., Selmar, J., & Soder, A. L. (1997). *Photo articulation test–3.* Austin, TX: Pro-Ed.

Logemann, J. A. (1994). Evaluation and treatment of swallowing disorders. *American Journal of Speech-Language Pathology, 3*(3), 41–44.

Logemann, J. A. (1996). Screening, diagnosis, and management of neurogenic dysphasia. *Seminars in Neurology, 16*(4), 319–327.

Logemann, J. A. (1997). Structural and functional aspects of normal and disordered swallowing. In C. T. Ferrand & R. L. Bloom (Eds.), *Introduction to organic and neurogenic disorders of communication: Current scope of practice.* Boston: Allyn and Bacon.

Logemann, J. A. (1998). *Evaluation and treatment of swallowing disorders* (2nd ed.). Austin, TX: Pro-Ed.

Lombardino, L. J., Bedford, T., Fortier, C., Carter, J., & Brandt, J. (1997). Invented spelling: Developmental patterns in kindergarten children and guidelines for early literacy intervention. *Language, Speech, and Hearing Services in Schools, 28,* 333–343.

Lord, C. (1988). Enhancing communication in adolescents with autism. *Topics in Language Disorders, 9*(1), 72–81.

Lotze, M. (1995). Nursing assessment and management. In S. R. Rosenthal, J. J. Sheppard, & M. Lotze (Eds.), *Dysphagia and the child with developmental disabilities: Medical, clinical, and family interventions.* San Diego, CA: Singular Publishing Group.

Love, R. J. (1992). *Childhood motor speech disability.* New York: Macmillan.

Lubinski, R., & Masters, M. G. (2001). Special populations, special settings: New and expanding frontiers. In R. Lubinski & C. Frattali (Eds.), *Professional issues in speech-language pathology and audiology* (2nd ed.). San Diego: Singular.

Lubker, B. B. (1997). Language learning disorders in children with chronic health conditions: Epidemiologic perspectives. *American Speech-Language-Hearing Association, Special Interest Divisions, Language Learning and Education, 4*(1), 2–5.

Lund, N., & Duchan, J. (1993). *Assessing children's language in naturalistic contexts* (3rd ed.). Englewood Cliffs, NJ: Prentice-Hall.

MacDonald, C. C. (1992). Perinatal cocaine exposure: Predictor of an endangered generation. *Infant-Toddler Intervention: The Transdisciplinary Journal, 2*(1), 1–12.

Mackay, L. E., Bernstein, B. A., Chapman, P. E., Morgan, A. S., & Milazzo, L. S.

(1992). Early intervention in severe head injury: Long-term benefits of a formalized program. *Archives of Physical Medicine and Rehabilitation, 73,* 635–641.

MacLachlan, B. G., & Chapman, R. S. (1988). Communication breakdowns in normal and language-learning-disabled children's conversation and narration. *Journal of Speech and Hearing Disorders, 53,* 2–9.

Mallette, B. (1994). *The effects of fetal alcohol syndrome on children.* Workshop presented at Buffalo Hearing and Speech Center, Buffalo, NY.

Mann, G., & Hankey, G. J. (2001). Initial clinical and demographic predictors of swallowing impairment following acute stroke. *Dysphagia, 16,* 205–216.

Manning Kratcoski, A. (1998). Guidelines for using portfolios in assessment and evaluation. *Language, Speech, and Hearing Services in Schools, 29,* 3–10.

Markel, N., Meisels, M., & Houck, J. (1964). Judging personality from voice quality. *Journal of Abnormal Social Psychology, 69,* 458–463.

Marshall, R. C. (1997). Aphasia treatment in the early postonset period: Managing our resources effectively. *American Journal of Speech-Language Pathology, 6*(1), 5–11.

Martin, B. J. (1994). Treatment of dysphagia in adults. In L. R. Cherney (Ed.), *Clinical management of dysphagia in adults and children.* Gaithersburg, MD: Aspen.

Martin, B. J., & Corlew, M. M. (1990). The incidence of communication disorders in dysphagic patients. *Journal of Speech and Hearing Disorders, 55*(1), 28–32.

Martin, F. N. (1994). *Introduction to audiology* (5th ed.). Englewood Cliffs, NJ: Prentice-Hall.

Martin, R. E., Neary, M. A., Diamant, N. E. (1997). Dysphagia following anterior cervical spine surgery. *Dysphagia, 12*(1), 2–10.

Marvin, C. A., & Wright, D. (1997). Literacy socialization in the homes of preschool children. *Language, Speech, and Hearing Services in Schools, 28,* 154–163.

Masterson, J., & Pagan, F. (1993). *Interactive system for phonological analysis: Version 1.0* (Macintosh Computer Program). San Antonio, TX: The Psychological Corporation.

Max, L., & Caruso, A. J. (1997). Contemporary techniques for establishing fluency in the treatment of adults who stutter. *Contemporary Issues in Communication Science and Disorders, 24,* 45–52.

McCarthy, J., & Light, J. (2001). Instructional effectiveness of an integrated theatre arts program for children using augmentative and alternative communication and their nondisabled peers: Preliminary study. *Augmentative and Alternative Communication, 17,* 88–98.

McCune, L., & Vihman, M. M. (2001). Early phonetic and lexical development: A productivity approach. *Journal of Speech, Language, and Hearing Research, 44,* 670–684.

McDearmon, J. R. (1968). Primary stuttering at the onset of stuttering: A reexamination of data. *Journal of Speech and Hearing Research, 11,* 631–637.

McDonald, E. T. (1964). *Articulation testing and treatment: A sensory-motor approach.* Pittsburgh: Stanwix House.

McDowell, F. H., & Cederbaum, J. M. (1988). The extrapyramidal system and disorders of movement. In R. J. Joynt (Ed.), *Clinical neurology* (vol. 3). Philadelphia: J. B. Lippincott.

McGregor, K. K. (2000). The development and enhancement of narrative skills in a preschool classroom: Toward a solution to clinician-client mismatch. *American Journal of Speech-Language Pathology, 9,* 55–71.

McKinlay, W. W., Brooks, D. N., Bond, M. R., Martinage, D. P., & Marshall, M. M. (1981). The short-term outcome of severe blunt head injury as reported by the relatives of the injured person. *Journal of Neurology, Neurosurgery, and Psychiatry, 44,* 527–533.

McNaughton, D., Light, J., & Groszyk, L. (2001). "Don't give up": Employment experiences of individuals with amyotrophic lateral sclerosis who use augmentative and alternative communication. *Augmentative and Alternative Communication, 17,* 179–195.

McWilliams, B. J., Morris, H. L., & Shelton, R. L. (1990). *Cleft palate speech* (2nd ed.). Philadelphia, PA: B.C. Decker.

Mentis, M., Briggs-Whittaker, J., & Gramigna, G. D. (1995). Discourse topic management in senile dementia of the Alzheimer's type. *Journal of Speech and Hearing Research, 38,* 1054–1066.

Mentis, M., & Lundgren, K. (1995). Effects of prenatal exposure to cocaine and associated risk factors on language development. *Journal of Speech and Hearing Research, 38,* 1303–1318.

Merrell, A. W., & Plante, E. (1997). Norm-referenced test interpretation in the diagnostic process. *Language, Speech, and Hearing Services in Schools, 28,* 50–58.

Meyers, P. S. (1999). *Right hemisphere damage.* San Diego: Singular.

Miccio, A. W., & Elbert, M. (1996). Enhancing stimulability: A treatment program. *Journal of Communication Disorders, 29,* 335–351.

Millar, J., & Whitaker, H. (1983). The right hemisphere's contribution to language: A review of the evidence from brain-injured subjects. In S. Segalowitz (Ed.), *Language functions and brain organization.* New York: Academic Press.

Miller, C. A., Kail, R., Leonard, L. B., & Tomblin, J. B. (2001). Speed of processing in children with specific language impairment. *Journal of Speech, Language, and Hearing Research, 44,* 416–433.

Miller, J. F. (1981). *Assessing language production in children: Experimental procedures.* Baltimore: University Park Press.

Miller, J. F., Chapman, R., & MacKenzie, H. (1981). Individual differences in the language acquisition of mentally retarded children. *Proceedings from the Second Wisconsin Symposium on Research in Child Language.* Madison: University of Wisconsin.

Miller, L. (1993, January). Testing and the creation of disorder. *American Journal of Speech Language Pathology, 2,* 13–16.

Miller, T. J. (2001). Professional liability in audiology and speech-language pathology: Ethical and legal considerations. In R. Lubinski & C. Frattali, (Eds.), *Professional issues in speech-language pathology and audiology* (2nd ed.). San Diego: Singular.

Miniutti, A. (1991). Language deficiencies in inner-city children with learning and behavioral problems. *Language, Speech, and Hearing Services in Schools, 22,* 31–38.

Molfese, V., Molfese, D., & Parsons, C. (1983). Hemisphere processing of phonological information. In S. Segalowitz (Ed.), *Language functions and brain organization.* New York: Academic Press.

Morgan, D. L., & Guilford, A. M. (1984). *Adolescent Language Screening Test.* Austin, TX: Pro-Ed.

Murray, L. L. (2000). Spoken language production in Huntington's and Parkinson's diseases. *Journal of Speech, Language, and Hearing Research, 43,* 1350–1366.

Murray, L. L., Holland, A. L., & Beson, P. M. (1997). Auditory processing in individuals with mild aphasia: A study of resource allocation. *Journal of Speech, Language, and Hearing Research, 40,* 792–808.

Murray, L. L., Holland, A. L., & Beson, P. M. (1998). Spoken language of individuals with mild fluent aphasia under focused and divided-attention conditions. *Journal of Speech, Language, and Hearing Research, 41,* 213–225.

National Joint Committee on Learning Disabilities. (1991). Learning disabilities: Issues on definition (A position paper). *Asha, 33* (Suppl. 5), 18–20.

Neilson, M., & Andrews, G. (1993). Intensive fluency training of chronic stutterers. In R. F. Curlee (Ed.), *Stuttering and related disorders of fluency* (pp. 139–165). New York: Thieme Medical Publishers.

Nelson, N. W. (1993). *Childhood language disorders in context: Infancy through adolescence.* Columbus, OH: Merrill.

Nelson, N. W. (1998). *Childhood language disorders in context: Infancy through adolescence* (2nd ed.). Boston: Allyn and Bacon.

Netsell, R. (1986). *A neurobiological view of speech production and the dysarthrias.* San Diego, CA: College Hill Press.

Nilsson, H., Ekberg, O., Olsson, R., & Hindfelt, B. (1998). Dysphagia in stroke: A prospective study of quantitative aspects of swallowing in dysphagic patients. *Dysphagia, 13*(1), 32–38.

Nippold, M. (2000). Language development during the adolescent years: Aspects of pragmatics, syntax, and semantics. *Topics in Language Disorders, 20*(2), 15–28.

Nippold, M. A., Moran, C., & Schwarz, I. E. (2001). Idiom understanding in preadolescents: Synergy in action. *American Journal of Speech-Language Pathology, 10,* 169–179.

Northern, J., & Downs, M. (1991). *Hearing in children* (4th ed.). Baltimore, MD: Williams and Wilkins.

Norton, S., & Stover, L. (1994). Otoacoustic emissions: An emerging clinical tool. In J. Katz (Ed.), *Handbook of clinical audiology* (4th ed., pp. 448–462). Baltimore, MD: Williams and Wilkins.

Odderson, M. D., Keaton, J. C., & McKenna, B. S. (1995). Swallow management in patients on an acute stroke pathway: Quality is cost effective. *Archives of Physical Medicine and Rehabilitation, 76*(12), 1130–1133.

Oetting, J. B., & Morohov, J. E. (1997). Past-tense marking by children with and without specific language impairment. *Journal of Speech, Language, and Hearing Research, 40,* 62–74.

Olivier, C., Hecker, L., Klucken, J., & Westby, C. (2000). Language: The embedded curriculum in postsecondary education. *Topics in Language Disorders, 21*(1) 15–29.

Oller, J. W., Kim, K., & Choe, Y. (2001). Can instructions to nonverbal tests be given in pantomime? Additional applications of a general theory of signs. *Semiotica, 133,* 15–44.

Olmsted, D. (1971). *Out of the mouth of babes.* The Hague: Mouton.

Olswang, L., Bain, B., & Johnson, G. (1990). Using dynamic assessment with children with language disorders. In S. Warren & J. Reichle (Eds.), *Causes and effects of communication and language intervention.* Baltimore, MD: Paul H. Brookes.

Olswang, L. B., Rodriguez, B., & Timler, G. (1998). Recommending intervention for toddlers with specific language learning difficulties: We may not have all the answers, but we know a lot. *American Journal of Speech-Language Pathology, 7*(1), 23–32.

Oram, J., Fine, J., Okamoto, C., & Tannock, R. (1999). Assessing the language of children with attention deficit hyperactivity disorder. *American Journal of Speech-Language Pathology, 8,* 72–80.

Orange, J. B., Lubinsky, R. B., & Higginbotham, D. J. (1996). Conversational repair by individuals with dementia of the Alzheimer's type. *Journal of Speech, Language, and Hearing Research, 39,* 881–895.

Orsolini, M., Sechi, E., et al. (2001). Nature of phonological delay in children with specific language impairment. *International Journal of Language and Communication Disorders, 36,* 63–90.

Owen, A. J., Dromi, E., & Leonard, L. B. (2001). The phonology-morphology interface in the speech of Hebrew-speaking children with specific language impairment. *Journal of Communication Disorders, 34,* 323–337.

Owen, R. M. (2001). A brief SETI chronology. [On-line]. http://www.setileague.org/general/history.htm

Owens, R. E., Jr. (1999). *Language disorders: A functional approach to assessment and intervention* (3rd ed.). Boston: Allyn and Bacon.

Owens, R. E., Jr. (2001). *Language development: An introduction* (5th ed.). Boston: Allyn and Bacon.

Patterson, J. L. (2000). Observed and reported expressive vocabulary and word combinations in bilingual toddlers. *Journal of Speech, Language, and Hearing Research, 43,* 121–128.

Paul, R. (1991). Outcomes of early expressive language delay. *Journal of Childhood Communication Disorders, 15,* 7–14.

Paul, R. (1995). *Language disorders from infancy through adolescence: Assessment and intervention.* St. Louis: Mosby.

Paul-Brown, D., & Goldberg, L. R. (2001). Current policies and new directions for speech-language pathology assistants. *Language, Speech, and Hearing Services in Schools, 32,* 4–17.

Peach, R. K. (2001). Clinical intervention for global aphasia. In R. Chapey (Ed.), *Language intervention strategies in aphasia and related neurogenic communication disorders* (4th ed.). Baltimore, MD: Lippincott, Williams, & Wilkins.

Peña, E., Iglesias, A., Lidz, C. S. (2001). Reducing test bias through dynamic assessment of children's word learning ability. *American Journal of Speech-Language Pathology, 10,* 138–154.

Peña, E. D., & Quinn, R. (1997). Task familiarity: Effects on the test performance of Puerto Rican and African American children. *Language, Speech and Hearing Services in Schools, 28,* 323–332.

Perez, I., Smithard, D. G., Davies, H., & Kaira, L. (1998). Pharmacological treatment of dysphagia in stroke. *Dysphagia, 13*(1), 12–16.

Perkins, W. (1992). *Stuttering prevented.* San Diego, CA: Singular Publishing Group.

Peterson-Falzone, S. J., Hardin-Jones, M. A., & Karnell, M. P. (2001). *Cleft palate speech* (3rd ed.). St. Louis, MO: Mosby.

Peterson-Falzone, S. J., & Imagire, R. (1997). Basic genetic concepts in cranial-facial anomalies. In K. R. Bzoch (Ed.). *Communicative disorders related to cleft lip and palate* (4th ed.). Austin, TX: Pro-Ed.

Pimental, P. A., & Kingsbury, N. A. (1989). *Mini inventory of right brain injury*. Austin, TX: Pro-Ed.

Porch, B. E. (1981). *Porch index of communicative ability* (3rd ed.). Palo Alto, CA: Consulting Psychologists Press.

Postma, A., & Kolk, H. H. J. (1993). The covert repair hypothesis: Prearticulatory repair processes in normal and stuttered disfluencies. *Journal of Speech and Hearing Research, 36,* 472–487.

Powell, T. W., Elbert, M., & Dinnsen, D. A. (1991). Stimulability as a factor in the phonological generalization of misarticulating preschool children. *Journal of Speech and Hearing Research, 34,* 1311–1328.

Powell, T. W., & Miccio, A. W. (1996). Stimulability: A useful clinical tool. *Journal of Communication Disorders, 29,* 237–253.

Poyatos, F. (1983). *New perspectives in nonverbal communication: Studies in cultural anthropology, social psychology, linguistics, literature and semiotics.* Oxford, England: Pergamon Press.

Prather, E., Hedrick, D., & Kern, C. (1975). Articulation development in children aged two to four years. *Journal of Speech and Hearing Disorders, 40,* 179–191.

Prelock, P. A. (2000). Prologue: Multiple perspectives for determining the roles of speech-language pathologists in inclusionary classrooms. *Language, Speech, and Hearing Services in Schools, 31,* 213–218.

Prins, D., Hubbard, C. P., & Krause, M. (1991). Syllabic stress and the occurrence of stuttering. *Journal of Speech and Hearing Research, 34,* 1011–1016.

Prontnicki, J. (1995). Presentation: Symptomatology and etiology of dysphasia. In S. R. Rosenthal, J. J. Sheppard, & M. Lotze (Eds.), *Dysphagia and the child with developmental disabilities: Medical, clinical, and family interventions.* San Diego, CA: Singular Publishing Group.

Raffaelli, M., & Duckett, E. (1989). "We were just talking . . . ": Conversation in early adolescence. *Journal of Youth and Adolescence, 18,* 567–582.

Rainforth, B., York, J., & MacDonald, C. (1992). *Collaborative teams for students with severe disabilities: Integrating therapy and educational services.* Baltimore: Brookes.

Ramig, L. (1986). Acoustic analysis of phonation in patients with Huntington's disease. *Annals of Otology, Rhinology, and Laryngology, 95,* 288–293.

Ramig, L. (1994). Voice disorders. In F. Minifie (Ed.), *Introduction to communication sciences and disorders* (pp. 481–520). San Diego, CA: Singular Publishing Group.

Ramig, L., & Ringel, R. (1983). Effects of physiologic aging on selected acoustic characteristics of voice. *Journal of Speech and Hearing Research, 26,* 22–30.

Ramig, L., & Verdolini, K. (1998). Treatment efficacy: Voice disorders. *Journal of Speech-Language-Hearing Research, 41,* S101–S116.

Redmond, S. M., & Rice, M. L. (2001). Detection of irregular verb violations by children with and without SLI. *Journal of Speech, Language, and Hearing Research, 44,* 655–669.

Reichle, J., Halle, J. W., & Drasgow, E. (1998). Implementing augmentative communication systems. In A. Wetherby, S. Warren, & J. Reichle (Eds.), *Transitions in prelinguistic communication* (pp. 417–436). Baltimore: Brookes.

Rescorla, L., & Alley, A. (2001). Validation of the Language Development Survey (LDS): A parent report tool for identifying language delay in toddlers. *Journal of Speech, Language, and Hearing Research, 44,* 434–445.

Rescorla, L., Roberts, J., & Dahlsgaard, K. (1997). Late talkers at 2: Outcome at age 3. *Journal of Speech, Language, and Hearing Research, 40,* 556–566.

Rescorla, L., & Schwartz, E. (1990). Outcome of toddlers with specific expressive language delay. *Applied Psycholinguistics, 11,* 393–407.

Reynolds, M. E., & Jefferson, L. (2000). Natural and synthetic speech comprehension: Comparison of children from two age groups. *Augmentative and Alternative Communication, 16,* 174–182.

Rhea, P. (1997). Facilitating transitions in language development in children who use AAC. *Augmentative and Alternative Communication, 13,* 141–148.

Rhyner, P. M., Kelly, D. J., Brantley, A. L., & Krueger, D. M. (1999). Screening low-income African American children using the

BLT-2S and the SPELT-P. *American Journal of Speech-Language Pathology, 8,* 44–52.

Rice, M. L., Cleave, P. L., & Oetting, J. B. (2000). The use of syntactic cues in lexical acquisition by children with SLI. *Journal of Speech, Language, and Hearing Research, 34,* 582–594.

Rieber, R. W., & Wollock, J. (1977). The historical roots of the theory and therapy of stuttering. *Journal of Communication Disorders, 10,* 3–24.

Riley, G., & Riley, J. (1981). *Stuttering prediction instrument for young children.* Tigard, OR: C.C. Publications.

Ringo, C. C., & Dietrich, S. (1995). Neurogenic stuttering: An analysis and critique. *Journal of Medical Speech-Language Pathology, 2,* 111–122.

Riski, J. E. (1995). Secondary surgical procedures to correct postoperative velopharyngeal incompetencies found after primary palatoplasties. In K. R. Bzoch (Ed.), *Communicative disorders related to cleft lip and palate,* (4th ed., pp. 121–152). Austin, TX: Pro-Ed.

Ritvo, E. R., & Freeman, B. J. (1978). National Society for Autistic Children definition of the syndrome of autism. *Journal of Autism and Childhood Schizophrenia, 8,* 162–167.

Roberts, J., & Schuele, C. (1990). Otitis media and later academic performance: The linkage and implications for intervention. *Topics in Language Disorders, 11*(1), 43–62.

Robey, R. R. (1994). The efficacy of treatment for aphasic persons: A meta-analysis. *Brain and Language, 47,* 585–608.

Robey, R. R. (1998). A meta-analysis of clinical outcomes in the treatment of aphasia. *Journal of Speech, Language, and Hearing Research, 41,* 172–187.

Rogers, B. (1996). Neurodevelopmental presentation of dysphasia. *Seminars in Speech Language Pathology, 17*(4), 269–281.

Rogers, B., Arvedson, J., Buck, G., et al. (1994). Characteristics of dysphagia in children with cerebral palsy. *Dysphagia, 9*(1), 69–73.

Romski, M. A., & Sevcik, R. A. (1996). *Breaking the speech barrier: Language development through augmented means.* Baltimore: Brookes.

Rosenbek, J. C., & LaPointe, L. L. (1985). The dysarthrias: Description, diagnosis, and treatment. In D. F. Johns (Ed.), *Clinical management of neurogenic communica-*

tion disorders (pp. 97–152). Boston: Little, Brown.

Rosenbek, J. C., LaPointe, L. L., & Wertz, R. T. (1989). *Aphasia: A clinical approach.* Austin, TX: Pro-Ed.

Rosenfeld, S. J. (1999). EDLAW, LLC, Section 504 and IDEA: Basic similarities and differences. [On-line] http://www.edlaw.net/service/504idea.html

Rosenfeld-Johnson, S., & Manning, D. (1997, August 4). Preventing oral-motor problems in Down syndrome. *Advance for Speech-Language-Pathologists, 20.*

Rosenfield, D. (1991). Pharmacologic approaches to speech motor disorders. In D. Vogel & M. Cannito (Eds.), *Treating disordered speech motor control.* Austin, TX: Pro-Ed.

Rosenthal, S. R., Sheppard, J. J., & Lotze, M. (1995). *Dysphagia and the child with developmental disabilities: Medical, clinical, and family interventions.* San Diego, CA: Singular Publishing Group.

Ross, M. (1994). Overview of aural rehabilitation. In J. Katz (Ed.), *Handbook of clinical audiology* (4th ed., pp. 587–595). Baltimore, MD: Williams and Wilkins.

Roth, F. P., & Worthington, C. K. (1996). *Treatment resource manual for speech-language pathology.* San Diego: Singular Publishing Group.

Rowland, C., & Schweigert, P. (1989). Tangible symbols: Symbolic communication for individuals with multisensory impairments. *Augmentative and Alternative Communication, 5,* 226–234.

Rowland, C., & Schweigert, P. (2000). Tangible symbols, tangible outcomes. *Augmentative and Alternative Communication, 16,* 61–78.

Runte, C., Lawerino, M., Dirksen, D., et al. (2001). The influence of maxillary central incisor position in complete dentures on /s/ sound production. *The Journal of Prosthetic Dentistry, 85,* 485–495.

Russell, N. (1993). Educational considerations in traumatic brain injury: The role of the speech-language pathologist. *Language, Speech, and Hearing Services in Schools, 24,* 67–75.

Ryan, B. P. (1974). *Programmed therapy for stuttering children and adults.* Springfield, IL: Charles C. Thomas.

Ryan, B. P., & Van Kirk Ryan, B. (1983). Programmed stuttering therapy for children:

Comparisons of four established programs. *Journal of Fluency Disorders, 8,* 291–321.

Ryan, B. P., & Van Kirk Ryan, B. (1995). Programmed stuttering treatment for children: Comparisons of two established programs through transfer, maintenance, and follow-up. *Journal of Speech and Hearing Research, 38,* 61–75.

Saint-Exupéry, A. de (1968). *The little prince.* New York: Harcourt Brace.

Sameroff, A., & Fiese, B. (1990). Transactional regulation and early intervention. In S. Meisels & J. Shonkoff (Eds.), *Early intervention: A handbook of theory, practice, and analysis.* New York: Cambridge University Press.

Sanders, E. (1972). When are speech sounds learned? *Journal of Speech and Hearing Disorders, 37,* 55–63.

Sanders, L. D., & Neville, H. J. (2000). Lexical, syntactic, and stress-pattern cues for speech segmentation. *Journal of Speech, Language, and Hearing Research, 43,* 1301–1321.

Sarno, M. T. (1969). *Functional Communication Profile.* Rehabilitation Monographs 42. New York: New York University Medical Center.

Sarno, M. T., Buonaguro, A., & Levita, E. (1986). Characteristics of verbal impairment in closed head injury. *Archives of Physical Medicine and Rehabilitation, 67,* 400.

Scarborough, H., Wyckoff, J., & Davidson, R. (1986). A reconsideration of the relationship between age and mean utterance length. *Journal of Speech and Hearing Research, 29,* 394–399.

Scheffner Hammer, C., & Weiss, A. L. (1999). Guiding language development: How African American mothers and their infants structure play interactions. *Journal of Speech, Language, and Hearing Research, 42,* 1219–1233.

Schow, R., & Nerbonne, M. (1980). Hearing levels among elderly nursing home residents. *Journal of Speech and Hearing Research, 45,* 124–132.

Schow, R., & Nerbonne, M. (1996). *Introduction to audiological rehabilitation* (3rd ed.). Boston: Allyn and Bacon.

Schraeder, T., Quinn, M., Stockman, I. J., & Miller, J. (1999). Authentic assessment as an approach to preschool speech-language screening. *American Journal of Speech-Language Pathology, 8,* 195–200.

Schreibman, L. (1988). *Developmental clinical psychology and psychiatry. Vol. 15: Autism.* Newbury Park, CA: Sage.

Schuell, H. (1972). *The Minnesota test for the differential diagnosis of aphasia.* Minneapolis: University of Minnesota Press.

Schwartz, H. (1993). Adolescents who stutter. *Journal of Fluency Disorders, 18,* 291–321.

Schwarz, S. M., Corredor, J., Fisher-Medina, J., et al. (2001). Diagnosis and treatment of feeding disorders in children with developmental disabilities. *Pediatrics, 108,* 671–676.

Scott, A. (1998). NICE and easy. *Advance for Speech-Language Pathologists and Audiologists, 8*(24), 16–17.

Seagle, M. B. (1997). Primary surgical correction of cleft palate. In K. R. Bzoch (Ed.), *Communicative disorders related to cleft lip and palate,* (4th ed., pp. 115–120). Austin, TX: Pro-Ed.

Segebart DeThorne, L., & Watkins, R. V. (2001). Listeners' perceptions of language use in children. *Language, Speech, and Hearing Services in Schools, 32,* 142–148.

Selley, W. G., Parrott, L. C., Lethbridge, P. C., et al. (2001). Objective measures of dysphagia complexity in children related to suckle feeding histories, gestational ages, and classification of their cerebral palsy. *Dysphagia, 16,* 200–207.

Seung, H., & Chapman, R. (2000). Digit span in individuals with Down syndrome and in typically developing children: Temporal aspects. *Journal of Speech, Language, and Hearing Research, 43,* 609–620.

Seymour, C. M. (1997). Research, graduate education, and the future of our professions. *Asha, 39*(3), 7.

Shadden, B. B., & Toner, M. A. (Eds.). (1997). *Aging and communication: For clinicians by clinicians.* Austin, TX: Pro-Ed.

Shapiro, B., & Danley, M. (1985) The role of the right hemisphere in the control of speech prosody in propositional and affective contexts. *Brain and Language, 25,* 19–36.

Shapiro, L., Swinney, D., & Borsky, S. (1998). On-line examination of language performance in normal and neurologically impaired adults. *American Journal of Speech-Language Pathology, 7*(1), 49–60.

Shaw, G. Y., & Searl, J. P. (2001). Botulinum toxin treatment for cricopharyngeal dysfunction. *Dysphagia, 16,* 161–167.

Shekim, L. (1990). Dementia. In L. L. LaPointe (Ed.), *Aphasia and related neurogenic language disorders* (pp. 210–220). New York: Thieme Medical Publishers.

Shekim, L., & LaPointe, L. L. (1984, February). *Production of discourse in patients with Alzheimer's dementia.* Paper presented at the International Neuropsychology Society meeting, Houston.

Sheppard, J. J. (1991). Managing dysphagia in mentally retarded adults. *Dysphagia, 6*(2), 83–87.

Sheppard, J. J. (1995). Clinical evaluation and treatment. In S. R. Rosenthal, J. J., Sheppard, & M. Lotze (Eds.), *Dysphagia and the child with developmental disabilities: Medical, clinical, and family interventions.* San Diego, CA: Singular Publishing Group.

Shipley, K. G. (1997). *Interviewing and counseling in communicative disorders: Principles and procedures* (2nd ed.). Boston: Allyn and Bacon.

Shipley, K. G., & McAfee, J. G. (1998). *Assessment in speech-language pathology: A resource manual* (2nd ed.). San Diego, CA: Singular Publishing Group.

Shipp, T., Qi, Y., Huntley, R., & Hollien, H. (1992). Acoustic and temporal correlates of perceived age. *Journal of Voice, 6*(3), 211–216.

Shprintzen, R. J. (1995). A new perspective on clefting. In R. J. Shprintzen & J. Bardach (Eds.), *Cleft palate speech management: A multidisciplinary approach.* St. Louis, MO: Mosby.

Shprintzen, R. J., & Goldberg, R. (1995). The genetics of clefting and associated syndromes. In R. J. Shprintzen & J. Bardach (Eds.), *Cleft palate speech management: A multidisciplinary approach.* St. Louis, MO: Mosby.

Shprintzen, R. J., McCall, G. M., Skolnick, L. (1975). A new therapeutic technique for the treatment of velopharyngeal incompetence. *Journal of Speech and Hearing Disorders, 40*, 69–83.

Shriberg, L. D., Aram, D. M., & Kwiatkowski, J. (1997a). Developmental apraxia of speech: II. Toward a diagnostic marker. *Journal of Speech, Language, and Hearing Research, 40*(2), 286–312.

Shriberg, L. D., Aram, D. M., & Kwiatkowski, J. (1997b). Developmental apraxia of speech: III. A subtype marked by inappropriate stress. *Journal of Speech, Language, and Hearing Research, 40*(2), 313–317.

Shriberg, L. D., Austin, D., Lewis, B. A., & McSweeney, J. L., & Wilson, D. L. (1997). The percentage of consonants correct (PCC) metric: Extensions and reliability data. *Journal of Speech, Language, and Hearing Research, 40*(4), 708–722.

Shriberg, L. D., & Kent, R. D. (1995). *Clinical phonetics* (2nd ed.). Boston: Allyn and Bacon.

Shriberg, L. D., & Kwiatkowski, J. (1994). Developmental phonological disorders. I: A clinical profile. *Journal of Speech and Hearing Research, 37*, 1100–1126.

Sigafoos, J. (2000). Creating opportunities for augmentative and alternative communication: Strategies for involving people with developmental disabilities. *Augmentative and Alternative Communication, 16*, 183–190.

Silverman, E. M., & Zimmer, C. H. (1975). Incidence of chronic hoarseness among school-aged children. *Journal of Speech and Hearing Disorders, 40*, 211–215.

Silverman, F. H. (1995). *Communication for the speechless* (3rd. ed.). Boston: Allyn and Bacon.

Simmons-Mackie, N. N., & Damico, J. S. (1996). The contribution of discourse markers to communicative competence. *American Journal of Speech-Language Pathology, 5*(1), 37–43.

Simmons-Mackie, N., Damico, J. S., & Damico, H. L. (1999). A qualitative study of feedback in aphasia treatment. *American Journal of Speech-Language Pathology, 8*, 218–230.

Singh, R., Cohen, S. N., & Krupp, R. (1996). Racial differences in cerebrovascular disease. *Neurology, 46*(Suppl. 2), A440–A441.

Skoner, D. (1998, July 17). The interplay between otitis media and rhinitis in children. *Medscape Respiratory Care* [On-line serial]. Available: www.medscape.com/ Medscape/RespiratoryCare/1998/v02.n02/ mrc3024.skon/

Skuse, D. H. (2000). Imprinting, the X-chromosome, and the male brain: Explaining sex differences in the liability to autism. *Pediatric Research, 47*(1), 9–16.

Small, L. H. (1999). *Fundamentals of phonetics: A practical guide for students.* Boston: Allyn and Bacon.

Snowling, M., & Frith, U. (1986). Comprehension in "hyperlexic" readers. *Journal of*

Experimental Child Psychology, 42, 392–415.

Sohlberg, M., & Mateer, C. (1989). *Introduction to cognitive rehabilitation: Theory and practice.* New York: Guilford Press.

Solomon, N. P., McKee, A. S., Larson, K. J., Nawrocki, M. D., Tuite, P. J., Eriksen, S., Low, W. C., & Maxwell, R. E. (2000). Effects of pallidal stimulation on speech in three men with severe Parkinson's disease. *American Journal of Speech-Language Pathology, 9,* 241–256.

Solomon, N. P., Robin, D. A., & Luschei, E. S. (2000). Strength, endurance, and stability of the tongue and hand in Parkinson's disease. *Journal of Speech, Language, and Hearing Research, 43,* 256–267.

Sommers, R. K., & Caruso, A. J. (1995). Inservice training in speech-language pathology: Are we meeting the needs for fluency training? *American Journal of Speech-Language Pathology, 4*(3), 22–28.

Sonies, B. C. (1997). Evaluation and treatment of speech and swallowing disorders associated with myopathies. *Current Opinion in Rheumatology, 9*(6), 486–495.

Sonies, B. C., & Frattali, C. M. (1997). Critical decisions regarding service delivery across the health care continuum. In B. C. Sonies (Ed.), *Dysphagia: A continuum of care.* Gaithersburg, MD: Aspen.

Soto, G., Muller, E., Hunt, P., & Goetz, L. (2001). Critical issues in the inclusion of students who use augmentative and alternative communication: An educational team perspective. *Augmentative and Alternative Communication, 17,* 62–72.

Sparks, R. W., Helm, N., & Albert, M. (1974). Aphasia rehabilitation resulting from melodic intonation therapy. *Cortex, 10,* 303–316.

Sparks, R. W., & Holland, A. L. (1976). Method: Melodic intonation therapy for aphasia. *Journal of Speech and Hearing Disorders, 41,* 287–297.

Spiegel, B., Benjamin, B. J., & Spiegel, S. (1993). One method to increase spontaneous use of an assistive communication device: A case study. *Augmentative and Alternative Communication, 9,* 111–117.

Starch, S., & Falltrick, E. (1990). The importance of home evaluation for brain injured clients: A team approach. *Cognitive Rehabilitation, 8,* 28–32.

Starkweather, W. (1987). *Fluency and stuttering.* Englewood Cliffs, NJ: Prentice-Hall.

Starkweather, W. (1997). Therapy for younger children. In R. F. Curlee & G. M. Siegel (Eds.), *Nature and treatment of stuttering: New directions* (2nd ed., pp. 143–166). Boston: Allyn and Bacon.

Stecker, N. A. (1998). Overview and update of central auditory processing disorders. In M. G. Masters, N. A. Stecker, & J. Katz (Eds.), *Central auditory processing disorders: Mostly management.* Boston: Allyn and Bacon.

Steele, C. M., Greenwood, C., Ens, I., et al. (1997). Mealtime difficulties in a home for the aged: Not just dysphagia. *Dysphagia, 12*(1), 43–51.

Stinneford, J. G., Keshavarzian, A., Nemchausky, B. A., Doria, M. I., & Durkin, M. (1993). Esophagitis and esophageal motor abnormalities in patients with chronic spinal cord injuries. *Paraplegia, 31*(6), 384–392.

Stoel-Gammon, C., & Dunn, C. (1985). *Normal and disordered phonology in children.* Austin, TX: Pro-Ed.

Strand, E. A., & McCauley, R. (1997, November). *Differential diagnosis of phonological impairment and developmental apraxia of speech.* Paper presented at the American Speech-Language-Hearing Association Annual Convention, Boston, MA.

Strange, W., & Broen, P. (1980). Perception and production of approximant consonants by 3-year-olds: A first study. In G. Yeni-Komshian, J. Kavanaugh, & C. A. Ferguson (Eds.), *Child phonology: Vol. 2. Perception.* New York: Academic Press.

Straus, D., Cable, W., & Shavelle, R. (1999). Causes of excess mortality in cerebral palsy. *Developmental Medicine and Child Neurology, 41,* 580–585.

Teasdale, G., & Jennett, B. (1974). Assessment of coma and impaired consciousness. *Lancet, ii,* 81–84.

Teele, D. W., Klein, J. O., & Rosner, B. (1989). Epidemiology of otitis media during the first seven years of life in children in greater Boston: A prospective cohort study. *Journal of Infectious Diseases, 160,* 83–94.

Thal, D., Jackson-Maldonado, D., & Acosta, D. (2000). Validity of a parent-report measure of vocabulary and grammar for Spanish-speaking toddlers. *Journal of Speech, Language, and Hearing Research, 43,* 1087–1100.

Thomas, L. (1979). *The medusa and the snail: More notes of a biology watcher.* New York: Viking.

Thompson, C. K. (1988). Articulation disorders in children with neurological pathology. In N. J. Lass, L. V. McReynolds, & D. E. Yoder (Eds.), *Handbook of speech-language pathology and audiology* (pp. 548–590). Burlington, Ontario, Canada: B. D. Decker.

Tierney, L. M., Jr. (1993). *Current medical diagnosis and treatment, 1994.* Los Altos, CA: Appleton & Lange.

Tierney, L. M., Jr., McPhee, S. J., & Papadakis, M. A. (2000). *Current medical diagnosis and treatment* (39th ed.). New York: Lange Medical Books/McGraw-Hill.

Titze, I. R. (1994). *Principles of voice production.* Englewood Cliffs, NJ: Prentice-Hall.

Tjaden, K. (2000). A preliminary study of factors influending perception of articulatory rate in Parkinson's disease. *Journal of Speech, Language, and Hearing Research, 43,* 997–1010.

Tjaden, K., & Turner, G. (2000). Segmental timing in amyotropic lateral sclerosis. *Journal of Speech, Language, and Hearing Research, 43,* 683–696.

Tomes, L. A., Kuehn, D. P., & Peterson-Falzone, S. J. (1995). Behavioral treatments of velopharyngeal impairment. In K. R. Bzoch (Ed.), *Communicative disorders related to cleft lip and palate* (4th ed., pp. 529–562). Austin, TX: Pro-Ed.

Tompkins, C. A. (1995). *Right hemisphere communication disorders: Theory and management.* San Diego: Singular.

Tompkins, C. A., Baumgaertner, A., Lehman, M. T., & Fassbinder, W. (2000). Mechanisms of discourse comprehension impairment after right hemisphere brain damage: Suppression of lexical ambiguity resolution. *Journal of Speech, Language, and Hearing Research, 43,* 62–78.

Toner, M. A. (1997). Targeting dysphagia in the elderly: Prevention, assessment, and intervention. In B. B. Shadden & M. A. Toner (Eds.), *Aging and communication: For clinicians by clinicians.* Austin, TX: Pro-Ed.

Tyler, A., & Watterson, K. (1991). Effects of phonological versus language intervention in preschoolers with both phonological and language impairment. *Child Language Teaching and Therapy, 7,* 141–160.

Uffen, E. (1998). So you want to go abroad? Here's how. *Asha, 40*(4), 43–46.

Ukrainetz, T. A., Harpell, S., Walsh, C., & Coyle, C. (2000). A preliminary investigation of dynamic assessment with Native American kindergarteners. *Language, Speech, and Hearing Services in Schools, 31,* 142–154.

U.S. Census Bureau. (1997). Americans with disabilities: 1997. [On-line] http://www.census.gov/hhes/www/disable/sipp/disabl97/asc97.html

U.S. Department of Health and Human Services. (1994). *International classification of diseases,* 9th revision. DHHS Publication No. (PHS) 94–1260. [On-line] http://cedr.lbl.gov/icd9.html)

U.S. Department of Justice, Civil Rights Division, Disability Rights Section. (2000). A Guide to Disability Rights Laws. [On-line] http://www.usdoj.gov/crt/ada/cguide.htm

Van Riper, C. (1982). *The nature of stuttering.* Englewood Cliffs, NJ: Prentice-Hall.

Van Riper, C. (1992). *The nature of stuttering* (2nd ed.). Prospect Heights, IL: Waveland Press.

Van Riper, C., & Erickson, R. (1996). *Speech correction: An introduction to speech pathology and audiology* (9th ed.). Englewood Cliffs, NJ: Prentice-Hall.

Venkatagiri, H. S. (2000). Efficient keyboard layouts for sequential access in augmentative and alternative communication. *Augmentative and Alternative Communication, 16,* 126–134.

Wagner, R. K., Torgesen, J. K., & Rashotte, C. A. (1999). *Comprehensive test of phonological processing (CTOPP).* Austin, TX: Pro-Ed.

Wallach, G. P., & Butler, K. G. (1995). Language learning disabilities: Moving in from the edge. *Topics in Language Disorders, 16*(1), 1–26.

Warburton, E., Price, C. J., Swinburn, K., & Wise, R. J. (1999). Mechanisms of recovery from aphasia: Evidence of positron emission tomography studies. *Journal of Neurology, Neurosurgery, and Psychiatry, 66,* 155–161.

Waterman, E. T., Koltai, P. J., Downey, J. C., & Cacace, A. T. (1992). Swallowing disorders in a population of children with cerebral palsy. *International Journal of Pediatric Otorhinolaryngology, 24*(1), 63–71.

Watson, B. C., & Freeman, F. J. (1997). Brain imaging contributions. In R. F. Curlee & G. M. Siegel (Eds.), *Nature and treatment of stuttering: New directions* (2nd ed., pp. 143–166). Boston: Allyn and Bacon.

Watzlawick, P., Beavin, J., & Jackson, K. (1967). Pragmatics of human communication: a study of interactional patterns, pathologies, and paradoxes. New York: W. W. Norton.

Weiner, F. (2000). *Diagnostic report writer, 2000.* West Bloomfield, MI: Parrot Software.

Weinstein, B. (1994). Presbycusis. In J. Katz (Ed.), *Handbook of clinical audiology* (4th ed., pp. 568–584). Baltimore, MD: Williams and Wilkins.

Weismer, S. E., Evans, J., & Hesketh, L. J. (1999). An examination of verbal working memory capacity in children with specific language impairment. *Journal of Speech, Language, and Hearing Research, 23,* 1234–1248.

Weismer, S. E., & Hesketh, L. J. (1996). Lexical learning by children with specific language impairment: Effects of linguistic input presented at varying speaking rates. *Journal of Speech and Learning Research, 39,* 177–190.

Weismer, S. E., Tomblin, J. B., Zhang, X., Buckwalter, P., Gaura Chynoweth, J., & Jones, M. (2000). Nonword repetition performance in school-age childen with and without language impairment. *Journal of Speech, Language, and Hearing Research, 43,* 865–878.

Weiss, B., Weisz, J., & Bromfield, R. (1986). Performance of retarded and nonretarded persons on information-processing tasks: Further tests of the similar structure hypothesis. *Psychological Bulletin, 100,* 157–175.

Wells, G. (1985). *Language development in the preschool years.* New York: Cambridge University Press.

Wertz, R. T. (1985). Neuropathologies of speech and language: An introduction to patient management. In D. F. Johns (Ed.), *Clinical management of neurogenic communicative disorders* (2nd ed.). Boston: Little, Brown.

Wertz, R. T., LaPointe, L. L., & Rosenbek, J. C. (1991). *Apraxia of speech in adults: The disorder and its management.* San Diego, CA: Singular Publishing Group.

Westby, C. E. (1997). There's more to passing than knowing the answers. *Language, Speech, and Hearing Services in Schools, 28,* 244–287.

Whitmire, K. A. (2000). Adolescence as a developmental phase: A tutorial. *Topics in Language Disorders, 20*(2), 1–14.

Wilcox, K., & Morris, S. (1999). *Children's speech intelligibility measure.* San Antonio, TX: Psychological Corporation.

Wilson, D. (1987). *Voice problems in children* (3rd ed.). Baltimore, MD: Williams and Wilkins.

Windsor, J., & Hwang, M. (1999). Testing the generalized slowing hypothesis in specific language impairment. *Journal of Speech, Language, and Hearing Research, 42,* 1205–1218.

Windsor, J., Scott, C. M., & Street, C. K. (2000). Verb and noun morphology in the spoken and written language of children with language learning disabilities. *Journal of Speech, Language, and Hearing Research, 43,* 1322–1336.

Wingate, M. E. (1969). Sound and pattern in "artificial" fluency. *Journal of Speech and Hearing Research, 12,* 677–686.

Wingate, M. E. (1970). Effect on stuttering of changes in audition. *Journal of Speech and Hearing Research, 13,* 861–873.

Witzel, M. A. (1995). Communicative impairment associated with clefting. In R. J. Shprintzen & J. Bardach (Eds.), *Cleft palate speech management: A multidisciplinary approach.* St. Louis, MO: Mosby.

Wolk, S., & Schildroth, A. N. (1986). Deaf children and speech intelligibility: A national study. In A. N. Schildroth & M. A. Karchmer (Eds.), *Deaf children in America* (pp. 139–159). San Diego: College-Hill.

Wood, P., & Emick-Herring, B. (1997). Dysphagia: A screening tool for stroke patients. *Journal of Neuroscientific Nursing, 29*(5), 325–329.

Woods, E. K. (1995). The influence of posture and positioning on oral motor development and dysphagia. In S. R. Rosenthal, J. J. Sheppard, & M. Lotze (Eds.), *Dysphagia and the child with developmental disabilities: Medical, clinical, and family interventions.* San Diego, CA: Singular Publishing Group.

Wooi, M., Scott, A., & Perry, A. (2001). Teaching speech pathology students the interpretation of videofluoroscopic swallowing studies. *Dysphagia, 16,* 32–39.

World Health Organization. (2001). *International classification of functioning, disability, and health.* Final draft, full version. Geneva: Author. [On-line] http://who

Wright, H. H., & Newhoff, M. (2001). Narration abilities of children with language-learning disabilities in response to oral and written stimuli. *American Journal of Speech-Language Pathology, 10*, 308–319.

Yairi, E. (1981). Disfluencies of normally speaking 2-year-old children. *Journal of Speech and Hearing Research, 24*, 301–307.

Yairi, E. (1982). Longitudinal studies of disfluencies in 2-year-old children. *Journal of Speech and Hearing Research, 25*, 402–404.

Yairi, E. (1983). The onset of stuttering in 2- and 3-year-old children: A preliminary report. *Journal of Speech and Hearing Disorders, 48*, 171–177.

Yairi, E., & Ambrose, N. (1992a). A longitudinal study of children: A preliminary report. *Journal of Speech and Hearing Research, 35*, 755–760.

Yairi, E., & Ambrose, N. (1992b). Onset of stuttering in preschool children: Selected factors. *Journal of Speech and Hearing Research, 35*, 782–788.

Yairi, E., & Ambrose, N. G. (2001). Recovery from early stuttering: Additional issues within the Onslaw & Packman–Yairi & Ambrose (1999) exchange. (Letter to the editor). *Journal of Speech, Language, and Hearing Research, 44*, 862–867.

Yairi, E., Ambrose, N., & Nierman, B. (1993). The early months of stuttering: A developmental study. *Journal of Speech and Hearing Research, 36*, 521–528.

Yairi, E., Watkins, R., Ambrose, N., et al. (2001). What is stuttering? (Letter to the editor). *Journal of Speech, Language, and Hearing Research, 44*, 585–592.

Yang, M. T., Ko, F. T., Cheng, N. Y., et al. (1996). Clinical experience of esophageal ulcers and esophagitis in AIDS patients. *Kao Hsiung I Hsueh Ko Hsueh Tsa Chih, 12*(11), 624–629.

Yaruss, J. S. (1997). Clinical measurement of stuttering behaviors. *Contemporary Issues in Communication Science and Disorders, 24*, 33–44.

Yavas, M. (1998). *Phonology: Development and disorders.* San Diego: Singular Publishing Group.

Yavas, M., & Goldstein, B. (1998). Phonological assessment and treatment of bilingual speakers. *American Journal of Speech-Language Pathology, 7*(2), 49–60.

Ylvisaker, M. (1994). Collaboration in assessment and intervention after TBI. *Topics in Language Disorders, 15*(1), 1–81.

Yoder, D., & Munson, L. (1995). The social correlates of co-ordinated attention to adults and objects in mother-infant interaction. *First Language, 15*, 219–230.

Yont, K. M., Hewitt, L. E., & Miccio, A. W. (2000). A coding system for describing conversational breakdowns in preschool children. *American Journal of Speech-Language Pathology, 9*, 300–309.

Yorkston, K. M., Beukelman, D. R., & Bell, K. R. (1988). *Clinical management of dysarthric speakers.* Boston: College Hill Press.

Yorkston, K. M., Miller, R. M., & Strand, E. A. (1995). *Management of speech and swallowing disorders in degenerative disease.* Tucson, AZ: Communication Skill Builders.

Yorkston, K. M., Smith, E., & Beukelman, D. R. (1990). Extended communication samples of augmentative communicators: I. A comparison of individualized versus standard single-word vocabularies. *Journal of Speech and Hearing Disorders, 55*, 217–224.

Yorkston, K. M., Strand, E. A., Miller, R. M., Hillel, A., & Smith, K. (1993). Speech deterioration in amyotrophic lateral sclerosis: Implications for the timing of intervention. *Journal of Medical Speech-Language Pathology, 1*, 35–46.

Zangari, C. (2001). Helping families gain acceptance of AAC strategies. *American Speech-Language Hearing Association Special Interest Division 1, Language Learning and Education Newsletter, 8*(1), 14–17.

Zangari, C., & Kangas, K. A. (1997). Intervention principles and procedures, In L. L. Lloyd, D. R. Fuller, & H. H. Arvidson (Eds.), *Augmentative and alternative communication: A handbook of principles and practices.* Boston: Allyn and Bacon.

Zantal-Wiener, K. (1988). Preschool Services for Children with Handicaps. ERIC Digest #450. ERIC Clearinghouse on Handicapped and Gifted Children, Reston, VA.

Zemlin, W. R. (1998). *Speech and hearing sciences: Anatomy and physiology.* Boston: Allyn and Bacon.

Zemlin, W. R. (1998). *Speech and hearing sciences: Anatomy and physiology* (4th ed.). Boston: Allyn and Bacon.

Zeuschner, R. (1997). *Communicating today* (2nd ed.). Boston: Allyn and Bacon.

Zitnay, G. A. (1995). Foreword. In D. G. Stein, S. Brailowsky, & B. Will (Eds.), *Brain repair* (pp. v–vi). New York: Oxford University Press.

Author Index

Subject Index

Omissions, 331
Open syllable, 313
Oral apraxia, 412
Oral cavity, 64
Oral-motor training, 342
Organic/somatogenic, 134
Organ of Corti, 459
Orthodontist, 366
Ossicles, 458
Ossicular discontinuity, 486
Otitis media, 320, 368
Otitis media with effusion (OME), 464
Otoacoustic emissions (OAEs), 476
Otosclerosis, 486
Ototoxic, 467

Palatal, 310
Palatal obturator, 449
Palatal shelves, 353
Palatoplasty, 365
Paralysis, 76
Paraphasia, 212
Paresis, 322
Parkinson's disease, dysphagia and, 430–431
Passive recoil forces, 60
Pausing/phrasing, 272
Pectoral girdle, 56
Pediatric dysphagia, 425–428
  cerebral palsy, 426–427
  HIV/AIDS, 428
  mental retardation and developmental delay, 427
  pervasive developmental disorder (PDD) and autism, 427–428
  spina bifida, 427
  structural and physiological abnormalities, 428
Percentile ranks, 141
Perceptual or ear training, 340
Perilymph, 459
Perseveration, 169, 222
Personal hearing aids, 487–488
Pervasive developmental disorder (PDD), 176–179
  and autism, dysphagia and, 427–428
  language characteristics, 178–179
  life span issues, 178
Pharyngeal cavity, 64
Pharyngeal flap, 365
Pharyngostomy, 449
Pharynx, 349
Phonation, 93

Phonemes, 89
Phonemic symbols for English speech sounds, table, 308
Phonetically balanced (PB) words, 485
Phonetically consistent forms (PCFs), 92
Phonological processes, 317
  of young children, table, 100
Phonology, 32, 313
  preschoolers, 106
  school-age children and adolescents, 113
Phonotactic rules, 32
Physiological tests, 476–478
Physiology, definition of, 56
Pictogram Ideogram Communication (PIC), 504
Picture Communication Symbols (PCS), 504
Pidgin signed English (PSE), 494
Pierre Robin syndrome (Robin sequence), 359
  dysphagia and, 428
Pinna, 457
Pitch, 36
Play audiometry, 479
Porch Index of Communicative Abilities, 228
Portfolio, 136
Portfolio evaluation, 199
Postlingual, 466
Post-therapy tests, 156
Prader-Willi syndrome, 427
Pragmatics, 33
  rules for speakers of American English, table, 34
Precipitating cause, 133–134
Predictors and risk factors of language change in toddlers, table, 190
Predisposing cause, 133
Prelingual, 466
Premaxilla, 350
Presbycusis, 469
Pressure consonants, 378
Pressure equalization (PE) tubes, 464
Prevalence, 49
Primary motor cortex, 69
Production training, 340
Professional organizations, 14–17
  American Speech-Language-Hearing Association (ASHA), 14–17
  advocacy, 16–17

clinical service in speech-language pathology and audiology, 15
maintenance of ethical standards, 15–16
scientific study of processes and disorders of human communication, 15
related organizations, 17
Prognosis, 135–136
Prolongations, 44
Prolonged speech, 272
Prosody, 35
Prosthodontist, 367
Proxemics, 37–38
Pseudobulbar palsy, 404
Pull-out therapy, 155
Pulmonary system, 57–58
Pure oralism, 493
Pure tone audiometry, 479
Pure tones, 127
Pure tone testing, 479–484
Pure word deafness, 218
Purulent otitis media, 464
Push-in therapy, 155
Pyloric stenosis, 428
Pyramidal tract, 75

Rate, 34
Raw score, 141
Rebus Symbols, 504
Reduplicated babbling, 94
Referrals, 125–127
Reflexes, 74, 87
Rehabilitation Institute of Chicago Evaluation (RICE) of Communicative Problems in Right-Hemisphere Dysfunction, 235
Reinforcement, 153
Reliability, 139
Repetitions, 44
Repetitive Oral Suction Swallow (ROSS), 434
Representation, 96
Resonance disorders associated with clefts, 373–377
Resonants, 310
Resonation, 93
Respiratory system, 56–62
Reverse swallow, 327
Rhotics, 310
Rib cage, 56
Right hemisphere injury (RHI), 232–235
Right Hemisphere Language Battery, 235